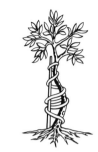

Orthopaedic
Dictionary

Orthopaedic Dictionary

Stanley Hoppenfeld, MD

Associate Clinical Professor of Orthopaedic Surgery
Albert Einstein College of Medicine
Bronx, New York

Attending Physician, Jack D. Weiler Hospital of the Albert Einstein College of Medicine
Montefiore Hospital and Our Lady of Mercy Medical Center
Bronx, New York

Associate Attending, Orthopaedic Institute of the Hospital for Joint Diseases and
Westchester County Medical Center
Westchester, New York

Michael S. Zeide, MD

Clinical Associate Professor of Orthopaedic Surgery
Department of Orthopaedics and Rehabilitation
University of Miami School of Medicine
Miami, Florida

Attending Orthopaedic Surgeon
J.F.K. Medical Center
Lake Worth, Florida

Illustrations by James Capizzuto

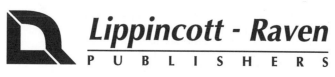

Lippincott - Raven
PUBLISHERS
Philadelphia • New York

Production Editors: Jim Slade and Sandra Cherrey
Designer: Doug Smock
Cover Designer: Tom Jackson
Production Manager: Helen Ewan
Production Coordinators: Sharon McCarthy
Compositor: CRWaldman Graphic Communications
Printer: R.R. Donnelley & Sons Company/Willard
Binder: R.R. Donnelley & Sons Company/Crawfordsville

Printed in the United States of America

6   5   4

Library of Congress Cataloging-in-Publication Data

Orthopaedic dictionary/edited by Stanley Hoppenfeld, consulting editor, Cheryl J. Rubin; illustrations by James Capizzutto.
    p.   cm.
  ISBN 0-397-51311-9
  1. Orthopedics—Dictionaries. I. Hoppenfeld, Stanley, 1934–
II. Zeide, Michael S.
  [DNLM: 1. Orthopedics—dictionaries. WE 13 077 1994]
RD723.076 1994
6171.3′003—dc20
DNLM/DLC
for Library of Congress   93-31209
                                            CIP

DEDICATIONS

To my wife, Norma, and my children, Jon-David, Robert, and Stephen,
who give my life special meaning.

S.H.

To our parents, Agatha and David Hoppenfeld
and Harold and Stella Zeide,
for providing us with a special education
that made this book possible.

S.H. *and* M.S.Z.

To my children, Elana and David,
and their dedicated mother, Suzanne.

M.S.Z.

To Dr. Peter Roget, an English physician and educator.
He is the founder of The Diffusion of Knowledge Society and is best known for his thesaurus.
His main interest in life was the transmission of knowledge.
In the same spirit, we dedicate this book to all the orthopaedic educators
who have participated in this great endeavor.

S.H. *and* M.S.Z.

EDITORIAL REVIEW BOARD

PUBLISHER'S FOREWORD

It was in the mid-1970s that Stanley Hoppenfeld and Michael Zeide first mentioned that they were working on an orthopaedic dictionary. What was a new interest then became an obsession by the end of that decade. In 1984, having enlisted the aid of the inimitable James Capizzuto, Jr., they reported that "we are diligently working on the dictionary. It takes time to fulfill the needs of our fellow professionals."

And time it continued to take. What was expected in the early 1980s we now present to you in the mid-1990s, a formal dictionary of orthopaedic terminology—anatomic, surgical, instrumental, eponymic—virtually any word or cluster of words particular to orthopaedic surgical practice. Over 1000 illustrations illuminate the definitions, and extensive cross-referencing further clarifies understanding of the terminology. We believe that the creation of such a work by full-time orthopaedic professionals has no parallel or equivalent in the literature. It is a unique accomplishment.

It is also a highly worthwhile and important accomplishment. In examining these pages, the orthopaedist will find that the words are defined and illustrated from the orthopaedist's point of view and that the definitions take on the flavor and relevance of a true orthopaedic lexicon.

These dictionary entries are carefully crafted definitions and explanations written by master surgeons and scholars in the field. All entries were reviewed by a specially convened board of 22 professional peers and recognized experts.

J.B. Lippincott is pleased to present to you a formal orthopaedic dictionary. We hope and expect that this once-in-a-lifetime accomplishment will stand as one of the truest and most useful milestones in the orthopaedic literature.

J. Stuart Freeman, Jr.
J.B. Lippincott Company

PREFACE

The purpose of the *Orthopaedic Dictionary* is to transmit orthopaedic information directly in a concise and orderly manner. A great number of illustrations have been included to clarify and give visual dimension to the definitions. Our efforts in developing this book span 18 years. We sometimes worked at night or in the early morning, exchanging information via the mail, the telephone, and personal meetings whenever possible.

This dictionary represents more than an orthopaedic lexicon. After the definitions were written, they were submitted to our editorial review board for their evaluation, suggestions, additions, and changes, which added further depth and scope to the project. The definitions presented are a consensus of the understanding of many orthopaedic surgeons of the terms.

The maintenance of a dictionary is an ongoing process. We hope that there will be an interchange of ideas between the entire orthopaedic world and ourselves. The readers and users of this volume are encouraged to communicate their thoughts to us, suggesting additions, corrections, deletions, and recommendations. With this spirit of cooperation, we will be able to continually improve information and provide an ongoing standard for our profession.

Stanley Hoppenfeld, MD
1180 Morris Park Avenue
Bronx, New York 10461

Michael Zeide, MD
2306 Embassy Drive
West Palm Beach, Florida 33401

ACKNOWLEDGMENTS

This book is written with the help of many very special people in diverse ways. We acknowledge them, express our appreciation, and ask for their continued guidance.

Rick Hutton—In appreciation of our long-term friendship and his great appreciation of the English language. He was kind enough to do the original work, placing the dictionary on the computer, providing the initial corrections, and giving us direction and organization.

Hugh Thomas—My long-term friend, whose knowledge of anatomy and professional artwork is always greatly appreciated. He has provided many artistic concepts in the production of all of our books.

James R. Capizzuto, who has worked on this book for the past 5 years. His artwork adorns the book. He has contributed over 1000 drawings, which have given the book its very special presence.

Alison Guss—For her professional editing of this book. Alison reviewed each of the definitions and brightened them with appropriate English.

Dr. Cheryl Rubin—With deep appreciation for her review of all of the definitions and her professional point of view. Most of this was done during her sports medicine fellowship.

Stuart Freeman, Senior Editor, Medical Books, at J.B. Lippincott Company—His long-term friendship and advice have always been appreciated. We especially appreciate that he believed that this work was worthwhile and that he was persistent and waited 13 years for us to deliver.

Dr. Alan Apley—In appreciation of his long-term friendship and setting high academic standards as Editor of the *Journal of Bone and Joint Surgery,* British edition.

Eileen Wolfberg—In appreciation for all her help in the production of this book.

Doug Smock—In appreciation for his work in the design of the dictionary.

Jim Slade, Project Editor—In appreciation for all his work.

Dr. John Feagin—For his long-term friendship and for the very special definitions he wrote in his book *The Crucial Ligaments.*

Dr. Herman Robbins—For his inspiring article on orthopaedic terminology in the bulletin of the Hospital for Joint diseases.

Dr. Linda Lane, Professor of American Languages, Columbia University—For her guidance in the use of The American Phonetic Alphabet (A.P.A.).

Marie Capizzuto—My long-term executive secretary and friend who helped in managing this book so that we could bring it to its proper fruition. She provided professional help so that there was enough time available for this major effort.

Donna Avacato—In appreciation of her professional help and preparing the phonetics of the orthopaedic terms.

Maxine Stevenson—For typing parts of the manuscript at night.

Mary Ann Becchetti—In appreciation for her long-term help in typing many of our manuscripts, including the dictionary.

Robert A. Hoppenfeld—For tallying our artwork and keeping the definition count accurate.

Roberta and **David Ozerkis,** my sister and brother-in-law, whose devotion and friendship made it possible to write this dictionary.

Frank Ferrieri, my long-term friend. His friendship is greatly appreciated. His loss is greatly felt.

Barbara and **James Sinclair,** who have been kind and supportive during the writing of this book, with special appreciation of our long-term friendship.

Mary and **Jim Wallach,** special friends, who have been there for all of our projects.

Arleen and **Shelley Weiner,** my friends—Some of the writing was done during two summers at their special camp "Winadu" in the Berkshires.

Abraham Irvings, a special friend who kept things going with good humor, professionalism, and economic guidance throughout the writing of this book.

Mimi and **Nat Shore,** who said it could be done and taught me how to do it. I'm grateful for their friendship.

Dr. Paula Neyman, who helped to define the postoperative care of patients with scoliosis.

Dr. Gabriel Molnar, my long-term friend and professional colleague, who has helped in defining pediatric rehabilitation.

Dr. Vasantha Murthy, my long-term colleague, who helped to define the care of scoliosis patients requiring bracing.

Dr. Mark Greenbaum—For the professional care given to the patients with scoliosis.

Dr. M. Donald Coleman—In appreciation for his help in defining my life and giving a very special lift.

Acknowledgments

Al Meier, former Editor-in-Chief of J. B. Lippincott Company—in appreciation for his encouragement, knowledge, and special understanding of an orthopaedic dictionary.

Hospital for Joint Disease, The Orthopaedic Institute, our parent institution—for providing our education in the field of orthopaedics; it has made this work possible.

The Albert Einstein College of Medicine and the Department of Orthopaedic Surgery, which through its great residency program and residents, has been a special stimulus in furthering all of our education, and to **Dr. Edward Habermann,** its Chairman.

The Gottesman Library of the Albert Einstein College of Medicine—Much of the work was done in this wonderful library, using its many reference books and computers. We express our appreciation to the librarians and their great dedication to detail and making information available to us.

Robert Schultz—For his book *The Language of Fractures.*

Sandra Cherrey, Project Editor—In appreciation for all of her work on the production of this book.

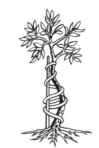

Orthopaedic
Dictionary

A

Abadie's Sign (ah-bah-dez'/sīn) (n.) An early sign of tabes dorsalis. On clinical examination, the Achilles tendon is insensitive to pressure.

A Band (A-Band) (n.) The dark-staining, birefringent transverse band that forms the broad middle segment of each sarcomere in striated muscle fibrils. It represents the zone occupied by thick myosin filaments interdigitated with thin actin filaments. It is so named because the band is **anisotropic** in polarized light. Each A band is divided by an **H zone**, with the **M band** at its center.

Abasia (ah-bā'zhe-ah) (n.) The inability to walk.

Abatement (ah-bāt'ment) (n.) The alleviation, termination, or decrease in severity and/or intensity of a symptom.

ABD Pads (ABD/padz) (n.) A bulky, absorbent bandage. Its name is derived from its original application, to cover abdominal wounds. Also known as **combines** or **combination pads**.

Abdominal Flap (ab-dom'ĭ-nal/flap) (n.) A type of distant flap graft used to provide subcutaneous tissue for coverage of deep soft-tissue defects. Used to cover hand defects, either with a distal flap based on the superficial epigastric or superficial circumflex iliac vessels or with a proximal flap based on the thoraco-epigastric vessels.

Abducens Nerve (ab-dū'senz/nerv) (n.) The sixth cranial nerve.

Abduction (ab-duk'shun) (n.) 1. The movement of a part away from the midline. 2. The position obtained by that movement. Compare **Adduction**.

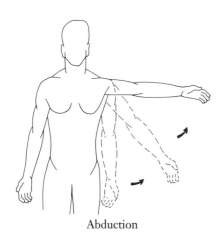

Abduction

Abduction Brace (ab-duk'shun/brās) (n.) A removable brace used to maintain a position of abduction at the hip.

Abduction Contraction (ab-duk'shun/kon-trak'shun) (n.) A contracture of a body part in which that part is fixed in abduction.

Abduction External Rotation Test (ab-duk'shun/eks-ter'nal/ro-ta'shun/test) (n.) A method of evaluating shoulder pain. With the patient upright, abduct the patient's shoulder 90 degrees, flex the elbow 90 degrees, and then gently externally rotate the shoulder by pushing the patient's hand posteriorly. If the patient experiences only pain, rotator cuff pathology is indicated. Apprehension or apprehension with pain suggests anterior shoulder dislocation.

Abduction Osteotomy (ab-duk'shun/os"te-ot'o-mē) See **Valgus Osteotomy**.

Abduction Stress Test (ab-duk'shun/stres/test) (n.) A procedure used to evaluate the integrity of the medial ligaments of the knee. Place the patient on an elevated examining surface. Abduct the hip so that the thigh rests on the table surface, and flex the knee to 30 degrees over the side of the table. Hold the patient's foot or ankle with one hand and place the other hand against the lateral aspect of the patient's knee. Gently apply an abduction stress to the knee. Compare the amount of "opening" of the medial joint line to that obtained on examination of the affected knee. Repeat the stress test with the knees in full extension. This is also known as the **Valgus Stress Test**. Compare **Adduction Stress Test**.

Abductor (ab-duk'tor) (n.) Any muscle that moves a body part into abduction.

Abductor Muscle(s) (ab-duk'tor/mus'el) See **Muscle**.

Aberrant (ab-er'ant) (adj.) A deviation from the standard in shape, form, structure, or course.

Ablate (ab-lāt') (v.) To remove. In surgical terms, excision, especially of abnormal growths, diseased organs or tissues, or harmful substances from the body.

Abnormal (ab-nòr'mal) (adj.) Differing from the usual or standard condition; not normal.

ABOS Abbreviation for American Board of Orthopaedic Surgery.

Above-Elbow Amputation (a-buv'/el'bo/am"pu-tā'shun) (n.) An ablative procedure of the upper extremity performed at a level above the elbow joint.

Above-the-Knee Amputation (a-buv'/ne/am"pu-tā'shun) (n.) An ablative procedure of the lower extremity performed at a level above the knee joint.

Abrasion (ah-bra'zhun) (n.) A lesion in which skin or a mucous membrane is scraped or rubbed away; this represents a split-thickness skin loss. The injury is considered an **avulsion** if the stratum germinatavum is lost.

Abrasion Arthroplasty (ah-bra'zhun/ar'thro-plas"tē) (n.) A debridement procedure for localized areas of articular cartilage degeneration, usually performed arthroscopically. Degenerative cartilage is abraded with curettage and high-speed burring down to the level of bleeding subchondral bone in an attempt to stimulate regeneration of fibrocartilage in this area.

Abscess (ab′ses) (n.) A localized collection of pus in a cavity. It is formed by tissue necrosis, usually the result of an infectious process.

Absorbed Dose (ab-sorbed′/dōs) (n.) In radiotherapy, the quantity of energy imparted to a mass of exposed material. One unit of absorbed dose is called a *rad.*

AC Joint (AC/joint) (n.) Abbreviation for Acromioclavicular Joint.

Acceleration (ak-sel″er-ā′shun) (n.) The rate of change of linear velocity. The unit of measure of magnitude is meters (or feet) per second squared (m/sec², or ft/sec²).

Accessory Bones of the Foot (ak-ses′o-re/bōnz/of the foot) (n.) Irregularly occurring supernumerary but well-defined bones found in an otherwise normal foot. Generally, these are easily differentiated from acute fractures by the presence of an intact, smooth cortical surface around the entire circumference. Some of the more commonly found accessory bones include:

Calcaneus secundarium, Cuboides secundarium, Os intermetatarseum, Os supranaviculare, Os sustenaculi, Os tibial externum, Os trigonum, Os vesalium, Pars peronaea metatarsalis primi.

Accessory Navicular Bone (ak-ses′o-re/nah-vik′u-lar/bōn) (n.) A bone in the foot resulting from an accessory ossification center at the medial end of the tarsal navicular to which the posterior tibial tendon has an aberrant attachment. It is present as a separate bone in about 10% of individuals. The accessory navicular is occasionally painful or tender over the instep. It may fuse with the main body of the navicular bone and create a medial prominence on the foot that will produce local symptoms. It must be differentiated from a sesamoid bone within the tibialis posterior tendon. It is also known as the **navicular secundum, os tibiale externum, prehallux, or accessory tarsal navicular.**

Accessory Nerve (ak-ses′o-rē/nerv) (n.) The eleventh cranial nerve.

Accreditation (a-kred′i-tā′shun) (n.) The formal process of evaluation and certification by which an institution or an educational or training program meets the standards of a governing organization.

Ace Bandage (ās/ban′dij) (n.) A proprietary name for a woven cotton elastic bandage. Obtainable in various widths; used to apply pressure or support or for splint application.

Acetabular ACM Angle of Idelberger and Frank (as″e-tab′u-lar /ACM /ang′g′l /of /Idelberger and Frank) (n.) A radiographic assessment of the potential sphericity of the growing acetabulum. The ACM angle is measured on an anteroposterior radiograph of the pelvis in the following manner:

Draw a line from A–D, locating Point A as the lateral rim of the acetabulum, while Point D is identical to the last point of the acetabular rim at the end of the facis lunata, which is where there is interruption by the incisura acetabuli. Point D may be difficult to find in children younger than 10 years of age. Then, bisect line A–D (point M). The point where this line crosses the bony acetabular roof is called C. The ACM angle is measured at the intersection of the A–C and C–M lines. With an ACM angle of 45 degrees, the acetabulum will be a full hemisphere, i.e., an acetabulum of 100% for an ACM angle of greater than 45 degrees means that there will be less than a 100% hemispheric acetabulum.

Acetabular Angle of Hilgenreiner (as″e-tab′u-lar/ ang′g′l/of hil′gen-răn′er) (n.) See **Acetabular Index.**

Acetabular Angle of Sharp (as″e-tab′u-lar/ang′g′l/of/ sharp) (n.) A method of evaluating acetabulum inclination on an anteroposterior radiograph of the pelvis. Draw a line between the lateral edge of the acetabular roof and the inferior tip of the teardrop. Draw a horizontal line between teardrops of both acetabuli; the angle between these two lines will be the measure of the angle of inclination of the acetabulum.

Acetabular Angle of the Weight-Bearing Area (as″e-tab′u-lar/ang′g′l/of/the/wāt/bār′ing/area) (n.) A radiographic measurement used in evaluating the shape of the acetabulum. It is similar to the acetabular index measurement, but it is used when the triradiate cartilage is no longer visible. On an anteroposterior radiograph of the pelvis, first determine the medial point as the beginning of the sclerotic line that marks the area of main weight-bearing. To define the angle, draw both a horizontal line and a line to the acetabular rim through this medial point.

Acetabular Component (as″e-tab′u-lar/kom-po′ nent) (n.) See **Acetabular Cup.**

Acetabular Coverage (as″e-tab′u-lar/kŭv′er-ĭj) (n.) The percentage of the femoral head covered by the acetabulum. This is measured on an anteroposterior radiograph of the pelvis as follows:

Draw a line perpendicular to the line connecting the teardrop figures from the lateral lip of the acetabulum. The widest extent of the femoral head is

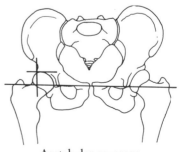

Acetabular coverage

measured perpendicular to this line. Calculate the percentage of the head medial to the lateral lip of the acetabulum along this line.

Acetabular Cup (as″e-tab′u-lar/kup) (n.) A prosthesis to replace the acetabular surface. These cups are made in a variety of sizes, materials, and external contours. Methods of fixation for different cups also vary. Also known as the **acetabular component**.

Acetabular Depth (as″e-tab′u-lar/depth) (n.) A radiographic method of evaluating the width or diameter of the acetabulum. It is measured on an anteroposterior radiograph of the pelvis from the lateral edge of the teardrop figure to a Perkin's line.

Acetabular Depth Index (as″e-tab′u-lar/depth/in-deks) (n.) A radiographic method of assessing acetabular development. Draw a line that extends from the superior rim of the acetabulum to its inferior rim. Draw a second line bisecting this to the bony rim of the acetabulum. Divide this second distance by half the length of the first line: this is the width of the acetabulum opening. In a spherical acetabulum, this index will be approximately 1.

Acetabular Fossa (as″e-tab′u-lar/fos′ah) (n.) The deep, central, nonarticular portion of the acetabulum. See **Acetabulum**.

Acetabular-Head Quotient (as″e-tab′u-lar/hed/kwō′shent) (n.) A mathematic expression of the size of the femoral head proportional to the acetabulum. On an anteroposterior roentgenogram of the pelvis, draw line A as a horizontal line extending from the most medial edge of the head to a vertical line projected from the lateral margin of the acetabulum. Line B is drawn as a horizontal line on the same level, extending from the medial edge of the head to a vertical line projected from the most lateral surface of the head. A/B × 100 = acetabular-head quotient.

Acetabular Index (as″e-tab′u-lar/in-deks) (n.) A measurement used to determine the shape of the growing acetabulum. An angle is formed between the Y line of Hilgenreiner and a line drawn from the lateral edge of the acetabulum to the triradiate cartilage. The index is normally less than 30 degrees. This is also known as **Acetabular Angle of Hilgenreiner**.

Acetabular Notch (as″e-tab′u-lar/noch) (n.) The

opening on the inferior margin of the acetabulum into which nerves and vessels pass into the joint. The notch is bridged by the transverse acetabular ligament.

Acetabular Quotient (as″e-tab′u-lar/kwo′shent) (n.) A mathematical expression of either the shallowness of the acetabulum or the obliquity of the acetabular roof. It is calculated on an anteroposterior radiograph of the pelvis, and represents the ratio of acetabular height (A) to width (B). Expressed as a percentage, A/B × 100.

Acetabuloplasty (as″e-tab′u-lō-plas″tē) (n.) 1. Any surgical reconstruction of the acetabulum. 2. Any operation intended to redirect the inclination of the acetabular roof by an osteotomy of the ilium superior to the acetabulum, followed by an inferior leveling of the roof.

Acetabulum (as″e-tab′u-lum) (n.) The hemispheric concavity on the anterolateral surface of the pelvis that articulates with the femoral head. It is formed superiorly by the ilium, posteroinferiorly by the ischium, and anteroinferiorly by the pubis. It has a semilunar articular portion (the lunate surface) and a deep, central, nonarticular portion (the acetabular fossa).

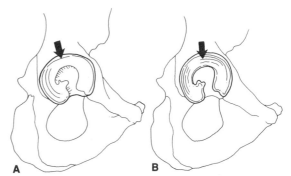

A, Acetabulum. B, Articular surface of acetabulum.

Acetaminophen (ah-sēt″ah-mǐ′no-fen) (n.) A generic medication used to relieve pain and reduce fever. Unlike aspirin, acetaminophen does not have anti-inflammatory effects. It is marketed under many proprietary names, including Tylenol, Datril, and Panadol.

Acetylcholine (as′e-til-ko′lēn) (n.) An acetic acid ester of choline. It is a neurotransmitter released by the preganglionic fibers of both the sympathetic and parasympathetic systems and all postganglionic parasympathetic nerve fibers. It is also the neuromuscular transmitter for skeletal muscle.

Acetylsalicylic Acid (ah-se′til-sal″ah-sil″ik/as′id) (n.) The chemical name for aspirin. See **Aspirin**.

Achilles Tendonitis (ah′kil′ēz/ten″do-nī′tis) (n.) An overuse syndrome in which local inflammation of the Achilles tendon occurs near its insertion into the

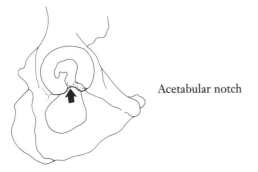

Acetabular notch

calcaneus. It is characterized by heel pain that increases with physical activity (particularly running) and decreases with rest. Physical findings include tenderness directly over the Achilles tendon, often with a palpable thickening of the tendon or peritendinous tissues, and visible soft-tissue swelling. Most symptomatic patients have some limitation of passive foot dorsiflexion as well.

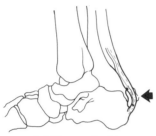

Achilles tendonitis

Achilles Tendon (ah-kil′ēz/ten′dun) (n.) The conjoined tendon of the gastrocnemius and soleus muscles of the calf, situated at the back of the ankle and inserting into the calcaneus. It is named after Achilles, the ancient Greek hero. According to legend, the infant Achilles was dipped headfirst into the magical river Styx by his mother, Thetis, to render him invulnerable. His heels, however, were not immersed. He was killed during the Trojan War by Paris, who shot an arrow into his heel. Also known as the *calcaneus tendon.*

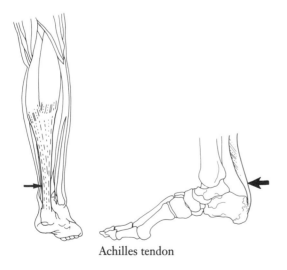

Achilles tendon

Achilles Tendon Lengthening (ah-kil′ēz/ten-dun/len′then-ing) (n.) A procedure for the correction of equinus deformity that allows the foot and the ankle

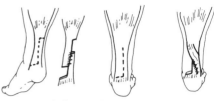

Achilles tendon lenthening

to become plantigrade (foot at right angle to the tibia). The tendon lengthening may be in the form of "Z" plasty or transposition.

Achilles Tendon Reflex (ah-kil′ēz/ten-dun/rē′fleks) (n.) A normal muscle stretch or deep tendon reflex of the ankle. It is mediated through the gastrocnemius-soleus muscles. To test the reflex, seat the patient in a passive position on the end of the examining table, and dorsiflex the ankle sufficiently to obtain optimal stretch of muscles to be tested. Alternatively, grasp the foot and passively dorsiflex it to produce proper stretch of the muscle while striking the tendon with a reflex hammer. Tapping the Achilles tendon results in plantar flexion at the ankle due to contraction of the soleus and gastrocnemius muscles. It is predominantly supplied by the S1 nerve root, although S2 makes a lesser contribution. Also known as **ankle jerk** or **triceps surae reflex.**

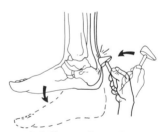

Achilles tendon reflex

Achondroplasia (ah-kon″dro-plā′ze-ah) (n.) A short-limbed, disproportionate dwarfism. It is an inherited disorder with an autosomal dominant mode of transmission, although spontaneous mutation resulting in achondroplasia is not uncommon. Some of the characteristic findings include frontal bossing, an inability to approximate the fingers when they are extended, mild thoracolumbar kyphosis with increased lumbar lordosis, and a waddling gait. Also known as **chondrodysplasia fetalis, dyschondroplasia fetalis,** and **chondrodystrophic dwarfism.**

Acid (as′id) (n.) 1. A substance that dissociates, releasing hydrogen (H+) ions but not hydroxyl (OH) ions. 2. An aqueous solution with a pH of less than 7. 3. A molecule or ion that liberates protons, usually in water.

Acid Dye (as'id/dī) (n.)   A dye whose actively stain-ing part consists of an acidic organic grouping of an-ions combined with a metal. An acid dye has an af-finity for cationic or basic substances.

Acid-Fast (as'id/fast) (adj.)   A property of certain bacteria to retain an initial stain after decolorization with acid alcohol. Only mycobacteria and a few no-cardia are acid-fast bacteria.

Acidic (ah-sid'ik) (adj.)   Of or pertaining to acids.

Acinetobacter (as"i-net"o-bak'ter) (n.)   A genus of nonmotile, aerobic, gram-negative coccobacilli.

ACL   Abbreviation for anterior cruciate ligament.

Acquired (ah-kwīrd) (adj.)   A condition or disorder contracted or developed after birth that is not hereditary.

Acral (ak-ral) (adj.)   Of or pertaining to the limbs or extremities.

Acrocephalosyndactyly (ak"ro-sef"ah-lo-sin-dak'ti-lē) (n.)   A syndrome of congenital facial deformities characterized by a high, broad forehead; wide-set eyes with the outer canthus lower than the inner; a prominent lower jaw; a sunken, small maxilla with crowded teeth; and a high, arched, and possibly cleft palate. Associated hand deformities are usually sym-metrical and consist of a complex syndactyly of the long, ring, and little fingers. This is also known as **Apert syndrome** or **Apert acrocephalosyndactyly**.

Acromegaly (ak"ro-meg'ah-lē) (n.)   A disorder marked by the progressive overgrowth of bone due to excess growth hormone; this is particularly seen in the jaw, the skull, the hands, and the feet. Acro-megaly is often caused by an eosinophilic adenoma in the anterior lobe of the pituitary gland.

Acromial Angle (ah-kro'me-al/ang'g'l) (n.)   The sub-cutaneous and palpable bony prominence at the most lateral aspect of the scapular spine. It is created by the sharp, forward turn of the acromion.

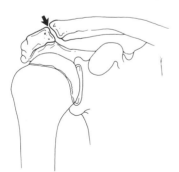
Acromioclavicular joint

Acromioclavicular Joint (ah-kro"mē-o-klah-vik'-u-lar/joint) (n.)   The diarthrodial joint formed be-tween the medial margin of the acromion process of the scapula and the lateral end of the clavicle. Ab-breviated **AC Joint**.

Acromioclavicular Joint Injuries (ah-kro"mē-o-klah-vik'u-lar/joint/in'ju-rēs) (n.)   Any of a spectrum of traumatic disorders of the AC joint that range from ligamentous sprains to subluxations to complete dis-locations. These injuries can result from either di-rect forces applied to the point of the shoulder or indirect forces applied through the upper extremity. A common classification of these injuries in current use rates them as types I–III; this rating is based on the degree of disruption of the acromioclavicular and coracoclavicular ligaments and the degree and direc-tion of clavicular displacement and associated injury to the deltoid and trapezius muscles.

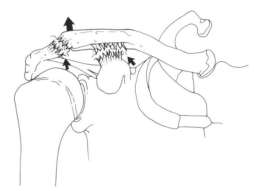
Acromioclavicular joint injuries

Acromioclavicular Ligaments (ah-kro"mē-o-klah-vik'u-lar/lig'ah-ments) (n.)   The ligaments that sur-round and stabilize the acromioclavicular articula-tion. There are inferior and superior ligaments and thin anterior and posterior ligaments.

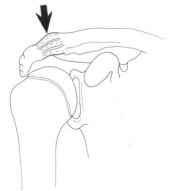
Acromioclavicular ligaments

Acromion (ah-kro'mē-on) (n.)   The flat, oblong, or triangular bony process formed by the lateral exten-sion of the spine of the scapula that overhangs the shoulder joint. It has a medially located smooth tract that articulates with the clavicle to form the acromioclavicular joint. Also called the "point of the shoulder" or the **acromion process**.

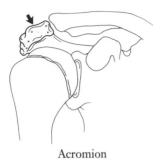

Acromion

Acromionectomy (ah-kro″mē-on-ek′to-mē) (n.) Resection of the acromion.

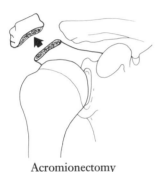

Acromionectomy

Acromioplasty (ah-kro″mē-o-plas′tē) (n.) A surgical procedure in which the anterior aspect of the acromion is resected in order to decompress impingement of the rotator cuff in the subacromial space. A resection of the coracoacromial ligament is usually performed simultaneously. This may be carried out either by open procedures or arthroscopically.

Acropathy (ah-krop′ah-thē) (n.) Any disorder or abnormal condition of the extremities.

Acrylic Cement (ă-kril′ik/se-ment) (n.) See **Polymethylmethacrylate**.

ACTH (n.) Abbreviation for adrenocorticotropic hormone.

Actin (ak′tin) (n.) A muscle protein which, combined with the protein myosin, is responsible for the shortening or contraction of the muscle. Localized in the I bands of myofibrils, actin consists of individual G (globular) actin units polymerized into an F (fibrous) actin strand. F-actin strands are wound into a double helix that attaches to or passes through Z lines. Actin has "reactive sites" on it where it may form bridges with the myosin heads.

Actinomyces (ak″ti-no-mī′sēz) (n.) A genus of anaerobic, gram-positive bacilli. It exhibits structural branching resembling that of a fungus.

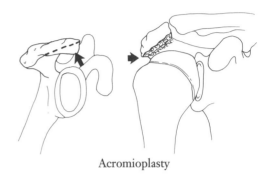

Acromioplasty

Actinomycosis (ak″ti-no-mī-ko′sis) (n.) The disease that results from infection with actinomyces, a fungus.

Action Potential (ak′shun/po-ten′shul) (n.) 1. The measurable electrical changes associated with the conduction of a nerve impulse or the contraction of a muscle. 2. The complete cycle of electric changes in transmembrane potential that occur with depolarization and repolarization of an excitable cell.

Active Acquired Immunity (ak′tiv/ah-kwīrd/i-mu′ni-tē) (n.) Immunity resulting from a subclinical or frank case of disease; injection of the infectious agent, either dead or attenuated; or injection of a product or component of the infectious agent.

Active-Assistive Exercise (ak′tiv/ah-sis′tiv/ek′ser-sīz) (n.) Movement of a muscle or part in which the patient is assisted. Assistance may be active or passive and provided by a therapist, a mechanical device, or the patient.

Active Exercise (ak′tiv/ek′ser-sīz) (n.) Voluntary muscle contractions performed by a patient.

Active Immunity (ak′tiv/i-mu′ni-tē) (n.) Immunity acquired as a result of the body's own reactions to pathogenic microorganisms or their products.

Active Range of Motion (ak′tiv/rănj/of/mō′shŭn) (n.) The range of joint motion achievable by voluntary and unassisted muscular activity.

Active Resistive Exercise (ak′tiv/re-zis′tiv/ek′ser-sīz) (n.) Movements performed by a patient in which voluntary muscle contractions are resisted by a therapist or mechanical device.

Active Transport (ak′tiv/trans′port) (n.) The process by which a substance moves across the cell membrane from a point of lower concentration to a point of higher concentration. This goes against the diffusion gradient and therefore requires an expenditure of energy.

Activities of Daily Living (ak′tiv′i-tēs/of daily living) (n.) Routine self-care, including dressing, eating, personal hygiene, transfer in and out of bed, ambulating or using a wheelchair, manual tasks, and job activities. Abbreviated ADL.

Actomyosin (ak″to-mī′ō-sin) (n.) The protein complex formed in muscle by actin and myosin during contraction.

Actual Leg Length (ak'chu-al/leg/length) (n.) The true measurement of the length of the lower limb. Clinically, the measured distance from the anterior-superior iliac spine to the medial malleolus. Radiographically, this can be measured on a scanogram. Actual leg-length measurement is important when differentiating apparent leg-length discrepancies, which may result from scoliosis or pelvic tilt, or from true leg-length discrepancies. Contrast **Apparent Leg Length**.

Acupressure (ak'ū-presh″er) (n.) A system of healing similar to acupuncture in which symptoms are relieved by exerting pressure on selected locations instead of by using needles.

Acupuncture (ak'u-pungk″cher) (n.) A traditional Chinese system of healing in which needles are inserted into the body to relieve symptoms. Stimulation is effected by rotating or twirling the needles, or by applying electric currents to very fine gauge needles. Locations known as meridian points are selected that are believed to produce analgesia or anesthesia in desired regions of the body.

Acute (ah-kūt) (adj.) 1. Sharp; severe. 2. A descriptive term used for a symptom or disease of severe, rapid onset, and/or brief duration.

Acute Care (ah-kūt/care) (n.) Treatment of the acute phase of an illness or disability.

Acute Osteomyelitis (ah-kūt/os″te-o-mī″e-lī′tis) (n.) Osteomyelitis of acute onset. Also known as acute hematogenous osteomyelitis. See **Osteomyelitis**.

Acute Pain (ah-kūt/pān) (n.) A complex constellation of unpleasant sensory, perceptual, and emotional experiences. It is accompanied by certain associated autonomic responses and psychologic and behavioral reactions. Acute pain may be caused by tissue damage induced by disease or trauma, or provoked by surgical operations or other therapeutic measures.

Psychologic factors often have a profound influence on the intensity, duration, and characteristics of acute pain. However, primary causation by psychopathology or severe emotional disorders is rare. Compare to **Chronic pain**.

Acute Polyradiculoneuritis (ah-kūt/pol″ē-ra-dik″u-lō-nu-rī′tis) (n.) See **Guillain-Barré Syndrome**.

ADA Abbreviation for Americans for Disability Act.

Adamantinoma (ad″ah-man″ti-nō′mah) (n.) A slow-growing, malignant neoplasm of bone. Usually seen in the jaw bones, it can occur in long bones—most commonly the tibia. Radiographically, one sees an osteolytic lesion that has a soap bubble-like appearance, along with surrounding sclerosis, cortical thinning, and expansion. Histologically, the lesion shows a characteristically biphasic appearance—a fibrous stroma alternating with cords or nests of epithelioid cells. Satellite lesions are not uncommon with this tumor. Also known as **Ameloblastoma**.

Adamkiewicz' Artery (ah-dam-ke′viks/ar′ter-ē) (n.)

The largest anterior radiculospinal artery in the thoracic region. It is the largest blood vessel feeding the lumbar spinal cord and the inferior thoracic spinal cords. Located on the left at the level of T9 to T11 in 80% of people. Synonyms: *great anterior medullary artery, great anterior radicular artery*.

Adaptation (ad″ap-tā′shun) (n.) The acquisition by an organism of characteristics that contribute to its environmental survival.

Adaptic Dressing (ah-dap′tik/dres′ing) (n.) A proprietary nonadhering mesh wound dressing.

Addison's Disease (ad-i-sonz/dĭ-zēz′) (n.) A syndrome involving a deficiency of adrenal steroid hormones; it is due to the primary inability of the adrenal gland to produce sufficient hormone. Known also as **Primary adrenocortical deficiency** or **Chronic glucocorticoid deficiency**.

Additional Diagnosis (a-dish′un-al/dī-ag-nō′sis) (n.) A diagnosis made after the initial principal diagnosis. It describes a condition for which a patient receives treatment or one that the physician considers of sufficient significance to warrant inclusion for further investigative medical studies even though it was not the primary reason for treatment.

Adduction (ah-duk′shun) (n.) 1. The movement of a part toward the midline of the body. Compare **Abduction**. 2. The position obtained by that movement.

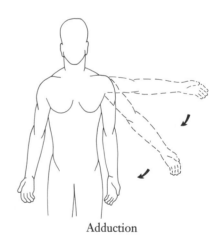

Adduction

Adduction Contracture (ah-duk′shun/kon-trak′tūr) (n.) A contracture of a body part that is fixed in adduction.

Adduction Osteotomy (ah-duk′shun/os″tē-ot′o-mē) (n.) See **Varus Derotation Osteotomy**.

Adduction Stress Test (ah-duk′shun/stres/test) (n.) A clinical examination used in the evaluation of the integrity of the lateral ligaments of the knee. Place one hand on the medial side of the knee and the opposite hand on the lateral aspect of the foot or ankle. Apply an adduction force across the knee and assess for laxity on the lateral knee. Check the knee both in full extension and 30 degrees of flexion. Compare these results with an examination of the opposite, normal knee. Also known as **Varus stress test**.

Adductor Brevis Muscle (ah-duk'tor/brev'is/mus'el) (n.) See **Muscle**.

Adductor Canal (ah-duk'tor/kah-nal') (n.) See **Hunter's Canal**.

Adductor Hallucis Muscle (ah-duk'tor/hal'ŭ-sis/mus'el) (n.) See **Muscle**.

Adductor Hiatus (ah-duk'tor/hi-ā'tus) (n.) A gap in the tendinous insertion of the adductor magnus muscle at a point just above the adductor tubercule through which the femoral vessels pass into the back of the knee. It is at this hiatus that the adductor (or Hunter's Canal) terminates.

Adductor Longus Muscle (ah-duk'tor/long'us/mus'el) (n.) See **Muscle**.

Adductor Magnus Muscle (ah-duk'tor/mag'nus/mus'el) (n.) See **Muscle**.

Adductor Pollicis Muscle (ah-duk'tor/pol'i-sis/mus'el) (n.) See **Muscle**.

Adductor Tenotomy (ah-duk'tor/ten-ot'ō-mē) (n.) A soft tissue release for the treatment of adduction contractures at the hip. The tight adductor muscle origin may be released percutaneously or through an open surgical procedure.

Adductor Tubercle (ah-duk'tor/too'ber'k'l) (n.) A bony projection on the medial epicondyle of the femur onto which the ischiocondylar portion of the adductor magnus muscle inserts. Also known as the **Adductor Tuberosity**.

Adductor Tuberosity (ah-duk'tor/too"be-ros'i-tē) (n.) See **Adductor Tubercle**.

Adenine (ad'e-nēn) (n.) A purine component of nucleosides, nucleotides, and nucleic acid.

Adenocarcinoma (ad"e-nō-kar"si-nō'mah) (n.) A malignant epithelial tumor that arises from glandular structures. There are histologic and histogenetic classifications: histologically, the term refers to a carcinoma in which the anaplastic parenchymal cells form glands; histogenetically, it refers to a carcinoma arising from the parenchyma of a gland.

Adenoma (ad"e-nō'mah) (n.) Any benign tumor of epithelial tissue in which the tumor cells form glands or glandlike structures.

Adenopathy (ad"e-nop'ah-thē) (n.) Enlargement of a gland, usually a lymphatic gland.

Adenosine Diphosphate (ah-den'o-sēn/dī-fos'fāt) (n.) A product of the hydrolysis of adenosine triphosphate that contains two phosphate groups. It is abbreviated ADP.

Adenosine Triphosphate (ah-den'o-sēn/trī-fos'fāt) (n.) An organic compound containing the purine adenine, the five-carbon sugar ribose, and three phosphate groups. ATP is a major carrier of phosphate and energy in biologic systems. On hydrolysis, ATP loses one phosphate and one hydrogen to become adenosine diphosphate (ADP), releasing energy in the process.

Adhesion (ad-hē'zhun) (n.) 1. The union or adherence of two normally separate surfaces. 2. The fibrous band formed from exudate on a serous membrane that causes adherence of two normally separate surfaces.

Adhesive Capsulitis (ad-hē'siv/kap"su-lī'tis) (n.) A clinical affection of the shoulder joint characterized by a chronic inflammatory process of the articular, capsular, and periarticular tissues. This results in pain, stiffness, and a loss of active and passive motion of the shoulder. The etiology is unknown, and the disorder may have a protracted clinical course. Arthrography of the affected shoulder demonstrates diminished joint capacity and a loss of the normal axillary fold. Also known as **Frozen Shoulder** or **Pericapsulitis**.

Adhesive Tape (ad-hē'siv/tāp) (n.) A strip of material evenly coated on one side with a pressure-sensitive adhesive.

Adipose Tissue (ad-i-pōs/tish'u) (n.) Fatty tissue.

Adjuvant (ad-joo'vant) (n.) Any agent or substance that, when used or mixed in conjunction with another, enhances the other substance's activity.

ADL (n.) Abbreviation for Activities of Daily Living.

Admission (ad-mish-en) (n.) Formal acceptance. There are various forms of patient admission:
Clinic Outpatient: A formal acceptance by a hospital of a patient who is to receive diagnostic services or treatment in a formally organized unit of a medical or surgical specialty or subspecialty but who is not to be lodged in the hospital's inpatient unit.
Inpatient: A formal acceptance by a hospital of a patient who is to receive health care services while lodged in an area of the hospital reserved for continuous nursing services.
Outpatient: A formal acceptance by a hospital of a patient who is to receive health care services but who is not to be lodged in an area of the hospital for continuous nursing services.
Preadmission Process: A formal acceptance by a hospital of a patient for preliminary tests on an outpatient basis prior to admission as an inpatient.

Adolescent Scoliosis (ad"ō-les'ent/skō"le-ō'sis) (n.) Lateral spinal curvature that appears before the onset of puberty and before skeletal maturity. It is more common in females.

ADP (n.) Abbreviation for adenosine diphosphate.

Adrenal Cortex (ah-drē'nal/kor'teks) (n.) The outer, cortical portion of the adrenal gland that produces and secretes steroid hormones.

Adrenaline (ah-dren'ah-lēn) (n.) See **Epinephrine**.

Adrenocorticotropic Hormone (ad-rē"no-kor"te-kō-trōp'ik/hor'mōn) (n.) A hormone secreted by the anterior lobe of the pituitary gland that stimulates the adrenal cortex to secrete hormones, such as steroids. Abbreviated ACTH.

Adrey-Vidal Apparatus (ad-rē/vē-dahl/ap-ă-rat'ŭs)

(n.) A device for external skeletal fixation; originally a French modification of the Hoffman Device. See **Hoffman External Fixator.**

Adson Test (ad'son/test) (n.) An evaluation of thoracic outlet syndrome. Elevate the patient's arm 90 degrees and externally rotate it while the elbow is flexed to a right angle. Turn the patient's head maximally to the unaffected side. If, in this position, the patient's radial pulse is diminished on the affected side, the test is considered positive, suggesting thoracic outlet syndrome. Accentuation of pain, obliteration or weakening of the pulse, and/or a drop of blood pressure when the head is turned toward the unaffected side support the diagnosis of thoracic outlet syndrome. Also known as the **Adson Maneuver.**

Adult Respiratory Distress Syndrome (ah-dult/respi'rah-to"re/distres'/sin'drom) (n.) A descriptive term for acute, diffuse, infiltrative pulmonary lesions of various etiologies that are associated with severe hypoxemia. In every case one sees increased liquid in the lungs without an increase in pulmonary capillary pressure along with the resultant alveolar collapse. Ventilation-perfusion imbalance also occurs, which results in decreased lung compliance. If the condition progresses one will see the classic radiographic appearance of diffuse, extensive bilateral interstitial and alveolar infiltrates. Treatment is directed toward respiratory support as well as therapy for the underlying cause. Abbreviated **ARDS.**

Adult Scoliosis (ah-dult/sko"le-o-sis) (n.) Scoliosis of any cause present after skeletal maturity.

Advancement (ad-vans'ment) (n.) A surgical technique in which a detached structure, such as a ligament or a tendon, is reattached to a more distal point.

Advancement Flap (ad-vans'ment/flap) (n.) A sliding technique of local skin flap grafts used frequently to cover terminal digital defects.

Adventitia (ad"ven-tish'e-ah) (n.) The outermost or external coat of the wall of an organ or structure that is not actually an integral part of that structure.

Adventitious Bursa (ad"ven-tish'us/ber'sah) (n.) Bursae not normally present that develop over bony prominences or prominent implants following repeated trauma or constant friction or pressure. These bursae do not have a true endothelial lining.

Adverse Drug Reaction (ad-vurs'/drug/re-ak'shun) (n.) A noxious and unintended reaction to a drug that occurs at doses normally used for prophylaxis, diagnosis, or therapy. Also known as an **Adverse Drug Experience** or **Adverse reaction.**

Adverse Reaction (ad-vurs/re-ak'shun) (n.) See **Adverse Drug Experience.**

Advil (ad-vil') (n.) A proprietary name for ibuprofen, a nonsteroidal, anti-inflammatory drug.

AEA (n.) Abbreviation for above-elbow amputation.

AE Amputation (AE/am"pu-ta'shun) (n.) Abbreviation for above-elbow amputation.

Aerobacter Aerogenes (ar"-o-bak'ter/ar'o-jenz) (n.) See enterobacter aerogenes.

Aerobe (a'er-ob) (n.) 1. Any organism that requires the presence of molecular oxygen for life and growth. 2. Any organism that can grow in the presence of air. Compare **Anaerobe.**

Aerobic Exercises (a-er-o'bik/ek'ser-siz-es) (n.) Organized movements intended to increase endurance and cardiovascular function by causing inhalation of oxygen at a rate sufficient for continuous energy production for muscle contraction.

Aerosol (a'er-o-sol") (n.) 1. A spray or mist. 2. A suspension of liquid or solid microscopic particles in a gas or atmosphere.

AFB (n.) Abbreviation for Acid-Fast Bacillus.

Afferent Nerve Fiber (af'er-ent/nerv/fi'ber) (n.) A nerve fiber that carries impulses from a receptor toward the central nervous system or a central ganglion. These are sensory nerve fibers. Also known as **Afferent Neuron.** Compare **Efferent Nerve.**

Afferent Neuron (af'er-ent/nu'ron) (n.) See **Afferent Nerve Fiber.**

AFO (n.) Abbreviation for ankle-foot orthosis.

AFP (n.) Abbreviation for alpha-fetoprotein.

Africoid Talus (a-fri-koyd/tal'us) (n.) A development anomaly in which the head and neck of the talus are tilted dorsally.

Agar-Agar (ag"ar-ag'ar) (n.) A dried polysaccharide extract of red algae (*Rhodophyceae*) used as the solidifying agent in the preparation of nutrient media for growing microorganisms. It is commonly referred to as agar.

Agglutination (ah-gloo"ti-na'shun) (n.) The aggregation of particles into clumps; specifically, the aggregation of a cellular antigen by antibody.

Agglutinin (ah-gloo'ti-nin) (n.) An antibody in the plasma capable of causing clumping of specific antigens on red blood cells.

Agility (a-jil'i-te) (n.) A person's ability to react quickly and to shift body position or direction rapidly while maintaining balance but not losing speed.

Agonist (ag'o-nist) (n.) In anatomy, a muscle that, when contracted, opposes the action of another muscle, which is known as its antagonist. This opposition simultaneously causes the antagonist to relax. For example, when the elbow is held extended, the triceps muscle is the agonist, while the relaxed biceps muscle is one of the antagonists. These muscles are also called **Prime Movers.**

A–G Ratio (A–G/ra'she-o) (n.) Abbreviation for the albumin to globulin ratio.

AHF (n.) Abbreviation for antihemophilic factor.

Ainhum (an'hum) (n.) A condition of unknown etiology characterized by the formation of a constricting ring around a digit, usually the fifth toe. Ultimately, spontaneous amputation occurs, usually after three to ten years. Synonyms include: **Dacty-**

lolysis Spontanea, **Banko-kereude**, and **Sukha Pokla Quijila**.

Air Bed (ār/bed) (n.)   A bed with an air-filled mattress.

Aircast (ār/kast) (n.)   1. A brace that is composed of contoured, molded plastic shells and inflated aircells that provide comfort, support, and gradual compression. This is a registered trademark of its manufacturer. The company is best known for its Air-Stirrup Ankle Brace; they also design braces for other body parts, including the patella and the upper extremity. 2. A commonly used term to refer to an **Air-Stirrup, Ankle Brace**.

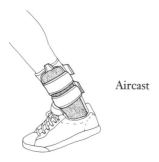

Aircast

Air Contrast Arthrogram (ār/kon′trast/ar′-thrō-gram) (n.)   A technique of injecting air and a radio-opaque dye, as contrast agent, into a joint. The knee, shoulder, and ankle are most commonly injected.

Air Contrast Myelography (ār/kon′trast/mi″e-log′ rah-fē) (n.)   A rarely used technique of myelography in which air is injected as the contrast agent.

Air Embolism (ār/em′bō-lism) (n.)   An obstructive bubble formed from a bolus of intravascular air.

Air Fluidized Bed (ār/flū′i-dīzed/bed) (n.)   A bed with a mattress containing hundreds of millions of small ceramic beads, each about 0.1 mm in diameter, that form a layer about 30 cm thick. The beads are suspended by a stream of warm air and covered with a polyester sheet; the patient then floats on this. Used for the treatment and prevention of decubitus ulcers.

Airplane Cast (ār′plān/kast) (n.)   A device that holds the thorax and the affected upper extremity in a position of abduction. It is called an "airplane cast" because the arm held in abduction looks like an extended wing. Used in the immobilization of the shoulder and shoulder girdle; also called a **Shoulder Spica**.

Airplane Splint (ār′plān/splint) (n.)   A removable device used to maintain the upper extremity in a position of abduction.

Airsplint (ār′splint)   An inflatable sleeve or stocking. It is used at the onset of injury as a first-aid device, providing support, pressure, and immobilization of the extremity during transport. See **Inflatable Splint**.

Aitken's Classification (ā-kenz/klas″sĭ-fĭ-ka′shun) (n.)   A descriptive system of physeal fractures. There are three types:

Type I: fractures that have traveled completely through the physis without exiting through the bone or metaphysis.

Type II: a fracture that has traversed the physis and epiphysis.

Type III: a fracture that has traversed the metaphysis, the physis, and the epiphysis. Contrast with **Salter Classification**.

Aitken Classification of Proximal Focal Femoral Deficiency (ā-ken/klas″sĭ-fĭ-ka′shun/of/prok′sĭ-mal/fo′kal/fem′or-al/de-fish′en-se) (n.)   A systematic division of proximal focal femoral deficiencies into four types:

Type A: The acetabulum is competent and contains an ossified femoral head. The proximal femur will usually ossify, but with severe subtrochanteric varus angulation and possible pseudoarthrosis formation.

Type B: The acetabulum is dysplastic but contains an ossified femoral head. The femoral shaft is displaced proximally so that its end is proximal to the femoral head. Ossification will not occur between the head and the shaft.

Type C: The acetabulum is dysplastic and does not contain an ossified femoral head. A small tuft of ineffective ossified tissue is present at the proximal end of the shaft.

Type D: The acetabulum is almost completely absent and contains no ossified femoral head. There is no tuft of ossified tissue at the proximal end of the femoral shaft.

AK (n.)   Abbreviation for above-knee amputation.

AKA (n.)   Abbreviation for above-knee amputation.

AK Prosthesis (n.)   Abbreviation for an above-knee prosthesis.

Akin Osteotomy (ā′kin/os″tē-ot′o-mē) (n.)   A technique for the surgical treatment of hallux valgus in which a closing wedge osteotomy at the base of the proximal phalanx is combined with resection of the medial eminence. An adductor tenotomy and/or lateral capsulotomy also may be performed simultaneously.

Alar Ligaments (ā′lar/lig′ah-mentz) (n.)   The paired fibrous bands that connect the superolateral aspect of the odontoid process of the second cervical vertebra to the medial sides of the occipital condyles. They present excessive rotation at the median atlanto-occipital joint.

Albers-Schonberg Disease (ahl-berz/shun-berg/di-sēz′)   Eponym for benign osteopetrosis, which is inherited as an autosomal dominant trait. See **Osteopetrosis**.

Albright's Disease (awl′brīts/di-sēz) (n.)   A syndrome resulting from hypothalamic-hypophyseal dysfunction. It consists of polyostotic fibrous dysplasia in the skeleton, segmental pigment disorders of the skin, premature skeletal maturation, precocious puberty, and/or hyperthyroidism. Synonyms: **Osteitis Fibrosa disseminata**; **Fuller-Albright syndrome**; **Albright-McCune-Sternberg syndrome**. See related term **Dysplasia**.

Albumin (al-bu′min) (n.) A simple protein that is soluble in water and coagulable by heat. It is found widely in the tissues and fluids of both plants and animals. In humans, serum albumin is the principal protein in blood plasma.

Alcaptonuria (al-kap″tō-nū′rē-ah) (n.) See **Alkaptonuria**.

Aldosterone (al′dō-ster-ōn) (n.) The most active mineralocorticoid hormone secreted by the cortex of the adrenal gland. Aldosterone functions in the regulation of salt metabolism.

Alignment (ah-līn′ment) (n.) 1. The act of bringing into line. 2. A term used in fracture management to refer to the position of one fracture fragment to the next fragment or the overall linearity of the involved limb. See **Apposition**.

Alignment Index of Garden (ah-līn′ment/in′deks/of/gar-den′) (n.) See **Garden's Alignment Index**.

Alivium (n.) The trademark name for a cobalt chromium molybdenum alloy that has been vacuum melted and casted. Used to make orthopaedic implants. Other brands include **Austenal** and **Vitallium**.

Alkali (al′kah-lī) (n.) 1. A substance that dissociates, releasing hydroxyl (OH−) ions but not hydrogen (H+) ions, and whose aqueous solution has a pH of greater than 7. 2. A molecule or ion that liberates electrons, usually in water.

Alkaline (al′kah-līn,lin) (adj.) Of or pertaining to an alkali.

Alkaline Phosphatase (al′kah-līn,lin/fos′fah-tās) (n.) An enzyme that liberates inorganic phosphate from phosphate ester by hydrolysis. It is produced by many tissues, especially bone, intestine, liver, and placenta; most normal serum alkaline phosphate, however, is produced by bone. Abbreviated **ALP**.

Alkaptonuria (al″kap-tō-nū′rē-ah) (n.) An inherited disorder of phenylalanine-tyrosine metabolism in which a deficiency of the enzyme homogentisic oxidase results in excessive excretion of homogentisic acid in the urine, along with the accumulation of oxidized homogentisic acid pigment in connective tissues. The darkened pigmentation is known as ochronosis. A distinct form of degenerative arthritis develops in these patients, with symptoms usually appearing in the fourth decade of life. See **Ochronosis**.

Allele (ah-lel′) (n.) One or more genes that occur at the same position on a specific pair of chromosomes; this means that these genes have the same locus on homologous chromosomes.

Allen's Test (al′enz/test) (n.) An evaluation of dual arterial supply to the hand. Instruct the patient to elevate the hand and to clench the fist several times to exsanguinate the hand. Simultaneously, use finger pressure to compress both the radial and the ulnar arteries. The patient should then lower the hand and open the fist while you release pressure from each artery separately. The patency of each artery is demonstrated by the immediate flush of blood into the pale skin of the palm supplied by that artery after pressure is removed from the vessel.

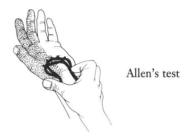

Allen's test

Allergen (al′er-jen) (n.) A substance, antigen, or hapten that incites hypersensitivity or allergy.

Allergic Reaction (ah-ler′jik/re-ak′shun) (n.) A tissue injury that is the manifestation of an interaction between an antigen and an antibody.

Allergy (al′er-jē) (n.) A state of specific increased reactivity of tissues to repeated contacts with an antigen or hapten.

Allis Maneuver (al′is/mah-noo′ver) (n.) A technique for the gentle reduction of both anterior and posterior hip dislocations. For both dislocations, place the patient supine and have an assistant stabilize the pelvis. In anterior hip dislocation, flex the knee to relax the hamstrings; then flex the hip slightly and apply longitudinal traction in line with the axis of the femur. Next, gently adduct and internally rotate the femur to achieve reduction. The assistant also may apply lateral traction to the inside of the thigh. In posterior dislocations, apply longitudinal traction in line with the deformity, with the knee flexed to 90°; then gently flex the hip to 90°. The hip is then gently rotated internally and externally to achieve reduction.

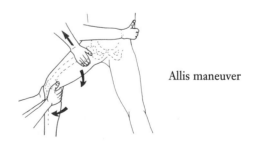

Allis maneuver

Allis Sign (al′is/sīn) (n.) 1. In congenital dislocation of the hip, this clinical sign indicates an apparent shortening of the femur due to superior migration of the proximal femur. Place the patient in a supine position with his knees flexed and his soles resting on the examining table. The knee on the affected side will be lower than the unaffected side. Also known as **Galeazzi's Sign**. 2. A clinical indication of a femoral neck fracture in which there is noted to be relaxation of the fascia between the crest of the ilium and the greater trochanter.

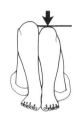

Allis sign

(handwritten margin note: alpha angle (in FAI) per insert)

Allogeneic (al″o-je-nē′ik) (adj.) Having different genetic constitutions within the same species; differing in genotype.

Allograft (al′ō-graft) (n.) A tissue graft from a donor of one genotype of a species to a host of another genotype of the same species. Synonym: **Homograft**.

Allopurinol (al″o-pūr′ĭ-nŏl) (n.) A drug used in the treatment of gout. It controls hyperuricemia by decreasing uric acid synthesis through the inhibition of xanthine oxidase. Marketed under the trade name **Zyloprim**.

Allowable Stress (ă-low′able/stress) (n.) In biomechanical terms, a stress value higher than that due to normal loads but lower than the yield stress of a material.

Alloy (al′loi) (n.) A substance composed of two or more metals intimately mixed by fusion, electrolytic deposition, or other processes.

Alphafetoprotein (al″fah-fē″tō-prō′tē-in) A protein derived from yolk and embryonic liver cells used in the prenatal diagnosis of neural tube defects. This protein is normally present in embryonic fluid from the sixth to the fourteenth week of gestation; it then drops to undetectable levels. If, upon amniocentesis at 16 to 18 weeks' gestation, a high level of AFP is found, this usually indicates an open neural tube defect.

ALRI (n.) Abbreviation for anterolateral rotatory instability.

Alsberg's Angle (alz-bergz/ang′g′l) (n.) An equilateral triangle whose apex points upward. It is formed by three lines, as follows: (1) Pass a line through the long axis of the femur, (2) Pass a second line through the long axis of the neck of the femur, and (3) Pass a third line on a plane through the base of the head of the femur. The angle of the apex is known as the angle of elevation.

Ambling Gait (am′bling/gāt) (n.) A type of walking in which both the upper and lower limbs of the same side advance at the same time.

Ambulation (am′bu-la′shun) (n.) Walking or moving about. Persons with impaired ability to ambulate may be divided into four functional levels:

1. **Community ambulators:** Patients able to walk indoors and outdoors for most of their activities. Crutches and/or braces may be needed. Wheelchairs are needed only for long distances.

2. **Household ambulators:** Patients able to walk only short distances indoors and only with the aid of an apparatus. They are capable of getting in and out of a chair and bed with little or no assistance. Wheelchairs may be used for some indoor activities at home or school and for all outside activities.

3. **Nonfunctional ambulators:** Patients able to walk in the context of therapeutic sessions at home, in school, or in the hospital. Wheelchairs are used to get from place to place and to satisfy all needs for transportation. These patients are also known as exercise ambulators.

4. **Nonambulators:** Wheelchair-bound patients who may be able to stand only for transfers from bed to chair.

Ambulatory Care (am′bu-lah-to″rē/care) (n.) The provision of health care services to outpatients and other patients who do not require hospital admission as inpatients.

Ambulatory Care Center (am′bu-lah-to″rē/care/center) (n.) A health facility with an organized professional staff providing various medical, surgical, and health-related services to patients who do not require hospital admission. Also known as **Ambulatory Care Institution**.

Ambulatory Care Institution (am′bu-lah-to″rē/care/in′sti-too′shun) (n.) See **Ambulatory Care Center**.

Amelia (ah-mē′lē-ah) (n.) A developmental anomaly characterized by the congenital absence of a limb or limbs.

American Academy of Orthopaedic Surgeons The purpose of the ACADEMY shall be to foster and assure the highest quality musculoskeletal health care through: education of orthopaedic surgeons, other health care professionals, and the public; promotion of research; communication with other professionals and the public; and provision of leadership in the development of health care policy. These and other purposes of the ACADEMY exclusively are to foster, develop, support, and augment charitable, scientific, or educational activities. 6300 North River Road, Rosemont, IL 60018. Abbreviated **AAOS**.

American Board of Orthopaedic Surgery The certifying board for American Orthopaedic Surgeons. 400 Silver Cedar Court, Chapel Hill, NC 27514.

Amikacin (am″i-ka′sin) (n.) An aminoglycoside antibiotic; a semisynthetic derivative of kanamycin. Active against *Pseudomonas*.

Amino Acid (ah-mē′no/as′id) (n.) An organic compound of the general formula $H_2N-CHR-COOH$, where R may be one of 20 or more different sidechains. Amino acids are known as the building blocks of proteins because the compound has both a basic amine group, $-NH_2$, and an acidic carboxyl group, $+COOH$. The linear order of the amino acids in a peptide or protein is called an amino acid sequence and is genetically determined.

Amipaque (am′ĭ-pāk) (n.) A proprietary brand of metrizamide; a nonionic, water-soluble iodinated contrast medium used for myelographic examinations.

Amniocentesis (am-nē-o-sen-tē-sis) (n.) Aspiration of amniotic fluid between the fourteenth and sixteenth week of pregnancy for the purposes of performing studies on the fluid. These tests are useful in the prenatal diagnosis of certain metabolic defects, chromosome abnormalities, neural tube defects, sex of the fetus, and other conditions.

Amoss' Sign (a′mos/sīn) (n.) An indication of painful flexure of the spine. Instruct the supine patient to rise to a sitting position. In a positive test, the patient supports the rise by placing the hands far behind the body.

Amoxicillin (ah-moks″i-sil′in) (n.) A derivative of ampicillin demonstrating better oral absorption and higher blood levels and urinary excretion levels than the parent drug.

Amphiarthrosis (am″fē-ar′thrō′sis) (n.) A joint in which there is little motion between the opposed surfaces of bones, which are united by cartilage. Types of amphiarthroses include synchondroses and symphyses. Also known as a **Junctura Cartilaginae**.

Amphotericin B (am″fo-ter′i-sin/B) (n.) A polyene antibiotic substance used as an antifungal agent.

Ampicillin (amp″i-sil′in) (n.) A semisynthetic aminobenzyl penicillin that is not penicillinase-resistant.

Amputation (am″pu-tā′shun) (n.) The removal of a limb, part of a limb, or any other protuberant body part. See also specific types of amputation.

Amputation Flap (am″pu-tā′shun/flap) (n.) A simple, broad-based skin or myocutaneous section remaining after amputation of a body part. It need not be advanced, but is contoured to provide proper coverage of the stump.

Amputation Neuroma (am″pu-tā′shun/nu-rō′mah) (n.) A benign, tumorlike mass of proliferating proximal nerve fibers and fibrous tissue that may develop in the stump of a severed nerve. This may be a painful condition. Also known as **Traumatic Neuroma**.

Amputation Stump (am″pu-tā′shun/stump) (n.) The rounded and shaped distal portion of an amputated limb or organ.

Amputee (am″pu-tē′) (n.) A person with one or more amputated limbs.

Amstutz Total Hip Arthroplasty (ahm-shtutz/tō′tal/hip/ar′thrō-plas″tē) (n.) A type of total hip prosthesis that contains a 28-mm head component and a collar and a curved stem that is inserted into the femur.

Amyloidosis (am″ĭ-loi-do′sis) (n.) A disorder characterized by the accumulation of amyloid, a unique,

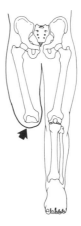

Amputation stump

extracellular, filamentous glycoprotein found in the connective tissues. It occurs as a primary or secondary disorder following chronic infections, inflammatory conditions, and neoplasms. Clinical manifestations are variable and depend on specific organ involvement and the infiltration of amyloid around nerves and vessels.

Amyotrophic Lateral Sclerosis (ah-mī″ō-trōf′ik/lat′er-al/skle-rō′sis) (n.) A progressive disorder of the motor neurons in which muscular atrophy and hyperreflexia are combined. It is of unknown etiology. Also known as **Lou Gehrig's disease**.

ANA Abbreviation for antinuclear antibody.

Anaerobe (an-a′er-ōb) (n.) An organism that survives and grows in the absence of molecular oxygen. Compare **Aerobe**.

Analgesia (an″al-jē′zē-ah) (n.) The absence of pain on noxious stimulation.

Analogous (ah-nal′ō-gus) (adj.) Of or pertaining to structures that are similar in function but of differing origin or structure.

Anal Wink (a′nal/wingk) (n.) A normal cord-mediated reflex elicited by gently pricking the perianal region with a pin, which should cause a contracture of the external anal sphincter.

Anaphylaxis (an″ah-fi-lak′sis) (n.) An acute, severe, systemic hypersensitivity reaction caused by the release of histamine and other mediators from basophils and mast cells. This is the result of an antigen–antibody reaction. The clinical picture of anaphylaxis can range from a local reaction to anaphylactic shock.

Anaplasia (an″ah-plā′ze-ah) (n.) A loss of differentiation that is characteristic of tumor cells. Also called **Undifferentiation**.

Anastomosis (ah-nas″tō-mō′sis) (n.) A connection or communication between tubular structures or vessels.

Anatomic Axis (an″-ah-tom′-ik/ak′sis) (n.) 1. The true axis of an extremity, which is measured by lines drawn parallel to the shaft of the bone. 2. To measure the anatomic axis of the lower extremity, obtain weight-bearing anteroposterior radiographs on a long cassette. Draw lines parallel to the midshaft of the femur and the tibia. The axis may be described in relationship to the transverse knee or ankle axes, the mechanical axis of the lower extremity, or the vertical axis of the body. The anatomic axis of the femur is normally in 6° valgus from the mechanical axis, and that of the tibia is in 2–3° of varus from the **Mechanical axis**.

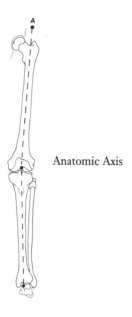

Anatomic Axis

Anatomic Neck of the Humerus (an″-ah-tom′-ik/ nek/of the/hu′mer-us) (n.)   The slight indentation along the humeral head margin to which the articular capsule is attached. It separates the articulating portion of the humeral head from the greater and lesser tubercles. Compare **Surgical Neck of Humerus**.

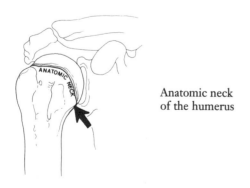

Anatomic neck of the humerus

Anatomic Position (an″-ah-tom′-ik/pō-zish′un) (n.) The position in which the body is erect and facing the observer, arms hanging at the sides and palms turned forward. All references to location of parts assume the body to be in anatomic position.

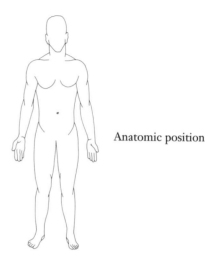

Anatomic position

Anatomic Triangle (an′-ah-tom′-ik/tri′ang-g′l) (n.) See **Ranawat's Triangle**.

Anatomic Snuff-Box (an″-ah-tomik/snuf/box) (n.)   A triangular depression formed on the radial aspect of the wrist when the thumb is extended and abducted. It is shaped by the arrangement of the extensor pollicis longus and the tendons of the extensor pollicis brevis and abductor pollicis longus. See **Snuff-Box**.

Anatomy (ah-nat′ō-mē) (n.)   The study of the structure of living organisms.

Anchoring Holes (ang′ker-ing/hōlz) (n.)   Drill holes made in the surface of bones to which a prosthetic implant is to be cemented. These holes are intended to improve cement fixation by creating areas of deeper penetration.

Ancillary Services (an′sil-lär″e/services) (n.)   Services provided to hospital patients in the course of care; those included are laboratory, radiology, pharmacy, and therapy services; excluded are room, board, and medical and nursing services.

Anderson and Fowler Calcaneal Osteotomy (an′der-son/and/fow′ler/kal-ka′ne-al/os″tē-ot′o-mē) (n.)   An operation to treat pes planus. The lateral column of the foot is lengthened by an opening wedge anterior calcaneal osteotomy and the tibialis posterior tendon is advanced plantar, medial, and distally. If necessary, a closing wedge osteotomy of the first cuneiform is performed to correct tarsometatarsal supination.

Anderson and Green Growth Prediction Chart (an′der-son / and / grēn / groth / prē″dik-shun / chart) (n.)   See **Green-Anderson Tables**.

Anderson Splint (an′der-son/splint) (n.)   See **Roger Anderson Device**.

Anderson Well-Leg Traction (an′der-son/well-leg/

trak'shun) (n.)   See **Roger Anderson Well-Leg Traction**.

Andrews Procedure (an-drooz/pro-sē'jur) (n.)   A technique for extra-articular reconstruction of anterior cruciate ligament insufficiency of the knee. In this technique, a tenodesis of the iliotibial band is performed through drill holes in the distal femur.

Androgen (an'drō-jen) (n.)   A general term for the steroid hormones of males, in which androgens promote the development of secondary sex characteristics and stimulate activity of accessory sex organs.

Android Pelvis (an'droyd/pel'vis) (n.)   A pelvic shape considered to be male. The inlet is wedge-shaped and the forepelvis narrowed. The anteroposterior and widest transverse diameters of the inlet may be roughly equivalent, but the posterior sagittal diameter at the inlet is much shorter than the anterior sagittal diameter. The sidewalls are typically convergent, and the ischial spines are prominent. The height of the symphysis is more than 6 cm; the transverse diameter of the outlet is less than 10 cm; and the subpubic arch is narrowed. The bone structure is also characteristically heavy, with the sacrum inclined forward, especially in its lower third.

Anemia (ah-nē'mē-ah) (n.)   A condition in which the hemoglobin concentration of blood decreases below normal levels.

Anergy (an'er-je) (n.)   Absence of a reaction when a hypersensitivity reaction would be expected in other subjects similarly sensitized to a specific antigen or allergen.

Anesthesia (an"es-the'ze-ah) (n.)   A partial or total loss of sensation, with or without the loss of consciousness. See specific types: bier block, caudal, epidural, general, local, nerve block, regional, and spinal.

Anesthesia Dolorosa (an"es-the'ze-ah/do-lo'rō-sa) (n.)   Pain in an area or structure that is anesthetic.

Anesthesia Screen (an"es-the'ze-ah/screen) (n.)   An adjustable frame that positions and supports drapes away from the patient's face; separates the nonsterile area from the sterile operating field.

Anesthesiologist (an"es-thē"zē-ol'o-gist) (n.)   A physician specializing in the field of anesthesiology.

Anesthesiology (an"es-thē"zē-ol-o-jē) (n.)   The study of anesthetics and anesthesia.

Anesthetic (an"es-thet'ik)   1. (n.) An agent or compound that produces anesthesia. 2. (adj.) Describing the loss of or decrease in sensation.

Anesthetist (ah-nes'thĕ-tist) (n.)   A person trained in administering anesthetics, but not necessarily a physician. Compare **Anesthesiologist**.

Aneurysm (an'u-rizm) (n.)   A circumscribed dilation of the wall of an artery. Aneurysms occur most commonly in the aorta, but many occur in any artery. They may be caused by trauma, congenital vascular disease, infection, or arteriosclerosis. Aneurysms can be both true and false: a **true aneurysm** results from degeneration of an arterial wall; a **false aneurysm** is caused by injury to the wall of an artery by direct trauma, such as a penetrating wound from a knife or bullet. This traumatic aneurysm is actually a pulsating, encapsulated hematoma that communicates with the lumen of the injured vessel.

Aneurysmal Bone Cyst (an"u-riz'mal/bōn/sist) (n.)   A benign, non-neoplastic cystic lesion of bone. Radiographically, it is characterized as an expansile, eccentric lesion; grossly, the lesion appears as a multiloculated cystic cavity. Microscopically, there are cystic spaces of various sizes that are filled with blood but not lined by vascular endothelium. These cysts are often found in the long bones and the spine. In some cases, the lesion may coexist with another benign tumor.

Angiography (an"jē-og'rah-fē) (n.)   The radiographic visualization of vessels obtained after intravascular injection of radiopaque contrast material. Also known as **arteriography**.

Angioma (an"jē-ō'mah) (n.)   A benign swelling or tumor due to the proliferation and enlargement of blood vessels (a hemangioma) or lymph vessels (a lymphangioma).

Angioplasty (an'jē-ō-plas"tē) (n.)   Surgical repair of injured or diseased blood vessels.

Angle of Depression (ang'g'l/of/de-presh'un) (n.)   An angle formed by the line of sight and the horizontal plane for any object below the horizon.

Angle of Elevation (ang'g'l/of/el"e-vā'shun) (n.)   An angle formed by the line of sight and the horizontal plane for any object above the horizon.

Angle of Femoral Torsion (ang'g'l/of/fem'or-al/tor'shun) (n.)   The angle formed in the sagittal plane by the projection of the longitudinal axis of the femoral neck on the transverse bicondylar axis of the knee. If this angle is projected anteriorly, it is referred to as **Anteversion**; if it projects posteriorly, the angle is called **Retroversion**.

Angle of Incidence (ang'g'l/of/in'si-dens) (n.)   The angle that a line meeting a surface makes with a line perpendicular to the surface at the point of incidence.

Angle of Inclination (ang'g'l/of/in"klĭ-na'shun) (n.)   See **Neck Shaft Angle** and **Angle of Thoracic Inclination**.

Angle of Inclination of the Humerus (ang'g'l/of/in"kli-nā'shun/of the/hū'mer-us) (n.)   As measured on a lateral radiograph, the relationship of the longitudinal axis of the humerus to the anterior tilt of the distal humeral articular surface. The normal value is approximately 40°.

Angle of Inclination of the Pelvis (ang'g'l/of/in"klĭ-nā'shun/of the/pel'vis) (n.)   1. The angle formed by the anterior wall of the pelvis and the anteroposterior diameter of the pelvic inlet. This may be measured on a lateral radiograph of the pelvis. 2. The angle formed either by the pelvis and the general line of the trunk, or by the plane of the outlet of the pelvis and the horizon.

Angle of Louis (ang'g'l/of Louis) (n.)   The angle formed by the manubrium and the body of the sternum. Synonyms: **Angulus Ludovici, Sternal Angle**.

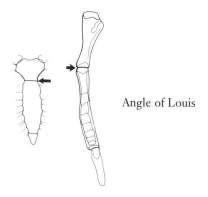

Angle of Louis

Angle of Thoracic Inclination (ang'g'l/of/tho-ras'ik/in"klĭ-na'shun) (n.)   In a standing patient whose trunk is flexed 90° at the hips, the angle formed between a line parallel to the ground and a plane across the trunk of the greatest thoracic prominence.

Angstrom (ang'strem) (n.)   Unit of measurement equal to 1/100,000,000 of a centimeter, or 1/10,000 of a micron. It is named for the Swedish physicist Anders John Ångström.

Angular Deformity (ang'gu-lar/dē-for'mi-tē) (n.)   Any deformity in which there is deviation from a straight line in a normally linear structure. In describing angulation, name the direction that the apex of the deformity points, for example, medial or lateral angulation. Angular deformities are measured in degrees.

Angulation (ang"gu-lā'shun) (n.)   1. The act of forming an angle. 2. An angular position, shape, or formation. 3. Deviation from the normal axis, as with a displaced fracture of a bone.

Anion (an'ī-on) (n.)   A negatively charged ion that is characterized by migration toward the positive electrode, or anode, in an electric field.

Anisocytosis (an-ī"so-sī-tō'sis) (n.)   Denotes variation in the size of cells that are usually uniform.

Anisotropic (an-i"so-trop'ik) (adj.)   Exhibiting directionality in mechanical properties according to direction of testing. For example, wood and bone are anisotropic materials.

Ankle (ang'k'l) (n.)   The hinge or ginglymus joint connecting the foot and leg. It is formed by the articulation of the tibia and fibula with the talus.

Ankle Clonus Test (ang'kl/klo'nus/test) (n.)   A test to evaluate the intactness of the spinal cord after the surgical correction of scoliosis. If ankle clonus is

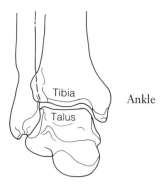

Tibia

Talus

Ankle

present as the patient is awakening from anesthesia, the spinal cord is intact. Described by S. Hoppenfeld.

Ankle-Foot Orthosis (ang'k'l/foot/or-thō'sis) (n.)   A device that supports the foot and extends over the malleoli of the ankle. Abbreviated **AFO**.

Ankle Jerk (ang'k'l/jerk) (n.)   See **Achilles Tendon Reflex**.

Anklet (ang'k'l-et) (n.)   A soft orthosis that embraces the ankle, offering support or protection.

Ankylosing Spinal Hyperostosis (ang"ki-lō-sing/spī'nal/hī"per-os-tō'sis) (n.)   See **DISH**.

Ankylosing Spondylitis (ang"ki-lō-sing/spon"di-lī'tis) (n.)   A chronic, progressive inflammatory disease of the spine, sacroiliac joints, and paravertebral soft tissues. It is characterized by early sacroiliac joint involvement, followed by ossification of the annulus fibrosus and surrounding connective tissue, along with arthritic changes in the intervertebral joints, which results in bony ankylosing of the spine. Peripheral joints also may be involved. The disease occurs predominantly in young adult males and is often associated with the presence of the HLA-B27 antigen, absence of rheumatoid factor in the serum, and lack of rheumatoid nodules. Synonym: **Marie-Strumpell Disease**. See **Bamboo Spine**.

Ankylosing Vertebral Hyperostosis (ang"ki-lō-sing/ver'tē-bral/hī"per-os-tō'sis) (n.)   See **DISH**.

Ankylosis (ang"ki-lō'sis) (n.)   Abnormal fixation, stiffness, immobility, and consolidation of a joint. This may result from bony, cartilagenous, or fibrous tissue overgrowth.

Annular Ligament (an'u-lar/lig'ah-ment) (n.)   A strong, circular band that encircles most of the head of the radius and attaches to the anterior and posterior margins of the radial notch of the ulna. It serves as a restraining ligament for the radial head.

Annulus (an'u-lus) (n.)   Any ring-shaped, circular structure.

Annulus Fibrosus (an'u-lus/fī-bro'sis) (n.)   The outer concentric layers of fibrous tissue in the intervertebral discs. It consists of laminated collagen fibers arranged obliquely, but in opposite directions, in adjacent layers, thus improving torsional resistance.

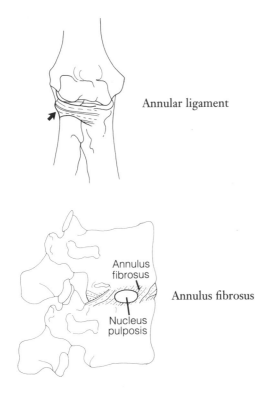

Annular ligament

Annulus fibrosus

brachioradialis muscle laterally. The floor of the fossa is formed by the brachialis and supinator muscles. Important neurovascular structures, such as the brachial artery and radial nerve, pass through this fossa over the elbow joint. Synonym: **Antecubital Space**.

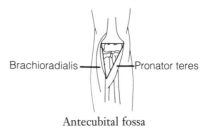

Antecubital fossa

Anterior (an-ter′e-or) (adj.)   1. Situated before, in front of. 2. The ventral surface of the body.

Anterior Atlanto-occipital Membrane (an-ter′e-or/at-lan″tō-ok-sip′i-tal/mem′brān) (n.)   A wide, dense, fibroelastic band that extends between the anterior margin of the foramen magnum and the upper border of the anterior arch of the atlas. It is reinforced in the midline by the proximal continuation of the anterior longitudinal ligament.

Anterior Cervical Cord Syndrome (an-ter′e-or/ser′vi-kal/kord/sin′drōm) (n.)   An incomplete spinal cord syndrome characterized by complete motor loss and loss of pain and temperature discrimination below the level of injury. Deep touch, position sense, and vibratory sensation remain intact throughout. Prognosis for significant neurologic recovery is poor. The syndrome may result from direct trauma to the anterior cord and from injury to the anterior spinal artery system.

Anterior Cruciate Ligament (an-ter′e-or/kroo′shē′āt/lig′ah-ment) (n.)   A ligament in the knee that extends from the nonarticular area in front of the intercondylar eminence of the tibia upward and backward to the posterior part of the medial aspect of the lateral femoral condyle. This ligament acts as the primary restraint to anterior translation of the tibia on the femur. See **Cruciate Ligament Anterior**.

Anode (an′ōd) (n.)   A positive electrode toward which negatively charged ions, known as anions, migrate.

Anomaly (ah-nom′ah-lē) (n.)   Any deviation from normal form, structure, function, or location.

Anostosis (an″ōs-tō′sis) (n.)   Any defective ossification of bone.

Ansaid (n.)   A proprietary brand of flurbiprofen, a nonsteroidal antiinflammatory drug.

Antagonist (an-tag′o-nist) (n.)   A muscle whose contraction opposes that of another muscle, which is called the agonist or prime mover. Antagonists must be relaxed if agonists are to contract effectively. See **Agonist**.

Antalgic (ant-al′jik) (adj.)   Of or pertaining to a gait, position, or posture assumed to avoid pain.

Antalgic Gait (ant-al′jik/gāt) (n.)   1. A painful limp. 2. Shortening of the stance phase on the affected side by quick, soft steps to avoid weight-bearing and to diminish pain.

Ante (an-te)   A prefix indicating before, anterior to, or in front of.

Antecubital (an″te-ku′bi-tal) (adj.)   Situated in front of the elbow.

Antecubital Fossa (an″te-ku′bi-tal/fos′ah) (n.)   A triangular anatomic space at the anterior aspect of the bend of the elbow. Its downward apex is bounded by a line connecting the humerus epicondyles superiorly, the pronator teres muscle medially, and the

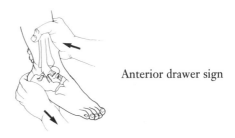

Anterior drawer sign

Anterior Drawer Sign (an-ter′e-or/drawer/sīn) (n.)   A method of evaluation of anterior talofibular ligament integrity. Hold the lower leg firmly and draw the foot anteriorly by pulling on the heel. Excessive forward talar displacement is pathologic, indicates ligamentous disruption, and should be compared with the opposite ankle. Actual talar subluxation may be measured on a lateral radiograph obtained while applying anterior stress to the ankle. Also known as the **Anteroposterior Stress Test**.

Anterior Drawer Test (an-ter′e-or/drawer test) (n.) A method of evaluation of the integrity of the anterior cruciate ligament of the knee. With the patient supine on an examining table, flex the hip to 45° and the knee to 90°, placing the foot on the tabletop. Sit on the dorsum of the patient's foot to stabilize it, and place both hands behind the knee to feel for the relaxation of the hamstring muscles. Gently and repeatedly pull and push the proximal part of the leg anteriorly and posteriorly, noting the movement of the tibia on the femur. Perform this test with the tibia in three positions of rotation: internally rotated 30°, externally rotated 15°, and in neutral rotation. Record the degree of displacement in each position of rotation, and compare it with the normal knee. See **Posterior Drawer Test**.

Anterior Funiculus (an-ter′e-or/fu-nik′u-lus) (n.) The anterior white matter of the spinal cord; it lies between the anterior median fissure and the ventral root on either side of the spinal cord.

Anterior Horn Cell (an-ter′e-or/horn/cell) (n.) A large, multipolar nerve cell in the anterior horn of the spinal cord whose axon functions as an efferent fiber innervating a muscle.

Anterior Interbody Fusion (an-ter′e-or/in″ter-bod′ē/fu′zhun) (n.) A technique of spinal arthrodesis performed through an anterior approach to the spine. In this technique, excision of the intervertebral disc and the cartilage end-plates is performed, followed by the insertion of bone graft between the two adjacent vertebrae.

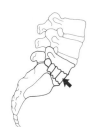

Anterior interbody fusion

Anterior Interosseous Nerve (an-ter′e-or/in″ter-os′e-us/nerv) (n.) A branch of median nerve originating an inch below the elbow. The nerve clings to the interosseous membrane in the forearm and supplies the flexor pollicis longus, the flexor digitorum profundus (radial half), and the pronator teres muscles.

Anterior Interosseous Nerve Syndrome (an-ter′e-

or/in″ter-os′e-us/nerv/sin′drōm) (n.) A compressive neuropathy of the anterior interosseous nerve in the forearm. The hand typically displays an inability to create an "OK sign" due to paralysis of the flexor digitorum profundus muscle of the index finger and the flexor pollicis longus muscle of the thumb. There are characteristically no sensory abnormalities.

Anterior Knee Pain Syndrome (an-ter′ē-or/nē/pān/sin′drōm) (n.) A frequently used term for anterior and peripatellar knee pain resulting from various causes, including chondromalacia patella.

Anterior Longitudinal Ligament (an-ter′ē-or/lon″ji-tu′di-nal/lig′ah-ment) (n.) A broad ligament that extends from the occipital bone to the sacrum. It supports the vertebral column and unites the vertebral bodies anteriorly.

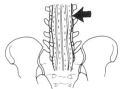

Anterior longitudinal ligament

Anterior Sacral Foramina (an-ter′e-or/sa′kral/foram′i-nah) (n.) Circular openings on either side of the midline of the front of the sacrum through which pass the anterior branches of the sacral nerves.

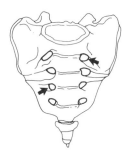

Anterior sacral foramina

Anterior Tibial Artery (an-ter′ē-or/tib′ē-al/ar-te′ry) (n.) A branch of the popliteal artery, enters the anterior compartment of the leg medial to the neck of the fibula and supplies all the muscles of the compartment.

Anterior Tibial Compartment Syndrome (an-ter′e-or/tib′e-al/com-part′ment/sin′drōm) (n.) A syndrome characterized by tender, swollen, and painful anterior tibial muscles, along with overlying skin that may be red and edematous. It occurs most frequently after strenuous training in young athletes or soldiers. The syndrome is thought to be caused by edema and small hemorrhages in the muscles of this compartment. Acute symptoms usually subside spontaneously after a few days; however, residual permanent muscular weakness or even paralysis and subsequent fibrosis and atrophy may result. In severe cases, surgical decompression by division of the fascia may be necessary. Also known as **traumatic necrosis of the pretibial muscles** or **march gangrene**.

Anterior Tibialis Muscle (an-tēr′e-or/tib″e-a′lis/mus′el) (n.)   See **Tibialis Anterior** under **Muscle**.

Anterior Triangle of the Neck (an-tēr′e-or/tri′ang-g′l/of the/nek) (n.)   A triangular anatomic area bordered superiorly by the mandible, laterally by the sternocleidomastoid muscle, and medially by the median line of the neck. It is subdivided into three small triangles: the submandibular (or gastric); submental; and carotid.

Antero (an″ter-o) (prefix.)   Anterior; in front of.

Anteroinferior (an″ter-o-in-fēr′e-or) (adj.)   Situated in front and below.

Anterolateral (an″ter-ō-lat′er-al) (adj.)   Situated in front and to the outer side of.

Anteromedial (an″ter-ō-mī′dē-al) (adj.)   Situated in front and to the inner side of.

Anteroposterior (an″ter-ō-pos-tēr′e-or) (adj.)   Directed from the front toward the back.

Anteroposterior Diameter of the Pelvis (an″ter-ō-pos-tēr′ē-or/di-am′e-ter/of the/pl′vis) (n.)   The depth of the pelvis. To measure the diameter of the pelvic inlet on a lateral radiograph, draw and measure a line that joins the sacrovertebral angle to the superior aspect of the pubic symphysis. To measure the diameter of the pelvic outlet, measure the distance between the lower margin of the symphysis pubis and the tip of the sacrum or the tip of the coccyx. Also call **Sacro Pubic Diameter**.

Anteroposterior Stress Test (an″ter-ō-pos-tēr′ē-or/stres/test) (n.)   See **Anterior Drawer Test**.

Anterosuperior (an″ter-ō-su-pēr′e-or) (adj.)   In front of and above.

Anteversion (an″te-ver′zhun) (n.)   The tilting or tipping forward of a part or organ. For example, the degree of forward projection of the femoral neck from the coronal plane of the femoral shaft.

Anthropoid Pelvis (an′thro-poid/pel′vis) (n.)   A type based on the Caldwell-Moloy classification. This pelvic shape is characteristic of the ape and monkey, but also occurs commonly in humans. The inlet is elongated anteroposteriorly, the widest transverse diameter being shorter than the anteroposterior diameter; the sidewalls are characteristically divergent; and the sacrum is inclined posteriorly.

Antibiotic (an′ti-bī-ot′ik) (n.)   A natural or synthetic chemical substance capable of destroying or inhibiting the growth of bacteria and other microorganisms. Antibiotics may be either broad-spectrum, affecting a wide range of organisms, or selective.

Antibody (an′ti-bod″ē) (n.)   A protein synthesized by β lymphocytes in response to and reacting specifically with a foreign substance or antigen, as in anti-body- or humoral-mediated immunity. Abbreviated as Ab. Also called **Immunoglobulin**.

Anticoagulant (an″ti-kō-ag′u-lant) (n.)   A substance that inhibits, prevents, or supresses clotting of blood.

Antidote (an′ti-dōt) (n.)   An agent that prevents, counteracts, or neutralizes the action of a poison.

Antiembolism Stocking (an″ti-em″bō-lizm/stok-ing) (n.)   An elastic dressing that compresses superficial veins, presumably improving deep venous circulation.

Antigen (an′ti-gen) (n.)   Any substance capable of stimulating the production of antibodies and reacting with them. The most strongly antigenic substances usually are proteins; their antigenic specificity depends on their chemical structure. Specific carbohydrates and lipids also may become antigens. Also called **Allergen**.

Antigravity Muscle (an-ti-grav′i-tē/mus′el) (n.)   In the erect body, a muscle that normally helps support or lift a body segment against gravity.

Antigravity Suit (an-ti-grav′i-tē/sōot) (n.)   A device using circumferential pneumatic compression to control hemorrhage, counteract postural hypotension, and maintain venous pressure. It is an inflatable vinyl envelope that is wrapped and laced about the patient from the ankles to the xiphoid process. It is very effective in controlling intra-abdominal pelvic and extremity bleeding during transport following trauma. Commonly known as the G-suit.

Antihemophilic Factor (an″ti-hē″mo-fil′ik/fak′tor) (n.)   One of the coagulation proteins, more commonly known as factor VIII. Deficiency of the procoagulant activity of factor VIII is the inherited defect in classic hemophilia.

Anti-inflammatory (an″ti-in-flam′ah-to″rē) (adj.)   Inhibiting or reducing inflammation.

Antimicrobial (an″tĭ-mi-kro′be-al) (n.)   A substance that inhibits or destroys microorganisms by biologic or chemical action.

Antineoplastic (an″ti-nē″o-plas′tik) (n.)   Agents that inhibit or destroy neoplastic cells or tumors.

Antinuclear Antibodies (an″ti-nū′kle-ar/an″ti-bod-ēz) (n.)   Antibodies directed against antigens in the cell nucleus. The presence of these antibodies is associated primarily with systemic lupus erythematosus and other rheumatic disorders. They are generally demonstrated by immunofluorescence; their clinical significance has been attributed to various fluorescent patterns. Abbreviated ANA. Also called **Antinuclear Fluorescent Factors (ANF)**.

Antipyretic (an″ti-pī-ret′ik) (n.)   An agent that reduces fever.

Antiseptic (an″ti-sep′tik) (n.)   An agent that inhibits or prevents the growth of microorganisms.

Antiserum (an″ti-se′rum)   Blood serum containing antibodies.

Antispasmodic (an″ti-spaz-mod′ik) (n.)   An agent

that relieves, prevents, or diminishes spasm in smooth and striated muscle.

Antitoxin (an″tĭ-tok′sin) (n.) An antibody capable of uniting with and neutralizing a specific toxin.

Anulus (an′u-lus) (n.) See **Annulus**.

AO Abbreviation for Arbeitsgemeinschaft Osteosynthesefragen, a nonprofit European research group of surgeons and engineers who study and design internal fixation techniques. In English, Association for the Study of Internal Fixation. Abbreviated **ASIF**.

AOA Abbreviation for American Orthopaedic Association.

AO Plates (ĀŌ/plātz) (n.) Plates designed following the techniques and principles of internal fixation developed by the AO/ASIF group. The varied sizes and shapes of these plates allow for their function as tension band plates, neutralization plates, or buttress plates.

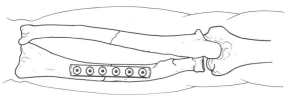

AO plate and screws

AO Screws (AO/skrūz) (n.) Screws designed following the techniques and principles of internal fixation developed by the AO/ASIF group. Most require a cutting tapper after drilling. They are available in a variety of sizes and designs, e.g., cortical, cancellous, and malleolar.

AO System (AO/sis′tem) (n.) Rigid fixation by screws, plates, and other implants designed to achieve stable internal fixation of bones. Developed by the **ASIF**.

Ape Hand (āp/hand) (n.) A deformity in which the thumb is extended and the hand flattened. Ape hand is caused by wasting of the abductor indicis, thenar and hypothenar, interosseii, and lumbrical muscles. It is seen in progressive spinal muscular atrophy or lesions of the median and ulnar nerve.

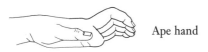

Ape hand

Apert's Syndrome (ah-parz/sin′drōm) (n.) A congenital disorder in which facial deformities occur in association with typical hand abnormalities, mental retardation, and anomalies of the lower extremity and the viscera. The hands are affected bilaterally, with a complex syndactyly of all the fingers often

associated with webbing of the thumb to the index finger. Also known as **Acrocephalosyndactyly**.

Apheresis (ah-fe-rē′sis) (n.) The removal of a component of the blood from intravascular circulation, depleting the intravascular compartment of either plasma constituents (plasmapheresis or cryoapheresis) or cellular elements (cytapheresis).

Apical Ligament (ap′i-kal/lig′ah-ment) (n.) A vestigial ligament connecting the tip of the dens to the basiocciput.

Apical Stitch (ap′i-kal/stich) (n.) Technique of repairing skin lacerations or incisions in which there is a sharp angle. The stitch is placed to hold the apex apposed without compromising the circulation.

Apical Vertebra (ap′i-kal/ver′te-brah) (n.) In spinal deformity, the vertebra that is most rotated or most deviated, thus forming the "apex" of the deformity.

Aplasia (ah-plā′zhe-ah) (n.) Defective development or absence of a part.

Apley Scratch Test (ap′lē/skratch/test) (n.) A clinical method of evaluating active ranges of shoulder motion. Several tests are involved: To test abduction and external rotation, have the patient reach behind his head and touch the superior medial angle of the opposite scapula. To evaluate internal rotation and adduction, have the patient reach in front of his head and touch the opposite acromion. To further test internal rotation and adduction, have the patient reach behind his back and touch the interior angle of the opposite scapula. Observe the patient's movement during all phases of testing for fluidity, limitation of motion, and asymmetry.

Apley Test (ap′lē/test) (n.) A technique used to differentiate knee joint line tenderness due to ligamentous injury from meniscal injury. Have the patient lie prone with his affected knee flexed to 90°. Grasp the patient's leg, apply weight to the foot, and then rotate the tibia internally and externally. Knee pain is present if the meniscus is injured. This is the **compression** or "grind" part of the test. Then exert pressure on the back of the patient's thigh while pulling on the tibia through the foot to distract the knee joint; again, rotate the tibia. Knee pain is present on this maneuver if there is injury to the collateral ligaments. This is the **distraction** part of the test.

Apley's Traction (ap′lēz/trak/shun) (n.) Skeletal traction used to achieve early motion following fractures of the tibial plateau.

Aponeurosis (ap″ō-nu-rō′sis) (n.) A flat sheet of fibrous connective tissue attaching muscle to bone or bone or other tissues at the points of origin or insertion.

Aponeurositis (ap″ō-nu-rō′sī′tis) (n.) Inflammation of an aponeurosis.

Apophyseal (ap″ō-fiz′ē-al) (adj.) Of or pertaining to an apophysis.

Apophyseal Joint (ap″o-fiz′e-al/joint) (n.) The true intervertebral joint between the articular process.

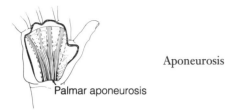

Aponeurosis

Palmar aponeurosis

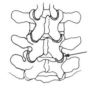

Apophyseal joint

Apophysis (ah-pof′i-sis) (n.) 1. A projection or outgrowth from a bone. 2. An accessory ossification center that develops late, forming a protrusion from the end or near the end of the shaft of a long bone. Apophyses usually serve as attachments for muscles or ligaments, and do not contribute significantly to the length of a long bone.

Apophysitis (ah-pof″i-zī′tis) (n.) Inflammation of an apophysis.

Apparent Leg Length (ah-par′ent/leg/length) An index of the functional length of the lower extremities, measured from the umbilicus to the lowest point of the medial malleolus. Compare to **Actual Leg Length.**

Apportionment (ah-por′shun-ment) (n.) The determination of the degree to which an occupational or nonoccupational factor may contribute to a particular impairment. For each alleged factor, two criteria must be met: 1. The alleged factor *could* have caused the impairment (a medical decision). 2. The factor *did* cause the impairment (a nonmedical determination).

Apposition (ap″o-zish′un) (n.) 1. In describing the positions of fractured or osteotomized bone fragments, the placement or positioning of fragments so that they are in contact at their ends. 2. The state of being fitted together. See **Alignment.**

Apprehension Sign (ap″rē-hen′shun/sīn) (n.) A voluntary or involuntary demonstration of anticipated fear. In the examination of a joint for instability, sometimes, the attempt of the examiner to reproduce the unstable position causes pain and apprehension. For example, in a patient with anterior shoulder instability, the apprehension sign is elicited when the shoulder is passively placed toward extremes of abduction and external rotation. See **Fairbank's Sign.**

Approach (ah-prōch′) (n.) In surgery, the technique of securing access to a part or structure using an incision through the overlying or neighboring structures.

Apraxia (ah-prak′sē-ah) (n.) A disorder of voluntary motor function in which power may be maintained but the ability to execute purposeful motion is lost.

Arachnodactyly (ah-rak″nō-dak′ti-l(ē)) (n.) Abnormally long and slender fingers and toes. See **Marfan's Syndrome.**

Arachnoid Mater (ah-rak′noid/ma′ter) (n.) The delicate membrane of the brain and spinal cord between the dura and pia maters.

Arachnoiditis (ah-rak″noid-ī′tis) (n.) A nonspecific inflammatory process of the arachnoid membrane of the spinal cord that may lead to fibrosis, resulting in scarring and compression of the roots of the cauda equina.

ARA Functional Class (ARA/funk′shun-al/klas) (n.) In the evaluation of disability, a classification of capacities, as follows:

  I. Complete functional capacity; able to carry on all usual duties without handicaps.

  II. Functional capacity adequate for normal activities, despite handicap, discomfort, or limited mobility of one or more joints.

  III. Functional capacity adequate to perform only a few or none of the usual duties or occupations of self-care.

  IV. Great or total incapacitation; patient is bedridden or confined to a wheelchair, permitting little or no self-care.

The American Rheumatism Association has changed its name to the American College of Rheumatology.

Arc of Motion (ark/of/mō′shun) (n.) See **Range of Motion.**

Arcade of Frohse (ar-kād′/of/frōz) (n.) An arch of tendinous tissue that runs along the proximal border of the superficial head of the supinator muscle in the forearm. It is significant in its relationship to the posterior interosseous nerve that passes directly beneath it.

Arcade of Struthers (ar-kād/of/struthers) (n.) A band of fibrous tissue that connects a supracondylar process on the medial aspect of the distal humerus to the medial epicondyle. It may be clinically important because the median nerve and the brachial artery pass directly beneath it. See **Ligament of Struthers.**

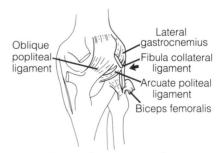

Arcuate ligament complex

Arcuate Ligament Complex (ar′ku-āt/lig′ah-ment/kom′pleks) (n.) A group of ligaments in the posterior lateral corner of the knee consisting of the arcuate ligament, the fibular collateral ligament, the tendoaponeurotic portion of the popliteus muscle and the lateral head of the gastrocnemius muscle. The stability of the posterolateral corner is provided by both the capsular and noncapsular ligaments that form this functional unit.

Area Moment of Inertia (a're-ah/mo'ment/of/in-er'she-ah) (n.) The biomechanical quantity that takes into account the area and distribution of material around an axis in bending. The larger the area moment of inertia, the stronger and stiffer the material.

Areflexia (ah"rē-flek'sē-ah) (n.) Absence of reflexes.

Areolar Tissue (ah"rē'-ō-lar/tissu) (n.) A meshwork of collagen, elastic tissue, and reticular fibers interspersed with numerous connective tissue cells.

ARIF Abbreviation for Arthroscopically-Assisted Reduction and Internal Fixation.

Arm (arm) (n.) Commonly used to refer to the entire upper extremity. More accurately, that part of the upper extremity between the shoulder and the elbow.

AROM Abbreviation for **Active Range of Motion.**

Arterial (ar-te'rē-al) (adj.) Of or pertaining to an artery.

Arteriogram (ar-te're-ō-gram") (n.) A roentgen study produced by arteriography.

Arteriography (ar"te-rē-og-rah-fē) (n.) A diagnostic technique in which a series of radiographs are taken of an artery previously outlined by injection of a radiopaque contrast medium.

Arteriovenous Aneurysm (ar-tē"rē-ō/vē'nus/an'u-rizm) (n.) A dilated vessel that occurs as a communication between an artery and a vein.

Arteriovenous Fistula (ar-tē"rē-ō-vē'nus/fis-tu-lah) (n.) An abnormal communication between an artery and a vein.

Arteritis (ar"te-rī'tis) (n.) Inflammation of an artery.

Artery of Adamkiecwicz (ar"ter-e/of/ah-dam-ke' viks) (n.) See **Adamkiewicz' Artery.**

Arthralgia (ar-thral'jē-ah) (n.) Pain in or affecting a joint.

Arthritic (ar-thrit'ik) 1. (adj.) Of, pertaining to, or affected by arthritis. 2. (n.) Colloquial term for an individual affected with arthritis.

Arthritis (ar-thrī'tis) (n.) Any inflammatory process in a joint. These disorders are classified by etiology or underlying rheumatic disease. The etiology is markedly variable. See under individual disorder.

Arthritis Deformans Juvenilis (ar-thrī'tis/dē-fōr-mans'/jōō've-nil-is) (n.) See **Osteochondritis Dissecans.**

Arthritis Foundation (ar-thrī'tis/fown-dā-shun) (n.) An American voluntary health organization devoted to the rheumatic diseases.

Arthro (ar-thrō) Prefix referring to the joints.

Arthrocentesis (ar"thrō-sen-tē'sis) (n.) The needle aspiration of fluid from a joint space through a puncture wound.

Arthrochalasis Multiplex Congenita (ar"thro-kal'ah-sis/mul'ti-pleks/kon-jen'i-tah) (n.) A variety of Ehlers-Danlos syndrome (EDS VII) notable for extreme joint laxity. It may result from an abnormal procollagen peptidase and/or an abnormal alpha-2 chain in collagen.

Arthrochondritis (ar"thrō-kon-drī'tis) (n.) Inflammation of the cartilage of a joint.

Arthroclasia (ar"thrō-klā'ze-ah) (n.) The surgical disruption of an ankylosis in order to produce increased joint motion.

Arthrodesis (ar"thrō-dē'sis) (n.) An operation to produce fusion of the opposing joint surfaces. Usually accomplished by resection of articular cartilage until subchondral bone is exposed, followed by apposition of bone surfaces and then immobilization using internal and/or external fixation techniques to achieve bony fusion. See **Charnley Arthrodesis, Fusion.**

Arthrodia (ar-thrō'dē-ah) (n.) A plane or gliding synovial joint. Also known as **Arthrodial Joint.**

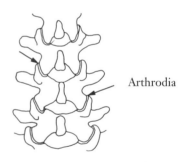

Arthrodia

Arthrodial Cartilage (ar-thrō'dē-al/kar'ti-lij) (n.) Cartilage that lines the articular surfaces of synovial joints.

Arthrodial Joint (ar-thrō'dē-al/joint) (n.) See **Arthrodia,** and **Gliding Joint.**

Arthrodynia (ar"thrō-dīn'e-ah) (n.) Arthralgia or pain in a joint.

Arthrodysplasia (ar"thrō-dis-plā'ze-ah) (n.) Any anomaly of joint development. See **Nail-Patella Syndrome.**

Arthroempyesis (ar"thrō-em"pī-ē'sis) (n.) Suppuration within a joint.

Arthrofibrosis (ar"thro-fi-brō'sis) (n.) Fibrotic scarring and adhesions in a joint, resulting in loss of motion.

Arthrogram (ar'thro-gram) (n.) A roentgen study obtained by arthrography.

Arthrography (ar-throg'rah-fe) (n.) Roentgenography of a joint space after injection of air or radio-paque contrast material.

Arthrogryposis Multiplex Congenita (ar″thrō-gri-pō′sis/mul′ti-pleks/kon-jen′i-tah) (n.) A congenital syndrome characterized by nonprogressive, multiple, and variable joint contractures. Sometimes associated with atrophy or absence of musculature, diminished skin creases, and subcutaneous tissues, and joint dislocations. Apparently nongenetic and related to neurogenic, myogenic, skeletal, and environmental factors. There is usually intact sensation and mental function. Also known as **Multiple Congenital Contractures, Amyoplasia Congenita, Myodystrophia Fetalis Deformans**, and **Multiple Congenital Articular Rigidities**.

Arthrokatadysis (ar″thrō-kah-tad′i-sis) (n.) An intrapelvic protrusion of the acetabulum, with displacement of the acetabulum medial to Köhler's line. Also known as **Otto Pelvis**.

Arthrokinematic Movement (ar″thrō-kin-e-ma′tik/mo͞ov′ment) (n.) Movement between joint surfaces. It includes the following:

Compression: approximation of joint surfaces. This always occurs when moving toward the close-packed position.

Roll: movement in which points at intervals on the moving joint surface contact points at the same intervals in the opposing surface.

Distraction: separation of joint surfaces.

Slide: movement in which a single contact point on the moving surface contacts various points on the opposing surface.

Spin: type of slide that accompanies spin of a bone. One half of the joint surface slides in one direction, while the other half slides in the opposite direction.

Arthrometer (ar-throm′ĕ-ter) (n.) A gauge that can apply stress across a joint and measure its translation in order to assess the degree of instability.

Arthro-onycho Dysplasia (ar″thrō-on″i-kō/dis-pla′zhah) (n.) See **Nail-Patella Syndrome**.

Arthropathy (ar-throp′ah-the) (n.) Any disease of, or involving, joints.

Arthroplasty (ar′thro-plas″te) (n.) The surgical reconstruction of a joint or joints in order to restore motion and function to its attached structures (muscles, ligaments, soft tissues). Choice of procedure used depends on the specific joint: Surgical procedures include resection arthroplasty, resurfacing arthroplasty, interpositional arthroplasty, and total or partial joint replacement arthroplasty.

Arthrosclerosis (ar″thro-skle-ro′sis) (n.) Any condition producing stiffening or hardening of the joints.

Arthroscope (ar′thro-skōp) (n.) An endoscope used for examination of the interior of a joint. Usually, a fiberoptic arthroscope consists of a rod-lens system surrounded by light-conducting glass fibrils enclosed in a rigid metal sheath.

Arthroscopic (ar′thrō-skop′ik) (adj.) Of, or pertaining to, use of an arthroscope.

Arthroscopically-Assisted Reduction and Internal

Fixation (ar′thrō-skop′ik′lē/ah-sis′ted/rē-duk′shun/and/in-ter′nal/fik-sā′shun) (n.) A surgical technique for repair of intra-articular fractures or carpal instabilities in which arthroscopic visualization is used for both direct observation of the restoration of articular surfaces and subsequent internal fixation with pins or screws. The latter may be accomplished percutaneously or may require an ancillary incision. Abbreviated **ARIF**.

Arthroscopically-Assisted Surgery (ar′thrō-skop′ik′lē/ah-sis′ted/ser′jer-ē) (n.) Any surgical procedure in which arthroscopic visualization is used to facilitate correction of intra-articular pathology in association with ancillary surgical incisions. One common procedure is arthroscopically assisted ACL reconstruction.

Arthroscopy (ar-thros′ko-pe) (n.) Examination or surgical repair of the interior of a joint with an arthroscope. Compared to arthrotomy, arthroscopy allows thorough joint examination with decreased postoperative morbidity, using multiple small incisions or portals around the joint. **Diagnostic arthroscopy** refers to a complete joint examination. **Surgical arthroscopy** refers to any operative procedure performed under arthroscopic visualization.

Arthrosis (ar-thro′sis) (n.) Any disease of the joint. Example: **Osteoarthrosis**.

Arthrostomy (ar-thros′to-me) (n.) The surgical creation of an opening in a joint, as for drainage.

Arthrosynovitis (ar″thro-sin″o-vi′tis) (n.) Inflammation of the synovial membrane of a joint.

Arthrotomy (ar″throt′o-me) (n.) Incision of a joint.

Arthroxesis (ar-throk′sĕ-sis) (n.) Scraping of an articular surface.

Articular (ar-tik′u-lar) (adj.) Of, or pertaining to, a joint articulation.

Articular Capsule (ar-tik′u-lar/kap′sūl) (n.) The saclike soft-tissue envelope that encloses the cavity of a synovial joint by attaching to the circumference of the articular end of each involved bone.

Articular Disc (ar-tik′u-lar/disk) (n.) A pad of fibrocartilage or dense fibrous tissue present in some synovial joints.

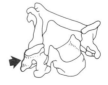

Articular pillar

Articular Pillar (ar-tik′u-lar/pil′ar) (n.) In the lower cervical spine, C3–C7, at the junction of the pedicles and laminae, this is a rhomboid-shaped pillar projecting laterally. The pillar supports the superior and inferior articular facets on each side.

Articular Process (ar-tik′u-lar/pros′es) (n.) Any

bony projection that has an articular facet. For example, the zygapophyses of the vertebrae.

Articular process

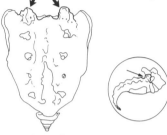

Articular process, superior

Articulation (ar-tik″u-lā′shun) (n.) 1. Any occurring union or junction between two or more bones; more commonly known as a joint. 2. Usually indicates motion between two or more bones. 3. A junction of prosthetic components. 4. See specific types of articulations: synarthroses—immovable; schindyleses—grooved; gomphoses—socket; suturae—sutures; diarthroses—movable; arthrodia—gliding; ginglymus—hinges; enarthroses—ball and socket; and amphiarthroses—mixed or combinations.

Articulotrochanteric Distance (ar-tik′u-lo-tro″kan-ter′ik/dis′tans) (n.) A measurement used to assess the position of the tip of the greater trochanter in relation to the femoral head. It is actually the longitudinal distance between the ossified greater trochanter and the ossified femoral head.

On an anteroposterior radiograph of the pelvis, measure the length of the ATD in millimeters from the articular surface of the femoral head to the tip of the greater trochanter. A positive value is given if the tip of the greater trochanter is distal to the center of the femoral head, neutral if the two are level, and negative if the greater trochanter is higher than the center of the femoral head. Abbreviated **ATD**.

Artifact (ar′ti-fakt) (n.) Anything, such as a structure or appearance, that is artificial or incidental; a product of technique; not occurring naturally. For example, on X-ray films, a foreign or artificial mark caused by improper processing, static electrical charge, or faulty equipment or technique.

Ascending Degeneration (ah-send′ing/dē-jen″er-a′shun) (n.) See **Wallerian degeneration**.

Ascorbic Acid (ah-skor′bik/as′id) (n.) Vitamin C.

Ase (ās) (suffix) Suffix used in forming the name of an enzyme. It is added to the name of the substance on which it acts.

Asepsis (a-sēp′sis) (n.) Absence of disease-producing microorganisms.

Aseptic (a-sep′tik) (adj.) Free of contaminating microorganisms capable of causing infection.

Aseptic Necrosis (a-sep′tik/ne-krō′sis) (n.) See **Avascular Necrosis**; **Osteonecrosis**.

Aseptic Technique (a-sep′tik/tek-nēk) (n.) Any method by which contamination with microorganisms is prevented.

ASIF Abbreviation for Association for the Study of Internal Fixation. See **AO**.

Asnis Screw (as′nis/skrū) (n.) An eponym and trademark of the Howmedica Company for a cannulated screw.

Aspiration (as″pi-rā′shun) (n.) The withdrawal of fluid from the body or a body cavity.

Aspiration Biopsy (as″pi-rā′shun/bī′op-se) (n.) Process by which tissue or fluid of a lesion is removed via suction through a needle attached to a syringe.

Aspirin (as′pi-rin) (n.) A drug that relieves pain and reduces inflammation and fever. Synonym: Acetylsalicylic acid. Abbreviated **ASA**.

Assisted Respiration (ah-sis′ted/res″pi-rā′shun) (n.) The use of an intermittent positive pressure breathing device or lung ventilator when deficiencies in respiratory rate and inspiration occur. It assures sufficient inspiratory volume and automatizes control of respiration.

ASTM Abbreviation for American Society for Testing and Materials. This society provides standards for the chemical characteristics of metals and alloys.

Astragalus (ah-strag′ah-lus) (n.) See **Talus**.

Astragalectomy (as″trag-ah-lek′tō-me) (n.) Surgical excision of part, or all, of the talus.

Astrocyte (as′trō-sīt) (n.) A star-shaped neuroglial cell attached to the blood vessels of the brain and spinal cord by perivascular feet.

Astroglia (as-trog′le-ah) (n.) Neuroglia composed of astrocytes.

Astrom Suspension Test (as-trom′/sus-pen′shun/test) (n.) A test used in evaluation of sciatica. Have the patient grasp the top of a door and suspend himself; tap the lumbar region. In sciatica, discomfort is not elicited. However, the same lumbar tapping will elicit discomfort and pain when the patient is standing erect.

Asynergia (a″sin-er′je-ah) (n.) Lack of coordination among parts or organs that normally act in harmony.

Ataxia (ah-tak′se-ah) (n.) Failure of muscular coordination.

Ataxic Gait (ah-tak′sik/gāt) (n.) An unsteady, uncoordinated gait, characterized by staggering and walking on a wide base, as though drunk. The legs are spread far apart, and in taking a step, the leg is lifted abruptly and too high, and then brought down with the whole sole of the foot striking the ground at once. Ataxic gait is usually caused by central nervous system diseases, especially of the cerebellum, rather than by a disorder of the extremities.

Atelectasis (at″e-lek′tah-sis) (n.) Collapse of the alveoli of the lungs as a result of failure of expansion or resorption of air. This is a not uncommon cause of fever postoperatively and in bedridden patients. Radiographically, it may appear as linear densities if a large enough area is involved.

Athetoid (ath′ĕ-toid) (adj.) 1. Of, pertaining to, or resembling athetosis. 2. Affected with athetosis.

Athetosis (ath″ĕ-to′sis) (n.) 1. A derangement marked by involuntary movements, usually resulting from a lesion of the basal ganglia, characterized by recurring slow, sinuous writhing movements of the hands and feet. 2. A fluctuation of posture superimposed upon a persistent attitude. It may be described as "swings" of movement from one posture to another, caused by release of two opposing actions. (One example is alternation from hyperextension of the fingers and wrist and pronation of the forearm to full flexion of the fingers and wrist and supination of the forearm.)

Athlete's Foot (ath′lētz/foot) (n.) A common name for tinea pedis fungal infection, usually of the interdigital areas of the toes.

Atlanta Brace (at-lan′ta/brās) (n.) An ambulation-abduction orthosis used in the treatment of Legg-Calvé-Perthes Disease that allows limited motion of the hip joint. Also called **Scottish Rite Hospital Orthrosis.**

Atlantoaxial (at-lan″to-ak′sē-al) (adj.) Of, or pertaining to, the joint or space between the first two cervical vertebrae.

Atlantoaxial Angle (at-lan″to-ak′sē-al/ang′g′l) (n.) The angle formed between the first two cervical vertebrae. It is determined on a lateral radiograph of the neck.

Atlantoaxial Dislocation (at-lan″to-ak′sē-al/dis″lo-kā′shun) (n.) Any dislocation of the first cervical vertebra on the second cervical vertebra. Traumatic dislocations may be anterior, posterior, or rotary in nature.

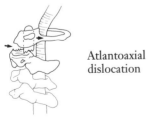
Atlantoaxial dislocation

Atlantoaxial Rotary Subluxation (n.) See **Rotary Subluxation of C₁ or C₂.**

Atlanto-occipital Dislocation (at-lan″tō-ok-sip′i-tal/dis″lō-kā′shun) (n.) A rare injury of the upper cer-

vical spine in which the atlas is dislocated from its articulation with the occiput. The diagnosis is evident on a lateral radiographic view of the skull or cervical spine.

Atlanto-odontoid (at-lan″tō-ō-don′toid) (adj.) Of, or pertaining to the joint formed between the dens of the axis and the atlas.

Atlas (at′las) (n.) The first cervical vertebra (C-1). It articulates with the condyles of the occipital bone of the skull superiorly and with the dens of the axis inferiorly.

Atony (at′o-nē) (n.) Absence of muscular tone.

ATP Abbreviation for adenosine triphosphate.

Atresia (ah-trē′ze-ah) (n.) Congenital absence or pathologic closure of a normal opening or lumen.

Atrophy (at′ro-fē) (n.) The wasting-away or decrease in size of a structure, organ, tissue or cell part. The defect may be congenital or acquired, or may occur from lack of nutrition, loss of nerve supply, aging, or disuse.

Attachment (ah-tach-ment) (n.) The location of fixation of one organ or tissue to another. For example, the origin or insertion of a muscle in a bone.

Attending (ah-tend′ing) (n.) A physician who has completed a postgraduate training program and is responsible for (or "attending to") patient care. This term is commonly used in teaching institutions to differentiate these physicians from interns or residents still in training.

Aufranc-Turner Prosthesis (aufranc-turner/pros-the′sis) (n.) A design of a total hip prosthesis in which the femoral component is similar to a Muller prosthesis except the head is more undercut, the neck is oval in cross section and the stem is slightly thicker and wider.

Austin-Moore Prosthesis (aws′tin/moor/pros-the′sis) (n.) An endoprosthesis commonly used for femoral head replacement after subcapital and femoral neck fractures. It consists of a metal ball connected to a stem, which is then inserted into the medullary canal of the proximal femur and then articulates with the patient's acetabular cartilage. The stem is either solid or fenestrated.

Australia Antigen (Aws-trā-lya/an′tĭ-jen) (n.) An older term for the hepatitis B surface antigen.

Authenticate (aw-then-ti′kāt) (v.) To validate authorship of an entry made in a patient's medical record by means of a written signature, identifiable initials, a computer key, or a personally used rubber stamp.

Autoantibody (aw″to-an′ti-bod″e) (n.) An antibody produced in response to, and reacting against, an antigenic constituent of the individual's own tissues.

Autoclave (aw′to-klāv) (n.) An apparatus that uses steam under pressure to sterilize, especially surgical instruments.

Autograft (aw′to-graft) (n.) Any tissue transplanted from one site to another on the same individual.

Autoimmune Disease (aw″to-i-mūn/di-zēz′) (n.) A disorder characterized by the mounting of an immune response against constituents of an individual's own tissues. Also known as **Autoallergy**.

Autologous (aw-tol′o-gus) (adj.) Derived from the same organism.

Autologous Blood (aw-tol′o-gus/blud) (n.) Blood collected from a person for later retransfusion to that person. This technique is often used prior to elective surgery if blood loss is expected to occur. This avoids the use of banked blood from unknown donors.

Autologous Graft (aw-tol′o-gus/graft) (n.) A graft taken from another area of the patient's own body. Synonym: **Autograft**.

Autolysis (aw-tol′i-sis) (n.) Digestion or disintegration of cells by the action of their own enzymes.

Autonomic Dysreflexia (aw″to-nom′ik/dis″rē-fleks-ē-ah) (n.) A syndrome that occurs in patients with spinal cord lesions at or above T6, characterized by exaggerated autonomic responses to stimuli that are innocuous in normal individuals. Characteristic symptoms and signs include excessive sweating, flushing of the face, congestion of the nasal passages, pilomotor erection, throbbing headache, paroxysmal hypertension, and bradycardia. Abbreviated **AD**.

Autonomic Ganglia (aw″to-nom′ik/gang′gle-ah) (n.) Aggregations of cell bodies of neurons of the autonomic nervous system. Includes both the parasympathetic and the sympathetic ganglia and their combinations.

Autonomic Nerve (aw″to-nom′ik/nerv) (n.) A nerve within the autonomic nervous system.

Autonomic Nervous System (aw″to-nom′ik/ner′vus/sis′tem) (n.) A division of the nervous system comprised of a series of reflex areas that control involuntary motor functions and innervate the heart, glands, viscera, and smooth muscle. It is subdivided into **sympathetic** and **parasympathetic** systems.

Autonomous Zone (aw-ton′ō-mus/zōn) (n.) In describing the sensory distribution of a peripheral nerve, this is the area supplied exclusively by that nerve in which sensation would be lost if the nerve were severed. Also known as the **Isolated Zone**.

Autophor Prosthesis (aw-tō′for/pros-thē′sis) (n.) A brand name for a ceramic total hip prosthesis. A ceramic cup is screwed into the pelvis. A ceramic head is pressed onto a post of a tapered metal stem.

Autopsy (aw′top-sē) (n.) A postmortem examination of the body. Also called **Necropsy** and/or **Postmortem Examination**.

Autoradiography (aw″to-ra″de-og′rah-fē) (n.) The detection of a radioactive compound or organelle in a cell by placing the compound in contact with a photographic emulsion, and allowing the compound to "take its own picture." The emulsion is developed, and the location of the radioactivity in the cell is recorded on a photographic plate.

Autosome (aw′to-sōm) (n.) Any chromosome other than the sex chromosomes. Each human has 22 pairs of autosomes and 1 pair of sex chromosomes.

Autotransfusion (aw″to-trans-fu′zhun) (n.) The practice and technique of transfusing previously drawn autologous blood back to the same patient.

Avascular (ah-vas′ku-lar) (adj.) Lacking blood vessels.

Avascular Necrosis of Bone (ah-vas′ku-lar/ne-krō′sis/of/bōn) (n.) 1. Cell death that occurs as a result of loss of blood supply. 2. A variety of disorders in which there is interruption of the blood supply to bone resulting in death of osteocytes. It may occur following trauma, dislocations, in association with certain systemic diseases, the use of certain drugs, radiation, rapid decompression (Caisson's disease), and idiopathically. If it occurs near an articular surface, the necrotic bone may fracture and collapse, resulting in arthritic changes. Abbreviated **AVN**. Also known as **Osteonecrosis, Aseptic Necrosis** and **Ischemic Necrosis of Bone**. Many types of idiopathic avascular necrosis of specific bones are more commonly known by an eponymic name. See also **Necrosis** and specific diseases.

Avascular Necrosis of Carpal Lunate Bone (ah-vas′ku-lar/ne-krō′sis/of/kar′pal/loo′nāt/bōn) See **Kienbock Disease**.

Avascular Necrosis of the Second Metatarsal Head (ah-vas′ku-lar/ne-krō′sis/of the second/met″ah-tar′sal/hed) (n.) See **Freiberg Disease**.

Average Dose (av′rij/dōs) (n.) A dose ordinarily expected to produce the therapeutic effect for which the ingredient or preparation is most commonly employed.

Aviator's Astragalus (ā′vē-a′terz/ah-strag′ah-lus) (n.) Fracture/dislocations of the talus. So named because of a high incidence described in pilots suffering hyperdorsiflexion of the foot when the sole of the foot is rested on the foot bar of the aircraft at the point of landing.

Avulsion (ah-vul′shun) (n.) The tearing-away or forceable separation of a part from a structure.

Avulsion Fracture (ah-vul′shun/frak′chur) (n.) The separation of a small piece of bone that has been pulled away from the shaft, typically at the attach-

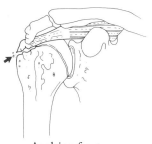

Avulsion fracture

ment of a ligament or tendons, and usually involving a tuberosity or bony process.

Awl (awl) (n.) An instrument with a sharp pointed tip used in orthopaedic surgery to initiate access through cortical bone.

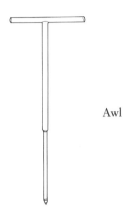

Awl

Axial Compression (ak′se-al/kom-presh′un) (n.) In mechanical terms, longitudinally directed compressive forces. This principle is utilized in the internal fixation of fractures by the application of plates under tension.

Axial Compression Test (ak′se-al/kom-presh′un/test) (n.) A clinical evaluation of pain in and about the carpometacarpal (C-M) joint of the thumb. Rotate the thumb as the C-M joint is compressed by the metacarpal. When pain is elicited by this maneuver, symptoms are mechanical and are located within the joint.

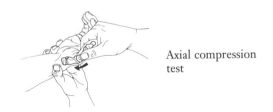

Axial compression test

Axial Line (ak′se-al/līn) (n.) The line separating the more rostral segmental dermatomes from the more caudal ones.

Axial Load Compression (ak′se-al/lōd/kom-presh′un) (n.) A mechanism of injury to the cervical spine in which an axially directed load exerts a longitudinally compressive force. This usually results in an explosive, comminuted fracture of a mid-cervical vertebral body.

Axial Pattern Flap (ak′se-al/pat′ern/flap) (n.) Free tissue flaps of distinctive vascularity. This pattern relies on a definite and usually consistent arterial supply centered on one or more arteries. Compared to random pattern flaps, these have no length-to-width requirements, thus decreasing the risk of failure.

Axial Tomography (ak′se-al/to-mog′rah-fē) (n.) Sectional radiography in which a series of cross-sectional images along an axis are combined to constitute a three-dimensional scan. See **Computerized Axial Tomography**. Abbreviated **CAT** and **CT**.

Axilla (ak-sil′ah) (n.) The region where the arm joins the chest at the shoulder. Hollow in appearance, the axilla is bounded anteriorly by the pectoralis major muscle, and posteriorly by the latissimus dorsi muscle. Also called the **Armpit** or **Axillary Fossa**.

Axillary (ak′si-lar″ē) (adj.) Of, or pertaining to the axilla.

Axillary Block (ak′si-lar″ē/blok) (n.) A type of regional anesthetic in which the brachial plexus is anesthesized to produce anesthesia of the hand and forearm.

Axillary Crutches (ak′si-lar″ē/kruch′es) (n.) An underarm crutch that should be maintained about 2 finger-breadths below the axilla. Body weight is borne through the hands.

Axillary Incision (ak′si-lar″ē/in-sizh′un) (n.) A technique for an anterior surgical approach to the shoulder in which the skin incision is placed over the anterior axillary fold so that the scar is not noticeable when the arm is held at the side. Skin and subcutaneous undermining then allows deeper dissection through the delto-pectoral interval.

Axillary Nerve (ak′si-lar″ē/nerv) A branch of the posterior cord of the brachial plexus. It innervates the deltoid muscle and supplies sensation to the skin overlying the lateral aspect of the muscle. Contains fibers of C-5.

Axillary Region (ak′si-lar″ē/rē′jun) (n.) A region on the lateral aspect of the thorax, extending from the axilla to a line drawn from the lower border of the mammary region to that of the scapular region.

Axillary View (ak′si-lar″ē/vū) (n.) A radiographic view of the shoulder that provides a true lateral image of the glenohumeral joint. It can be made with the patient prone, supine, or standing, and with minimal abduction of the arm.

Axis (ak′sis) (n.) 1. The second cervical vertebra (C-2). From the body of the axis, a long, pointed projection directed cranially, called the dens or odontoid process, articulates with the atlas, allowing cervical rotation. It articulates with C-3 inferiorly. 2. An imaginary line passing through the center of a body or organ around which parts are symmetrically aligned. 3. The fulcrum or center of a joint, determined for a certain movement. It is that point that does not move in relation to either of the two bones involved in the movement. The axis may sometimes be at the geometric center of the convex head of the proximal bone of the joint. In other cases, if the convex head of the bone is not a true circle, the axis may change its position as the joint goes from extension into flexion. At any one position, the axis is called the "instant center."

Axis of Rotation (ak′sis/of/ro-ta′shun) (n.) A line of right angles to the plane in which adjacent limb segments move, and about which all moving parts of the segments describe circular arcs.

Axon (ak′son) (n.) The long cytoplasmic process of a neuron through which nerve impulses are conducted away from the cell body. It may be myelinated or nonmyelinated.

Axon Reflex (ak′son/re′fleks) (n.) A nervous response occurring without involvement of a nerve cell body or a synapse; therefore, not a true neurologic reflex. It occurs when a stimulus is applied to a terminal branch of a sensory nerve, giving rise to an impulse that ascends to a collateral branch of the same nerve fiber, down which it is conducted antidromically to an effector organ. This reflex is believed to be important in the local regulation of blood vessel caliber, especially in the skin.

Axonotmesis (ak′son-ot-me′sis) (n.) Damage and injury to nerve fibers resulting in loss of axon continuity. Wallerian degeneration occurs distal to the site of the lesion. The epineurium and intimate supporting structures of the nerve remain intact, so that regeneration of nerve fibers and spontaneous recovery should occur.

Axoplasm (ak′so-plazm) (n.) The cytoplasm of an axon.

Azotemic Osteodystrophy (az-ō-tē′mik/os″te-o-dis′tro-fē) (n.) See **Renal Osteodystrophy**.

B

Baastrup Disease (bah-strup/dĭ-zēz′) (n.) A lumbar interspinous bursitis seen in degenerative joint disease. It is characterized by a bridging between adjacent osteophytes. Synonyms: **Kissing Osteophytes; Michotte Disease**.

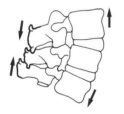

Baastrup disease

Babbitt (bab′it) (n.) 1. The surface lining of a bearing. It is usually made of a soft, low melting-point alloy or mixture of metals. 2. In orthopaedics it is used to describe the hyaline cartilage layer in a joint, which truly is a surface lining of a bearing.

Babcock's Triangle (bab′koks/trī′ang′l) (n.) A relatively radiolucent triangle seen on an anteroposterior radiograph of the hip in the subcapital region of the femoral head. It is an area of loosely arranged trabeculae noted between the more radiodense lines of the normal bony trabeculae groups.

Babinski Sign (bah-bin′skē/sīn) (n.) A pyramidal tract response elicited by a tactile stimulus to the lateral aspect of the sole and directed from the heel toward the metatarsophalangeal joint. When present, the response consists of dorsiflexion of the great toe and fanning of the lesser toes. This indicates disruption of the pyramidal tract. In normal adults, the response is plantar flexion of the toes. A Babinski sign is considered normal in infants younger than 18 months. Modifications include **Chaddock's Sign**, **Gordon's Sign**, and **Oppenheim's Sign**. Also known as **Babinski response**.

Back (bak) (n.) 1. Dorsum 2. Used commonly in reference to the posterior aspect of the torso, from the neck to the coccyx.

Backbone (bak′bōn) (n.) The vertebral or spinal column.

Backfire Fracture (bak′fir/frak′chur) (n.) A fracture of the radial styloid. See **Chauffeur's fracture**.

Background Radiation (bak′grownd/ra-de-a′shun) The sum total of radioactivity measured in a given area. This includes emissions from cosmic radiation, terrestrial radiation of natural radioactive materials, and all other sources.

Back-Knee (bak-nē) (n.) See **Genu recurvatum**.

Backpart (bak′part) (n.) In shoe terminology, the portion of the last that extends from the ball of the shoe to the posterior edge.

Back-Scatter (bak′skat-er) (n.) Radiation generated when x-rays capable of penetrating an object strike the surface upon which the film-holder lies.

Back School (bak/skool) (n.) Formal instruction in body mechanics and back care intended to educate the patient about back disorders. It is used in both the treatment and prophylaxis of back injuries.

Although there are many different types of back schools, the common, underlying philosophy is that the education of patients will lead to both a greater willingness to accept responsibility for sustaining health through prevention, and active participation in the healing process, as opposed to passive observance of treatment. These are usually outpatient education programs, although in-hospital programs exist. Both involve the participation of physicians, physical therapists, and other health-care professionals.

Back Seam (bak/sēm) (n.) In shoe terminology, a posterior seam joining the quarters of the uppers.

Bacteremia (bak-tēr″ē′me-ah) (n.) A condition in which viable bacteria are present in the blood stream.

Bacteria (bak-te′rē-ah) (n.) The plural of bacterium.

Bactericidal (bak-tēr′i-sī′dal) (adj.) Capable of killing bacteria.

Bacteriology (bak-te′rē-ol′ō-jē) (n.) The study of bacteria.

Bacteriophage (bak-te′rē-ō-fāj) (n.) A virus that infects bacteria. They are named for the bacterial species or strain for which they are specific.

Bacteriostatic (bak-te′rē-ō-stat′ik) (adj.) Capable of preventing or inhibiting the growth of bacteria.

Bacterium (bak-te′re-um) (n.) A prokaryotic microorganism that is typically unicellular. It is differentiated from blue-green algae by the absence of a photosynthesis pigment system.

Bacteriuria (bak-te′rē-ū′rē-ah) (n.) Bacteria in the urine. If more than 100,000 colonies of a single bacterial species are grown in a urine culture, urinary tract infection is present.

Bacteroides (bak′te-roi′dēz) (n.) A genus of anaerobic, nonsporeforming, gram-negative rods. They are normally found in the oropharynx and constitute a large part of the fecal flora.

Baer's Sacroiliac Point (bārz/sa″kro-il′ē-ak/point) (n.) An area of elicited tenderness that indicates a nonspecific back injury. With the patient supine, palpate each lower quadrant of the abdomen. Baer's point is situated two inches from the umbilicus on a line between it and the anterior superior spine. Baer's point presumably overlies the sacroiliac joint.

Bag of Bones (bag/of/bōnz) (n.) Descriptive term applied to severely comminuted and displaced intercondylar fractures of the distal humerus.

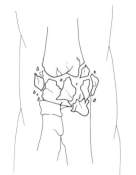

Bag of bones

Bailey Rod (bā′lē/rod) (n.) A telescoping intramedullary nail used in the fixation of corrective osteotomies for long bone deformities in growing children with osteogenesis imperfecta.

Baker's Cyst (bā′kerz/sist) (n.) A distended bursa in the popliteal space. There are numerous bursae in the region that are potentially affected, but symptoms most commonly develop in the semimembranous bursa or the medial gastrocnemius bursa. The cyst may also result from herniation of the synovial membrane through the posterior capsule of the knee. Occasionally, aspiration is necessary. Ultrasound or MRI may help differentiate the causes of popliteal swelling.

In children, the typical cyst occurs on the medial side of the popliteal space, just lateral to the semitendinosus muscle. Many of these cysts regress or remain asymptomatic. An enlarging, symptomatic cyst will respond well to simple excision. In adults, these cysts are usually associated with such intra-articular disorders as degenerative joint disease, rheumatoid arthritis, or meniscal tears. Frequently, the cyst will disappear after the intra-articular pathology is corrected. If only the cyst is excised, recurrence is common if the associated intra-articular disorder persists. Also known as a **Popliteal Cyst**.

Baker's Test (bā′kerz/test) (n.) A method of evaluation of contractures of the gracilis and medial hamstring muscles. Place the patient supine with knees fully flexed and both hips held firmly in 90° of flexion and as much abduction as possible. This position will stabilize the pelvis. Extend the knee on the side to be tested as far as possible, or to the point where it is necessary to adduct the hip to allow further extension of the knee. If the gracilis or one of the medial hamstrings prevents extension of the knee unless the hip is adducted, the tendon or muscle most involved in the knee contracture will be the first to stand out as a taut band. If it is necessary to extend but not adduct the hip in order to extend the knee, the test is not considered positive for the gracilis-hamstring contracture. If there is no contracture, it will be possible, without undue force, to take the knee of the side tested into full extension without a loss of abduction.

Balanced Anesthesia (bal′ans′d/an′es-thē′ze-ah) (n.) A technique widely used for general anesthesia. A combination of inhalation and intravenous agents are used to provide hypnosis, analgesia, muscle relaxation, and the depression of reflexes. Physiologic functions are minimally disturbed.

Balanced Traction (bal′ans′d/trak′shun) (n.) A type of traction produced by balancing or "treating" the extremity in a traction apparatus against a counterforce other than the patient's body weight. When a balanced or suspension apparatus is used in conjunction with skin or skeletal traction, the patient is able to move about in bed freely without disturbing the line of traction. The extremity is balanced with countertraction, and any slack in the traction caused by the patient's movement is taken up by the suspension apparatus. The use of balanced traction facilitates nursing care. Also known as **Balanced Suspension Traction**.

Baldwin Aeroplane Splint (bald-win/ār'o-plān/ splint) (n.) A shoulder abduction orthosis that is secured to the body by a half pelvic band and posterior upright.

Balkan Frame (bawl'kan/frām) (n.) An overhead quadrilateral frame made of metal tubing that is fastened to a hospital bed. It is used for suspending limbs, applying traction, and facilitating the mobility of bedridden patients. It is manufactured under various brand names.

Ball 1. In shoe terminology, the widest part of the sole of a shoe; this normally corresponds to the area beneath the metatarsal heads. 2. A colloquial term used in reference to the area of the foot beneath the metatarsal heads, as in the "ball of the foot."

Ball and Socket Joint (bawl/and/sok'et/joint) (n.) A type of synovial joint in which a convex, rounded head—the ball—moves within a concave surface or a cup-shaped depression—the socket. An example of this is the hip joint. Also known as a **Sphenoidal Joint** or **Enarthrosis**.

Ball Girth (bawl/ġerth) (n.) In shoe terminology, the widest circumference of the last that exists at the ball of the shoe.

Ballottable (bah-lot'ah-bl) (adj.) Capable of exhibiting ballottement.

Ballottement (bah-lot'-ment) (n.) A clinical test for fluid or floating objects by palpation. This is elicited by a flicking motion of the hand or fingers on the surface of the area to be tested and the palpation with the opposite hand for the transmission of a fluid wave or the bouncing back of a solid organ. For example, in ballottement of the knee joint, place one hand on the medial joint compartment, and with the other hand, make quick thrusts up on the lateral joint compartment to feel for fluid or floating loose bodies.

Bamberger-Marie Syndrome (bahm'ber-ger-mah' rē/sin'drōm) (n.) See **Hypertrophic Pulmonary Osteoarthropathy**.

Bamboo Spine (bam-bū' spīn) (n.) The appearance of the vertebral column on an anteroposterior radiograph in advanced cases of ankylosing spondylitis. This appearance results from extensive soft tissue calcification or ossification within the outer fibers of the annulus fibrosus and the fibers of the anterior longitudinal ligament. It also results from syndesmophytes, which create new bone bridges across the intervertebral spaces. See **Ankylosing Spondylitis**.

Bandage (ban'dij) (n.) A strip or roll of gauze, fabric, or other material used to dress or cover a wound or to wrap, support, or bind any part of the body.

Bankart Lesion (bank-art/lē'zhun) (n.) A traumatic detachment of the fibrocartilaginous labrum from the anterior rim of the glenoid. This may occur with anterior dislocation of the glenohumeral joint.

Bankart Procedure (bank-art/pro-sē'jur) (n.) A surgical technique for the treatment of recurrent ante-

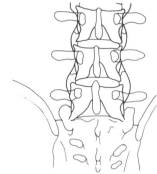

Bamboo spine

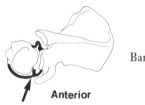

Bankart lesion

Anterior

rior dislocation of the shoulder. The detached anterior labrum and the anterior joint capsule are reattached to the glenoid rim.

Barlow's Disease (bar'lōz/dĭ-zēz') (n.) See **Scurvy**.

Barlow Splint (bar'lo/splint) (n.) A type of immobilization used in the treatment of congenital dislocation of the hip. After reduction of the hip, the lower ends of the splint are molded around the thighs, with the hips positioned in 90° of abduction and flexion.

Barlow's Test (bar'lōz/test) (n.) A provocative maneuver used to detect congenitally dislocatable hips. If the femoral head is in the acetabulum during examination, the test will detect instability.

To perform the examination, lay the infant supine with knees and hips flexed. The hips are placed in abduction; then, the thigh is grasped and the hip is adducted while gentle downward pressure is applied. The femoral head can be palpated as it slips out of the acetabulum if the hip is dislocatable. The diagnosis is confirmed with the Ortolani or reduction test. Also known as the **Dislocation Test**.

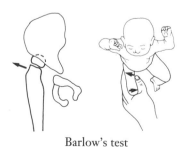

Barlow's test

Barr's Triad (bahrz/trī′ad) (n.)   A decrease in the height of the intervertebral space, lumbar scoliosis, and absence of normal lumbar lordosis.

Barre-Liéou Syndrome (bar-ra′-lē-ū″/sin′drōm) (n.)   A cervical syndrome that is characterized by headaches and otolabyrinthine involvement such as vertigo, nausea, and tinnitus; visual problems, such as spots before the eyes and burning feeling in the eyes; and laryngeal phenomena, such as dysphonia, or a lump in the throat. Psychologic components include anxiety and loss of memory. All of the symptoms are rarely present simultaneously; rather, they are most often isolated or diversely grouped. The symptoms frequently manifest following incorrect manipulation or minor cervical trauma. Synonyms: **Bartschi-Rochain's**, **Chronic Cervical Arthritis**, **Sympathetic Posterior Cervical Arthritis**, **Sympathetic Cervical Arthritis**.

Barton's Fracture (bar′tunz/frak′chur) (n.)   An eponym for a fracture of the dorsal rim of the distal end of the radius. This is an intra-articular fracture that is propagated to the dorsum of the distal radius and is associated with tearing of the palmar radiocarpal ligaments and dorsal subluxation of the carpus. This is also known as a **Dorsal Rim Fracture Dislocation**.

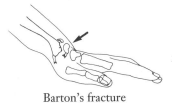

Barton's fracture

Barton's Tongs (bar′tunz/tongz) (n.)   A metallic clamp that attaches to the parietal bones of the skull 1 inch above the external ear and provides skeletal traction to the cervical spine. Chiefly used in the treatment of injuries of the neck.

Base (bās)   1. A substance having a pH greater than 7 that, on dissociation, releases hydroxyl (OH−) ions but not hydrogen (H+) ions. 2. A common reference to the bottom or root of a body part; for example, the base of the skull.

Baseball Elbow (bās′bawl/el′bō) (n.)   A commonly used term for the characteristic arthritic changes seen in the elbows of veteran baseball pitchers. These changes include olecranon and distal humeral hypertrophy, joint space narrowing, loose bodies, and calcification at the flexor muscle origin. These changes are believed to result from chronic medial tension, lateral compression, and extension injuries inherent to the pitching motion.

Baseball Finger (bās′bawl/fing′ger) (n.)   A colloquial term for an avulsion of the common extensor tendon, usually with a fragment of bone, from its insertion at the base of the distal phalanx of a finger. It is

called this because it may be caused by a baseball striking the fingertip, suddenly forcing the tip into flexion. See **Mallet Finger**.

Baseline Film (bās′līn/film) (n.)   Radiographs taken prior to or at an initial examination, which are then compared with films taken later to evaluate treatment and recovery.

Basement Membrane (bās′ment/mem′brān) (n.)   An extracellular filamentous layer of material that parallels the cell membrane of cells that are in juxtaposition to tissue.

Basic Dye (ba′sik/dī) (n.)   A dye consisting of a basic organic grouping of cations as the actively staining material, which are then combined with an acid, usually inorganic. Basic dye has an affinity for acidic compounds.

Basket Forceps (bas′ket/for′seps) (n.)   A surgical instrument commonly used in arthroscopic surgery. The base of the basket is open to allow each bite of tissue to fall freely within the joint, so the instrument need not be removed after each bite. These instruments may be straight or angled, and the jaws may be straight or hooked. Also known as **Punch Biopsy Forceps**.

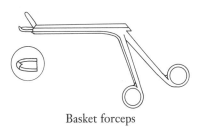

Basket forceps

Basketball Foot (bas′ket-bawl/foot) (n.)   A colloquial term applied to medial subtalar dislocations. It is so-named because a fall on a basketball court is not an uncommon mechanism of injury for this dislocation.

Basilar Impression (bas′i-lar/im-presh′un) (n.)   An anomaly of the cervicobasilar junction characterized by cephalad displacement of the cervical spine into the skull and an occipital indentation of the posterior foramen magnum. This is seen as a congenital anomaly or as a result of ligamentous instability, such as that which occurs in rheumatoid arthritis.

The diagnosis is made on a lateral radiograph of the cervicobasilar junction. Chamberlain's line is drawn from the hard palate to the inner aspect of the posterior rim of the foramen magnum, or alternatively, McGregor's line is drawn from the hard palate to the outer cortex of the posterior rim of the foramen magnum. The level of the dens with respect to these lines is then evaluated. In symptomatic basilar impression there is usually significant dens protrusion.

This anomaly is sometimes erroneously called **pla-**

tybasia, which is really just a benign flattening of the base of the skull.

A basilar impression is also known as a **Basilar Invagination**.

Batchelor Plasters (bach'-e-lor/plas'terz) (n.) Casts applied to hold the hips in abduction and medial rotation. Only the lower limbs are encircled, with the casts extending from the groin to the ankles. They are joined by a crossbar to maintain position. The knees are held at 15–20° of flexion to prevent rotation of the limbs within the plaster.

Bateman Prosthesis (bāt'man/pros-the'sis) (n.) A bipolar femoral head prosthesis. It has three components: a metallic femoral component, a polyethylene bearing, and an outer metallic cup.

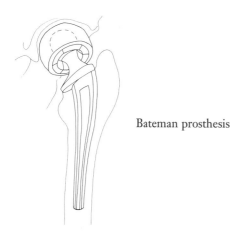

Bateman prosthesis

Batson's Plexus (bat'sunz/plek'sus) (n.) A complex network of nonvalvular veins in and around the vertebral column. This system of vertebral veins plays a significant role in the spread of tumor and infection from the systemic and portal areas to the vertebrae, the spinal cord, and the brain or skull.

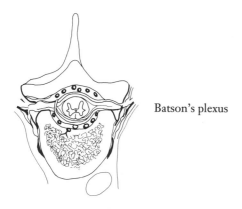

Batson's plexus

Battered-Child Syndrome (bat'er'd/chīld/sin'drōm) (n.) A complex of conditions that may cause permanent injury or death in young children following physical abuse or neglect. The syndrome should be considered in any child exhibiting evidence of unusual or multiple fractures, subdural hematoma, soft tissue swellings, skin bruising or burns, or failure to thrive, especially when the degree and type of injury is at variance with the history given; or in any child who dies suddenly. If a high index of suspicion for child abuse exists, the case must be reported for further investigation.

Battle's Sign (bat't'lz/sīn) (n.) A clinical sign indicative of basilar skull fractures. The accumulation of blood beneath the deep fascia produces postauricular discoloration and ecchymosis. This first appears near the tip of the mastoid process.

Baumann's Angle (bō'manz/ang'g'l) (n.) A radiographic measurement used in the evaluation of the angulation of the distal humerus. It is the angle formed by the intersection of a line perpendicular to the humerus and a line drawn along the physeal line of the lateral condyle. The angle is measured on the roentgenogram of the elbow, with the x-ray beam neutral and the cassette placed parallel to the humerus. This is a consistent angle when both elbows are compared and when the x-ray beam is not deviated from the perpendicular. This angle does not equal the carrying angle in the older child.

Bayonetted (ba'yo-net-ed) (adj.) Descriptive term used for fracture fragments that are opposed and overlapped.

BE Amputation; BEA (b-e/am"pu-ta'shun) (n.) Abbreviation for below-the-elbow amputation.

Beat Knee (bēt/nē) (n.) See **Prepatellar Bursitis**.

Beau's Lines (bōs/līnz) (n.) Transverse furrows that occur on the fingernails and toenails following wasting diseases.

Beaver's Blade (bē'verz/blād) (n.) A brand name for a thin, disposable, somewhat flexible knife that is used in meniscal surgery, both open and arthroscopic.

Bechterew's Test (bek-ter'yewz/test) (n.) A method used to detect sciatica. Have the patient sit; then simultaneously extend both knees. If sciatica is present, the patient will be able to straighten each knee in turn, but not both at one time.

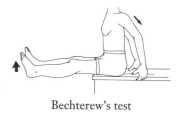

Bechterew's test

Becker's Type Muscular Dystrophy (bek'erz/tīp/mus'ku-lar/dis'trō-fē) (n.) A type of sex-linked muscular dystrophy similar to Duchenne's dystrophy in clinical appearance but with a much more benign clinical course. Compared with Duchenne's, the age of onset is usually later, about age 7, and the progress is slower, with the patient remaining ambulatory until teenage or adult life.

Bed Count (bed/kownt) (n.) The number of beds regularly maintained by a hospital for inpatients.

Bedside X-Ray Examination (bed'sīd/x-rā'/eg-zam"i-nā'tion) (n.) A radiographic examination that uses a portable x-ray apparatus and is conducted while the patient remains in bed.

Beevor's Sign (be'vorz/sīn) (n.) A clinical sign of asymmetrical paralysis of the rectus abdominus and paraspinal muscles. Have the supine patient perform a quarter sit-up, with arms crossed on the chest. While the patient holds this position, observe the umbilicus. Normally, it will not move. Umbilical movement indicates a weak segmental portion of these muscles. The umbilicus is drawn toward the stronger or uninvolved side.

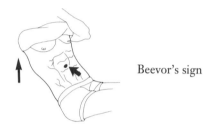

Beevor's sign

Behavior Modification (be-hāv'yor/mod"i-fi-kā'shun) (n.) The use of one or more of a number of techniques based on learning theory and the principles of learning to effect specific changes in behavior.

Behcet's Syndrome (bā'sets/sin'drōm) (n.) A disease complex characterized by both recurrent ulcerations of the mouth and genitalia and by iritis. Also, one often sees the presence of articular disease. Initially the syndrome is limited to arthralgias, but ultimately it becomes an irregularly intermittent or chronic periarticular inflammation. Less commonly associated features include thrombophlebitis, erythema nodosum, and the involvement of the gastrointestinal and central nervous systems. Synonyms: **Mucocutaneous Oral Syndrome, Triple Symptom Complex.**

Bell's Law (belz/law) (n.) The law describing nerve functions—the anterior roots of spinal nerves are motor nerves, and the posterior roots are sensory nerves.

Belly of Muscle (bel'e/of/mus'el) (n.) The prominent, fleshy, central portion of a muscle.

Below-the-Elbow Amputation (bē'lō/the/el-bō/am'pu-ta'-shun) (n.) Any ablative procedure of the upper extremity performed distal to the elbow.

Below-the-Knee Amputation (bē'lō/the/nē/am'pu-ta'shun) (n.) Any ablative procedure of the lower extremity performed distal to the knee.

Bence-Jones Protein (bens-jōnz/pro'tēn) (n.) An abnormal protein found in the urine of patients with multiple myeloma. Its distinguishing characteristic is precipitation from the urine at a temperature between 50 and 56° Celsius. The protein redissolves at boiling temperatures and then reprecipitates on cooling.

Bending (bend'ing) (n.) In biomechanics, a type of load that may be applied to a structure. In three-point bending, loads are applied to either end of a structure in the same direction while a centrally applied load is placed in the opposing direction.

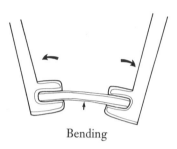

Bending

Bending Pliers (bend'ing/plī'erz) (n.) A hand-held instrument used to contour plates for internal fixation.

Bending Press (bend'ing/pres) (n.) A large metallic instrument that rests upon a table and is used in conjunction with twisting irons to contour plates for internal fixation.

Bending Rigidity (bend'ing/rĭ-jid'ĭ-te) (n.) A biomechanic term used to describe the deflection of a structure per unit of bending load.

Bending Strength (bend'ing/strength) (n.) A biomechanic term used to describe a structure's ability to resist bending loads. Proportional to the area's moment of inertia.

Benediction Sign (ben'-e-dik-shun/sīn) (n.) See **Bishop's Hand.**

Benign Tumor (be-nīn/too'mor) (n.) A nonmalignant neoplasm, or one that does not have the potential for uncontrollable growth and metastasis.

Bennett's Fracture (ben'ets/frak'chur) (n.) An intra-articular fracture subluxation at the base of the

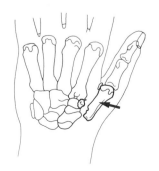

Bennett's fracture

first metacarpal. The fracture produces a small volar lip fragment that remains attached to the trapezium and trapezoid bones by means of the strong oblique ligament, while the shaft is displaced by the deforming pulls of the adductor pollicis and abductor pollicis longus muscles.

Betadine (bā′tah-dīn) (n.)   The trade name for a solution of povidone-iodine used as an antiseptic.

Biceps Brachii Muscle (bi′seps/bra′ke-i/mus′el) (n.) See **Muscle**.

Biceps Femoris Muscle (bi′seps/fem′or-is/mus′el) (n.)   See **Muscle**.

Biceps Reflex (bi′seps/re′fleks) (n.)   A muscle-stretch reflex characterized by contraction of the biceps muscle, with resulting flexion of the elbow. The reflex center is at the 5th and 6th cervical segments. Synonym: **Biceps Jerk**.

Biceps Tendonitis (bi′seps/ten″do-ni′tis) (n.)   See **Bicipital Tendonitis**.

Bicipital (bī sip′i-tal) (adj.)   Having two heads.

Bicipital Groove (bi sip′i-tal/groov) (n.)   A shallow linear depression on the anterior surface of the proximal humerus, between the greater and lesser tubercles. The groove lodges the tendon of the long head of the biceps. Also called **Intertubercular Groove**.

Bicipital Syndrome (bī-sip′i-tal/sin′drōm) (n.)   A symptom complex produced by a dislocation of the tendon of the long head of the biceps brachii from the intertubercular or bicipital groove.

Bicipital Tendonitis (bi-sip′i-tal/ten″do-nī′tis) (n.)   A painful affliction of the tendon of the long head of the biceps muscle in which the tendon is affected by an inflammatory process involving both the tendon and its sheath. Also known as **Bicipital Tenosynovitis** or **Biceps Tendonitis**.

Bicipital Tenosynovitis   See **Bicipital Tendonitis**.

Bicipital Tuberosity (bī sip′i-tal/too″bĕ-ros′ĭ-tē) (n.)   The prominence on the neck of the radius for attachment of the biceps tendon.

Bicycle Spoke Injury (bi-sikl/spōk/injerē) (n.)   An injury to the lower extremity seen in children when a foot is caught between the spokes of a bicycle wheel. Initially, the appearance of the extremity often is normal, with only minor abrasions noted. However, because of the shearing and crushing components of the injury, about 24 to 48 hours after the accident one will see edema of the foot and leg and areas of skin loss; even full thickness skin loss may occur. The most common sites of necrosis are over the malleoli, on top of the Achilles tendon, or on the top of the lateral aspect of the foot.

BID   Abbreviation for *bis in die,* the Latin meaning twice a day.

Bier Block (bēr/blok) (n.)   A method of intravenous regional anesthesia. In this technique, a catheter or needle is placed into a superficial vein of the extremity to be anesthetized. The limb is then exsanguinated with elevation and/or a pressure bandage, and a pneumatic tourniquet is inflated to a pressure appropriate for that limb. A solution of lidocaine or another anesthetic agent at recommended volume is injected. Anesthesia is usually seen after five minutes. For the patient's comfort, a second tourniquet should be inflated distal to the first on anesthetized skin; then the original tourniquet, which is on unanesthetized skin, may be deflated.

Bifid (bi′fid) (adj.)   Divided into two parts.

Bifurcation (bi″fur-ka′shun) (n.)   The site of division of a structure into two branches.

Bigelow Maneuver (big′e-lō/mah-noo′ver) (n.)   A technique for the reduction of a posterior hip dislocation. In this maneuver, the patient lies supine, and countertraction is applied as downward pressure on both anterosuperior iliac spines. Longitudinal traction is applied to the affected limb in line with the deformity; then the hip is flexed. While maintaining traction, gently lever the femoral head into the acetabulum by abduction, external rotation, and extension of the hip.

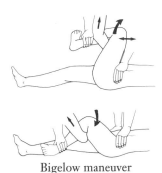

Bigelow maneuver

Bigelow Y Ligament (big′e-lō/y/lig′ah-ment) (n.)   The iliofemoral ligament.

Bilateral (bi-lat′er-al) (adj.)   1. Occurring on both sides of the midline. 2. Of or pertaining to both sides of the body. Example: bilateral total knee replacements.

Bimalleolar Angle (bi″mal-e′o-lar/ang′g′l) (n.)   An angle that demonstrates fibula shortening following fracture of the distal fibula. Draw a vertical line par-

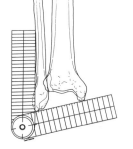

Bimalleolar angle

allel to the fibula that extends to the tip of its malleolus. Intersect this line with one drawn from the tip of the fibula malleolus to the tip of the medial malleolus. The average angle is 24°. The angle obtained from the injured ankle must be compared with the opposite ankle because there is variability between patients. Every degree of angle difference is equal to 1 mm of fibular shortening.

Bimalleolar Ankle Fracture (bī′mal-e′o-lar/ang′k′l/frak′chur) (n.) A fracture of the ankle in which both the distal fibula and the medial malleolus are broken. See also **Pott's Fracture**.

Bimalleolar Equivalent (bī′mal-e′o-lar/ē-kwiv′ah-lent) (n.) An injury to the ankle in which either the medial or lateral malleolus is fractured and there is significant ligamentous damage on the opposite side of the ankle.

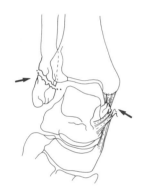

Bimalleolar equivalent

Biologic Dressings (bī-o-loj′ik/dres′ingz) (n.) The use of homologous or heterologous skin for wound coverage.

Biologic Fixation (bi-o-loj ik/fik-sa′shun) (n.) The progressive incorporation of bone into the surface porosity of an implant resulting in an intrical bone—implant interface that confers increased implant support and fixation.

Biomechanics (bī″o-me-kan′iks) (n.) The study of the relationship between forces and motion in biologic systems.

Biopsy (bī′op-sē) (n.) To obtain a piece of tissue for histologic evaluation, especially when there is a suspected tumor. The techniques include needle aspiration, the use of a cutting needle, or an open procedure for incisional or excisional biopsy.

Bipartite Patella (bī-par′tīt/pah-tel′ah) (n.) A congenital anomaly of the patella in which an accessory ossification center gives the patella the appearance of being in two pieces. This variation is benign and is usually bilateral and symmetrical. The accessory center is most commonly in the superolateral quadrant.

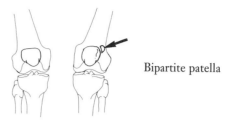

Bipartite patella

Bipolar Prosthesis (bī-po′lar/pros-thē′sis) (n.) Any femoral head replacement device that is composed of a metallic shaft and a metallic acetabular cup with an interposed polyethylene liner. There is potential motion at two "poles"—the inner bearing between the metal head and the polyethylene liner and the outer bearing between the acetabulum and the metallic cup. These prostheses were intended to decrease acetabulum erosion and protrusion. They are convertible to total hip arthroplasties by removing the polyethylene liner and metallic outer bearing cup and fitting an acetabulum component compatible with the size of the metal head. Synonym: **Universal Proximal Femoral Endoprosthesis**.

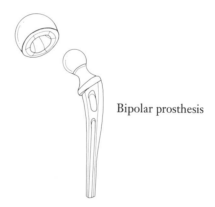

Bipolar prosthesis

Birefringent (bi″re-frin′jent) (n.) The property of a substance of doubly refracting a beam of light.

Bishop's Hand (bish′ups/hand) (n.) A low ulna nerve palsy (involves the muscles of the hand only) that causes clawing of the ring and small fingers. This

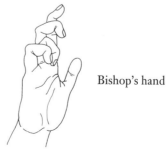

Bishop's hand

results in hyperextension of the metacarpophalangeal joint and flexion of the proximal and distal interphalangeal joints. It does not affect the thumb, index, and long fingers. This results in the appearance of the hand, as in the sign of benediction.

BKA Abbreviation for below-the-knee amputation.

Blade Plate (blād/plāt) (n.) A fixed, right-angle metallic device used in the internal fixation of supracondylar and proximal femur fractures. The blade portion is U-shaped in cross-section, and the fixed plate is secured to the diaphysis with screw fixation.

Blair Fusion (blār/fū′zhun) (n.) A technique of ankle repair intended for patients with avascular necrosis of the talar body or loss of the talar body. This procedure uses a sliding anterior tibial corticocancellous graft that fits into a quadrilateral hole in the talar head.

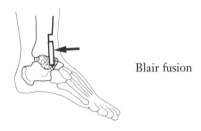

Blair fusion

Blastomycosis (blas″to-mī-kō′sis) (n.) An infection caused by the fungus *Blastomyces dermatitides*.

Bleeding (blēd′ing) (n.) Hemorrhage. The escape of blood from blood vessels.

Block Vertebra (blok/ver′tĕ brah) (n.) A congenital defect in which two or more vertebral bodies are fused without an intervening disk.

Blood Vessels (blud/ves′elz) (n.) The endothelial lined conduits through which blood is transported. These include arteries, arterioles, veins, venules, and capillaries.

Blount's Disease (blunts/di-zēz′) (n.) Tibia vara that occurs secondary to a growth disturbance of the medial aspect of the proximal tibial epiphysis. The diagnosis is made radiographically. The treatment and prognosis are based on radiographic appearance and the patient's age. Also known as **Tibia Vara** and **Osteochondrosis Deformans Tibia**.

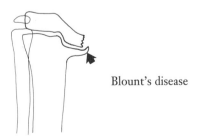

Blount's disease

Blumensaat's Line (blū-men-zahts/līn) (n.) A radiodense line seen on a lateral radiograph of the knee. It represents the bony roof of the intercondylar notch of the femur. It is identified on lateral x-ray by increased density of cortical bone at the roof of the notch. With the knee flexed to 30° this line normally touches the inferior pole of the patella.

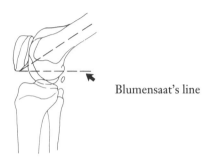

Blumensaat's line

BOA Abbreviation for British Orthopaedic Association.

Board Certified (bord/ser″ti-fid) (n.) A physician or other health profession who has passed an examination given by a medical specialty board and who has been certified by the board as a specialist in that particular field. The examination cannot be taken until the professional meets the requirements set by the specialty board. In orthopaedics the certification is by the American Board of Orthopaedic Surgery.

Board Eligible (bord/el′-e-je-bel) (n.) A physician or health professional who is eligible for a specialty board examination. Each of the specialty boards has requirements that must be met before the examination can be taken for specialty board certification.

Bobath Method (bō bath/meth′ud) (n.) A system of therapeutic exercises for patients with lesions of the central nervous system. Example: For adults with hemiplegia and children with cerebral palsy.

Body Cast (bod′ē/kast) (n.) A plaster or plastic cast that encompasses the body. It extends from the manubrial notch to the pubis and is molded over the iliac crests. Also known as a **Body Jacket**.

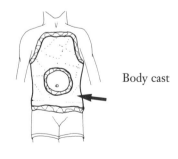

Body cast

Body Jacket (bod′ē/jak′et) (n.) See **Body Cast**.

Body-Powered Prosthetic Device (bod′ē/pow′er′d/ pros-the′tik/de′vīs) (n.) One that is manipulated by the patient's remaining functioning muscle groups. This is in contrast to electrically-powered prostheses.

Böhler-Braun Frame (bō-ler-brown/frām) (n.) An apparatus used for the application of skeletal traction to the lower extremity. It may be used with transcondylar, tibial or calcaneal pins. Also known as **Böhler Frame**.

Böhler Clamp (bō-ler/klamp) (n.) An apparatus designed to apply lateral compression to the calcaneus to effect closed reduction of calcaneal fractures. This clamp is applied under the medial and lateral malleoli.

Böhler Frame (bō-ler/frām) (n.) See **Böhler-Braun Frame**.

Böhler Splint (bō-ler/splint) (n.) A hand splint designed for the immobilization of phalangeal fractures. It consists of a wire outrigger attached to a dorsal slab across the wrist.

Böhler Tuber Joint Angle (bō-ler/too′ber/joint/ ang′g′l) (n.) A radiographic measurement of the normal anatomic relationships of the calcaneus. On the lateral radiograph of the ankle, it is the angle formed by the intersection of a straight line drawn along the upper surface of the tuber calcanei with a straight line connecting the highest point of the anterior upper joint surface of the calcaneus and the highest point of its posterior joint surface.

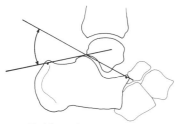

Böhler tuber joint angle

Bologna Cast (bō-lō′-nyah/kast) (n.) A technique of plaster cast application in which generous amounts of cotton padding are applied to the limb and then compressed with a plaster bandage to achieve appropriate tension.

Bolt (bolt) (n.) A metallic device used in internal fixation that resembles a screw. It crosses both cortices and is fixed with a nut on the side opposite the bolt head.

Bone (bōn) (n.) 1. The hard, connective tissue that forms the body's skeleton. Bone functions as a structural support, a hematopoietic repository, and a mineral reserve for calcium and phosphorus. 2. Bone is composed of minute hexagonal crystal-lattice structures containing calcium, phosphate ions, hydroxyl ions, and many trace minerals enmeshed in an or-

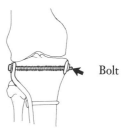

Bolt

ganic collagenous matrix. New bone formation proceeds with the crystallization of amorphous calcium phosphate and its subsequent maturation into hydroxyapatite crystals down to the matrix.

Bone Age (bōn/āj) (n.) The age of a patient based on the degree of skeletal maturation. The most common method of determining this age is by comparing a radiograph of the patient's left hand and wrist with a series of films typical of various age groups. These latter films may be found in texts such as the **Greulich-Pyle Atlas**.

Bone Bank (bōn/bank) (n.) A place in which homogenous bone is preserved and stored for use as allograft.

Bone Block (bōn/blok) (n.) 1. A segment of bone that is surgically transposed to create bony impingement and thus block motion at a joint. 2. A segment of bone that is transposed with its attached soft tissues to allow more secure reattachment of the soft tissues through actual bone healing.

Bone Cell (bōn/sel) (n.) See **Osteocyte**.

Bone Cement (bōn/se′ment) (n.) See **Polymethylmethacrylate**.

Bone Cyst (bōn/sist) (n.) 1. Any saclike abnormality in a bone. See also specific cysts. 2. A commonly used term for a unicameral bone cyst.

Bone Graft (bon/graft) (n.) 1. The transplantation of bone. Inserted bone tissue intended to become an integral part of the bone into which it is grafted. Bone for grafting can be taken from many places—from another body part (autogenous bone); from another member of the same species (homogenous bone); or even from a different species; xenograft. 2. (v.) To perform a bone graft.

Bone-holding Forceps (bōn/hōld′ing/fōr′seps) (n.) A device for holding a bone.

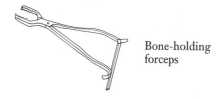

Bone-holding forceps

Bone Infarct (bōn/in-fahrkt) (n.) An area of localized bone necrosis. Radiographically, these lesions typically show interspersed irregular calcifications and ossifications with areas of intramedullary radiolucencies. Often seen in specific clinical situations that include caisson workers, divers in pressurized atmospheres, patients with sickle cell disease, and patients on prolonged steroid therapy. Idiopathic infarcts are also seen.

Bone Island (bōn/ī′land) (n.) An asymptomatic bone lesion noted radiographically as a sclerotic density. Usually clinically significant only in the differential diagnosis of radiodense lesions. See **Enostosis**.

Bone Marrow (bōn/mar′o) (n.) The soft, fatty material found in the intramedullary cavities and cancellous regions of long bones. The bone marrow is essentially a hematopoietic organ. See **Marrow Cavity**.

Bone Peg (bōn/peg) (n.) A bone-grafting technique in which a cylindrical peg of bone is used for internal fixation as well as osteogenesis. Also known as a **Peg Graft**.

Bone Scan (bōn/skan) (n.) A scintigraphic study in which radiopharmaceutical agents are injected that are localized to the skeleton. Localization of these agents, most commonly Tc^{99} (technetium pertechnetate), depends on blood and osteoblastic activity.

Bone Spur (bōn/spur) (n.) Any small bony projection.

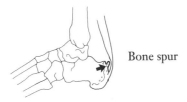

Bone spur

Bone Wax (bōn/waks) (n.) A refined bee's wax used to stop bleeding from bony surfaces.

Bony Bridge (bōn′ē/brij) (n.) See **Physeal Bar**.

Boot (boot) (n.) In shoe terminology, a high-quarter shoe in which the quarters cover the malleoli to any point up to the hip.

Boot Cast (boot/kast) (n.) A cast extending from just below the knee to the base of the toes. Also known as a short leg cast.

Boot-Top Fracture (boot-top/frak′chur) (n.) A transverse fracture of the distal one-third of the tibia. Is is so-named because it frequently occurred just above the top of a skier's boot when those boots were low, ending at the level of the distal tibia.

Booth Test (booth/test) (n.) A clinical examination to assess the integrity of the transverse humeral ligament. Apply pressure to the bicipital groove while rotating the patient's arm internally and externally. During external rotation, abduct the arm. Pain with an audible snap or pop is indicative of rupture of the

transverse ligament with bicipital tendon subluxation. Synonym: **Marvel Test**.

Boss (bos) (n.) A rounded or knoblike protuberance from the surface of a bone.

Bosworth Fracture (bos′werth/frak′chur) (n.) A fracture and dislocation of the ankle, with entrapment of the fibula behind the tibia.

Bosworth Procedure (bos′werth/pro-se′jur) (n.) A technique for the reduction and fixation of acromioclavicular dislocation. In addition to the ligamentous repairs, a Bosworth screw is placed from the clavicle into the base of the coracoid to hold it in reduction.

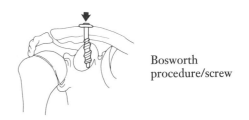

Bosworth procedure/screw

Bosworth Screw (bos′werth/skrū) (n.) A screw designed for the internal fixation of the clavicle to the base of the coracoid. This is a lag screw with a broad head. See **Bosworth Procedure**.

Bottom Filler (bot″m/fil′er) (n.) In shoe terminology, the material used for filling the cavity between the insole and outsole of shoes. Granulated cork in a resinous binder is the most widely used bottom filler. Other fillers contain rubber latex, cork sheet, impregnated felt, or laminated wood cut to shape.

Bouchard's Nodes (boo′sharz′/nōdz) (n.) Firm, nontender cartilaginous and bony enlargements on the dorsal surface of the proximal interphalangeal joints of the finger, as seen in osteoarthritis.

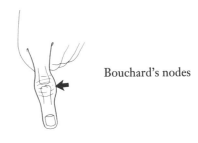

Bouchard's nodes

Boundary Layer Lubrication (bownd′rē/la′er/loo′ bri-ka′shun) (n.) A technique used when each bearing surface is coated or impregnated with a layer of a "slipper" film. This allows the applied surface to slide on the opposing surface with easy motion and little stress-concentration effect.

Boutonnière Deformity (bū-tōn-jayr/de-for′mĭ-te) (n.) A deformity of the finger that results from disruption or attenuation of the central slip of the extensor expansion of the fingers. As a result, the lateral bands subluxate volarward, and the finger assumes a position of flexion at the proximal interphalangeal joint and hyperextension of the distal interphalangeal joint. Hyperextension of the metacarpophalangeal joint is also often seen. Also known as **Buttonhole Deformity**.

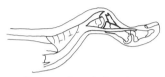

Boutonnière deformity

Bow Sign (bō/sīn) (n.) A radiographic sign indicative of severe spondylolisthesis, usually of L5 on S1. On an AP roentgen view of the lumbosacral spine, a density that gives the appearance of a bow with its convex surface downward. It is seen as a result of the overlap of the vertebral bodies.

Bowing Fracture (bō′ing/frak′chur) (n.) A traumatic injury seen in growing bones in which the bone is deformed beyond full elastic recoil into a phase of permanent plastic deformation.

Bowleg (bō′leg) (n.) See **Genu Varum**.

Bowler's Thumb (bō′lerz/thum) (n.) A perineural fibrosis of the ulnar digital nerve of the thumb caused by the repetitive compression that occurs while grasping a bowling ball. Symptoms include tingling and hyperesthesia around the pulp space of the thumb; usually there is a palpable, exquisitely tender lump, sometimes accompanied by distal skin atrophy.

Bowstring Sign (bō′string/sīn) (n.) A sign elicited on examining for radiculopathy. Have the patient sit on a chair with the knee extended to a little more than right angle, and the body bent forward to flex the hips so as to lengthen the course of the sciatic nerve at the hip and knee joints. Then press your finger into the popliteal space to increase tension across the nerve. The test is positive if pain is felt in the course of the nerve at the back of the thigh or above the sciatic notch. Synonym: **Cram Test**.

Box Toe (boks/tō) (n.) In shoe terminology, the reinforced portion over the toes; also called the tip of a shoe. A stiffener is used to maintain the shape of a shoe toe, preserve the toe room, and protect the toes from blows.

Boxer's Fracture (boks′erz/frak′chur) (n.) A common name for a fracture of the neck of the 5th metacarpal, usually associated with volar displacement of the metacarpal head. This fracture is seen in boxers and others who strike a firm object with a clenched fist.

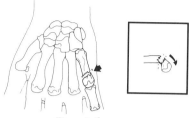

Boxer's fracture

Boyd and Anderson Technique (boid/and/an′der-son/tek′nēk) (n.) A method used to attach distal ruptures of the biceps tendon. It involves the use of two surgical incisions, thus reducing the risk of neurovascular damage associated with a repair through a simple anterior approach.

Boyd and Griffith Classification (boid/and/grif′ith/klas″si-fi-kā′shun) (n.) An arrangement of intertrochanteric femur fracture into four types:

Type I: Fractures extending along the intertrochanteric line.

Type II: Comminuted fractures in which the main fracture is along the intertrochanteric line.

Type III: Fractures that are basically subtrochanteric, with at least one fracture line passing or just distal to the lesser trochanter.

Type IV: Fractures of the trochanteric region and the proximal shaft, with a fracture in at least two planes.

Boyd-Sisk Procedure (boid-sisk/pro-se′jur) (n.) A surgical technique for the repair of recurrent posterior shoulder dislocation. A posterior capsulorrhaphy is performed with a posterior transfer of the long head of the biceps to the posterior glenoid rim.

Brace (brās) (n.) 1. An orthosis; 2. An apparatus or appliance applied to the body to correct or prevent deformities, support the weight of the body, assist or aid function, or control involuntary movements. 3. (v.) To support or make more rigid.

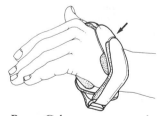

Brace, Galveston metacarpal

Brachial Plexus (brā′kē-al/plek′sus) (n.) A large nerve network in the neck and axilla formed from the ventral rami of the lower four cervical (C5–8) and the first thoracic (T1) spinal nerves. These roots unite to form three trunks—the superior trunk from C5 and C6, the middle trunk from C7, and the inferior trunk from C8 and T1. Each trunk separates into four anterior and posterior divisions. All the posterior divisions unite to form the posterior cord. The anterior divisions of the superior and middle trunk form the lateral cord; that of the inferior trunk continues as the medial cord. The cords give off terminal branches that regroup to form the terminal nerves that supply the upper extremity. These terminal nerves include the musculocutaneous, axillary, radial, median, and ulnar nerves.

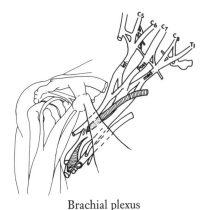

Brachial plexus

Brachial Plexus Block (brā′kē-al/plek′sus/blok) (n.) Regional anesthesia of the arm, forearm, and hand. It may be administered as a supraclavicular or axillary injection.

Brachial Plexus Palsy (brā′kē-al/plek′sus/pawl′zē) (n.) Paralysis that results from injury to part or all of the brachial plexus. An upper plexus injury is called **Erb's palsy**; a lower plexus injury is **Klumpke's palsy**. This is known as **Brachial Paralysis**.

Brachioradialis Muscle (brā″kē-ō-rā″dē-a′lis/mus′el) (n.) See **Muscle**.

Brachioradialis Reflex (brā″kē-ō-rā″dē-a′lis/re′fleks) (n.) An involuntary muscle stretch of the upper extremity. With the patient's forearm midway between pronation and supination and with the hand hanging loosely, strike the radial styloid process with a reflex hammer. This normally produces dorsiflexion of the wrist and supination of the forearm. This reflex primarily indicates neurologic integrity of C6, although it also has a C5 component. Also known as **Periosteoradial Reflex**, **Radial Reflex**, **Supinator Reflex**.

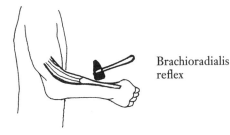

Brachioradialis reflex

Brachymelia (brāk″ē-mē′lē-ah) (n.) A short limb. See **Mesomelia**.

Brachypelvic (brak″e-pel′vik) (adj.) Pertaining to or having an oval type of pelvis, in which the transverse diameter exceeds the anteroposterior diameter.

Bracing (brās′ing) (n.) The act of applying a brace.

Bradford Frame (brad′ford/frām) (n.) A canvas bed suspended from rectangular poles that has an opening for the buttocks. It allows bed-pan placement or a bed-liner change with minimal disturbance of the patient's position. Initially, this was designed to facilitate the care of patients confined to bed in traction apparatuses.

Bradykinin (brād″ē-kī′nin) (n.) A potent vasodilator released from alpha-2-globulin by kallikrein, a proteolytic enzyme. This is one of a number of so-called "kinins."

Bragard's Sign (brā-ġerdz/sīn) (n.) A test for the presence of lumbosacral radiculopathy. With the patient supine, raise the extended leg to a point just short of producing pain; then dorsiflex the foot. In a positive test, this will bring out sciatic pain. If there is no increase in pain by this maneuver, the problem is unlikely to be neurologic irritation. Similar to **Lasègue test**.

Brailsford Syndrome (brīlz-ferd/sin′drōm) (n.) See **Morquio Syndrome**.

Brand Slipper Sock Test (brand/slip′er/sok/test) (n.) A method for semiquantitative dynamic pressure assessment inside a shoe. Use a polyurethane foam sock impregnated with microcapsules of blue dye. Sprinkle sodium bicarbonate in the sock prior to the test so that the acid brompherol dye will develop in this alkaline medium. Instruct the patient to put on the sock and test shoe and to walk 30 paces. As pressure and shearing forces develop, more microcapsules are broken, releasing dye. Pressure distribution can be assessed by evaluating the dye pattern and intensity.

Break (brāk) (n.) 1. A colloquial term for a fracture. 2. In shoe terminology, the wrinkle or crease formed across the vamp of a shoe when the shoe is flexed at the ball.

Breast (brest) (n.) In shoe terminology, the anterior surface of the heel.

Breastbone (brest′bōn) (n.) The sternum.

Breastline (brest′līn) (n.) In shoe terminology, an arbitrary line defining the forward boundary on the heel of a shoe.

Breaststroker Knee (brest′strōk-er/nē) (n.) A painful affection of the medial side of the knee that occurs in swimmers who do the breaststroke. It is attributed to injury or strain of the tibial collateral ligament and related to improper use of the whipkick while swimming.

Brevicollis (brev″e-kōl′is) (n.) A congenital deformity characterized by shortness of the neck. See **Klippel-Feil Syndrome**.

Brim Sign (brim/sīn) (n.) A thickening of the pelvic brim seen radiographically in Paget's disease of the pelvis.

Brisement (brēz-maw′) (n.) A closed manipulation of a stiff shoulder, usually performed for frozen shoulder or adhesive capsulitis.

Bristow-Helfet Procedure (bris-tō-help-et/pro-se′jur) (n.) See **Bristow Procedure**.

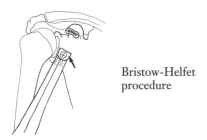

Bristow-Helfet procedure

Bristow Procedure (bris-tō/pro-se′jur) (n.) A technique for the repair of recurrent anterior shoulder dislocation. The coracoid process is transferred through the subscapularis tendon and fixed to the anterior glenoid rim with a screw. Also known as the **Bristow-Helfet Procedure**.

Brittain Arthrodesis (brit-tun/ar″thrō-dē′sis) (n.) A technique of extra-articular hip fusion. A broad tibial cortical graft is inserted through a subtrochanteric femoral osteotomy into a cleft made in the ischium below the acetabulum.

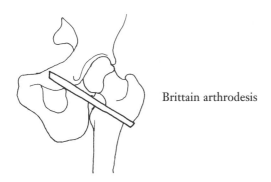

Brittain arthrodesis

Brittle Bones (brit″l/bōnz) (n.) The result of pathologic affections of bone in which ductility is lost. For example, this may occur in osteopetrosis and osteogenesis imperfecta.

Brittle Failure (brit″l/fāl′yer) (n.) A material distortion by fracture before permanent deformation occurs.

Brittleness (brit″l-nes) (n.) A material property that implies that no significant permanent deformation has occurred prior to fracture of that material. Methylmethacrylate and most ceramics are brittle materials.

Broach (brōch) (n.) Any one of a variety of barbed, tapered instruments used to enlarge the medullary canal, where there is cancellous bone to prepare for the insertion of implants such as arthroplasty components.

Broad-Based Cane (brod-bās′d/kān) (n.) A cane with three or four tips designed to provide a relatively wide base of support. Also called a three- or four-point cane, or a three- or four-legged cane.

Brodie's Abscess (bro′dēz/ab′ses) (n.) A chronic abcess seen most commonly in the metaphysis of a long bone.

Brooks and Jenkins Technique (brooks/and/jen′kinz/tek′nēk) (n.) A surgical method of atlantoaxial fusion. This procedure uses two full thickness rectangular bone grafts from the iliac crest which are placed in the vertebral column between the arch of the atlas and the lamina of the axis on either side of the midline. Wires placed beneath the atlas and axis secure the grafts in place.

Brooks and Seddon Procedure (brooks/and/sed-un/prō-sē′jur) (n.) A technique for the restoration of elbow flexion when the biceps is completely paralyzed. The entire pectoralis major muscle is transferred by using the long head of the biceps brachii to prolong its tendon distally.

Broomstick Cast (broom′stik/kast) (n.) A cast used to maintain abduction of the hips. Cylinder casts are applied from groin to ankle, with the knees slightly flexed. Two cross-bars, which may be made from broomsticks, are incorporated to hold the cast rigidly together, with each hip abducted as desired. This cast permits free flexion and extension of the hips, and controls abduction.

Brown Dermatome (brown/der′mah-tōm) (n.) An electrically powered instrument used for cutting skin grafts.

Brown-Séquard Syndrome (brown/sā-kar/sin′drōm) (n.) A spinal cord syndrome that results from a hemispinal cord injury. It is characterized by a loss of pain and temperature sensation on the contralateral side of the injury and a loss of motor function as well as position and vibratory sensation ipsilateral to the injury. Also known as **Hemicord Syndrome**.

Brown Tumor (brown/too′mor) (n.) A localized lytic lesion seen in the bones of patients with hyperparathyroidism that suggests a tumor. On histologic examination, there are numerous giant cells on a fibrocellular stroma, with interstitial hemorrhage noted. This results from a markedly focal variation of the usually diffuse demineralization seen in the skeleton. Also known as the **Brown Tumor of Hyperparathyroidism**.

Bryant's Traction (bri′ants/trak′shun) (n.) A technique for the application of vertical skin traction for infants and young children with femur fractures. The patient is supine, and the hips are flexed to a right angle.

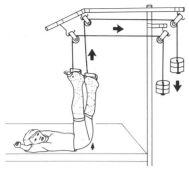

Bryant's traction

Buck's Traction (buks/trak′shun) (n.) A method of applying longitudinal skin traction to the lower extremity, with the use of weights and pulley, by means of longitudinal adhesive strips, held in place by an encircling bandage. This method is commonly used in patients with hip fractures, prior to surgical intervention, to make them more comfortable. Also called **Buck's Extension Traction.** See **Skin Traction**.

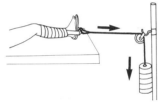

Buck's traction

Bucket Handle Tear (buk′et/hand′l/tār) (n.) A complete longitudinal tear of a meniscus of the knee that is displaced or that can be displaced into the joint.

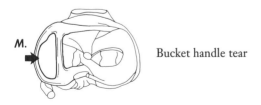

Bucket handle tear

Buckle Fracture (buk′l/frak′chur) (n.) See **Torus Fracture**.

Buddy Taping (bud′ē/tāp′ing) (n.) A technique for the dynamic splinting of a digit. The injured digit is simply taped to an adjacent normal digit; then the patient is encouraged to move the fingers or toes. The injured digit is thus passively moved along with the normal one.

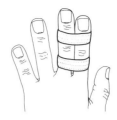

Buddy taping

Bulbocavernosus Reflex (bul′bo-kav′er-no′sus/rē′fleks) (n.) A normal cord-mediated involuntary reaction in which compression of the glans penis results in anal sphincter contraction. The return of this reflex is useful in determining the end of spinal shock after spinal cord injury.

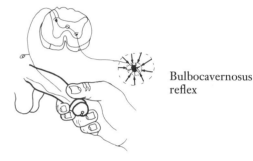

Bulbocavernosus reflex

Bumper Fracture (bum′per/frak′chur) (n.) A compression fracture of the lateral tibial plateau. Also called **Fender Fracture**.

Bunion (bun′yun) (n.) 1. The medial eminence associated with hallux valgus seen on the first metatarsophalangeal joint. 2. The commonly used layman's term for the spectrum of deformity associated with hallux valgus. 3. The complex of bunion deformity comprises hallux valgus, osteophyte formation, soft tissue contractures, and metatarsus primus varus. See **Hallux Valgus**.

Bunionette (bun′yun-et) (n.) 1. A bony prominence on the lateral side of the fifth metatarsal head. Also known as **Tailor's Bunion**. 2. The varus angulation of the fifth toe at the metatarsophalangeal joint, associated with an adventitious bursa on the lateral aspect of the fifth metatarsal head and a hard corn on the dorsal lateral aspect of the proximal interphalangeal joint of the fifth toe.

Bunnel Stitch (bun′el/stich) (n.) A technique for the end-to-end suture of tendons. A criss-crossing stitch.

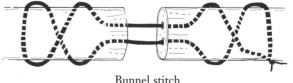

Bunnel stitch

use "e" per DIMD, other sources

e

Bunnell-Littler Test (bun'el-lit'ler/test) (n.) See **Intrinsic Tightness Test**.

Bunnell Pullout Suture (bun'el/pul'out/su'chur) (n.) See **Pullout Suture**.

Bupivacain (bu-pīv'ah-kān) (n.) A long-acting local anesthetic agent. Marketed as Marcaine.

Burn (bern) (n.) An injury that results from thermal insult or other cauterizing injury, as from chemicals, irradiation, or electricity. Burns are graded by severity, based upon depth of injury. First-degree burns exhibit redness. Second-degree burns show blisters. Third-degree burns reveal necrosis through the entire skin. First- and second-degree burns involve partial skin thickness. Third-degree burns involve full skin thickness.

Burnett's Syndrome (bur'nets/sin'drōm) (n.) See **Milk-Alkali Syndrome**.

Burns Bench Test See **Chicago Test**.

Burr (bur) (n.) A high-speed surgical instrument useful in drilling and enlarging holes in bones or teeth. The shaft has a rounded tip with cutting or fluting planes.

Bursa (ber'sah) (n.) A sac lined with a synovial-like membrane normally present around joints or in other areas subject to friction, e.g., where a tendon moves over a bony prominence. Bursae serve to reduce friction and protect underlying structures from excessive pressure. Adventitial bursae may form over aberrant bony prominences such as exostoses or even prominent screw heads or metal plates. See **Adventitious Bursa**.

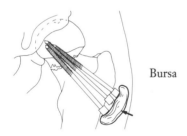

Bursa

Bursitis (ber-sī'tis) (n.) The inflammation of bursa. Example: **Deltoid Bursitis**.

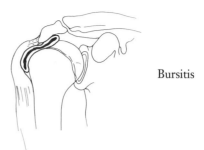

Bursitis

Burst Fracture (berst/frak'chur) (n.) A disruption of a vertebral body resulting from axial loading of the spine. In this fracture there is disruption of both the superior and inferior vertebral end-plates, as well as vertical fracture lines. Often there is retropulsion of bony fragments into the spinal canal. These fractures may be stable or unstable.

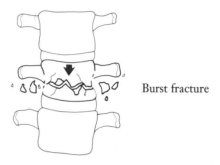

Burst fracture

Butterfly Fragment (but'-er-fli'/frag'-ment) (n.) A comminuted wedge-shaped fracture that has split off from the main fragment.

Butterfly Vertebra (but'-er-fli'/ver'te-brah) (n.) A radiographic finding of a biconcave vertebra characterized by notching of the endplates by the nucleus pulposus. The central part of the vertebral body is narrowed, creating the shape of a butterfly. Frequently seen after spinal fractures.

Buttonhole Deformity (but'n-hōl/de-for'mĭ-te) (n.) See **Boutonnière Deformity**.

Buttress Plate (but'res/plāt) (n.) A plate used in internal fixation to protect a thin cortex or to prevent a cancellous bone defect from collapsing. It is most often used around joints, such as the tibial metaphysis, for tibial plateau fracture fixation.

C

C-1 Abbreviation for the first cervical vertebra or nerve root.

C-2 Abbreviation for the second cervical vertebra or nerve root.

C-3 Abbreviation for the third cervical vertebra or nerve root.

C-4 Abbreviation for the fourth cervical vertebra or nerve root.

C-5 Abbreviation for the fifth cervical vertebra or nerve root.

C-6 Abbreviation for the sixth cervical vertebra or nerve root.

C-7 Abbreviation for the seventh cervical vertebra or nerve root.

C-8 Abbreviation for the eighth cervical nerve root.

C3-4 The space between the third and fourth cervical vertebrae.

C4-5 The space between the fourth and fifth cervical vertebrae.

C5-6 The space between the fifth and sixth cervical vertebrae.

C6-7 The space between the sixth and seventh cervical vertebrae.

C7-T1 The space between the seventh cervical and first thoracic vertebrae.

CA Ligament (C-A/lig′ah-ment) (n.) Abbreviation for coracoacromial ligament.

C-Arm (C-arm) (n.) A colloquial term for a portable image intensifier fluoroscopic unit.

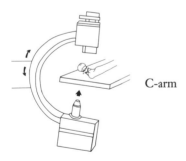

C-arm

C-Bar (C-bahr) (n.) A component of a hand orthosis, shaped like the letter C. The bar is placed between the second metacarpal bone and the opposed thumb to maintain the webspace open. An adduction stop maintains the thumb in abduction.

C-Cane (C-kān) (n.) A standard cane with a C-shaped, curved handle.

C-Spine (C-spīn) (n.) Abbreviation for cervical spine.

Ca (n.) 1. Chemical symbol for Calcium. 2. Abbreviation for cancer.

Cable Graft (kā′bel/graft) (n.) A procedure in which strands of a donor nerve are bundled together and the ends sutured to the larger proximal and distal stumps. This is useful when the nerve to be grafted is wider than the nerve to be used as a graft.

Cable Twister Orthosis (kā′bel/twis′ter/or-tho′sis) (n.) An orthotic device intended to control hip rotation and tibial torsion. It consists of a cable spring, pelvic belt, free-motion hip and ankle joint, connecting joints, stirrup, and shoe attachments.

Cadence (kād′ens) (n.) In gait analysis, a measurement of pace. It records the number of steps per minute. Average walking 90—100 steps per minute.

Café-au-lait Spots (ka-fā′ō-lā′/spots) (n.) Light yellowish brown, irregular areas of skin pigmentation with smooth margins. These macules are seen in the normal population but may be markers of neurofibromatosis or polyostotic fibrous dysplasia. If six or more café-au-lait spots measuring 1.5 cm or more in diameter are present, neurofibromatosis is suggested. When the circumference of the spots is smooth (described as resembling the coast of California) they also may be associated with neurofibromatosis. If the circumference is irregular (described as resembling the coast of Maine) they are likely to be associated with Albright's disease or Caffey's disease. See **Infantile Cortical Hyperostosis**.

Caffey's Sign (kaf-fēz/sīn) (n.) A radiographic change seen in patients with Legg-Calvé-Perthes disease. On an anteroposterior radiograph of the pelvis or, more commonly, on a frog lateral radiograph, a subchondral strip of decreased density is seen in the epiphysis. This is believed to represent early segmental fracture and to define the extent of avascularity in the femoral head. Also known as the **Crescent Sign of Caffey**.

Caisson Disease (kā′san/di-zēz′) (n.) Aseptic necrosis of bone, caused by sudden decrease of the atmospheric pressure. Synonyms: **Decompression Sickness** or **Diver's Disease**.

Calcaneal (kal-kā′nē-al) (n.) Of or pertaining to the calcaneus, or heel.

Calcaneal-Fifth Metatarsal Angle (kal-ka′ne-al/fifth/met″ah-tar′sal/ang′g′l) (n.) A measurement used in the evaluation of foot deformities on a lateral radiograph of the foot and formed by a line passing through the inferior cortex of the calcaneal body and another passing through the inferior cortex of the fifth metatarsal. Normal values vary from 150 to 175°.

Calcaneal Index (kal-kā′nē-al/in′deks) (n.) Method used in diagnosing and grading osteoporosis, based on the trabecular pattern of the calcaneus.

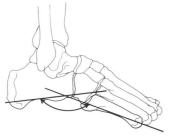

Calcaneal-fifth metatarsal angle

Grade V: The normal trabecular pattern of the calcaneus in a healthy young adult. The compression and tensile trabeculae are uniformly present and cross one another. The bone appears to be packed with cancellous tissue. The foramen calcanei shows a few thick dense trabeculae comparable in density with those in other parts of the bone.

Grade IV: The posterior compression trabeculae are seen as two pillars separated by a well-marked radiolucent area; this is due to recession and disappearance of the middle part of the posterior compression trabeculae.

Grade III: The borderline between a normal and an osteoporotic bone. In addition to the changes noted in Grades IV and V, there is recession and disappearance of the posterior tensile trabeculae, which stop short at the anterior pillar of the posterior compression trabeculae.

Grade II: Bone is definitely osteoporotic. The changes have progressed still further, with disappearance of the anterior tensile trabeculae. A thin sheath of the posterior tensile trabeculae can still be seen, crossing the anterior pillar of the posterior compression trabeculae.

Grade I: An advanced stage of osteoporosis. Both sets of tensile trabeculae have disappeared completely. There is generalized thinning, disappearance, and reduction in the number of compression trabeculae. The bone appears empty and not much denser than the soft tissues.

Calcaneal Spur (kal-kā′nē-al/spur) (n.)   An exostosis projecting on the plantar surface of the calcaneus near the origin of the plantar fascia. It is seen on a lateral roentgenogram of the heel. The exostosis may be associated with periosteal thickening and chronic bursitis. See **Heel Spur**.

Calcaneal Tendon (kal-kā′nē-al/ten′dun) (n.)   The common tendon of the gastrocnemius and soleus muscles that inserts into the heel. See **Achilles Tendon**.

Calcaneo (kal-kā′nē-ō)   Combining form for calcaneus.

Calcaneoapophysitis   (kal-kā′nē-ō-ah-pof″ĕ-zi′tis) (n.)   See **Sever's Disease**.

Calcaneocuboid Joint   (kal-kā″nē-ō-ku′boid/joint) (n.)   The articulation between the calcaneus and the cuboid bone in the foot.

Calcaneometatarsal Angle   (kal-kā″nē-ō-met″ah-tar′sal/ang′g′l) (n.)   See **Hibbs Angle**.

Calcaneonavicular Bar   (kal′kā″nē-ō-nah-vik′u-lar/bar) (n.)   A form of tarsal coalition in which a fibrous, cartilaginous, or osseous bridge, complete or incom-

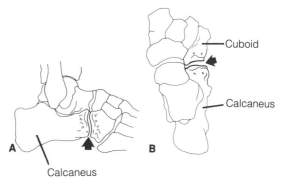

Calcaneocuboid joint

plete, forms between the os calcis and the tarsal navicular. This is a congenital anomaly that almost always produces a rigid flatfoot. It is best seen on oblique radiographs of the foot or with tomography.

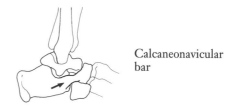

Calcaneonavicular bar

Calcaneovalgus (kal-kā″nē-ō-val′gus) (n.)   A foot deformity in which there is increased dorsiflexion of the ankle and lateral deviation of the foot. Usually seen in association with paralytic disorders.

Calcaneus (kal-kā′nē-us) (n.)   1. The heelbone. It is the large bone in the tarsus of the foot forming the projection of the heel behind the foot. The calcaneus articulates with the cuboid bone in front and with the talus above. Also known as the **Os Calcis**. 2. (adj.) A description of a deformation in which the foot is fixed in relative dorsiflexion to the tibia. This is the opposite of an equinus deformity.

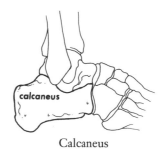

Calcaneus

Calcaneus Gait (kal-kā′nē-us/gāt) (n.)   The characteristic walk of a patient with paralyzed gastrocnemius-soleus muscles. The gait results from a lack of push-off, so that the tibia shifts posteriorly over the talus in the final portion of the stance phase when the extremity is trying to take off.

Calcaneus Secundarium (kal-kā″nē-us/sek′un-dar″-i′um) (n.) An accessory bone of the foot. It projects from the dorsal and distal end of the calcaneus, where it articulates with the cuboid and navicular bones. It is best seen in oblique roentgenograms of the foot.

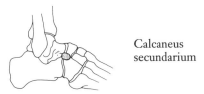

Calcaneus secundarium

Calcar (kal′kar) (n.) The thickened plate of cortical bone at the medial inferior edge of the femoral neck. Also called **Os calcar femorale**. Named by the Flemish medical illustrator Calcar.

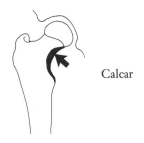

Calcar

Calcareous (kal-kā′rē-us) (adj.) Relating to or containing calcium, lime or calcific material that imports a chalky character.

Calciferol (kal-sif′er-ol) (n.) See **Vitamin D**.

Calcific Tendinitis (kal-sif′ik/ten″di-nī′tis) (n.) Any inflammatory condition of a tendon associated with calcium deposits that are visible radiographically.

Calcification (kal-si-fi-kā′shun) (n.) The deposition of calcium salts or calcareous matter within a tissue or structure.

Calcified Cartilage (kal-sif′īed/kar′ti-lij) (n.) Hyaline cartilage in which mineral salts have been deposited. Normally found in the growth plate at the junction of the hypertrophic zone and the metaphysis. Also in articular cartilage; the deepest zone, adjacent to the subchondral bone, is formed by calcified cartilage.

Calcify (kal-sif′ī) (v.) To deposit or lay down calcium salts.

Calcinosis (kal″si-nō′sis) (n.) A disorder characterized by the abnormal deposition of calcium salts in the tissues, particularly in or under the skin. It is often seen in association with progressive systemic sclerosis and dermatomyositis.

Calcinosis Universalis (kal″si-nō′sis/yū-ni-ver′sā-lis) (n.) Diffuse calcinosing in the skin, subcutaneous tissues, and connective tissue sheaths around muscles.

Dermal Calcinosis: Calcinosis localized to the skin and characterized by palpable, intracutaneous and/or subcutaneous deposits, usually located on digits or over large proximal joints or extensor surfaces of distal extremities. These masses are rock-hard and may ulcerate through the skin, draining gritty calcareous material.

Calciphylaxis (kal″sĭ-fi-lak′sis) (n.) A condition of induced systemic hypersensitivity in which tissues respond to various challenging agents with a precipitous (either evanescent or dense) deposit of calcium salts. The term denotes the defensive or phylactic response by the selective deposition of calcium in a challenged area.

Calcitonin (kal″sĭ-to′nin) (n.) A calcium-regulating hormone secreted by the parafollicular cells of the thyroid gland. Its production is stimulated by an elevated serum calcium level; it is known to inhibit osteoclastic resorption of bone. Its action results in a transient decrease in serum calcium, but its role in normal physiology has not been clearly defined. Synonym: **Thyrocalcitonin**.

Calcium (kal′se-um) (n.) A chemical element, atomic number 20, atomic weight 40.08, symbol Ca. Calcium is the most abundant mineral in the body. Serum calcium normally ranges from 8.5 to 10.5 mg/dL.

Calcium Carbonate (kal′se-um/kar′bon-āt) (n.) A crystalline compound, $CaCO_3$, occurring naturally in bone, shells, and so on, as calcite. It is used as both an astringent and an antacid.

Calcium Chloride (kal′se-um/klo′rīd) (n.) A calcium salt, $CaCl_2$, used in solution to restore electrolyte balance in alkalosis and to acidify urine.

Calcium Hydroxide (kal′se-um/hī-drok′sīd) (n.) An astringent compound, $CaOH_2$, used topically in solution or lotions.

Calcium Lactate (kal′se-um/lak′tāt) (n.) A preparation of calcium used for dietary supplementation.

Calcium Oxalate (kal′se-um/ok′sah-lāt) (n.) A compound occurring normally in the urine as a crystal sediment and abnormally in certain renal calculi.

Calcium Oxide (kal′se-um/ok′sīd) (n.) Chemical name for quicklime.

Calcium Phosphate (kal′se-um/fos′fāt) (n.) One of three salts containing calcium and the phosphate radical: dibasic and tribasic calcium phosphate are used as sources of calcium; monobasic calcium phosphate is used in fertilizer, and as a calcium and phosphorus supplement.

Calcium Pyrophosphate Dihydrate Deposition Disease (kal′sē-um/pī″rō-fos′fāt/dī-hī′drāt/de-poz′i-shun/di-zēz′) (n.) This is an arthropathy that involves the deposition of calcium pyrophosphate dihydrate crystals. It commonly presents clinically in a manner similar to osteoarthritis, or it may appear rheumatoid-like with symmetrical joint involvement, rapidly degenerating joint disease, or stiffness of the spine. Radiographically, chondrocalcinosis is seen. This disease accounts for about one-quarter of patients who present with chondrocalcinosis. Abbreviated as **CPDD disease.** Also called **Pseudogout.**

Calcium Sulfate (kal'se-um/sul'fāt) (n.) A compound of calcium and sulfate, occurring as gypsum or as plaster of Paris. Used in making plaster casts, splints, or other rigid dressings.

Calculus (kal'kū-lus) (n.) Any abnormal concretion, usually composed of mineral salts. Commonly called a stone, as in gallstones or kidney stones.

Caldwell-Moloy Classification (kald'wel-mo-loī'/klas"sĭ-fĭ-ka'shun) (n.) The system that designates the four types of pelves in terms of the configuration of pelvic inlet. It is based on normal variations in the following features:

Shape of inlet (width of forepelvis, ratio of widest transverse to longest anteroposterior diameter, ratio of anterior sagittal to posterior sagittal diameter), splay of sidewalls, prominence of spines, height of symphysis, transverse diameter of outlet (bituberous), width of subpubic arch, and curvature and inclination of sacrum.

The four basic types of pelves are: (1) Gynecoid, (2) Android, (3) Anthropoid, and (4) Platypelloid.

Calf (kaf) (n.) A popular name for the prominent muscle mass in the back of the leg, below the knee, composed mainly of the gastrocnemius and soleus muscles. Also known as the **Sura.**

Caliper (kal'ĭ-per) (n.) 1. An instrument with two prongs or "legs" used to measure thickness and diameter of objects. 2. The British term for a brace or splint.

Caliper Brace (kal'i-per/brās) (n.) An orthosis for the lower limb, with two upright bars attached to a shoe at the level of its sole. See **Long Leg Brace.**

Callaway's Test (kal'a-wāz/test) (n.) An examination used in obese patients to detect swelling in the shoulder by measuring the girth of the two shoulder joints. Loop a tape measure through the axilla, and measure the girth at the acromial tip. In a positive test, the girth of the affected joint is greater.

Callosity (kah-los'i-tē) (n.) Callus.

Callus (kal'us) (n.) 1. An acquired, circumscribed area of the skin, thickened by hypertrophy of the horny layer of the epidermis that is produced at a point of intermittent pressure, friction, or irritation. Also spelled callous. Also known as **Callosity, Callositas, Tyloma, Tylosis.** 2. The woven bone material that forms around bone ends following a fracture as part of the repair process. Initially, soft callus formation follows the inflammatory phase of bone healing and is a fibrocartilaginous stage that unites the bony fragments. Subsequently, this converts to fiber bone or the hard callus stage. The hard callus is eventually remodelled into lamellar bone.

Calorie (kal'o-rē) (n.) A unit of heat or energy.

Small Calorie: The amount of energy required to raise the temperature of 1 g. of water 1°C. Abbreviated cal or gram c.

Large Calorie: The amount of energy required to raise the temperature of 1 kg of water 1°C. It is abbreviated Cal or Kcal. This is the more commonly used unit in measurement of heat production in chemical reactions of biologic systems.

Camptocormia (kamp"to-kor'mē-ah) (n.) A deformity characterized by extreme flexion of the spine and hips associated with normal orthopaedic and neurologic findings. This is not a fixed deformity and usually can be corrected on recumbency or by suggestion. Often believed to have a hysterical etiology.

Camptodactyly (kamp"to-dak'ti-lē) (n.) A condition characterized by a flexion deformity of the proximal interphalangeal joint, usually of the little finger alone. Typically, camptodactyly is progressive, painless, and apparently hereditary.

Camurati-Engelmann Disease (kahm-oo-rahtē/eng'el-mahn/di-zēz') See **Diaphyseal Dysplasia.**

Canadian Crutch (ka-nā'dē-an/kruch) (n.) A lightweight crutch that resembles the axillary crutch but is shorter. It terminates in a cuff at or slightly above mid-arm level, thus preventing buckling of the elbow. Also called **California Crutch.**

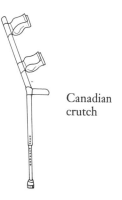

Canadian crutch

Canadian Orthopaedic Association The association that represents the majority of Canadian Orthopaedic Surgeons. Abbreviated **COA.**

Cancellous Bone (kan'se-lus/bōn) (n.) A type of structural organization of woven or lamellar bone; it is characterized by a reticular, spongy, or latticelike structure. The lattice work is aligned along lines of stress. This type of bone is subjected mainly to compressive forces. Also known as **Trabecular Bone.**

Cancellous Bone Graft (kan'se-lus/bōn/graft) (n.) Any bone graft, autologous or otherwise, in which cancellous bone is used in blocks, strips, or morselized. These grafts are most useful for their osteogenic potential. Compare **Cortical Bone Graft.**

Cancellous Screw (kan'sĕ-lus/skrū) (n.) Threaded

screws used for internal fixation. They have larger threads than cortical screws and are intended to provide more purchase in soft cancellous bone. They are frequently used in the metaphyseal areas. Selecting the proper drill size and tapping the drill hole are essential for secure purchase.

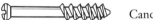

Cancellous screw

Cancer (kan′ser) (n.) Any malignant neoplasm.

Candida (kan′di-dah) (n.) Genus of yeastlike fungi capable of causing candidiasis, which may be manifested as an acute, chronic, or disseminated mycosis. Candida may be part of the normal body flora.

Candida Albicans (kan′di-dah/al′bi-kanz) (n.) The most common of the yeastlike fungus, **Candida**, that results in candidiasis. Cutaneous, oral, and vaginal infections are most commonly encountered. In very rare instances, disseminated disease results in osteomyelitis, arthritis, or other visceral lesions.

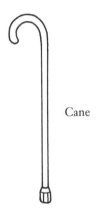

Cane

Cane (kān) (n.) A type of walking aid held in one hand; used to add stability in walking or to relieve weight from one limb. Also called **walking cane** or **walking stick**. In most cases, the appropriate cane size is found when the top curve of the hand-held piece of the cane is even with the hip joint. The correct length for a cane can be determined by flexing the elbow to 20° and placing the cane tip approximately 6 inches lateral to the base of the fifth toe.

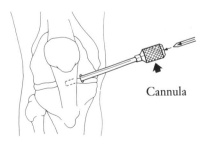

Cannula

Cannula (kan′u-lah) (n.) A hollow tube designed for insertion into a body cavity. It is usually used to aspirate fluid or to introduce medication. In arthroscopy, cannulae are placed into the joints through small portals and instrumentation can then be passed in and out of the joint.

Cannulated Drill (kan′u-lā-ted/dril) (n.) Any bit with a central lumen that is used to drill a hole in a bone over a guidewire.

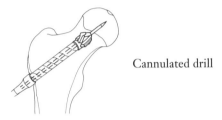

Cannulated drill

Cannulated Nail (kan′u-lā-ted/nāl) (n.) A general class of nail, having a lumen or hole in the center.

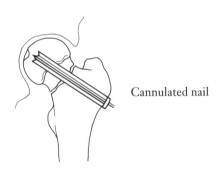

Cannulated nail

Cannulated Screw (kan′u-lā-ted/skru) (n.) A threaded screw that has a central lumen and is seated into bone over a previously placed guidewire.

Cantilever Fatigue (kan′ti-lē′ver/fah-tēg) (n.) A type of bending fatigue seen in femoral components of total hip or hemiarthroplasties. It is caused by loss of stem support proximally while the distal stem remains securely fixed in the canal.

Cape Bossa (kāp/bos′ah) (n.) See **Carpometacarpal boss**.

Capener's Method (kāp-nerz/meth′ud) (n.) A method of measuring the degree of spondylolisthesis. On a lateral radiograph of the spine, compare anteroposterior diameters of the spondylolytic vertebra with the normal vertebra above it.

Capillary (kap′i-lar″ē) (n.) A small, thin-walled blood vessel connecting arteries and veins through which diffusion and filtration into the tissues can occur.

Capillary Fragility Test (kap′i-lar″ē/frah-jil′i-tē/test) (n.) See **Rumpel-Leede Tourniquet Test**.

Capital Epiphysis (kap′i-tal/e-pif′i-sis) (n.) The proximal epiphysis of the femur. It ossifies at approximately 4 months in girls and 5 to 6 months in boys. It fuses at about 16 to 18 years of age in both sexes. Also known as **Capital Femoral Epiphysis** or **Subcapital Epiphysis**.

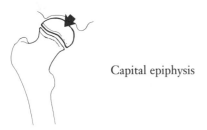

Capital epiphysis

Capitate (kap′i-tāt) (n.) One of the bones of the carpus. It articulates with the scaphoid and lunate bones proximally, predominantly the third metacarpal distally, the trapezoid laterally, and the hamate medially.

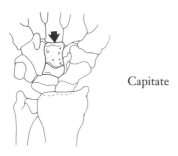

Capitate

Capitellum (kap″i-tel′um) (n.) The rounded, bony prominence on the lateral aspect of the distal humerus that articulates with the radial head. It is separated from the medial articular surface, the trochlea, by the capitulotrochlear groove. Also called **Capitulum**.

Capitulum (kah-pit′u-lum) (n.) See **Capitellum**.

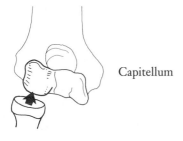

Capitellum

Capitulotrochlear Groove (kah-pit′u-lo-trok′lē-ar/grōōv) (n.) The indentation on the articular surface of the distal humerus that separates the trochlea from the capitellum.

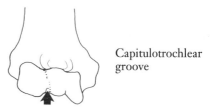

Capitulotrochlear groove

Capsule (kap′sūl) (n.) 1. A membrane made of collagen bundles that envelopes an organ or other body part. 2. In orthopaedics, generally used to describe the membrane that encloses a joint to form a closed cavity. See **Joint Capsule**.

Capsulectomy (kap″su-lek′to-mē) (n.) Any surgical procedure for the excision of all, or part of, a capsule.

Capsulitis (kap″su-lī′tis) (n.) Inflammation of a capsule.

Capsuloplasty (kap′su-lo-plas″tē) (n.) Surgical repair of a capsule. Example: **Putti-Blatt Procedure**.

Capsulorrhaphy (kap″su-lor′ah-fē) (n.) Suture of a capsule.

Capsulotomy (kap″su-lot′o-mē) (n.) Incision into a joint capsule.

Caput Index (kap′ut/in′deks) (n.) A radiographic technique used to determine femoral head sphericity, using arthrographic measurements. Measure the greatest breadth of the arthrographic outline of the femoral head. Construct a perpendicular line from the center of this line to the articular surface of the femoral head. The caput index is determined by calculating the relationship of this height of the femoral head to half of its greatest width. This index measures 1 in a perfectly spherical head.

Caput Quadratum (kap′ut/kwod-ra′tum) (n.) A clinical manifestation of rickets in which the cartilaginous components of the suture lines of the skull are enlarged. Also called **Hot-cross-bun Skull**.

Caput Ulnae Syndrome (kap′ut/ul′nae/sin′drōm) (n.) A descriptive term for an affection of the distal radioulnar joint in the rheumatoid hand in which the ulnar head is dorsally subluxated and the carpus subluxates volarly and rotates into supination. The major symptom is pain at the ulnar aspect of the wrist and forearm, aggravated by pronation and supination.

Carbenicillin (kar″ben-i-sil′in) (n.) A broad-spectrum penicillin, similar chemically to ampicillin but with greater activity against gram-negative bacterial strains, especially **Pseudomonas**, **Proteus** and some **Enterobacter**.

Carbohydrates (kar″bo-hī′drāts) (n.) Organic compounds with the general formula $(CH_2O)n$. Examples include sugars, starch, and cellulose.

Carbon Fiber (kar′bon/fī′ber) (n.) A fibril composed of pure carbon in a graphite structure. It has been used as an orthopaedic implant to provide biodegradable scaffolding for an artificial soft tissue implant.

Carbuncle (kar′bung-kl) (n.) A cluster of contiguous hair follicle infections with multiple, interconnecting drainage channels or sinuses.

Carcinogen (kar-sin′o-jen) (n.) Any substance that induces or produces cancer.

Carcinoma (kar″si-nō′mah) (n.) Any malignant neoplasm derived from epithelial tissue in any body site.

Carcinomatosis (kar″si-nō-mah-tō′sis) (n.) A condition in which there is disseminated carcinoma at multiple body sites or is widespread in a given body area.

Cardinal Symptoms (kar′di-nal/simp′tums) (n.) In establishing the identity of any medical disorder, those characteristics of greatest significance.

Cardiopulmonary Resuscitation (kar″dē-ō-pul′mo-ner′ē/re-sus″ĭ-tā′shun) (n.) A technique for basic lifesaving that attempts to restore respiratory and cardiovascular function after acute failure.

Care Plan (kār/plan) (n.) Formal written plan of activities to be conducted by personnel of a long-term care facility, home health agency, hospital, or other health facility on behalf of a patient. It is used to evaluate that patient's needs and progress. See **Nursing Care Plan**.

Carotid Triangle (kah-rot′id/trī′ang′g′l) (n.) An anatomic area in the anterior portion of the neck, useful for surgical approaches. Its borders are: cephalically, posterior belly of digastric and stylohyoid muscles; caudally, superior belly of omohyoid muscle; dorsally, sternocleidomastoid muscle. Compare **Anterior Triangle of the Neck**.

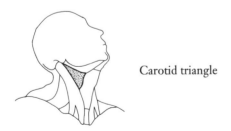

Carotid triangle

Carpal (kar′pal) (adj.) Of or in reference to the wrist, or carpus. See **Carpus**.

Carpal Bones (kar′pal/bōns) (n.) The eight small bones of the wrist, known collectively as the carpus. The carpal bones are the navicular or scaphoid, the lunate, the triquetrum, the greater and lesser multangulars (the trapezium and trapezoid), the capitate, the hamate, and the pisiform. See **Carpus**.

Carpal Boss (kar′pal/bos) (n.) See **Carpometacarpal Boss**.

Carpal Height (kar′pal/hīt) (n.) The distance between the distal cortex of the capitate and the prominent proximal lunate, as measured along the long axis of the third metacarpal. It is measured on a posteroanterior radiograph of the wrist. Decreases in carpal height, known as carpal collapse, are measured as the difference between pre- or postinjury or postoperative heights or by comparison to the unaffected side.

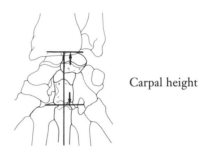

Carpal height

Carpal Tunnel (kar′pal/tun′el) (n.) The space between the flexor retinaculum of the wrist and carpal bones, through which pass the flexor tendons of the fingers and the flexor pollicis longus, and the median nerve.

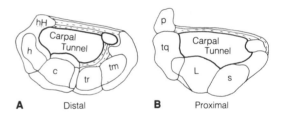

hH = Hook of Hamate; h = Hamate; c = Capitate;
tr = Trapezoid; tm = Trapizeum; p = Pisiform;
tq = Triquetrium; L = Lunate; s = Scaphoid

Carpal tunnel

Carpal Tunnel Syndrome (kar′pal/tun′el/sin′drōm) (n.) An entrapment or compression neuropathy of the median nerve in the carpal tunnel. The patient usually complains of paresthesias in the median nerve sensory distribution. Typically, the symptoms awaken the patient at night and are relieved by shaking the hand.

Carpal tunnel syndrome may be idiopathic or spontaneous. It can also result from any space-occupying lesion in the carpal tunnel (e.g., synovitis, edema, granulomatous tissue, or amyloid). Commonly associated diseases include rheumatoid arthritis, diabetes mellitus, degenerative joint disease, hypothyroidism, and acromegaly. This syndrome may occur during pregnancy, but usually disappears after delivery. Aberrant muscles of the forearm are another cause of median nerve compression. The diagnosis of a carpal tunnel syndrome is suggested by the history and confirmed by the presence of a spectrum of signs and symptoms. These include numbness of the radial 3½ digits, atrophy of the thenar muscles, a positive Tinel sign at the wrist, a positive Phalen sign, increased symptomatology on application of an arm tourniquet, and motor and sensory nerve electromyographic abnormalities. Also known as **Tardy Median Nerve Palsy**.

Carpectomy (kar-pek′to-mē) (n.) Literally, "removal of a body"; used in orthopaedics to describe a surgical procedure in which a carpal bone is excised.

Carpet Layer's Knee (kar′pet/la′erz/nē) (n.) See **Pre-Patellar Bursitis**.

Carpometacarpal Boss (kar″po-met″ah-kar′pal/bos) (n.) A bony prominence on the dorsum of the hand at the level of the base of the second and third metacarpals. It is usually visible on a tangential roentgenogram of the hand. Pain may appear on local pressure or on forced dorsiflexion of the wrist. Symptoms may result from subluxation or inflammation of the overlying extensor tendon. For some patients, it may present a cosmetic problem. Also known as **Carpal Boss**.

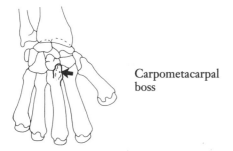

Carpometacarpal boss

Carpus (kar′pus) (n.) The eight small bones of the wrist, situated between the metacarpals distally and the radius and ulna proximally. See also **Carpal Bones**.

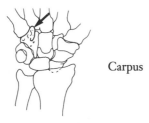

Carpus

Carr Splint (kar/splint) (n.) A splint used for the first-aid treatment of distal upper extremity injuries, including fractures. It consists of a straight dorsal splint and a palmar splint hollowed out for the thenar eminence. An oblique rounded bar is fixed to the lower end of the palmar splint to allow the fingers to grip the bar. To apply, the splints are bandaged to the hand and forearm.

Carrier (kar′ē-er) (n.) 1. An apparently well individual who, without signs of illness, harbors microor-

ganisms that may be disseminated to others. 2. An individual heterozygous for a recessive gene, who may be a normal phenotype. 3. Insurance company, prepayment plan, or government agency that, under a health insurance or prepayment program, administers claims submitted for or by its beneficiaries and, in certain cases, directly provides services. See also **Intermediary**.

Carrier State (kar′ē-er/stāt) (n.) The state of persistent colonization or asymptomatic infection of a host by a specific microbial species. That species usually has a significant pathogenic potential.

Carrying Angle (kar′ē-ing/ang′g′l) (n.) In the elbow, this is the normal valgus angle formed between the arm and the forearm when the elbow is fully extended and the forearm is fully supinated. There is controversy as to the true value of this angle and as to whether there is a significant difference between the value for males and females. In general, the normal angle measures from 0 to 20°; on the average, it is slightly greater in females.

One technique for measuring this angle is described by Bials, using an A-P roentgenogram of the elbow in complete extension and supination. Draw two midpoints in the distal humerus—one at the distal metaphyseal flare and one at the distal third of the diaphyses. Similarly, draw two midpoints in the proximal ulna—one at the level of the radial tuberosity and one at the most proximal ossification of the ulna. The carrying angle is formed by lines drawn through these points.

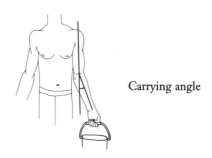

Carrying angle

Carter Rowe View (kar-ter/rō/vū) (n.) A radiographic visualization of the hip, taken at a 45° oblique angle. Used to determine the size of the bony fragments in a posterior fracture-dislocation of the hip.

Cartilage (kar′ti-lij) (n.) A specialized connective tissue composed of a homogeneous, highly polymerized hyaline matrix containing nucleated cells and chondrocytes, that lie in cavities or lacunae in the matrix. The matrix is white or gray, semiopaque, and nonvascular, consisting chiefly of proteoglycans and collagen fibers. The matrix is produced by cells called chondroblasts, which become embedded in the matrix as chondrocytes.

Although all cartilage matrix has a similar histologic appearance on light microscopy, there are significant differences in the microarchitecture and the function of different cartilaginous tissues. The mechanical properties of cartilage are due primarily to the properties of the complex extracellular matrix.

Articular Cartilage: A specialized type of hyaline cartilage that provides the self-lubricating, low-friction gliding and load-distributing surface of synovial joints. The complex microstructure of this type of cartilage, which is divided into four zones (based on the distribution of cells, proteoglycans, and orientation of collagen fibers) allows it to carry out these functions.

Costal Cartilage: The cartilage that forms the more anterior continuation of the bony rib.

Elastic Cartilage: A type of cartilage in which a large number of elastic fibers are contained in the extracellular matrix. Elastic cartilage is found in the auricles, nose, epiglottis, trachea, and eustachian tubes.

Fibrocartilage: A variety of cartilage in which large numbers of interlacing fibrous tissue strands are found throughout the matrix. It is found at tendon–bone interfaces, the menisci, and the intervertebral disks.

Fibroelastic Cartilage: Fibrocartilage that contains some elastic fibers.

Growth Plate Cartilage: A highly organized tissue that produces bone by endochondral ossification. It is found at the ends of the epiphysis and the physeal plate in growing bones. See **Physeal Plate**.

Hyaline Cartilage: Any cartilage that has a smooth and homogeneous appearance on gross examination or by light microscopy. The chondromucoid ground substance tends to obscure the actual fibrillar structure of the matrix.

Cartilage Hair Dysplasia (kar′ti-lij/hār/dis-pla′sē-ah) (n.)   A type of metaphyseal chondro-osseous dysplasia. It is possibly noted at birth, inherited as an autosomal recessive trait, and presents as a short-limbed stunting of growth. Also known as **Metaphyseal Chondrodysplasia, McKusick Type**.

Cartilaginous (kar″ti-laj′i-nus) (adj.)   Consisting of or pertaining to cartilage.

Cartilaginous Joint (kar″ti-laj′i-nus/joint) (n.)   A joint in which the bones are united by cartilage, providing only slight flexible movements. This includes symphysis and synchondrosis.

Cartwheel Fracture (kart′hwēl/frak′chur) (n.)   A fracture of the distal femoral epiphysis.

Caseation (ka″sē-a′shun) (n.)   The breakdown and necrosis of diseased tissue into a dry, amorphous, cheeselike mass. This type of coagulation necrosis is seen mostly in tuberculosis.

Cassette (kah-set) (n.)   In radiology, a thin, light-proof housing, in which a piece of x-ray film is placed for the taking of a radiograph. The tube side is composed of a radiolucent substance; the back side contains a thin lead sheet. The back is hinged and fits into the tube side, sealing out all light. Two intensifying screens are mounted inside, one on each side, between which the film is sandwiched. Cassettes come in various sizes.

Cast (kast) (n.)   A rigid circular dressing or casing used to encase or immobilize body parts. It functions to support and immobilize a part in optimal position until healing takes place. To be effective, a cast usually covers the joints above and below the affected area. In the past, casts were typically made of plaster-of-Paris. Currently, casts are also fabricated from various synthetic materials. See specific types of casts.

Cast Bender (kast/bend′er) (n.)   A heavy, forceps-type instrument used to bend a small portion of the edge of a cast away from an area to prevent impingement and allow freer movement.

Cast Boot (kast/bo͞ot) (n.)   A substitute for a shoe or heel that fits over the end of a lower-extremity cast. It is usually made of rubber and canvas.

Cast Brace (kast-brās) (n.)   A fracture orthosis that is intended to provide immobility for the fractured bone while permitting functional rehabilitation of the neighboring joint through the use of hinged joints incorporated into the cast.

Originally, these were described for use in supracondylar femur fractures to allow early ambulation, continued immobilization of the fracture, and early mobilization of the knee joint after the fracture became "sticky" with an initial period of traction. This lower extremity cast brace was composed of a thigh cuff molded into a quadrilateral socket, a short-leg walking cast, and a set of polycentric hinges connecting these across the knee. Currently, similar cast braces are applied to the upper extremity or across the ankle joint. There are also many commercially available prefabricated hinged cast braces. May be referred to as **Hinged Cast Brace**.

Cast Cutter (kast/kut′er) (n.)   See **Cast Saw**.

Cast Saw (kast/saw) (n.)   An electrically powered vibrating saw used to cut through plaster or synthetic casts. Referred to commonly as a **Cast Cutter**.

Cast Spreader (kast/spred′er) (n.)   A long-handled metal apparatus with short thin jaws; the jaws are inserted in the cutting line to pry open a cast for removal.

Cast Syndrome (kast/sin′drōm) (n.)   Acute obstruc-

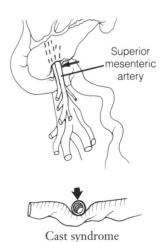

Cast syndrome

tion of the third portion of the duodenum, resulting from constriction of the superior mesenteric vessels following the application of a body cast. Symptoms include vomiting, which may be pernicious or projectile, abdominal distention, and pain. It may result in potentially dangerous fluid and electrolyte imbalances. Also known as **Superior Mesenteric Artery Syndrome**, **Body Cast Syndrome**.

CAT   Abbreviation for computerized axial tomography.

CAT Scan (kat/skan) (n.)   An acronym for the images produced by computerized axial tomography.

Catecholamines (kat″e-kol′ah-mēnz) (n.)   A group of physiologically important sympathomimetic substances, including epinephrine, norepinephrine, and dopamine. They have different roles, mainly as neurotransmitters, in the functioning of the sympathetic and central nervous systems.

Catheter (kath′e-ter) (n.)   A tube for insertion into body channels and spaces so that fluids may be introduced or removed.

Catheterization (kath″e-ter-i-zā′shun) (n.)   The introduction of a catheter into a body channel or cavity.

Cation (kat′ī-on) (n.)   A positively charged ion that migrates toward the negative electrode or cathode in an electric field. Contrast **Anion**.

Catterall Classification (kat-er-al/klas″sĭ-fĭ-ka′shun) (n.)   A prognostic classification of Legg-Calvé-Perthes disease based on the degree of involvement of the femoral head.

Group I: Less than 25 percent of the femoral head is involved, with avascularity of only the anterior portion of the epiphysis. No collapse occurs.

Group II: As much as 50 percent of the head is involved. The anterior portion of the femoral head is sequestrated, but this portion is between medial and lateral pillars of uninvolved, viable bone so that regeneration may occur without much loss of epiphyseal height.

Group III: As much as 75 percent of the femoral head is

involved and there is collapse of the head. The metaphysis and the physes are also usually involved.

Group IV: The entire proximal femoral epiphysis is involved.

Cauda Equina (kaw′dah/ē′kwīn-ah) (n.)   The terminal portion of the roots of the spinal nerves and spinal cord below the first lumbar nerve. It is named by the Latin for **Horse's Tail**, which it resembles.

Cauda Equina Syndrome (kaw′dah/ē-kwīn′-ah/ sin′drōm) (n.)   The clinical result of compression due to extrinsic pressure on the caudal sac. It usually results from a large, centrally herniated disc. Signs and symptoms include low back pain, bilateral lower extremity weakness, bilateral radiculopathy, saddle anesthesia, and bowel and bladder incontinence. The diagnosis is confirmed by myelography. Treatment requires prompt surgical decompression. Synonym: **Pseudo-intermittent Claudication**.

Caudad (kaw′dad) (adj.)   Toward the tail or inferior point of reference. Opposite of **Cephalad**.

Caudal Anesthesia (kaw′dal/an″es-thē′ze-ah) (n.)   Anesthesia induced by injection of a local anesthetic agent into the sacral canal at the level of the cauda equina.

Causalgia (kaw-zal′jē-ah) (n.)   1. Sustained burning pain after a peripheral nerve injury. 2. An intense and unpleasant burning pain that may be associated with trophic skin changes in the affected part of the body. The pain may be aggravated by the slightest stimuli (light touch, pressure, and movement), or it may be intensified by the emotions.

Cauterization (kaw″ter-i-zā′shun) (n.)   Destruction of tissue with a cautery.

Cauterize (kaw′ter-īz) (v.)   To destroy tissues by direct application of a heated instrument or electrical current.

Cautery (kaw′ter-ē) (n.)   The application of a caustic agent, an electric current, or other agent to destroy tissue.

Cavernous Hemangioma (kav′er-nus/hē-man″jē-

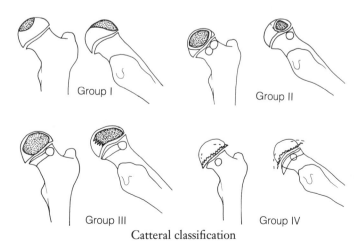

Catteral classification

ō′mah) (n.) A tumor of newly formed capillaries consisting of widely dilated, thickened vessels. These can occur in skeletal muscle or other soft tissues of the extremities. Surgical excision is usually curative.

Cavity (kav′i-tē) (n.) A hollow or space, or a potential space, within the body or a body organ.

Cavus (kāv′us) (n.) An increase in the height of the longitudinal arch of the foot. It gives the appearance of an equinus deformity of the forepart of the foot in relation to the hindfoot.

CDH Abbreviation for Congenital Dislocation or Dysplasia of the Hip. DDH, **Developmental Dysplasia of the Hip** is the preferred term.

C/E Angle (c-e/ang′g′l) (n.) Abbreviation for Center-Edge Angle.

C-E Angle of Wiberg (c-e/ang′g′l/of/wī-berg) (n.) A roentgenographic assessment of the width of the roof of the acetabulum in relation to the center of the femoral head. This is assessed on an AP radiograph of the pelvis.

Using the center of the femoral head, C, and the edge of the acetabulum, E, as reference points, draw a line between the points. Then draw a perpendicular to a horizontal line connecting the two femoral head centers from the center, C. The C-E angle is the angle subtended by these two lines, and is normally greater than 20°. If it is less than 20°, normal seating of the femoral head in the acetabulum is unlikely. Synonym: **Center-Edge Angle of Wiberg.**

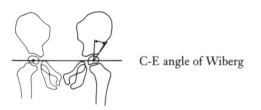

C-E angle of Wiberg

Cell (sel) (n.) The structural unit of protoplasm, composed of cytoplasm and one or more nuclei and surrounded by a plasma membrane. In plants, there is a cell wall outside the membrane.

Cell Membrane (sel/mem′brān) (n.) The outermost membrane of most animal cells. Also known as the **Plasma Membrane.**

Cellulitis (sel″u-li′tis) (n.) A diffuse inflammatory process of the connective tissue between adjacent tissues and organs.

Cement (se-ment′) (n.) 1. Any plastic material capable of becoming hard and binding together objects that are contiguous to it. 2. Commonly used shortened reference to polymethylmethacrylate, or bone cement.

Cement Gun (se-ment′/gun) (n.) An apparatus used for the introduction of low and medium viscosity bone cement.

Center-Edge Angle (sen′ter-ej/ang′g′l) (n.) See **C-E Angle of Wiberg.**

Center of Gravity (sen′ter/of/grav′i-tē) (n.) The central point of a body's mass. Also known as **center of mass.** The center in humans is 2 cm in front of the sacrum.

Centimeter (sen′ti-mē″ter) (n.) One-hundredth of a meter, approximately 0.3937 inch. Abbreviated **cm.**

Central Cord Syndrome (sen′tral/kord/sin′drōm) (n.) The most common incomplete spinal cord syndrome, consisting of gray matter destruction and central spinothalamic and pyramidal tract destruction. The prognosis is variable, but more than 50 percent of patients will have return of bowel and bladder control, become ambulatory, and show improved hand function. In this syndrome, upper extremity involvement is greater than that of the lower extremities. It usually results from hyperextension of the cervical spine in a patient with preexisting osteoarthritis.

Central Core Disease (sen′tral/kōr/di-zēz′) (n.) A form of congenital myopathy that presents in infancy. The lower extremities are more involved than the upper extremities, and the myopathy is generally nonprogressive. Diagnosis is based on muscle biopsy evaluation. Patients frequently improve with maturity.

Central Fracture Dislocation (sen′tral/frak′chur/dis″lō-kā′shun) (n.) Any intra-articular fracture with simultaneous displacement of the opposing articular surface into this central fracture. Most often seen in the hip joint with a central fracture of the acetabulum and dislocation of the femoral head into the defect.

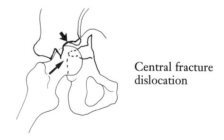

Central fracture dislocation

Central Nervous System (sen′tral/ner′vus/sis′tem) (n.) That part of the nervous system that is condensed and centrally located, e.g., the brain and spinal cord. Abbreviated **CNS.**

Central Pain (sen′tral/pān) (n.) Any pain associated with a lesion of the central nervous system.

Central Paralysis (sen′tral/pah-ral′i-sis) (n.) Any paralysis due to a lesion of the brain or spinal cord, i.e., within the central nervous system.

Central Ray (sen′tral/ra) (n.) 1. The center of a beam of x-rays emitted from an x-ray tube. 2. The middle digit and its associated metacarpal or metatarsal bone in the hand or foot.

Central Venous Catheter (sen′tral/vē′nus/kath′e-ter) (n.) A long intravenous catheter that is inserted either peripherally through an antebrachial vein, or centrally through the internal jugular or subclavian vein, whose tip is in or near the right atrium. These catheters are used as access routes for the administration of parenteral fluids through a large blood vessel and for the measurement of central venous pressure.

Central Venous Pressure (sen′tral/vē′nus/presh′ur) (n.) A measurement of ventricular end-diastolic pressure assessed with a central venous catheter-transducer system. Normally, it measures 5 to 12 cm of water. Abbreviated as **CVP.**

Centrifuge (sen′tri-fūj) (n.) An apparatus that uses centrifugal force to separate or remove particulate matter suspended in a liquid.

Cephalad (sef′ah-lad) (adv.) In a direction toward the head or most superior point of reference. Opposite of caudad.

Cephalic (se-fal′ik) (adv.) Situated toward the head or superior point of reference; opposite of caudal.

Cephalic Index (se-fal′ik/in′deks) (n.) The ratio of the breadth to the length of the skull multiplied by 100. For the **mesocephalic skull,** the index is 76.0 to 80.9; for the **brachycephalic skull,** 81.0 or more; and for the **dolichocephalic skull,** 95.9 or less.

Cephalosporin (sef″ah-lo-spōr′in) (n.) Any one of a group of semisynthetic antibiotics, derived from the natural antibiotic cephalosporin that contains a six-membered dihydrothiazine ring fused to the beta-lactam ring. These are broad-spectrum antibiotics whose first, second, and third generation derivatives have a sequentially increased spectrum of effectiveness.

Ceramics (se-ram′iks) (n.) Substances made of aluminum oxide and vitreous carbon. They have been used in arthroplasty and as a porous coating for the ingrowth of tissue. Ceramic components with highly polished surfaces are chemically inert and therefore well tolerated by the body, have a low coefficient of friction, and high resistance to wear. However, ceramic components are brittle, have a low tensile strength, and a high modulus of elasticity. Combinations of ceramic on ultra-high molecular weight polyethylene, ceramic on ceramic, and ceramic on metal have been used for implants.

Cerclage (ser′klaj) (n.) Encircling of a part with a ring or loop of wire to affix the adjacent ends of a fractured bone.

Cerclage Wire (ser′klaj/wīr) (n.) A wire or cable used to perform cerclage fixation.

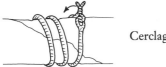

Cerclage wiring

Cerclage Wiring (ser′klaj/wīr′ing) (n.) A surgical technique in which circumferential wires or bands are placed around a bone.

Cerebellar Gait (ser″ĕ-bel′ar/gāt) (n.) An uncoordinated gait due to cerebellar degeneration. This gait manifests as an abnormal stance and an unsteady gait that is wavering and lurching in character.

Cerebral Concussion (ser′e-bral/kon-kush′un) (n.) An injury to the brain due to a blow or violent shaking. The resultant clinical syndrome is characterized by immediate and transient impairment of brain function, such as alteration of consciousness and disturbances of vision and equilibrium.

Cerebral Palsy (ser′e-bral/pawl′zē) (n.) A nonprogressive disorder that results from a static injury to the developing brain, producing permanent abnormalities in posture and movement. The insult may occur during gestation, perinatally, or postnatally. The association with mental retardation is high. The disorder may be classified by the geographic distribution of weakness, e.g., hemiplegia, diplegia, or it may be described by physiologic type.

Cerebrospinal Fluid (ser″ĕ-bro-spi′nal/floo′id) (n.) The clear fluid within the arachnoid space surrounding the brain and spinal cord. Cerebrospinal fluid circulates in the ventricles of the brain and in the central canal of the spinal cord. The total volume of the spinal fluid in the normal adult is about 150 mL. Abbreviated **CSF.**

Cerebrovascular Accident (ser″e-brō-vas′kū-lar/ak′si-dent) (n.) An interruption of blood flow to the brain resulting in cerebral damage. More commonly known as a stroke, it can result from an embolism, a thrombus, or a hemorrhage.

Certificate of Need (ser-tif′i-kit/of/nēd) (n.) A certificate of approval, usually issued by a state health planning agency to health care facilities that propose to construct or modify a health care facility, incur a major capital expenditure, or offer a new or different health service.

Cervical (ser′vĭ-kal) (adj.) Of or pertaining to the neck.

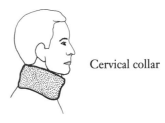

Cervical collar

Cervical Collar (ser′vĭ-kal/kol′ler) (n.) A basic type of cervical orthosis that wraps around the neck and is adjustable circumferentially. It can be soft (fabricated from polyethylene foam, rubber, and felt) or hard (fabricated from light polyethylene or other plastic). See **Soft Cervical Collar**.

Cervical Curve (ser'vĭ-kal/kurv) (n.)   Spinal curvature with an apex from C1 to C6. See **Cervical Scoliosis**.

Cervical Orthosis (ser'vĭ-kal/or-thō'sis) (n.)   A device prescribed for the neck intended to control and restrict head and neck motions and to reduce the load on the cervical spine by supporting some of the weight of the head. These devices are categorized as skin-contact, or soft-tissue, devices and bony-contact, or skeletal, devices. The soft-tissue devices may be collars or post appliances. The skeletal devices may be of the halo or tong type.

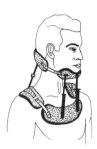

Cervical orthosis

Cervical Plexus (ser'vĭ-kal/plek'sus) (n.)   A network of nerve fibers supplying structures in the region of the neck. The cervical plexus is formed by the ventral rami of the first four cervical spinal nerves.

Cervical Rib (ser'vĭ-kal/rib) (n.)   A supernumerary rib arising from the seventh cervical vertebra. Typically, cervical ribs originate from the transverse process of the seventh cervical vertebra and attach directly or by ligaments to the first rib. They are usually unilateral. This is the most common congenital bony anomaly associated with the thoracic outlet syndrome, although fewer than 10 percent of these patients will have symptoms.

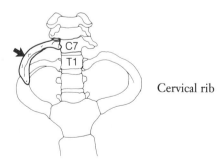

Cervical rib

Cervical Scoliosis (ser'vĭ-kal/skō"le-ō'sis) (n.)   Scoliosis having its apex between C1 and C6.

Cervical Spine (ser'vĭ-kal/spīn) (n.)   That portion of the vertebral column contained in the neck, consisting of seven cervical vertebrae.

Cervical Spondylosis (ser'vĭ-kal/spon"di-lō'sis) (n.)   Degenerative disease of the intervertebral discs and the zygapophyseal joints, occurring in the cervical spine.

Cervical Traction (ser'vĭ-kal/trak'shun) (n.)   Any type of traction, skin or skeletal, that applies distraction forces across the cervical spine. Skin traction, generally applied with a halter-like sling, is used in the treatment of painful muscular conditions or cervical nerve root irritation conditions. Skeletal traction is used to reduce and maintain positioning of cervical spine fractures, subluxations, and dislocations.

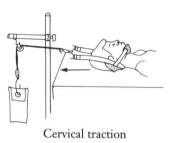

Cervical traction

Cervical Vertebrae (ser'vĭ-kal/ver'tĕ-bre) (n.)   The upper seven vertebrae that form the skeleton of the neck.

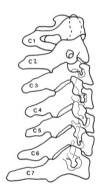

Cervical vertebrae

Cervico-Obturator Line (ser"vi-ko-ob'too-ra"tor/līn) (n.)   See **Shenton's Line**.

Cervicothoracic Curve (ser'vĭ-ko-tho-ras'ik/kurv) (n.)   Spinal curvature with an apex at C7 or T1.

Cervicothoracic Ganglion (ser'vi-kō-tho-ras'ik/gang'glē-on) (n.)   A ganglion on the sympathetic trunk anterior to the lowest cervical or the first thoracic vertebra, formed by a union of the seventh and eighth cervical and first thoracic ganglia. See **Stellate Ganglion**.

Chaddock's Sign (chad'oks/sīn) (n.)   A pyramidal tract sign elicited by stimulating the lateral aspect of the foot with a blunt object, such as a key, in a circular direction under and around the lateral malleolus. In a positive response, there is dorsiflexion of the great toe and fanning of the other toes. See related term, **Babinski Sign.**

Chairback Brace (chār'bak/brās) (n.)   See **Knight Brace.**

Chamberlain's Line (chām-ber-linz/līn) (n.)   A line used to assess basilar impression. On a true lateral radiograph of the skull, draw a line from the posterior margin of the hard palate to the posterior margin of the foramen magnum. This line will normally lie just above the odontoid process.

Chance Fracture (chans/frak'chur) (n.)   A fracture in the horizontal plane of the neural arch and vertebral body produced by acute spinal flexion, or distraction, over a fulcrum anterior to the spine. A horizontal splitting through both the vertebral body and posterior elements. Diagnosis is made radiographically by the characteristic appearance of the lesion, usually occurring in the upper two or three lumbar vertebra. Attention focused on the AP view of the lumbar spine will reveal the ovoid and tear-shaped appearance of the pedicles and spinous processes, respectively.

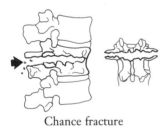

Chance fracture

Chandler Disease (chand'lėr/dĭ-zēz') (n.)   Idiopathic aseptic necrosis of the femoral head. Synonyms: **Femoral Head Idiopathic Necrosis, Osteochondritis Dissecans of the Hip.**

Chapple's Sign (chap-lz/sīn) (n.)   A radiologic sign of hip dislocation in newborns. There is blurring of the acetabular margin, a widened space between the femur and the acetabulum, alignment of the femur with a point lateral to the socket instead of the socket itself, and an iliac flare smaller than its normal counterpart.

Chapple Test (chap-l/test) (n.)   A method of evaluating congenital dislocation of the hip. With the infant supine, abduct the flexed thigh. The test is positive if it is not possible to abduct more than 45° from the perpendicular of the median raphe.

Charcot Joint (shar-kō/joint) (n.)   A rapidly progressive degeneration of a joint characterized by degeneration of the cartilage with formation of spurs and debris, bone fragmentation, spontaneous subluxation, or dislocation and swelling. Also known as **Neuropathic Joint.** This condition occurs as an abnormal response to trauma with decreased or absent sensation in the injured limb. Since a normal pain response to trauma does not occur, the patient continues to stress the affected area, with resultant destructive changes that produce permanent deformity and instability. Charcot joints have been described in association with tabes dorsalis, diabetes mellitus, syringomyelia, leprosy, peripheral nerve lesions, and congenital indifference to pain syndromes. Also known as **Charcot Arthropathy, Neuropathic Joint,** and **Neuropathic Arthropathy.**

Charcot-Marie Tooth Disease (shar-ko'-ma-rē/tōōth/di-zēz') (n.)   A form of hereditary motor and sensory neuropathy. See **Peroneal Muscular Atrophy.**

Charge-Covered (charj/kuv'erd) (n.)   The charge for services provided to an insured patient that is payable by a third party.

Charge-Daily Service (charj-dā'lē/ser'vis) (n.)   Dollar amount charged by a hospital for a day's stay in an inpatient care unit.

Charley-Horse (char'le-hors) (n.)   1. A colloquial term referring to a soreness, cramping, and stiffness of a muscle, especially the quadriceps, due to overstrain, contusion, or injury. 2. An intramuscular hemorrhage resulting from a direct blow to a muscle.

Charnley Arthrodesis (charn'-lē/ar"thro-dē'sis) (n.)   A technique for intra-articular fusion of a joint, using a temporary external fixation apparatus. Also referred to as **Compression Arthrodesis.**

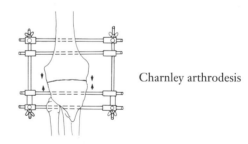

Charnley arthrodesis

Charnley Clamps (charn'-lē/klampz) (n.)   A simple external fixation frame used for stabilization of ankle and knee arthrodeses and certain fractures. Parallel pins are placed through the bones and connected on either side of the extremity by a rod and screw assembly. Tightening of the screws and clamps results in compression across the affixed bones or joint to be fused.

Charnley Low Friction Arthroplasty (charn'-lē/lō/frik-shun/ar'thrō-pla-stē) (n.)   The classic procedure for arthroplasty of the hip joint, combining a 22-mm femoral head and a high-density polyethylene acetabular cup. Commonly known as a **Charnley Total Hip Prosthesis.** Abbreviated as **LFA.**

Charnley Prosthesis (charn'-lē/pros-the'sis) (n.)

The classic standard for a cemented total hip arthroplasty.

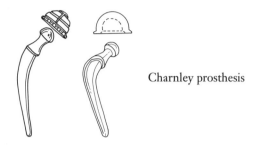

Charnley prosthesis

Charnley Retractor (charn'-lē/re-trak'tor) (n.) A large, U-shaped, self-retaining surgical retractor. Designed originally for maintaining exposure during total hip arthroplasty but useful in various surgical procedures.

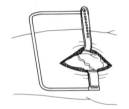

Charnley retractor

Chassaignac's Tubercle (shahs-ān-yaks/too'ber-k'l) (n.) The anterior tubercle on the transverse process of the sixth cervical vertebra.

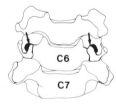

Chassaignac's tubercle

Chauffeur's Fracture (shō'ferz/frak'chur) (n.) A common name for a fracture of the radial styloid. Also called **Backfire Fracture, Truck Drivers' Fracture,** or **Lorry Drivers' Fracture**.

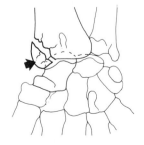

Chauffeur's fracture

Cheilectomy (kī-lek'to-mē) (n.) The surgical excision of bony protuberances from the edges of an articular surface that interfere with joint motion.

Cheilotomy (kī-lot'o-mē) (n.) Surgical procedure by which spurs, osteophytes, and bones are removed from the periarticular region.

Cheiralgia Paresthetica (kī-ral'jē-ah/par"as-the'tika) (n.) An isolated neuritis of the superficial radial nerve.

Chemonucleolysis (kē"mō-nū"klē-ōl'i-sis) (n.) The dissolution of extruded nucleus pulposus by injection of a proteolytic enzyme, such as chymopapain or collagenase. The enzyme dissolves the mucopolysaccharides of the nucleus, reduces its size, and decreases the water content, thereby lessening the pressure in the disc and decreasing its influence on the nerve root. See **Chymopapain**.

Chemoreceptor (kē"mō-rē-sep'tor) (n.) A receptor that detects substances according to their chemical structure. This includes smell and taste receptors.

Chemotaxis (kē"mo-tak'sis) (n.) A positive directional response to a chemical stimulus.

Chemotherapy (kē"mo-ther'ah-pē) (n.) The treatment of disease by the use of chemical substances or drugs.

Chevron Osteotomy (shev'ron/os"te-ot'ō-mē) (n.) 1. Any V-shaped osteotomy. 2. A V-shaped osteotomy in the coronal space of the first metatarsal head used to correct hallux valgus deformity. The advantages of this osteotomy are its inherent stability, the maintenance of length of the metatarsal, and its traversal of cancellous bone.

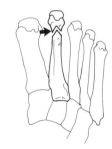

Chevron osteotomy

Chiari Shelf Procedure (kē-ar'ē/shelf/pro'sē'jur) (n.) An extra-articular osteotomy of the innominate bone at the upper margin of the acetabulum with medial displacement of the hip joint along with the femur. It is useful in those cases of congenital dysplasia of the hip in which the femoral head will not center on abduction due to a major abnormality of the acetabulum. The proximal segment of the osteotomy serves as an acetabular roof, with the capsule interposed between it and the femoral head, thus creating an arthroplasty. The procedure consists of the construction of a congruent shelf above the intact hip joint without bone grafting.

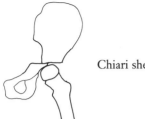

Chiari shelf procedure

Chicago Test (shi-ka′-gō/test) (n.) A clinical test used in differentiation of disc disease and back strain. The patient kneels on a chair and is asked to touch the floor with outstretched hands. Assist by applying pressure over the heels. With disc disease, the patient should be able to perform this test without pain. With back strain, he either will not be able to perform the test or will have considerable pain. Also called **Burn's Bench Test** and **Bench Test**.

Chief of Service (chēf/of/ser′vis) (n.) Member of a hospital medical staff who is elected or appointed to serve as the medical and administrative head of a clinical department.

Chief of Staff (chēf/of/staf) (n.) Member of a hospital medical staff who is elected, appointed, or employed by the hospital and who serves as the medical and administrative head of the medical staff.

Chiene's Line (shēnz/līn) (n.) A line used in evaluation of a femoral neck fracture. The level of the greater trochanter on one side may be compared with that of the other side by drawing two lines: one between the anterior superior spines; the other between the greater trochanter summits. Normally they are parallel.

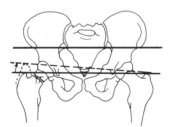

Chiene's line

Child Abuse (chīld/ah-būs′) (n.) A condition in which physical abuse, emotional or physical neglect, and/or psychologic or sexual abuse is inflicted on a child by any person.

Childress' Duck Waddle Test (child-res/duk/ wad′d′l/test) (n.) A clinical test used to evaluate knee meniscal lesions. Have the patient assume a squatting position and then waddle back and forth across the floor, moving from side to side before rising. A positive sign is indicated by clicking at the posteromedial aspect of the joint, usually accompa-

nied by localized pain. This snapping is fairly constant and is produced in the last 10 to 20° of flexion during the early phase of extension from the fully flexed position. A negative reaction may eliminate the possibility that a posterior medial meniscal lesion is present. Also called **Duck Waddle Test**.

Chin-to-Chest Distance (chin/to/chest/dis′tans) (n.) A measure of cervical spine flexibility. While nodding the head, the patient brings the chin down. Normally, it is possible to touch the chin to the sternum. If the patient is unable to do this, the distance between the sternum and the chin should be measured to the nearest 0.1 cm.

Chinese Fingertraps (chī′nēz/fin′ger-traps) (n.) See **Fingertraps**.

Chip Fracture (chip/frak′chur) (n.) A type of small, avulsion fracture in which only a fragment or a piece of the cortex has been separated from the main body of the bone by forcible tearing of the ligament, tendons, or muscle attachments. Also called **Corner Fracture**.

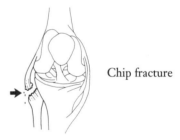

Chip fracture

Chiropodist (kī-rop′ō-dist) (n.) Podiatrist.

Chiropractor (kī″rō-prak′tor) (n.) Person qualified in chiropractic and licensed by the state to treat disease primarily by adjustment of the spinal column or mechanical therapeutics.

Chisel (chis″l) (n.) A single-bladed, bevelled on one side, surgical instrument used for cutting and contouring bone. Compare **Osteotome**.

Chisel Fracture (chis″l/frak′chur) (n.) Common name for an incomplete fracture of the medial portion of the radial head, with the fracture line extending distally about 1 cm.

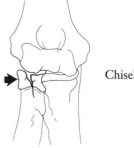

Chisel fracture

Chloramphenicol (klo″ram-fēn-i-kol) (n.) A broad-spectrum antibiotic, available for oral use and by injection, with an antimicrobial activity similar to the tetracyclines. Not commonly used.

Cholecalciferol (kō″le-kal-sif′er-ol) (n.) Vitamin D$_3$.

Chondral (kon′dral) (adj.) Of or pertaining to cartilage.

Chondralgia (kon-dral′je-ah) (n.) Pain in a cartilage. Also known as **Chondrodynia**.

Chondritis (kon-drī′tis) (n.) Inflammation of a cartilage.

Chondro (kon′dro) (n.) Prefix referring to cartilage.

Chondroblast (kon′drō-blast) (n.) An immature cartilage cell, found in growing cartilage, that synthesizes and deports extracellular matrix.

Chondroblastoma (kon″drō-blas-tō′mah) (n.) A benign, cartilaginous tumor that occurs in the epiphysis of long bones, usually presenting in the second decade of life. The most common sites for this tumor are the proximal tibia, proximal and distal femur, and proximal humerus. The symptoms are usually pain and swelling about the adjacent joint, frequently of several months' duration. The roentgenographic appearance is characteristic: there is an eccentric, lucent lesion in the epiphysis with a sclerotic margin and mottled calcifications. Histologically, the tumor consists of rounded or polyhedral cells with large nuclei. Irregular islands of chondroid tissue are present in the intercellular ground substance, with focal areas of calcification. Multinucleated giant cells are commonly present. Diagnosis is confirmed by biopsy. The treatment of choice is either curettage or local excision. Rarely, lung metastases have been reported. Also known as **Benign Chondroblastoma** and **Codman's Tumor**.

Chondrocalcinosis (kon″drō-kal″si-nō′sis) (n.) The radiographic or histologic evidence of cartilage calcification. The term is often used synonymously with **calcium pyrophosphate dihydrate (CPPD)** crystal deposition disease because pyrophosphate crystals are by far the most common form of calcium salts found. Cartilage calcification is also seen in association with gout, rheumatoid arthritis, osteoarthritis, ochronosis, hemachromatosis, and oxalosis. Depending on the underlying cause, the calcification forms within articular hyaline cartilage or meniscal fibrocartilage. Radiographically, this calcification can be linear, speckled, faint, or consolidated. Also called **Pseudogout**.

Chondroclasis (kon′drō-klā-sis) (n.) The resorption or crushing of cartilage.

Chondroclast (kon′drō-klast) (n.) A giant cell implicated in the resorption of cartilage.

Chondrocostal (kon″drō-kōs′tal) (adj.) Of or pertaining to the ribs and costal cartilages.

Chondrocyte (kon′drō-sīt) (n.) A mature cartilage cell that occupies a lacuna within the extracellular matrix.

Chondrodynia (kon″dro-dīn′e-ah) (n.) See **Chondralgia**.

Chondrodysplasia (kon″dro-dis-plā′ze-ah) (n.) An hereditary disorder of cartilage formation. See **Chondrodystrophy**.

Chondrodysplasia Fetalis (kon″drō-dis-plā′ze-ah/fe′tal-is) (n.) See **Achondroplasia**.

Chondrodysplasia Punctata (kon″drō-dis-plā′ze-ah/pungk′ta-tah) (n.) An osteochondrodysplasia, present at birth, that results in short-limbed, disproportionate dwarfism. It is usually inherited as an autosomal dominant trait, but there is a type with a poor prognosis that is an autosomal recessive trait. This disorder primarily affects the epiphyses. Radiographically, the ossification centers appear stippled or punctate. The epiphyses become confluent when ossification is completed, but there is usually limb length inequality and marked irregularity of joint surfaces, leading to early arthritis. Commonly known as **Stippled Epiphysis Disease**. Also known as **Conradi-Hunerman Disease**, **Chondrodystrophia Calcificans**, and **Punctate Epiphyseal Dysplasia**.

Chondrodystrophia Fetalis (kon″drō-dis-trō′fē-ah/fē′tal-is) (n.) See **Achondroplasia**.

Chondrodystrophic Dwarfism (kon″drō-dis-trō′fik/dwarf′izm) (n.) See **Achondroplasia**.

Chondrodystrophy (kon″drō-dis′trō-fē) (n.) Any of a heterogeneous group of disorders due to defective cartilage formation that results in disproportionately short stature. Synonym: **Osteochondrodysplasia**. See also specific diseases.

Chondroectodermal Dysplasia (kon″drō-ek′tō-derm′al/dis-plā′se-ah) (n.) A rare disorder of cartilaginous bone growth. It is transmitted by autosomal recessive inheritance that is manifested at birth and results in short-limbed, disproportionate dwarfism. Usually associated with polydactyly, hypoplasia of the teeth, nails, and hair, and congenital heart disease. There is mesomelic shortening of the extremities, and often deformities and shortening of the feet. Also known as **Ellis-van Crevald Syndrome**.

Chondroepiphysitis (kon″dro-ep″i-fiz′ī′tis) (n.) Inflammation of the epiphyseal cartilages.

Chondrogenesis (kon″drō-jen′e-sis) (n.) Formation of cartilage.

Chondroid (kon′droid) (adj.) Resembling or pertaining to cartilage.

Chondroitin Sulfate (kon-drō′i-tin/sul′fāt) (n.) One of the glycosaminoglycans, or sulfated mucopolysaccharides. These are an important constituent of cartilage, bone, and other connective tissues, and contribute to the formation of proteoglycans. Composed of repeating units of glucuronic acid and N-acetyl-D-galactosamine.

Chondrolysis (kon-drol′i-sis) (n.) 1. Degeneration of cartilage cells, resulting in cell death. 2. A disorder that results from acute cartilage necrosis in the femoral head as a complication of a slipped capital femoral epiphysis. Clinically, patients present with pain and a decreased range of motion. Radiographically, there is periarticular osteopenia, rapid progressive narrowing of the joint space, and erosive changes in the subchondral bone. Early closure of the capital femoral and greater trochanteric epiphyses may occur. Factors contributing to the occurrence of chondrolysis include increased severity of the slip, degree of manipulation for reduction, extent of immobilization if casted, and pin penetration for internal fixation. However, chondrolysis has been seen prior to any treatment in some patients and also occurs more commonly in black patients.

Chondroma (kon-drō'mah) (n.)   1. A benign cartilage tumor. The central form of chondroma is more commonly known as **Enchondroma**. See **Enchondroma**; see also related term, **Juxtacortical Chondroma**. 2. A rare, slow growing, locally invasive neoplasm believed to arise from notochondral remnants. Most commonly found in the sacrococcygeal and spheno-occipital regions. Radiographically, these tumors are lucent with irregular margins and calcification. Histologically, the characteristic cell is physaliphorous, large, and vacuolated, with a soap-bubble appearance. The intracellular matrix is mucinous. These tumors are radiosensitive but, if possible, complete surgical resection is the treatment of choice.

Chondromalacia (kon″drō-mah-lā′she-ah) (n.)   A pathologic state of softening with subsequent fibrillation, fissuring, and erosion of articular cartilage.

The pathoanatomic changes may be classified as follows:

Group I: There is swelling and softening of the articular cartilage but the surface remains intact. Also known as **Closed Chondromalacia**.

Group II: There is fissuring in the softened areas.

Group III: There is fibrillation or fasciculation of the articular cartilage.

Group IV: There is complete erosion of articular cartilage, with exposed subchondral bone.

Chondromalacia Patella (kon″drō-mah-lā′she-ah/pah-tel′ah) (n.)   Pathologic changes in the articular cartilage of the undersurface of the patella. Clinically, this may be associated with a syndrome of anterior knee pain in which the patient complains of persistent pain behind the patella, especially after sitting with knees flexed for a period of time or when the knee is loaded in a flexed position. The degree of clinical symptoms does not always correlate well with the extent of pathologic changes. Asymptomatic chondromalacia patella is often noted during arthroscopic examination.

Chondromatosis (kon″drō-mah-tō′sis) (n.)   1. Formation of multiple chondromas. See **Enchondromatosis**. 2. Shortened term for synovial chondromatosis. See **Synovial Chondromatosis**.

Chondromucin (kon″drō-mū′sin) (n.)   See **Chondromucoprotein**.

Chondromucoid (kon″drō-mū′koid) (n.)   See **Chondromucoprotein**.

Chondromucoprotein (kon″drō - mu″kō - prō′te - in) (n.)   A principal constituent of the ground substance of cartilage. It is a copolymer of a mucoprotein and chondroitin sulfate. Also known as **Chondromucoid** or **Chondromucin**.

Chondromyoma (kon″drō-mī-ō′mah) (n.)   A benign tumor with myxomatous and cartilaginous elements.

Chondromyxoid Fibroma (kon″drō-mik-soid/fi-brō′mah) (n.)   A benign tumor of bone that exhibits chondroid and myxoid features. It is usually discovered in patients in the second and third decades of life. The upper tibia and the femur are most commonly affected. Pain and local swelling are common symptoms, but complaints are generally mild.

Radiologically, the lesion usually appears as an eccentric, ovoid, radiolucent defect with a thin, well-defined, scalloped, sclerotic border. It is characteristically found at the end of the diaphysis of a long bone. Grossly, the tumor is usually firm, lobulated, and pearly-white, with small, scattered areas of yellow, gritty, calcified cartilage and hemorrhage. Microscopically, there is a lobulated pattern of sparsely cellular chondromyxoid tissue areas separated by cellular fibrous tissue septa. Also known as **Chondromyxoma**. Abbreviated **CMF**.

Chondromyxoma (kon″drō-mik-sō′mah) (n.)   See **Chondromyxoid Fibroma**.

Chondromyxosarcoma (kon″drō-mik″sō-sar-kō′mah) (n.)   A tumor whose parenchyma is composed of myxoid and cartilaginous elements.

Chondro-osteodystrophy (kon″drō-os″te-ō-dis′trō-fē) (n.)   See **Morquio Syndrome**.

Chondropathy (kon-drop′ah-thē) (n.)   Any disease of cartilage.

Chondroplasty (kon′drō-plas″tē) (n.)   Plastic or reparative surgery of cartilage.

Chondrosarcoma (kon″drō-sar-kō′mah) (n.)   A malignant tumor whose cells produce a cartilage matrix. This tumor most commonly occurs in adults. The most common sites are the femur, humerus, pelvis, scapula, and ribs. They may occur centrally, i.e., intramedullary, or peripherally, and may be primary or secondary in a pre-existing lesion. The patients usually have a prolonged history of pain and/or a mass. Radiologically, a radiolucent defect with calcifications. Grossly, these tumors are lobulated, grayish- or bluish-white, and with focal areas of calcification, mucoid degeneration, and necrosis. Microscopically, there are cartilaginous cells with increased cellularity and pleomorphism in comparison to benign tumors. The tumors are graded based on the degree of differentiation of cells, variation in nuclear size, number of mitoses, and multiple nuclei. Treatment and prognosis vary with the tumor grade.

Chopart's Amputation (shō-parz′/am″pu-tā′shun) (n.)   An amputation of the foot through the midtarsal joint.

grade in arabic numerals; 1–3 or, alternatively, 1–4

Chopart's Fracture-Dislocation (shō-parz'/frak' chur-dis"lo-kā'shun) (n.) A dislocation of the foot through the talonavicular and calcaneocuboid joints and the associated fractures.

Chopart's Joint (shō-parz'/joint) (n.) The midtarsal joint of the foot, consisting of the talonavicular and calcaneocuboid joints.

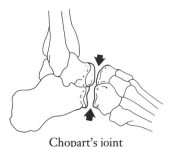

Chopart's joint

Chordoma (kor-do'mah) (n.) A locally aggressive tumor arising from remnants of the embryonal notocordal cells and large physaliphorous and small vacuolated cells. It occurs in the vertebral column, usually in the sacrum or the base of the skull.

Chrisman-Snook Procedure (chris-man/snook/pro-se'jur) (n.) A technique for the treatment of chronic lateral instability of the ankle, in which the anterior talofibular and calcaneofibular ligaments are reconstructed using half of the peroneus brevis tendon. Compare **Evans Procedure**.

Christie, Tables of (kris-tē/tā'b'lz) (n.) Tables of skeletal development in the neonate of the femoral head, neck, and trochanteric area.

Christmas Disease (kris'mas/di-zēz') (n.) Hemophilia B, an inherited factor IX deficiency, that has a sex-linked recessive mode of inheritance. See **Hemophilia B.**

Chromatin (krō'mah-tin) (n.) The darkly staining substance within the nucleus of most cells. It consists mainly of deoxyribonucleic acid combined with a basic protein.

Chromatography (krō"mah-tog'rah-fē) (n.) The process of separating chemical substances and particles of a mixture by their differential absorption to an insoluble matrix (e.g., paper) as the mixture is passed through the matrix.

Chromosome (krō'mō-sōm) (n.) A gene-containing filamentous structure in a cell nucleus. The number of chromosomes per cell nucleus is constant for each species. There are normally 46 chromosomes in a human cell.

Chromosome Abnormalities (krō'mō-sōm/ab"normal'i-tēz) (n.) Any addition or loss of genetic material sufficient to create a detectable abnormality by routine chromosome analysis. For example, any duplication of a chromosome resulting in trisomy.

Chronaxie (krō-nak'sē) (n.) 1. A value expressing sensitivity of nerve or muscle fibers to stimulation.

2. The duration of flow of a current twice the intensity of rheobase required to stimulate muscle contraction.

Chronic (kron'ik) (adj.) Of long duration. Opposite of **Acute**.

Chronic Fibrous Rheumatism (kron'ik/fī'brus/roo'mah-tizm) (n.) See **Jaccoud's Arthritis**.

Chronic Pain (kron'ik/pān) (n.) 1. A pain that either persists beyond the usual course of an acute disease or the expected time for an injury to heal, or that recurs and persists for months or years. 2. A pain that represents a useless, malevolent, and destructive force. Not a symptom of an underlying acute somatic injury, it must be considered a pathologic disorder in its own right. Tissue damage, often trivial at its inception, generally has healed and no longer serves as an underlying generator of pain. Frequently referred to as *chronic intractable pain* or *chronic benign pain*. Compare with **Acute Pain**.

Chronic Pain Patient (kron'ik/pān/pā-shent) (n.) A patient whose persistent pain is either resistant to indicated medical treatments and surgical procedures or is not associated with any clearly defined physiologic or anatomic disorders.

Chvostek's Sign (vos'/teks/sin) (n.) A clinical sign of tetany. Tap over the facial nerve just anterior to the ear. If positive, all the facial muscles supplied by the ipsilateral facial nerve will contract briskly.

Chymopapain (kī"mō-pah-pā'in) (n.) An enzyme used for chemonucleolysis.

Cicatrix (sik-ā'triks) (n.) The fibrous tissue that forms over and remains after the healing of a wound; commonly known as a scar.

Cidex (sī'deks) (n.) Proprietary name for activated glutaraldehyde, a liquid solution used for cold sterilization of surgical equipment, especially fiberoptic scopes.

Cincinnati Incision (sin-sin-at'-tē/in-sizh'un) (n.) A transverse foot incision that is extensible medially and laterally from the posterior aspect of the foot. It was described for use in a one-stage posteromedial release for clubfoot deformities.

Circoelectric Bed (serk-ō-elek-trik/bed) (n.) The proprietary name of an electrically operated frame in which the mattress may be turned around its transverse axis together with the patient it supports. This allows for positional and postural changes of an immobilized patient.

Circumduction Gait (ser"kum-duk'shun/gāt) (n.) Gait in which one lower limb is swung forward in a hemicircular fashion, with knee extended. It is characteristic of patients with spastic hemiplegia.

Circumferential Wiring (ser"kum-fer-en'shal/wīr'ing) (n.) A technique for internal fixation of fractures in which wire is threaded through the soft tissues around the bone at a point midway between the anterior and posterior surfaces and as close to the bone as possible. Used for fixation of patella fractures.

Citrobacter (sit″ro-bak′ter) (n.) Genus of gram-negative rods of the family *Enterobacteriaceae*. Seen as the causative agent in enteritis, septicemia, urinary tract infections, and burn wounds. *C. freundii* is the most common species.

Claims-Made Policy (klāmz/mād/pol′i-sē) (n.) A form of liability insurance that protects the insured against claims made against the insured for the limited period during which the policy is in effect.

Class (klas) (n.) In taxonomy, the category below the phylum and above the order. It therefore contains a group of related, similar orders.

Claudication (klaw″di-kā′shun) (n.) Limping due to muscle cramp or pain associated with activity or exertion. Usually implies intermittent claudication, which may be due to ischemia or neurologic impairment in the involved limb.

Clavicle (klav′ik′l) The collarbone. This bone forms the anterior aspect of the shoulder girdle. It articulates with the sternum medially and the acromion laterally.

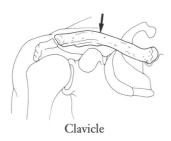

Clavicle

Clavus (klā′vus) (n.) A circumscribed, cone-shaped hyperkeratotic lesion of the skin. Also known as **Heloma** or **Corn**. **C. Dorum:** See hard corn. **C. Mollum:** See soft corn.

Claw Foot (klaw-fut) (n.) Common name for **Pes Cavus**.

Claw Hand (klaw-hand) (n.) A deformity of the hand that has a clawlike appearance. It results from paresis of the ulnar and/or median nerves, in which there is extension of the metacarpophalangeal joints and flexion of the interphalangeal joints, with associated flattening of the hand due to musculotendinous imbalance.

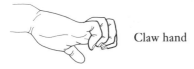

Claw hand

Claw Toes (klaw/tōz) (n.) A descriptive term for a foot deformity characterized by hyperextension of

the metatarsophalangeal joint and flexion of interphalangeal joints. This deformity may be fixed or flexible. Corns may appear on the dorsum of the proximal interphalangeal joint; frequently, an end corn may occur. Contrast with **Hammer and Mallet Toe**.

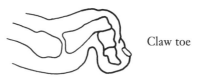

Claw toe

Clay-Shoveler's Fracture (klā/shuv′e-lerz/frak′chur) (n.) A familiar term for an avulsion fracture of a cervical spinous process, usually C-7. This results from avulsion by spine extensor and scapular elevator muscles. This fracture was seen in clay shovelers, in Australia, who would put sudden and great strain on their necks, thus the name. This fracture is also described in firemen who, in attempting to control whipping water hoses, have great stress placed suddenly on their necks. Synonym: **Schmitt-Weiser Syndrome**.

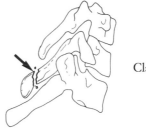

Clay-shoveler's fracture

Clean Area (klēn/a′re-ah) (n.) An area free of contaminants or pollutants.

Clean Technique (klēn/tek-nēk′) (n.) Medical asepsis.

Cleeman's Sign (klē′-munz/sīn) (n.) Creasing of the skin just above the patella. This clinical sign indicates that a fracture of the femur with overriding of the fragments has occurred.

Cleft Foot (kleft/fut) (n.) A congenital anomaly of the foot in which a single cleft extends proximally from the digits into the midfoot. The deformity varies in degree and type, but the first and fifth rays are usually present. Also known as **Lobster Foot** and **Partial Adactylia**.

Cleft Hand (kleft/hand) (n.) See **Lobster-Claw Hand**.

Cleidocranial Dysplasia (klī″do-krā′nē-al/dis-plā′se-ah) (n.) See **Cleidocranial Dysostosis**.

Cleidocranial Dysostosis (klī″dō-krā′ne-al/dis″os-tō′sis) (n.) An osteochondrodysplasia present at birth that results in a proportionate stunting of growth. It is transmitted as an autosomal dominant trait. Primarily involves defective bone formation of the calvarium and clavicles. At birth, the fontanelles are enlarged, and the cranial sutures widened. Occasionally, only isolated areas of the calvarium are calcified. The clavicles may be defective or entirely absent. Often, this occurs unilaterally. Usually, the lateral portion of the clavicle is absent. Defective mineralization of the pubis is also a frequent occurrence. Longevity is normal.

Cleland's Ligament (klē′-landz/lig′ah-ment) (n.)   A fibrous tissue band on the lateral side of the fingers that helps stabilize the skin during movement. This septum forms a common encircling sheath around the digital arteries and nerves; it then passes to the skin dorsal to the artery and nerve.

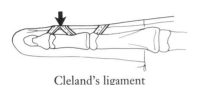

Cleland's ligament

Clinical Clerk (klin′ik′l/klerk) (n.)   Student of a medical or dental school who, as part of the school's curriculum, receives clinical experience by performing specific, supervised duties in a hospital.

Clinical Clerkship (klin′ik′l/klerk′ship) (n.)   Undergraduate clinical experience provided to a student of a hospital-affiliated medical or dental school as part of the school's curriculum.

Clinical Death (klin′ik′l/deth) (n.)   The absence of peripheral pulse, heartbeat, and effective circulation, with dilated pupils nonresponsive to light, and absence of breathing.

Clinical Evaluation (klin′ik′l/ē-val′yoo-ā′shun) (n.)   The collection of data by a health professional for the purpose of determining the health status of an individual. Data include patient history, clinical findings from a physical examination, laboratory tests (including radiographs, electrocardiograms, blood tests, and other special tests and diagnostic procedures), and measurements of anthropometric attributes and physiologic and psychophysiologic functions.

Clinical Laboratory (klin′ik′l/lab′o-rah-to″rē) (n.)   Laboratory for the examination of material derived from the human body by means of bacteriologic, biochemical, cytologic, hematologic, histologic, and serologic tests.

Clinoril (klī′nō-ril) (n.)   The proprietary name for Sulindac, a nonsteroidal anti-inflammatory drug.

Clipping Injury Fracture (klip′ing/in′ju-rē/frak′chur) (n.)   A fracture involving the distal femoral or proximal tibial epiphysis occurring in skeletally immature football players. In "clipping," impact is applied to the lateral surface of the knee while the foot is firmly planted.

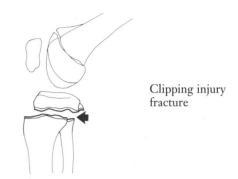

Clipping injury fracture

Clonus (klō′nus) (n.)   A characteristic movement often found in upper motor neuron disorders. It consists of rapid, repetitive, altered muscular contractions and relaxations. Clinically, clonus is elicited when muscles are suddenly stretched, resulting in alternate spasm and relaxation of agonist and antagonist muscles.

Closed Amputation (klōsd/am″pu-tā′shun) (n.)   Flap amputation in which flaps are made from skin and subcutaneous tissue and are sutured over the bone end of the stump.

Closed Anesthesia (klōsd/an″es-thē′ze-ah) (n.)   Anesthesia produced by the continuous rebreathing of a small amount of anesthetic gas in a closed system, with an apparatus removing carbon dioxide.

Closed Fracture (klōsd/frak′chur) (n.)   A fracture that does not communicate with the outside air. Formerly called a **simple fracture**.

Closed Reduction (klōsd/rē-duk′shun) (n.)   Manipulation or setting, without open surgical correction, of a fracture to bring the bony fragments into apposition and proper alignment.

Clostridium (klō-strid′ē-um) (n.)   Genus of anaerobic, spore-containing, gram-positive rods from the family of Bacillaceae. Clostridium usually decompose protein and/or form toxins. Those associated with causing human disease are described below.
  C. botulinum: The toxin of this species can contaminate food, resulting in botulism.
  C. tetani: This species' exotoxin results in tetanus.
  C. perfringens: Produces gas gangrene infections.
  C. welchii: Another name for *C. perfringens*, Type A, which causes gas gangrene.

Clot (klot)   1. (n.) The semisolid mass of fibrin threads and trapped blood cells that forms when blood coagulates. 2. (v.) To coagulate.

Cloverleaf Nail (klō′ver-lēf/nāl) (n.)   An intramedullary nail that in cross-section is shaped like a cloverleaf. One example is the **Kuntscher rod**.

Cloward Procedure (klow'-erd/pro-se'jur) (n.) A technique for anterior cervical discectomy and fusion utilizing an anterior cyclindrical opening into the spinal canal to remove osteophytes and disc fragments, followed by placement of a dowel-shaped bone graft in the opening to add stability postoperatively.

Clubbed Finger (klub'd/fing'ger) (n.) A finger with bulbous enlargement of the terminal phalanx, and a convexly curved nail so that the digit end looks like a club or drumstick. Clubbing may be a harmless congenital anomaly, or may be associated with serious pulmonary diseases and congenital heart diseases.

Clubfoot (klub'foot) (n.) The common name for *congenital Talipes Equinovarus*. This deformity has a multifactorial inheritance pattern in which there is forefoot adduction combined with inversion and supination of the forefoot, as well as hindfoot varus, where the talus is in equinus and the calcaneus is inverted beneath the talus. In unilateral cases there is some shortening of the involved foot and extremity. Often, the calcaneus is smaller than normal. Clubfoot varies widely in severity. Treatment and prognosis depend on the degree of deformity and the suppleness of the foot, and may range from conservative treatment with serial casting to operative management.

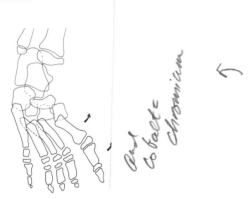

Clubhand (klub'hand) (n.) A congenital deformity of the hand. It is analogous to clubfoot in that the deformity may involve the palmar displacement, with or without radial or ulnar deviation, or dorsal displacement, with or without radial or ulnar deviation. Clubhand may be due to contracture of ligaments and muscles, or it may be caused by defective development of the radius, the ulna, or the carpal bones. See related **Radial Clubhand**, **Ulnar Clubhand**.

Clutton's Joints (klut'unz/jointz) (n.) A symmetrical, relatively painless, bilateral arthrosis resulting from congenital syphilis. It is usually seen in people 8 to 18 years old.

CMF Abbreviation for **chondromyxoid fibroma**.

Coach's Finger (kōch'ez/fing'ger) (n.) The clinical entity of finger pain with stiffness and deformity following athletic injury to the proximal interphalangeal joint. These joints are frequently injured in athletic competition, and the initial reduction and management are usually performed on the field by coaches or other supervisory personnel.

Coagulase (ko-ag'u-lās) (n.) An enzyme produced by pathogenic staphylococci that cause coagulation of blood plasma. It may be a determinant of pathogenicity.

Coagulation (ko-ag″u-la'shun) (n.) Formation of a solid from a liquid, especially in blood, where it is known as clotting.

Coagulation Factors (kō-ag″u-la'shun/fak'torz) (n.) A group of substances present in blood plasma that, under certain circumstances, undergo a series of chemical reactions that result in the conversion of blood from a liquid to a solid state. Also known as **Clotting Factors**.

Coagulation Time (kō-ag″u-la'shun/tīm) (n.) Measurement of the time required for blood or blood plasma to coagulate. Also known as **Clotting Time**.

Coagulopathy (kō-ag″u-lop'ah-thē) (n.) Any disorder of blood coagulation.

Coaptation Splint (kō-ap'ta-shun/splint) (n.) A type of splint applied to an injured extremity in which two slabs of plaster are molded on either side of the limb and held together with an outer dressing, typically an Ace bandage or a Kling bandage. In this manner the potential complications of a circumferential plaster cast may be avoided. A **sugar-tong splint** is one example.

Cobalt-Based Alloy (kō'bawlt/bāsd/al'loi) (n.) Any alloy whose principal component is cobalt. These alloys have significant resistance to fatigue and corrosion cracking and are not brittle. They are commonly used for orthopaedic implants. Examples include **Cobalt-Chrome-Molybdenum** and **Cobalt-Nickel-Chrome-Molybdenum Alloys**.

Cobb Elevator (kob/el'e-va″tor) (n.) A surgical instrument for periosteal stripping with a flattened, spoon-shaped elevating surface attached to a straight handle.

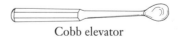
Cobb elevator

Cobb's Method (kobz/meth'ud) (n.) A technique for measuring the angle of the scoliotic curve on an anteroposterior radiograph of the spine.

First, determine the superior and inferior end vertebrae. The **superior** end vertebra is the last one in which the superior border points to the concavity of the curve to be measured. The **inferior** end vertebra is the last one whose inferior border still points toward the concavity of the curve to be measured. Then, draw intersecting perpendicular lines from the superior surface of the superior and the inferior surface of the inferior vertebra. The angle formed by these perpendicular lines is the angle of the curve. Also called **Cobb-Lippmann Method**.

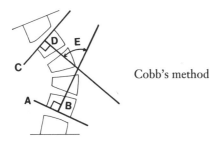

Cobb's method

Coccidioidomycosis (kok-sid″ē-oi″do-mī-kō′sis) (n.) A systemic disease caused by the fungus coccidioides immitis. Infection may be asymptomatic, producing an influenza-like illness, or less commonly, become hematogenously disseminated to skin, subcutaneous tissues, bone, central nervous system, and other organs.

Coccus (kok′us) (n.) A spherical or ovoid bacterium.

Coccygalgia (kok″se-al′je-ah) (n.) Pain in the coccyx region. More commonly known as **coccydynia**. Also known as **coccyalgia**.

Coccydynia (kok″se-dīn′e-ah) (n.) Pain in the most distal aspect of the spine, the coccygeal region.

Coccygeal Plexus (kok″sij′e-al/plek′sus) A small nerve plexus formed by the anterior primary rami of the coccygeal and fifth sacral nerves, with a communication from the fourth sacral nerve giving off the anococcygeal nerves.

Coccygectomy (kok″se-gek′tō-mē) (n.) Surgical excision of the coccyx.

Coccyx (kok′-six) (n.) The lowermost element of the backbone. It is considered to be the vestigial tail in humans; it consists of four rudimentary coccygeal

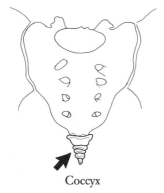

Coccyx

vertebrae fused to form a triangular bone that articulates with the sacrum.

Cockup Wrist Splint (kok-up/rist/splint) (n.) An orthosis used to support the wrist in mild dorsiflexion. It consists of a straight metal gutter, the concave side of which fits the flexor aspect of the forearm and continues distally into a dorsiflexed palmar piece, which extends to the distal palmar skin crease. The thumb remains free of the splint. Abbreviated as **CUWS**.

Codivilla's Extension (kod-i-vē′-laz/ek-sten′shun) (n.) A type of extension traction for fractures: a weight pulls on either calipers or a nail passed through the lower end of the bone.

Codman Exercises (kod′man/ek″ser-sīz-ez) (n.) Shoulder mobilization exercises. The patient is instructed to bend over from the trunk with the arm hanging, pendulumlike, toward the floor. The patient should then move the arm and shoulder in arcs or circles to increase shoulder range of motion. Also called **Pendulum** or **Circumduction Exercises**.

Codman Incision (kod′man/in-sizh′un) (n.) An eponym for a saber-cut approach to the shoulder; especially useful in acromioplasty and rotator cuff surgery.

Codman's Sign (kod′manz/sīn) (n.) A clinical sign of rotator cuff injury. The patient is noted to hunch the shoulder up when the deltoid contracts during abduction, owing to absence of adequate rotator cuff function. There should be no pain when the arm is passively abducted, but when support of the arm is removed and the deltoid contracts suddenly, pain will occur.

Codman's Triangle (kod′manz/tri′ang-g′l) (n.) A roentgenographic manifestation in malignant bone tumors of a type of periosteal reaction. This appears as a trumpet-shaped area in which the elevated periosteum meets the intact cortex at the apex. The base of the triangle is perpendicular to the shaft and is formed by the tumor mass.

Codman's Tumor (kod′manz/too′mor) (n.) An older eponym for chondroblastoma. See **Chondroblastoma**.

Coefficient of Friction (kō″e-fish′ent/of/frik′shun) (n.) A dimensionless, proportional constant that relates normal force to friction force between two bodies.

Coenzyme (kō-en′zīm) (n.) An organic compound that is made active when combining temporarily with an enzyme.

Cofactor (kō′fak-tor) (n.) A metallic ion necessary for enzyme activity (e.g., magnesium, zinc, copper, iron).

Coil Spring Brace (koil/spring/brās) (n.) A lower extremity orthosis with a single or double coil spring hinge, designed to support the foot in dorsiflexion.

Coinsurance (ko-in-shur′ans) (n.) The requirement in an insurance policy or prepayment plan that a predetermined portion or percentage of the provider's charges be paid by the beneficiary.

Colchicine (kol′chĭ-sēn) (n.) An anti-inflammatory agent used to relieve pain in acute attacks of gout. May be used as chronic prophylaxis against further acute attacks.

Cold Intolerance (kōld/in-tol′er-ans) (n.) A clinical condition, usually described in reference to the distal aspect of the extremities, especially the digits, in which there is marked sensitivity exposure to cold. There may be a neurologic or vascular etiology.

Coleman Block Test (kōl-man/blok/test) (n.) A clinical test in the evaluation of fixed heel varus in a cavovarus foot deformity. The weight-bearing foot is placed on a 1-cm thick wood block with the first ray hanging free on the medial side. If heel varus is not fixed, the calcaneus should return to neutral or slight valgus when weight-bearing in this position. The heel varus is fixed if the calcaneus does not realign.

Coliform (kō′li-form) (n.) An enterobacterium that resembles *Escherichia coli*. This excludes Shigella, Salmonella, and Proteus.

Collagen (kōl′ah-jen) (n.) A crystalline, biologic, solid protein of fixed chemical composition that is the major constituent of all connective tissues. At least 11 types of collagen have been identified. All molecules contain three polypeptide alpha chains that are wrapped around each other into a tight helix. Collagen structures are then formed by cross-linking of adjacent collagen molecules.

Collagen Diseases (kōl′ah-jen/di-zēz′ez) (n.) See **Connective Tissue Diseases**.

Collagen Vascular Diseases (kōl′ah-jen/vas′ku-lar/di-zēz′ez) (n.) An older term for a group of diseases now known as Connective Tissue Diseases. See **Connective Tissue Diseases**.

Collagenase (kōl-laj′e-nās) (n.) An enzyme that hydrolyzes peptides containing proline, including collagen and gelatin.

Collar (kol′ler) (n.) In shoe terminology, a band of leather stitched to and encircling the top of the quarter of a shoe.

Collar bone (kol′ler/bōn) (n.) See **Clavicle**.

Collar Button Abscess (kol′ler/but′n′/ab′ses) (n.) See **Web Space Infection**.

Collar and Cuff (kol′ler/and/cuf) (n.) A simple bandage used to support the upper extremity in which a cloth strap around the forearm is attached to a similar strap around the neck.

Collateral Ligament (kō-lat′er-al/lig′ah-ment) (n.) A ligament that runs on the medial or lateral side of a joint to check varus or valgus stresses applied across that joint. These ligaments are specifically named for their position and the joint they stabilize. For example, the Ulnar Collateral Ligament of the thumb or the Medial Collateral Ligament of the knee.

Colles' Fracture (kol′ēz/frak′chur) (n.) An eponym

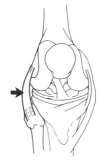

Collateral ligament

for a common fracture of the distal radius. Clinically, a "silver-fork" deformity results from the displacement. There may be an associated fracture of the styloid process of the ulna. There is usually comminution and impaction at the fracture site, with shortening of the radius and dorsal displacement of the articular surface, resulting in volar angulation. The fracture line may extend through the distal radioulnar joint proximally or the articular surface distally.

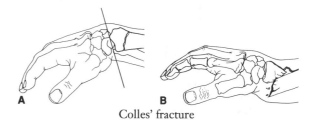

Colles' fracture

Collimator (kol″i-ma′tor) (n.) 1. An arrangement of openings or slits that limits a stream of particles to a beam in which all particles move in nearly the same direction. 2. A device to shield a detector, so that a particular region being scanned may be preferentially measured for radioactivity. Collimators may be of the parallel channel or tapered focused type.

Collodion (ko-lō′dē-on) (n.) A liquid substance that leaves a contractile, glossy film on drying. It is used as an impermeable barrier for cuts or surgical incisions or for the local application of medicinal substances.

Colloid (kol′oid) (n.) Aggregates of molecules, ranging from 1 nm to 100 nm in size, dispersed in a gaseous, liquid, or solid medium that resists sedimentation, diffusion, and filtration.

Colonization (kol′on-i-zā′shun) (n.) The superficial populating of body areas (e.g., skin or mucous membranes) by microbes, without tissue invasion or production of clinical disease.

Colonna Arthroplasty (kŏ-lōn′ah/ar′thro-plas″te) (n.) A type of interpositional arthroplasty of the hip now rarely used. The hip joint capsule is interposed between the femoral head and an enlarged acetabulum that has been denuded of articular cartilage.

Comma Bar (kom′ah/bar) (n.) In shoe terminology, metatarsal bar applied to the outer sole, just posterior to the metatarsal heads.

Comminuted Fracture (kom′i-nūt″ed/frak′chur) (n.) A descriptive term for any fracture in which the bone is broken into more than two distinct fragments.

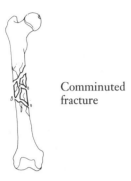

Comminuted fracture

Commissure (kom′i-shūr) (n.) A group of nerve fibers that cross the midline in the brain or spinal cord. Also spelled **commissura**.

Communicable Disease (ko-mū′ni-kah-b′l/di-zēz′) (n.) An illness caused by a specific infectious agent or its toxic products, transmitted directly or indirectly from an infected person or animal to a susceptible host.

Comolli's Sign (kom-ōl′ēz/sīn) (n.) A clinical sign of a scapula fracture. A triangular swelling over the region of the scapula reminiscent of the shape of the body of the scapula.

Compact Bone (kom-pakt′/bōn) (n.) Dense or cortical bone.

Comparison Film (kom-par′i-son/film) (n.) A radiograph of the uninvolved opposite extremity intended as a guide to baseline normalcy.

Compartment Syndrome (kom-part′ment/sin′drōm) (n.) A condition in which increased tissue pressure within a limited anatomic space compromises the local circulation and, therefore, the neuromuscular and vascular function of the contents within that space. This is seen to occur in any closed fascial space of the upper or lower extremity. The diagnosis is initially based on clinical suspicion. Signs and symptoms include pain out of proportion to physical examination, pain with passive stretch of the compartment, palpable swelling and tension in the compartment, paresthesias and paresis. Pulselessness and pallor are very late signs that may never occur. Compartmental pressure measurements are used to help confirm the diagnosis. See **Volkmann's Ischemic Contracture**.

Compartmental Knee Prosthesis (kom-part′ment′l/nē/pros-thē′sis) (n.) An implant that replaces only a compartment of the knee. Also known as **Unicompartmental Prosthesis**.

Compensation (kom″pen-sa′shun) (n.) 1. In scoliosis, when the thoracic cage is centered over the pelvis and the inion (the posterior occipital protuberance) is centered over the mid-sacrum. This usually results from development of a secondary curve. 2. Shortened reference to **Workman's Compensation**.

Compensation Neurosis (kom″pen-sa′shun/nu-rō′sis) (n.) The tendency of individuals to maintain various symptoms that occurred originally as the result of mishap; used as a defense against losing the various secondary gains obtained as a result of the original mishap, particularly monetary. Motivation to maintain symptoms must be unconscious, otherwise it is malingering.

Compensatory Curve (kom-pen′sah-to″rē/kurv) (n.) In spinal curvature, a secondary curve located above or below a major curve that develops in order to maintain normal body alignment.

Complement (kom′ple-ment) (n.) A thermolabile substance found in serum that participates in immunologic reactions, such as cytolysis and phagocytosis. It is actually composed of at least nine serum proteins, named C1 through C9, that interact sequentially and mediate aspects of antigen–antibody reactions.

Complete Fracture (kom′plēt/frak′chur) (n.) A fracture involving the entire cross-section of the bone.

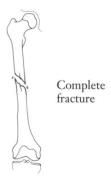

Complete fracture

Compliance (kom-plī′ans) (n.) A measure of the response of a material to stress; inverse of stiffness.

Complicating Disease (kom″pli-kā-ting/di-zēz′) (n.) A disease, foreseen or unforeseen, that occurs in the course of the development or treatment of another disease.

Complication (kom″pli-kā′shun) (n.) An additional diagnosis describing a condition arising after the beginning of hospital observation and treatment, thus modifying the course of the patient's illness or the medical care required. Used in a narrower sense to describe an undesired result or misadventure in the medical care of a hospital patient or, in a broader sense, to denote any condition concurrent with the principal diagnosis, regardless of the time of onset.

Compound (kom'-pownd) (n.) A complex substance. For example, a chemical compound is formed from the bonding of simple elements. A pharmaceutical compound is prepared from two or more simple ingredients.

Compound Fracture (kom'-pownd/frak'chur) (n.) A term formerly used for an open fracture, designating a fracture of a bone in which penetration of the skin has occurred and there is communication with the outside air. See **Open Fracture**.

Comprehensive Health Care (kom-prē-hen'siv/helth/kār) (n.) Services that meet the total health care needs of a patient.

Comprehensive Quotient (kom-prē-hen'siv/kwo'shent) (n.) A numerical expression of the overall shape of the femoral head: the mean of the epiphyseal quotient, acetabular quotient, head–neck quotient, and acetabulum–head quotients.

Compress (kom'pres) 1. (n.) A piece of gauze or similar dressing used in application of pressure or medication to a restricted area or local application of heat or cold. 2. (kom-pres') (v.) To squeeze together.

Compression (kom-presh'un) (n.) The pressing together of a structure by opposing forces that results in a decreased size and an increased density of that structure.

Compression Arthrodesis (kom-presh'un/ar"thrō-dē'sis) (n.) A technique for achieving bony fusion in which compression forces are applied across the denuded joint surfaces, usually with an external compression device. See **Charnley Arthrodesis**.

Compression Bandage (kom-presh'un/ban'dij) (n.) Any dressing meant to apply pressure to prevent or reduce swelling and check bleeding or to route absorption without interfering with the general circulation of the limb. This may be applied by alternating layers of cotton or cotton-wool wrapped with an elastic bandage around an extremity or locally with fluffed-up gauze pads held in place with elastic or foam adhesive tape. See **Jones Dressing** for related term.

Compression Fracture (kom-presh'un/frak'chur) (n.) A fracture due to impact loading in which the cancellous bone has been crushed. Seen, for example, in the vertebral bodies of osteopenic patients.

Compression Hip Screw (kom-presh'un/hip/skru) (n.) A self-impacting implant for compression and stabilization of fractures about the hip, used mostly for the treatment of intertrochanteric hip fractures and less commonly for appropriate subtrochanteric and basicervical fractures. These are actually screw and side-plate assemblies in which a large, cancellous threaded compression screw is placed across the femoral neck into the femoral head. The base of the screw is attached to a side plate through a barrel,

in which it may slide, and the side-plate is affixed to the proximal femoral shaft.

Compression Paralysis (kom-presh'un/pah-ral'i-sis) (n.) Partial or complete paralysis caused by pressure on a nerve or the spinal cord.

Compression Screw (kom-presh'un/skru) (n.) The large diameter, threaded screw part of a dynamic hip screw or dynamic condylar screw device that is fitted into the side-plate for internal fixation of proximal or distal femur fractures.

Computerized Axial Tomography (kom-pū'ter-īzed/ak'se-al/tō-mog'rah-fē) (n.) A noninvasive, radiologic method of imaging in which a computer graphically reconstructs the anatomic features registered by axial tomography. It produces highly contrasted, detailed cross-sectional studies of normal and pathologic anatomy in which structures are identified by differences in density. The computer also prints out numerical density values related to the radiation-absorption coefficients of the substances in the area scanned as the x-ray beam moves back and forth across the body. Abbreviated as **CAT Scan** or **CT Scan**.

Concentric Muscle Contraction (kon-sen'trik/mus'el/kon-trak'shun) (n.) Any contraction in which a muscle shortens while tension is generated.

Concussion (kon-kush'un) (n.) See **Cerebral Concussion**.

Condensation (kon"den-sā'shun) (n.) In orthopaedics, an area of increased bone density due to abnormal bone deposition that may occur in response to inflammation.

Conditioned Reflex (kon-dish'un'd/rē'fleks) (n.) A habitual response to a particular stimulus, determined by the previous experience of the organism.

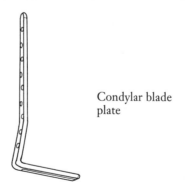

Condylar blade plate

Condylar Blade Plate (kon'di-lar/blād/plāt) (n.) An implant for the internal fixation of intercondylar femur fractures. It is a fixed angle device with a side plate attached at a 95° angle to the blade portion that is inserted across the condyles. The distal hole of the plate is designed for insertion of a cancellous screw to add stability to the femoral condyles.

Condyle (kon'dīl) (n.) Any rounded projection or

eminence of bone that functions in joint articulation. Examples: femur, humerus, and mandible.

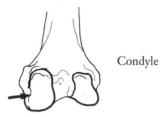

Condyle

Condylocephalic Nail (kon″di-lō′se-fal′ik/nāl) (n.) A flexible rod used for the intramedullary fixation of femur fractures. It is inserted in a retrograde fashion from the femoral condyle across the femoral neck into the femoral head.

Condyloid (kon′di-loid) (adj.) Of or resembling a rounded articular surface at the extremity of a long bone.

Condyloid Joint (kon′di-loid/joint) (n.) A type of synovial joint in which the rounded condyles of one bone articulate with a shallow elliptical cavity of another, permitting all movements except axial rotation. An example is the radiocarpal joint.

Cone (kōn) (n.) 1. A funnel-shaped attachment or tubular extension on the x-ray tube housing aperture; used to control the scattering of x-rays in the air and to limit the x-rays in any given area. 2. In shoe terminology, the curved upper surface of the backpart of the last, divided by a V-cut into a front and back cone.

Coned-Down View (kōn′d/down/vū) (n.) In radiology, a close-up view of a localized area obtained by using a cone attachment.

Confusion (kon-fū′zhun) (n.) 1. A mental state in which reactions to environmental stimuli are inappropriate. 2. Disorientation.

Congenital (kon-jen′i-tal) (adj.) Existing at birth. Refers to anomalous mental and physical conditions due either to inherited disorders or to intrauterine events.

Congenital Absence of the Radius (kon-jen′i-tal/ab′sens/of/the/rā′de-us) (n.) A congenital failure of formation in the upper extremity that presents with absence of all, or part of, the radius, shortening of the forearm, radial deviation of the hand, and generalized underdevelopment of the upper extremity. There are usually associated muscle and nerve anomalies in the affected extremity and often other associated deformities without a set pattern.

Congenital Absence of the Ulna (kon-jen′i-tal/ab′sens/of/the/ul′nah) (n.) A congenital failure of formation in the upper extremity in which all or part of the ulna does not form. There is a characteristic ulnar deviation of the hand, radial bowing of the radius, and dislocation of the radial head.

Congenital Amputation (kon-jen′i-tal/am″pu-tā′shun) (n.) Absence of all or part of a limb at birth. Attributed to constriction of the part by an encircling band of amniotic strings during intrauterine development.

Congenital Analgia (kon-jen′i-tal/an-al′jē-ah) (n.) See **Congenital Indifference to Pain**.

Congenital Brevicollis (kon-jen′i-tal/brev″e-kōl′is) (n.) See **Klippel-Feil Syndrome**.

Congenital Clasped Thumb (kon-jen′i-tal/klasp′d/thumb) (n.) A congenital anomaly that presents with the thumb clasped in a flexed position into the palm. It results from multiple defects in the extensors and flexors as well as from skin contractures and joint instability. Classification is based on the underlying contributing causes and associated anomalies.

Congenital Convex Pes Planus (kon-jen′i-tal/kon′veks/pes/plā′nus) (n.) See **Congenital Vertical Talus**.

Congenital Curly Toe (kon-jen′i-tal/cur-le/tō) A congenital deformity in which one or more of the lateral toes are in plantar flexion, medial deviation, and supination. The twisted terminal pulp may curl under the adjacent medial toe. This affection is usually bilateral and symmetrical, with a high familial incidence.

Congenital Digitus Minimum Varus (kon-jen′i-tal/dij′i-tus/min′i-mum/va′rus) (n.) A common familial deformity in which the fifth toe is hyperextended and adducted, overlapping the fourth toe. The capsule of the metatarsophalangeal joint is contracted on its dorsomedial aspect, the extensor tendon is shortened, and the skin between the fourth and fifth toes is contracted. Also known as **Congenital Overriding of Fifth Toe**.

Congenital Dislocation of the Elbow (kon-jen′i-tal/dis″lō-kā′shun/of/the/el′bō) (n.) A congenital dislocation of the humeroulnar articulation. It rarely occurs as an isolated deformity but usually results from a failure of formation of the proximal ulna or distal humerus.

Congenital Dislocation of the Hip (kon-jen′i-tal/dis″lo-kā′shun/of/the/hip) (n.) A congenital condition in which the femoral head is dislocated from the acetabulum. Used generally to include subluxation and hip dysplasia, as well as true dislocations. Diagnosis in the newborn must be based on a careful clinical examination; roentgenograms are unreliable because of lack of ossification of the femoral head. The most important clinical tests in this time period are the reduction test of Ortolani and the provocative test of Barlow. In the older infant, at about 3 to 6 months of age, the diagnosis may be easier, owing to secondary changes in surrounding soft tissue. In the child of walking age, gait abnormalities are seen. Also, as the child ages, roentgenographic changes become more clear. Treatment and prognosis depend on the age at the time of diagnosis and the degree of bone dysplasia and soft tissue contracture. Abbreviated as **CDH**. Also known as **Congenital Hip Disease**. The preferred term is **Developmental Dysplasia of the Hip**. Abbreviated **DDH**.

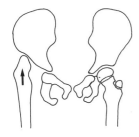

Congenital dislocation of the hip

Congenital Dislocation of the Radial Head (kon-jen′i-tal/dis″lo-kā′shun/of/the/rā′dē-al/hed) (n.) A congenital dislocation of the radiocapitellar joint that may occur as an isolated deformity. There may be some limitation of motion or a prominence at the elbow with a posterior dislocation, but usually few symptoms are associated with this anomaly. The disorder is usually differentiated radiographically from a traumatic dislocation by the presence of a flattened, deformed capitellum and a rounded, dome-shaped radial head. If symptoms warrant, resection of the radial head may be considered after completion of growth.

Congenital Elevation of the Shoulder (kon-jen′i-tal/el″e-vā′shun/of/the/shōl′der) (n.) An uncommon, congenital disorder characterized by malformation and malposition of the scapula. There is elevation and medial rotation of the inferior pole of the scapula. The bone is usually small, decreased in length, and often with anterior bending of the superior aspect. There may be a bony, cartilaginous, or fibrous tether between the scapula and the spine. Clinically, shoulder abduction is limited in proportion to the severity of angulation and elevation of the scapula. The treatment of choice is usually surgery. Commonly known as **Sprengel's Deformity**. Also known as **Congenital High Scapula**.

Congenital High Scapula (kon-jen′i-tal/hī/skap′u-lah) (n.) See **Congenital Elevation of the Shoulder**.

Congenital Hip Disease (kon-jen′i-tal/hip/di-zēz′) (n.) See **Congenital Dislocation of the Hip**.

Congenital Hip Subluxation (kon-jen′i-tal/hip/sub″luk-sā′shun) (n.) A type of developmental dysplasia or congenital dislocation of the hip in which the femoral head is only partly displaced from the acetabulum. Term also used when the hip is subluxatable at birth, so that, with provocation, the femoral head can be significantly, but not completely, displaced from the acetabulum.

Congenital Indifference to Pain (kon-jen′i-tal/in-di″fa-rens/to/pān) (n.) Lack from birth of appropriate response to painful stimuli. Seen in: Congenital Insensitivity to Pain, Congenital Sensory Neuropa-

thy, Hereditary Sensory Radicular Neuropathy, Familial Dysautonomia, and Familial Sensory Neuropathy with Anhidrosis. Also called **Riley-Day Syndrome**.

Congenital Insensitivity to Pain (kon-jen′i-tal/in-sen′si-tiv′i-tē/to/pān) (n.) A rare form of congenital indifference to pain in which the patient can perceive ordinary painful stimuli but does not respond to them as being harmful. The distribution of sensory loss is universal.

Congenital Metaphyseal Dysostosis (kon-jen′i-tal/met″ah-fiz′ē-al/dis″os-tō′sis) (n.) See **Jansen's Metaphyseal Dysostosis**.

Congenital Metatarsus Varus (kon-jen′i-tal/met″ah-tar′sus/va′rus) (n.) A fairly common congenital foot deformity in which the forefoot is adducted and supinated. It is sometimes associated with internal tibial torsion. The treatment is usually nonoperative with manual stretching and serial casting. Surgical correction may be indicated in the child over 6 years of age. Because it represents only one of the three deformities that make up a clubfoot, it has been called "one-third of a club foot." Because of its appearance, it has also been referred to as "skewfoot." Also called **Metatarsus Adductus**.

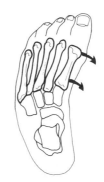

Congenital metatarsus varus

Congenital Overriding of the Fifth Toe (kon-jen′i-tal/o″ver-rīd′ing/of/the/fifth/tō) (n.) A familial disorder in which the fifth toe is in varus and therefore overlaps the fourth toe dorsally. Nonoperative treatment with passive stretching and splinting is usually unsuccessful. Operative treatment should be considered in symptomatic cases.

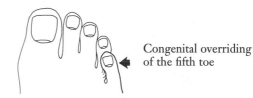

Congenital overriding of the fifth toe

Congenital Pseudoarthrosis of the Clavicle (kon-jen′i-tal/soo″dō-ar-thrō′sis/of/the/klav′i-k'l) (n.) A congenital anomaly in which there is a proximal and distal clavicle present with absence of the bone centrally. Usually it is the central one-third of the clavicle that is deficient. There may be symptoms of pain and instability that require surgical intervention.

Congenital Radioulnar Synostosis (kon-jen'i-tal/rā″dē-o-ul'nar/sin″os-tō'sis) (n.) A congenital anomaly due to failure of separation of the proximal radius and ulna, resulting in a fixed positioning of the forearm, usually in pronation.

Congenital Scoliosis (kon-jen'i-tal/skō″lē-ō'sis) (n.) Scoliosis due to congenitally anomalous vertebral development. These anomalies are classified as failure of vertebral formation and/or failure of segmentation. Prognosis and treatment depend on severity of the curve and presence or absence of progression.

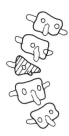

Congenital scoliosis

Congenital Sensory Neuropathy (kon-jen'i-tal/sen'so-re/nu-rop'ah-thē) (n.) A form of congenital indifference to pain inherited with an autosomal recessive pattern. All sensory modalities are affected, with an incomplete distribution. On skin biopsy, there is an absence of myelinated fibers and dermal nerve networks. This disease is usually manifested clinically in late infancy.

Congenital Short First Metatarsal (kon-jen'i-tal/short/first/met″ah-tar'sal) (n.) A congenital foot deformity that probably is a variation of normal, not associated with a true increase in foot complaints. Also known as **Metatarsus Atavicus**.

Congenital Synostosis (kon-jen'i-tal/sin″ōs-tō'sis) (n.) A congenital fusion of two or more bones.

Congenital Torticollis (kon-jen'i-tal/tor″ti-kōl'is) (n.) A congenital condition characterized by shortening and contracture of the sternocleidomastoid muscle, causing the head to be inclined toward the affected side and the chin to be deviated toward the opposite shoulder. Palpation of the muscle may reveal generalized firmness or a localized soft, nontender, mobile, tumorous enlargement. It is usually discovered within the first few weeks of life. Excellent results are usually obtained with conservative measures consisting of passive stretching, traction, and positioning. If torticollis persists beyond infancy, surgical intervention may be appropriate. Also known as **Congenital Wryneck** or **Congenital Muscular Torticollis**.

Congenital Vertical Talus (kon-jen'i-tal/ver'ti-kal/ta'lus) (n.) An uncommon, congenital deformity of the foot, with a characteristic appearance described as a **rocker-bottom flatfoot**. The talus is vertical and in marked equinus, with its head palpable medially and at the sole. The hindfoot is in valgus and equinus, and the midfoot is abducted and dorsiflexed. These clinical findings are confirmed radiographically. The navicular, when ossified, is seen to lie on the neck of the talus and may create notching there. The calcaneal lateral deviation results in an increased talocalcaneal angle on an anteroposterior view. With early diagnosis and initiation of treatment, an acceptable result may be achieved with manipulation and serial casting. Often, surgical intervention is required to reestablish and maintain talonavicular and talocalcaneal relationships. Also known as **Congenital Convex Pes Planus** and **Vertical Talus**.

Congenital Wryneck (kon-jen'i-tal/rī'neck) (n.) See **Congenital Torticollis**.

Congruence Angle (kong'grōō-ens/ang'g'l) (n.) An angle measured on a Merchant's view of the knee to reflect the relationship of the patella to the intercondylar sulcus. Draw the sulcus angle and bisect this to establish a 0 reference line. Project a second line from the apex of the sulcus angle to the lowest point on the articular ridge of the patella. The angle measured between these two lines is the congruence angle. If the apex of the patellar articular ridge is lateral to the 0 line, the congruence angle is designated positive; if it is medial, the congruence angle is negative. The normal value of the congruence angle is $-8°$ (range -24 to $+8°$, SD = 6°). An increasingly positive congruence angle is noted in chondromalacia patella and, more so, in recurrent patella subluxators. See **Sulcus Angle**.

Conical Reamers (kon'e-kal/rē'merz) (n.) Any surgical instrument for intramedullary reaming with a cone-shaped head.

Connective Tissue (ko-nek'tiv/tish'ū) (n.) A type of interstitium that forms the framework or supporting tissue throughout the body. It is found between groups of nerves, glands, and muscle cells, and beneath epithelial cells. Connective tissues are derived from the mesenchyme and tend to have cells that are irregularly distributed through a relatively large amount of intercellular material. Examples include bone, cartilage, blood, and lymph tissue.

Connective Tissue Disease (ko-nek'tiv/tish'ū/di-zēz) (n.) A group of disorders either hereditary (primarily affecting connective tissue structure, such as Marfan's Syndrome or Ehlers-Danlos Syndrome) or acquired, due to immunologic or inflammatory reactions. These latter disorders used to be referred to us collagen-vascular diseases, but this term has been changed, since collagen itself does not appear to be specifically affected. Acquired disorders include rheumatoid arthritis, systemic lupus erythematosus, scleroderma, polymyositis, dermatomyositis, Sjögrens' Syndrome, Amyloidosis, rheumatic fever, and some vasculitides.

Conoid Ligament (ko'noid/lig'ah-ment) (n.) A triangular-shaped ligament, with its apex inferiorly, that forms the posteromedial portion of the coracoclavicular ligament, extending from the coracoid process to the inferior surface of the clavicle. With the trapezoid ligament it forms the coracoclavicular ligament.

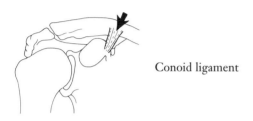

Conoid ligament

Conscious (kon'shus) 1. (adj.) Aware. 2. (n.) A characterization of thoughts, ideas, or decisions that occur when one is aware; in contradistinction to reflexive or automatic responses.

Consciousness (kon'shus-nes) (n.) Awareness or a state of general wakefulness and responsiveness to the environment. Consciousness may be impaired in any degree of severity. Terms such as lethargy, drowsiness, stupor, semicoma, and coma are commonly used to describe lower levels of consciousness.

Constitutional Disease (kon"sti-tū'shun-al/di-zēz') (n.) A systemic disease, or a disease that involves multiple body systems instead of strictly local involvement.

Constitutional Growth Delay (kon"sti-tū'shun-al/grōth/de'lā) (n.) A growth disturbance of unknown etiology in which there is normal early growth followed by a deceleration for a period, with subsequent reestablishment of a normal pattern.

Constitutional Symptoms (kon"sti-tū'shun-al/simp' tumz) (n.) Any untoward symptoms that beset the body in a generalized manner. Examples include fever, malaise, or unintended weight loss.

Constrained Knee Prosthesis (kon-strān'd/nē/prosthē'sis) (n.) A total knee implant that provides its own inherent stability. It may be partly or totally constrained. See **Guépar Knee Prosthesis**.

Constriction (kon-strik'shun) (n.) Narrowing. Usually refers to the narrowing of a lumen or a tubular structure.

Contact Dermatitis (kon'takt/der"mah-tī'tis) (n.) An inflammation of the skin due to external agents and mechanical irritants that touch it.

Contagious Disease (kon-tā'jus/di-zēz') (n.) A communicable disease transmitted by contact with the sick.

Contamination (kon-tam"i-nā'shun) (n.) 1. The presence of pathogenic microorganisms on animate or inanimate objects. The term contamination is often used to indicate the possible rather than the known presence of microorganisms. 2. Entry of undesirable organisms into some material or object. 3. Process by which an organic or inorganic material or object is rendered unclean or unsterile.

Continuous Passive Motion (kon-tin'ū-us/pas'iv/mō'shun) (n.) The application of passive exercise to joints. This is accomplished with a variety of devices that put a joint through a preset arc of motion with a variable speed control.

Contraction (kon-trak'shun) (n.) 1. A shortening or increase in tension such as occurs in normal muscle function. 2. A reduction in size.

Contracture (kon-trak'tūr) (n.) 1. A permanent shortening of a soft tissue, for example, a muscle-tendinous unit, so that it cannot passively attain its normal length. 2. A disorder in which limitation of the range of motion of a part is due to contracture.

Contraindication (kon"trah-in"di-kā'shun) (n.) Any factor or condition that renders a particular line of treatment improper or undesirable.

Contralateral (kon"trah-lat'er-al) (adj.) Of or pertaining to the opposite side. Contrast with **Ipsilateral**.

Contrast Medium (kon-trast/me'de-um) (n.) A liquid radiopaque substance given parenterally or orally and intended to improve visibility and interpretation of structures during radiography by providing greater contrast between structures.

Contrecoup (kon-tr-koo) (n.) Injury or damage to a body part resulting from a blow delivered to the side opposite the injured side.

Contusion (kon-tū'zhun) (n.) A bruise or injury to the soft tissue in which the skin is not broken. Usually produced by a blunt force, blow, or fall.

Conus Medullaris (kō'nus/med'u-lar-us) (n.) The distal termination of the spinal cord proper in an adult, usually at the $T_{12} = L_1$ level. Compare **Tethered Cord Syndrome**.

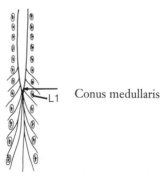

Conus medullaris

Conversion Reaction (kon-ver'zhun/rē-ak'shun) (n.) A disorder characterized by physical symptoms that do not have an organic basis but are judged to be the result of psychologic factors. There is usually a temporal relationship between a psychologic conflict or need and the initiation or exacerbation of the symptoms. The symptoms usually enable the individual to avoid some noxious activity or to get support from the environment that otherwise might not be forthcoming. For diagnosis, it must be established that the symptoms are not under voluntary control. Also known as **Conversion Hysteria** or **Hysterical Neurosis**.

Conversion Valley (kon-ver′zhun/val′ē) (n.) A specific response pattern on a psychologic test profile (**MMPI**) believed to be correlated with an emotional component in an individual with physical complaints. The patient emphasizes but fails to display real concern about somatic symptoms. Depression or anxiety is conspicuously absent. The patient is self-centered and demanding, yet independent.

Convulsion (kon-vul′shun) (n.) A motor seizure.

Cookie (kook′ē) (n.) A familiar term for a wafer-shaped leather shoe insert used as a longitudinal arch support. See **Navicular Pad**.

Coombs' Test (kōōmz/test) (n.) An antiglobulin test used in the diagnosis of immune hemolysis. The test relies on the ability of prepared animal antibodies directed against specific human serum proteins to agglutinate red blood cells if these proteins are present on the cell surface. This can be done directly or indirectly.

Coonrad Prosthesis (kūn′-rad/pros-the′sis) (n.) A semiconstrained hinged prosthesis used as an implant in total elbow arthroplasty.

Coopernails' Sign (koo′per-nālz/sīn) (n.) A clinical sign of fracture of the pelvis where ecchymosis is present on the perineum and scrotum or labia.

Copayment (ko′pā-ment) (n.) Specified share of total liability for which the insured is responsible. For example, a specific amount per hospital day, or a percentage of the total bill.

Coracoacromial (kor″ah-ko-ah-krō′mē-al) (adj.) Referring to the area between the coracoid process of the scapula and the acromion.

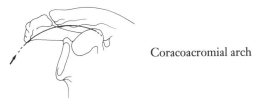

Coracoacromial arch

Coracoacromial Arch (kor″ah-ko-ah-krō′mē-al/arch) (n.) The archlike structure located between the subacromial bursa and the acromioclavicular joint; it is formed by the coracoid process, the coracoacromial ligament, and the acromion.

Coracoclavicular Ligament (kor″ah-kō-klah-vik′ū-lar/lig′ah-ment) (n.) The ligament that runs from the undersurface of the lateral clavicle to the medial aspect of the coracoid process. It consists of the conoid ligament medially and the trapezoid ligament laterally; it provides stability to the acromioclavicular joint.

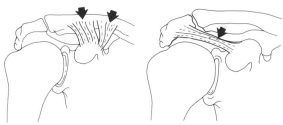

Coracoclavicular ligament   Coracoacromial ligament

Coracohumeral Ligament (kor″ah-ko-hu′mer-al/lig′ah-ment) (n.) A ligament of the shoulder that runs from the lateral border of the coracoid process medially to the greater and lesser tuberosities and capsule laterally. It strengthens the superior glenohumeral ligament, acting as a suspensory ligament of the humeral head and a checkrein to external rotation.

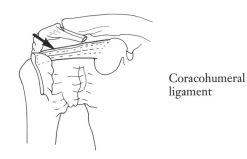

Coracohumeral ligament

Coracoid Process (kor′ah-koid/pros′es) (n.) A beak-shaped or hooklike process that projects superiorly, then forward and laterally from the neck of the scapula. The pectoralis minor muscle attaches here, and the short head of the biceps muscle and the coracobrachialis muscle originate at this point.

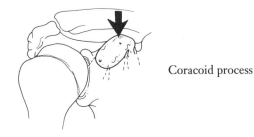

Coracoid process

Cord Injury (kord/in'ju-rē) (n.) Any complete or partial injury to the spinal cord resulting in neurologic deficit.

Cord Traction Syndrome (kord/trak'shun/sin'drōm) (n.) See **Tethered Cord Syndrome**.

Cordotomy (kor-dot'o-mē) (n.) A surgical procedure in which a tract of the spinal cord is divided by various techniques, including incision and cold cautery.

Core Decompression (kor/dē"kom-presh'un) (n.) A surgical procedure for the early treatment of avascular necrosis of the femoral head. It consists of removing an 8- to 10-mm core of bone from the anterolateral aspect of the femoral head through a lateral approach to the proximal femur. This procedure allows for bony biopsy to confirm the diagnosis and may be effective in pain relief and in halting progression of changes in the femoral head.

Corkscrew (kork'skrū) (n.) A surgical instrument with a conical, threaded tip attached to a T-shaped handle used to extract a fractured or osteotomized femoral head from the acetabulum.

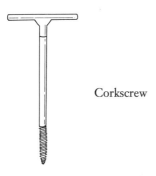

Corkscrew

Corn (korn) (n.) A circumscribed, conical area of hyperkeratosis on the foot produced by excessive extrinsic or intrinsic pressure. It is formed by proliferation of the stratum germinale (horny layer of epidermis). From within, the pressure is usually from an osseous condyle, resulting in soft corn formation between the toes. Extrinsic factors, such as shoe pressure, can result in hard corn formation. Seen on the heel, sole, or toes. Also known as **Clavus** or **Heloma**.

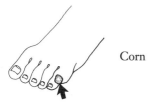

Corn

Corner Fracture (kor'ner/frak'chur) (n.) See **Chip Fracture**.

Coronal (ko-ro'nal) (n.) A reference plane at right angles to sagittal, dividing a structure into anterior and posterior portions.

Coronoid (kor'o-noid) Shaped like a crow's beak or crown.

Coronoid Fossa (kor'o-noid/fos'ah) (n.) The depression in the anterior surface of the distal end of the humerus into which the coronoid process of the ulna fits during elbow flexion.

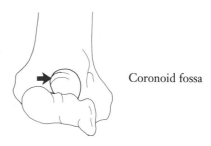

Coronoid fossa

Coronoid Process (kor'o-noid/pros'es) (n.) A triangular projection on the proximal, anterior end of the ulna; it forms the anterior part of the trochlear notch that articulates with the humerus. The tendon of the brachialis muscle inserts at this process.

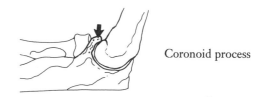

Coronoid process

Corrosion (ko-rō'zhun) (n.) The breakdown of materials, especially in regard to orthopaedic implants placed in an active physiologic environment in vivo.

Corrosion Fatigue (ko-rō'zhun/fah-tēg') (n.) A biomechanical term for fatigue failure of a structure caused by surface imperfections resulting from corrosion.

Corset (kor'set) (n.) 1. An orthosis that encircles all or part of the trunk. May also encompass a segment of a limb. Named specifically for the body part such as **Lumbosacral** or **Thoracolumbar Corsets**. 2. Any garment that goes around the trunk. 3. In shoe terminology, reinforcement in the upper with firm leather or stays to support or restrict ankle motion.

Cortex (kor'teks) (n.) 1. The outer part of an organ (e.g., cerebral cortex). 2. The dense bone that forms the external surface of a bone.

Cortical (kor'ti-kl) (adj.) Referring to the cortex.

Cortical Bone Graft (kor'ti-kl/bōn/graft) (n.) Any autogenous or other bone graft composed of dense, cortical bone. The primary advantage of these grafts is for fixation. They show limited osteogenic potential. Compare **Cancellous Bone Graft**.

Cortical Desmoid (kor′ti-kl/des′moid) (n.) A localized, asymptomatic irregularity along the posteromedial aspect of the distal femoral metaphyseal cortex near the insertion of the adductor magnus muscle. It is usually seen in adolescent males and may represent a periosteal reaction to muscular stress in this area. Also known as **Periosteal Desmoid**.

Cortical Screw (kor′ti-kl/skrū) (n.) A type of screw used for internal fixation of bone. These screws are usually fully threaded and not self-tapping. They can function either as positional screws or as lag screws for interfragmentary compression if the proximal cortex is overdrilled.

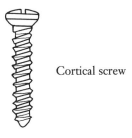

Cortical screw

Corticosteroid (kor″ti-ko-stē′roid) (n.) Any steroid hormone produced by the adrenal cortex. There are two main groups: glucocorticoids and mineralocorticoids.

Cortisone (kor′tĭ-sōn) (n.) A naturally occurring corticosteroid.

Cosmetic Hand (koz-met′ik/hand) (n.) An artificial hand in which appearance is emphasized. It is usually covered with a thin plastic glove that resembles skin, but its prehensile function is generally limited.

Costal Angle (kōs′tal/ang′g′l) (n.) The angle formed by the right and left costal cartilages at the xiphoid process.

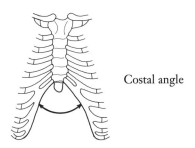

Costal angle

Costal Cartilage (kōs′tal/kar′ti-lij) (n.) The cartilage occupying the interval between the ribs and the sternum or adjacent cartilages. In true ribs, it is a bar of hyaline cartilage that attaches a rib to the sternum. In false ribs, this bar attaches a rib to the rib immediately above it.

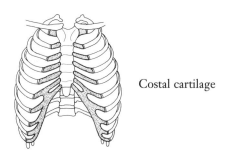

Costal cartilage

Costo (kōs′tō) Prefix for rib.

Costochondral Junction Syndrome (kōs″tō-kon′dral/junk′shun/sin′drōm) (n.) See **Tietze's Syndrome**.

Costochondritis (kōs″tō-kon′drī-tis) (n.) Inflammation of a costal cartilage. See **Tietze's Syndrome**.

Costoclavicular (kōs″tō-klah-vik′u-lar) (n.) Of or pertaining to the ribs and the clavicle.

Costoclavicular Maneuver (kōs″tō-klah-vik′u-lar/mah-noo′ver) (n.) A clinical technique used in the evaluation of neurovascular compression in the thoracic outlet syndrome. Instruct the patient, sitting upright, to thrust the shoulders backward while the hands rest on the thighs. This movement narrows the space between the clavicle and first rib. In a positive test, this maneuver reproduces the patient's symptoms. See **Addson Test** and **Wright's Hyper Abduction Maneuver**.

Costophrenic Angle (kōs″tō-frēn′ik/ang′g′l) (n.) The angle formed by the ribs and diaphragm.

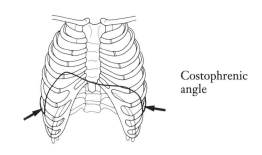

Costophrenic angle

Costotransversectomy (kōs″tō-trans″ver-sek′tō-mē) (n.) A technique for a lateral approach to the thoracic spine in which the transverse process and the posterior extent of the rib at the same level are resected. It is useful for the excision of predominantly laterally herniated thoracic discs and in the evacuation of paravertebral abscesses in this region.

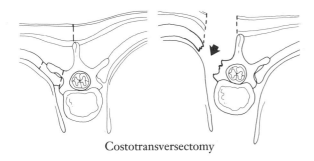

Costotransversectomy

Costovertebral (kōs″tō-ver′te-bral) (adj.) Of or pertaining to the ribs and vertebrae.

Costovertebral Angle (kōs″tō-ver′te-bral/ang′g′l) (n.) Angle formed by the articulation of the ribs with the bodies of the thoracic vertebrae.

Cotrel Cast (kō′-trel/kast) (n.) A technique for application of a body cast during cephalopelvic traction while the patient is suspended by derotation slings applied to the outside of the cast. It was developed for the treatment of scoliosis by Cotrel and others in France. Also called **EDF cast**, for Elongation, Derotation, and (lateral) Flexion.

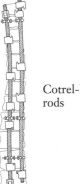

Cotrel-Dubousset rods

Cotrel-Dubousset System (kō′-trel/du-bōsēy/sys′tem) (n.) Stainless steel rods, hooks, and screws used for internal fixation and segmental treatment of scoliosis, dorsum rotundum, and spinal fractures. Distraction, compression, and derotation forces can be applied over a length of the spine. A spinal fusion that spans the distance from the uppermost to the lowermost hook or screw usually accompanies this form of spinal fusion. Abbreviated **CD**.

Cotrel Dynamic Traction (kō′-trel/dī-nam′ik/trak′shun) (n.) Traction involving the application of a head halter, pelvic apparatus, and foot stirrups to allow for preoperative stretching of paraspinal tissues in spinal curvature, especially scoliosis. Surgical correction may then be carried out with less po-

tential damage to the nervous system. Traction is usually applied 7 to 10 days preoperatively.

Cotton's Fracture (kot′nz/frak′chur) (n.) An eponym for a **trimalleolar fracture** of the ankle.

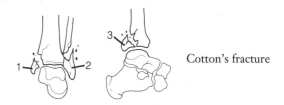

Cotton's fracture

Cough Fracture (kawf/frak′chur) (n.) A common name for bilateral fractures of the axillary segments of the sixth to ninth ribs. These fractures are usually nondisplaced and are so called because they may result from violent coughing in patients with osteopenic bone.

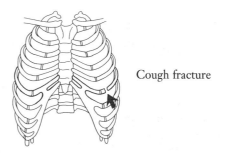

Cough fracture

Coumadin (koo′mah-din) (n.) An oral anticoagulation agent generically called **Warfarin**.

Counter (kown′ter) (n.) In shoe terminology, rigid reinforcement that preserves the shape of the shoe in the area of the anatomic heel. The long counter on the medial longitudinal arch area forms the basic design for the orthopaedic shoe through its extension to the navicular area.

Counterextension (kown″ter-eks-ten′shun) (n.) A technique consisting of traction on one part of the limb while the remainder of the limb is held steady.

Counterpressure (kown″ter-presh′ur) (n.) Manipulation to counterbalance pressure by the exercise of force in the opposite direction.

Countertraction (kown″ter-trak-shun) (n.) The use of a balancing opposing force during traction. A strong, continuous pull may be applied to a limb to maintain fracture alignment. A more sudden application of opposing traction forces is used for immediate fracture reduction.

Couple (kup′l) (n.) In biomechanics, a pair of equal and opposite parallel forces acting on a body and separated by a distance. The moment, or torque, of a couple is defined as a quantity equal to the product of one of the forces and the perpendicular distance between the forces. Also known as a **Force Couple**.

Coxa (kok′sah) (n.)   Hip or hip joint.

Coxa Magna (kok′sah/mag′nah) (n.)   An older term for osteoarthritis of the hip where osteophyte formation and loss of joint space result in an apparently enlarged femoral head. See **Femoral Head Size**.

Coxa Plana (kok′sah/plā′nah) (n.)   Literally, flat hip, referring to femoral head shape. See **Legg-Calvé Perthes Disease**.

Coxa Senilis (kok′sah/se′nil-is) (n.)   Descriptive term for degenerative hip disease concomitant with old age.

Coxa Valga (kok′sah/val′gah) (n.)   Hip deformity in which the femoral neck–shaft angle is increased. This position may contribute to instability of the femoral head in the acetabulum.

Coxa Vara (kok′sah/va′ra) (n.)   Hip deformity in which the femoral neck–shaft angle is reduced. It usually results in shortening of the affected limb. It may be a congenital anomaly, occurring as an isolated deformity or in association with femoral bowing, proximal femoral focal deficiency, or other congenital limb deficiency. It may be seen in association with other systemic congenital disorders, or it may be an acquired deformity.

Coxalgia (kok-sal′je-ah) (n.)   Pain in the hip.

Coxarthropathy (koks″ar-throp′ah-thē) (n.)   Any disease of the hip joint.

Coxarthrosis (koks-ar-thrō′sis) (n.)   Degenerative joint disease of the hip.

Cozen's Test (ko-zenz/test) (n.)   1. A variation of the sciatic stretch test. With the patient lying supine on the examining table, instruct him to sit up. When the patient attempts this, use pressure to keep the knees extended against the table, and give him some assistance in coming to the seated position. A patient with a normal spine can sit erect easily and flex forward at his hips. When sciatic pain and unilateral spinal muscle spasm are present, the patient will not be able to come to the erect position without flexing the knee on the affected side. Also known as the **Straight-leg Sitting Test**. 2. A maneuver used in the evaluation of lateral epicondylitis. Instruct the patient to clench the fist and dorsiflex the wrist. The examiner applies a flexing force opposing the dorsiflexion force of the patient. If positive, the characteristic pain is reproduced in the region of the lateral epicondyle.

CP   Abbreviation for **Cerebral Palsy**.

CPK   Abbreviation for **Creatinine Phosphokinase**.

CPM   Abbreviation for **Continuous Passive Motion**.

CPO   Abbreviation for **Certified Prosthetist and Orthotist**.

CPR   Abbreviation for **Cardiopulmonary Resuscitation**.

CPT   Abbreviation for **Current Procedural Terminology**.

Crab Cane (krab/kān) (n.)   Cane with three or more tips.

Crab Crutch (krab/kruch) (n.)   A crutch with three or more tips.

Craig Needle (krāg/nēd′l) (n.)   A needle used for obtaining biopsies of tissues, including bone. It consists of a guide, a cannula, and a sharp cutting needle to obtain a specimen. Most frequently used on the spine.

Craig Splint (krāg/splint) (n.)   A modification of the Ilfeld splint used in the treatment of Legg-Calvé-Perthes disease.

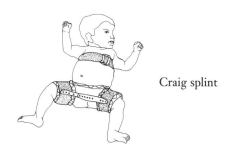

Craig splint

Cram Bowstring Test (kram/bō′string/test) (n.)   A clinical test used to indicate the presence of lumbar radiculopathy. With the patient supine, passively flex the hip with the knee fully extended to raise the leg in a straight position, first on the affected side and then on the opposite side. When the limb has been raised to the point of pain, flex the knee 20° and then raise the limb farther to a point just short of that which again causes pain. Then, apply firm pressure over the posterior tibial nerve in the popliteal space. In a positive test, this pressure will cause a sharp pain in the lower lumbar region or in the affected buttock. In the sound limb, the test causes no pain at all or causes pain in the lumbar region or in the opposite buttock. The mild local tenderness of a normal posterior tibial nerve is overshadowed by the gluteal pain when the sign is positive. Also called **Bowstring Test**.

Cramer Wire Splint (kra′mer/wīr/splint) (n.)   A conventional, flexible splint used for the emergency immobilization of an injured extremity. It consists of two stout parallel wires with fine crosswires, resembling a ladder.

Cramp (kramp) (n.)   A painful muscular contraction or spasm resulting from a disturbance within the peripheral neuromuscular system. Electromyographically, a cramp is characterized by large numbers of motor units firing synchronously and spontaneously at high frequency. Cramps tend to occur in response to a strong contraction of an already shortened muscle and are relieved by maneuvers that stretch the affected muscle. The exact cause of cramping is not known, but cramps are frequently associated with fatigue, salt deprivation, or other electrolyte imbalances.

Cranial Nerves (kra′nē-al/nervz) (n.) The 12 pairs of nerves that arise directly from the brain and leave the skull through separate apertures. The cranial nerves are assigned the following Roman numbers and names:

I, olfactory nerve; II, optic nerve; III, oculomotor nerve; IV, trochlear nerve; V, trigeminal nerve; VI, abducens nerve; VII, facial nerve; VIII, vestibulocochlear nerve; IX, glossopharyngeal nerve; X, vagus nerve; XI, accessory nerve; XII, hypoglossal nerve.

Creatinine-Height Index (kre-at′i-nin/hīt/in′deks) (n.) An index of skeletal muscle catabolism. It is measured as the urinary creatinine excretion for 24 hours, divided by the expected creatinine excretion in a normal adult of the same height.

Creatinine Phosphokinase (kre-at′ĭ-nin/fos-fō-kī′ nās) (n.) An enzyme that catalyzes the transfer of phosphate groups from phosphocreatine to ADP to form creatine and ATP. This reaction is important in muscle contraction; thus this enzyme is present in high levels in muscle mass. Elevation of serum CPK levels occurs following muscle injury, and isoenzyme measurements are required to differentiate skeletal muscle CPK from myocardial or other types. More commonly known by its abbreviation, **CPK**.

Creep (krēp) (n.) In biomechanics, a term for time-dependent stress-strain behavior.

Creeping Substitution (krēp′ing/sub″sti-tū′shun) (n.) The method by which avascular cortical bone grafts are incorporated. In this process, osteoclasts resorb the graft, bringing in granulation tissue and osteoblasts to lay down new bone, using the graft material as a scaffolding.

Crepitus (krep′i-tus) (n.) The audible or palpable transmitted grating or crackling sensation of bone or cartilage rubbing on bone or on each other.

Crescent Sign (kres′ent/sīn) (n.) 1. A radiographic sign of cubitus varus deformity seen on a lateral view of the elbow. In this deformity, part of the ulnar overlies the distal humeral epiphysis, producing a crescent sign. 2. See **Caffey's Sign**.

Crest (krest) (n.) 1. A sharp ridge, as occurs on bone. For example, the tibial crest along its subcutaneous border. 2. The surface along the outermost edge of a screw thread. 3. In shoe terminology, a ridge or prominence. For example, a cushion or filling in the space under the phalanges.

CREST Syndrome (krest/sin′drōm) (n.) An acronym for a form of systemic sclerosis with prominent Calcinosis, Raynaud's phenomenon, Esophageal dysfunction, Sclerodactyly, and Telangiectasia.

Crevice Corrosion (krev′is/ko-rō′zhun) (n.) A type of corrosion that occurs locally if there are differences in oxygen tension or pH changes in a confined space, resulting in an accelerated local corrosion reaction. One example is that occurring in the area between a bone screwhead and plate. Stainless steel is susceptible to crevice corrosion with cobalt. Chrome and titanium generally are not.

Cricoid Cartilage (krī′koid/kar′ti-lij) (n.) A partially ossified, ringlike cartilage that forms the lower part of the larynx.

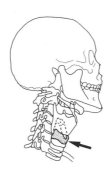

Cricoid cartilage

Critical Area of Pulleys (krit′i-kl/a′rē-ah/of/pul-ēz) (n.) The flexor zone of the hand, known as Zone II, between the distal palmar crease and the insertion of the sublimus tendon. In this zone, both the flexor digitorum profundus and flexor digitorum sublimus tendons run in the flexor tendon sheath. Also known as "**No-Man's Land**." See **Flexor Zones of the Hand**.

Cross-Finger Flap (kros/fing′ger/flap) (n.) A technique of local flap grafting most useful for coverage of a volar surface defect of one finger with a laterally based pedicle flap from the dorsum of an adjacent finger.

Cross-Infection (kros/in-fek′shun) (n.) Infection contracted by a patient from another patient or staff member, and/or contracted by a staff member from a patient.

Cross-Leg Flap (kros/leg/flap) (n.) A type of flap graft used for soft tissue coverage in lower extremity defects. Owing to the potential morbidity of the previously well leg and to advancements in microsurgical techniques, this technique is not commonly used today.

Cross-legged Gait (kros-leg′ged/gāt) (n.) See **Scissors Gait**.

Cross-Over Test (kros/o′ver/test) (n.) A clinical procedure used to document anterior cruciate ligament instability. With the patient standing, immobilize the affected extremity on the ground by standing on the patient's foot. Then instruct him or her to rotate his or her upper body, crossing the unaffected leg over the fixed foot until he or she faces approximately 90° in the opposite direction. In a positive test, this will result in discomfort and a sense of the knee "wanting to go out" of place.

Cross-Shaped (kros/shāp′d) (adj.) A description of the X-shaped, or cruciate, screws.

Crouch Gait (krowch/gāt) (n.) Gait with exaggerated flexion of the hips and knees. May often be seen in spastic paraplegia (e.g., in cerebral palsy).

Crouch Position (krowch/po-zish′un) (n.) Position of stooping, or low bending, of the trunk and flexion of the hips, with the feet on the ground. The knees are only partly flexed in contrast to a squat, where the knees are completely flexed.

Crown (krown) (n.) In shoe terminology, the lateral curvature of the bottom of the last.

Crucial Angle (kroo′shal/ang′g′l) (n.) An angle formed between the posterior and middle calcaneal facets. The lateral process of the talus is situated just superior to this angle. It is measured on a lateral radiograph of the foot. Also known as the **Crucial Angle of Gissane**.

Cruciate Ligament (kroo′she-āt/lig′ah-ment) (n.) Any paired set of ligaments that cross over each other, forming an "X." Usually, this term is used to refer to the anterior and posterior cruciate ligaments of the knee. Other examples are the cruciate ligaments of the occipitoaxial joint.

Cruciate Ligament, Anterior (kroo′she-āt/lig′ah-ment/an-ter′ē-or) (n.) A ligament that acts as the primary stabilizer to anterior translation of the tibia on the femur. It courses from the posterior aspect of the medial surface of the lateral femoral condyle to an area on the proximal tibial surface, just anterior and lateral to the anterior tibial spine. Abbreviated **ACL**. See **Anterior Cruciate Ligament**.

Cruciate Ligament, Posterior (kroo′she-āt/lig′ah-ment/pos-ter′e-or) (n.) A ligament that acts as the primary stabilizer to posterior translation of the tibia on the femur. It courses from the posterior aspect of the lateral surface of the medial femoral condyle to a depression in the posterior aspect of tibia, just behind the proximal articular surface. Abbreviated **PCL**. See **Posterior Cruciate Ligament**.

Crural Fascia (kroōr′al/fash′ē-ah) (n.) The superficial investing fascia of the leg.

Crush Fracture (krush/frak′chur) (n.) A type of comminuted fracture seen in a distal phalanx, so named for the mechanism of injury in which the finger is crushed in a door or between heavy objects.

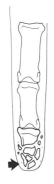

Crush fracture

Crush Syndrome (krush/sin′drōm) (n.) A severe, sometimes fatal condition that follows a severe crushing injury, particularly one involving large muscle masses. Owing to extensive soft tissue damage, it is characterized by extensive fluid and blood loss in the injured part with resultant hypovolemic shock, hematuria, myoglobinuria, renal tubular necrosis, and renal failure. Also known as **Compression Syndrome** or **Bywaters' Syndrome**.

Crust (krust) (n.) A mass of dried exudate.

Crutches (kruch-es) (n.) An ambulation aid composed of wood or metal with a single rubberized tip distally and a variable shape proximally.

Crutch Paralysis (kruch/pah-ral′i-sis) (n.) Paralysis due to excessive pressure on the brachial plexus caused by the axillary piece of a crutch.

Crutchfield Tongs (kruch-fēld/tongs) (n.) Hinged, metal tongs, whose points engage the parietal bone of the skull. They are used to provide cervical traction in the treatment of fractures and fracture-dislocations of the cervical spine and to form intraoperative neck stabilization.

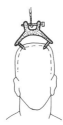

Crutchfield tongs

Cryosurgery (krī″o-sur′jer-ē) (n.) The destruction of tissue by application of extreme cold. Also known as **cold cautery**.

Cryptococcus Neoformans (krip″to-kok′us/ne″o-for′mans) (n.) A fungus that causes cryptococcosis. It may be introduced into the skin, causing local lesions, or it may be inhaled, producing pulmonary infection. Less often, it may cause granulomatous bone lesions, endocarditis, and various visceral lesions.

Crystal (kris′tal) (n.) A solid with characteristic, regular shapes and angles for a given compound that forms after freezing or precipitation out of solution.

Crystalline Arthropathy (kris′tah-līn/ar-throp′ah-thē) (n.) Any joint disease that results from the deposition of crystals within the joint. The diagnosis is made by the recognition of crystals in the synovial fluid, which can be identified by polarized light microscopy. Crystals can be differentiated by their characteristic appearance. Examples include urate crystal deposition, causing gout, and calcium pyrophosphate dihydrate crystals, resulting in pseudogout.

C & S Abbreviation for culture and sensitivity.

CSF Abbreviation for cerebrospinal fluid.

C-Spine (C-spīn) (n.) Abbreviation for cervical spine.

CT Scan (CT-skan) (n.) Abbreviation for computerized axial tomographic study.

Cuban Heel (kū-ban/hēl) (n.) In shoe terminology, a broad, high heel. It is higher than the heel of an Oxford shoe, approximately 3 to 5 cm, but less broad. Usually used only in women's shoes, the Cuban heel is still large and low enough to admit a standard ankle-foot orthosis.

Cubital Fossa. See Antecubital Fossa.

Cubital Tunnel Syndrome (ku'bī-tal/tun'el/sin' drōm) (n.) A compression neuropathy of the ulnar nerve at the elbow. The entrapment may occur at the groove posterior to the medial epicondyle, at the area where the nerve passes between the two heads of the flexor carpi ulnaris muscle, at the arcade of Struthers or by a supracondylar process, if present. The diagnosis may be clarified by electromyography and nerve conduction velocity studies.

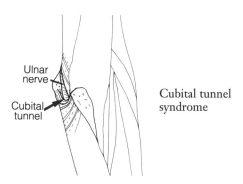

Ulnar nerve

Cubital tunnel

Cubital tunnel syndrome

Cubitus Valgus (ku'bi-tus/val'gus) (n.) An abnormal increase in the carrying angle or usual valgus inclination of the extended elbow. See **Carrying Angle.**

Cubitus Varus (ku'bi-tus/va'rus) (n.) A decrease, or reversal, of the normal carrying angle of the elbow. Also known as a **Gun Stock Deformity.** It may occur after a supracondylar fracture.

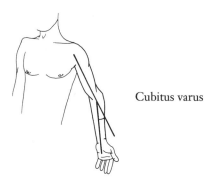

Cubitus varus

Cuboid (ku'boid) (n.) One of the tarsal bones. It is found on the lateral side of the foot between the anterior aspect of the calcaneus and the basis of the fourth and fifth metatarsals.

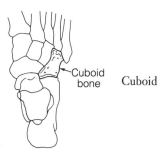

Cuboid bone   Cuboid

Cuboid Sign (ku'boid/sīn) (n.) On the anteroposterior radiograph view of the foot, an inverted "cuboid sign" shows that the nuclear center of the cuboid falls medial and inferior to the midcalcaneal long-axis line. On the lateral view, an everted "cuboid sign" demonstrates that the nuclear center is located lateral and superior to the midcalcaneal long-axis line. As noted, a normal "cuboid sign" shows no deformity in either view, with the nuclear center of the cuboid positioned on the midcalcaneal long-axis line.

Cuboides Secundarium (ku'boid es/sek'un-der"ium) (n.) An inconsistent accessory bone of the foot. It appears as a large ossicle on the plantar and medial aspect of the cuboid, articulating with the navicular. Also called **Secondary Cuboid.**

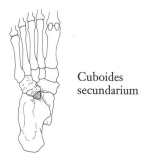

Cuboides secundarium

Cuff (kuf) (n.) Colloquiallism for **Rotator Cuff.**

Cuff-Tear Arthropathy (kuf/tār/ar-throp'ah-thē) (n.) Degenerative changes of the shoulder joint that result from a massive, untreated rotator cuff tear.

Culture (kul-tūr) (n.) A population of microorganisms cultivated in a medium.

Cumulative Dose (ku'mu-la"tiv/dōs) (n.) A term used in radiation medicine to describe the total dose resulting from repeated exposure of the same region or of the whole body to radiation.

Cuneiform (ku-nē'i-form) (n.) One of three wedge-shaped tarsal bones on the medial aspect of the foot. Proximally, each bone articulates with the tarsal navicular. Distally, each bone articulates with the first, second, or third metatarsal base to form the tarsometatarsal joints. There are also articular surfaces between the adjacent cuneiforms and between the lateral cuneiform and the cuboid. They are named by their location as medial, middle (or intermediate), or lateral.

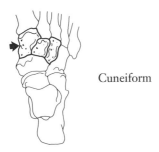

Cuneiform

Cuneiform Osteotomy (ku-nē′i-form/os″te-ot′ō-mē) (n.) 1. Any osteotomy in which a wedge of bone is removed. 2. An osteotomy of one or more of the cuneiforms.

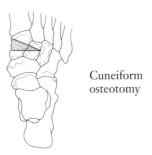

Cuneiform osteotomy

Cuneonavicular Joint (ku″ne-o-nah-vik′u-lar′/joint) (n.) The joint in the foot between the cuneiform bones and the navicular bone.

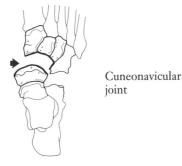

Cuneonavicular joint

Cup (kup) (n.) A familiar term for the acetabulum component of a total hip arthroplasty.

Cup Arthroplasty (kup/ar′thro-plas″tē) (n.) Remodeling of the femoral head and acetabulum via the insertion of a metal cup; this procedure has been supplanted by total hip and resurfacing procedures. The most common cups used were Aufranc, Crawford-Adams, and Smith-Petersen.

Curettage (ku″re-tahzh′) (n.) The removal of material from the walls of cavities and other surfaces by scraping with a curette.

Curette (ku-ret′) (n.) A spoon, ring, or looped surgical instrument with sharp edges used to remove material from the walls of cavities and other surfaces by scraping.

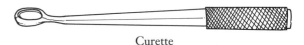

Curette

Curie (ku′re) (n.) A unit of measure of radioactivity. One curie is defined as the amount of radioactivity emitted by 1 g of radium^{226}. Abbreviated **Ci**.

Curvature (kur′vah-tūr) (n.) A bending.

Curve (kurv) (n.) 1. A continuous bend. 2. A colloquial term for a spinal curvature. 3. A graphic representation of measurement over time, for example, a temperature curve, created by a linear connection of regular temperature measurements.

Current Procedural Terminology (ker′ent/prose′jur al/ter″mĭ-nol′o-je) (n.) A copyrighted system of terminology and coding developed by The American Medical Association (AMA) used for describing, coding, and reporting medical services and procedures. Abbreviated **CPT**. See **ICD-9-CM**.

Cushing's Syndrome (kush′ingz/sin′drōm) (n.) A systemic disorder resulting from inappropriately elevated levels of glucocorticoids. Endogenous causes include excessive ACTH secretion from pituitary or occasionally, nonpituitary neoplasms or from excessive secretion of corticosteroids in adrenal hyperplasia or tumor. It can be caused by exogenous administration of ACTH or steroids. Clinical characteristics include truncal and facial adiposity, purple cutaneous striae, osteoporosis, hypertension, diabetes mellitus, weakness, and personality changes.

Custodial Care (kus-tō′dē-al/kār) (n.) Provision of board, room, and other nonmedical personal assistance to a physically and/or mentally incapacitated individual, generally on a long-term basis.

Custom Molded Shoe (kus′tom/mōld-ed/shoo) (n.) A shoe made from a cast of the foot, thereby conforming to any and all of the deformities of that foot. Also called *space shoes*.

Cutaneous (kū-tā′nē-us) (adj.) Of or pertaining to the skin.

Cutaneous Axon Reflex (kū-tā′nē-us/ak′son/rē′fleks) (n.) A reflex used to differentiate preganglionic intraspinal lesions from postganglionic extraspinal lesions. It is elicited by placing a drop of histamine on the skin along the cutaneous distribution of the nerve to be tested. If the skin is then scratched in this region, a normal response of vasodilatation, wheal formation, and flare is seen. A negative axonal response is suggested by the absence of a flare and implies that the injury is distal to the ganglion.

Cutaneous Flap (kū-tā′nē-us/flap) (n.) Any local, remote, or free-tissue flap composed of a vascularized cutaneous segment for coverage of soft-tissue defects.

Cutaneous Nodules (kū-tā′nē-us/nod′ūlz) (n.) Dermal neurofibromas seen in adults or adolescents with neurofibromatosis. Also known as **Fibroma Molluscum**.

CVA Abbreviation for cerebrovascular accident.

Cyanosis (si″ah-no′sis) (n.) A bluish discoloration of the skin and mucous membranes resulting from an inadequate level of oxygen in the blood.

Cybex Machines (sī′-beks/ma-shēnz′) (n.) The proprietary name for an isokinetic exercise machine. It allows the performance of reciprocal concentric contractors throughout the full range of motion, thereby encouraging simultaneous strengthening and coordination of reciprocal muscle groups at a wide range of speeds. The incorporation of a dual channel recorder—dynamometer and electrogoniometer—provides a continuous print-out curve of the range of joint angles and peak torque across the entire range of motion of the limb being tested. This system can generate torque-motion curves and allow the calculation of total work performed and power scores for different muscle groups.

Cylinder Cast (sil′in-der/kast) (n.) A circular cast used for immobilization in a number of injuries about the knee joint. It extends from just above the ankle to the proximal thigh.

Cyst (sist) (n.) An abnormal, closed, epithelium-line sac or cavity containing a liquid or semisolid substance. See also specific cysts.

Cystinosis (sis″ti-nō′sis) (n.) A rare, inherited metabolic disorder characterized by accumulation of free cystine in tissues. This disease must be considered in the differential diagnosis of any child with vitamin D-resistant rickets, the Fanconi syndrome, or glomerular insufficiency.

Cytolysis (si-tol′i-sis) (n.) Dissolution or disintegration of a cell.

Cytoplasm (sī′tō-plazm″) (n.) The protoplasm of a cell between its membrane and nucleus.

Cytosine (sī′tō-sēn) (n.) A nitrogen base present in nucleotides and nucleic acids.

D

D-Spine (d-spīn) (n.) Abbreviation, refers to the dorsal or thoracic spine.

Dactyl (dak′til) (n.) A digit of the hand or foot (i.e., a finger or toe).

Dactylitis (dak″ti-lī′tis) (n.) 1. An inflammatory condition of the digits. Seen diffusely in sickle cell disease, it can be confused with an infectious process. 2. Tuberculous dactylitis is also known as **spina ventosa**.

Dakin's Solution (dā′kinz/so-lū′shun) (n.) A solution for cleansing wounds composed of sodium hypochlorite and sodium bicarbonate.

Dalton (dawl-tun) (n.) A unit of weight equal to 1/12th the weight of 1 atom of carbon.

Damping (damp′ing) (n.) The dissipation of mechanical energy.

Dancer Pad (dans′er/pad) (n.) In footwear, a relatively thick metatarsal pad that reaches across the entire width of the sole. Also called **Buttons.**

Dark-Field Microscopy (dark/fēld/mi-kros′kō-pē) (n.) A type of microscopic examination. The microscopic field is dark; a peripheral light source brightly illuminates objects such as organisms (e.g., spirochetes).

Darrach Procedure (da′rak/pro-sē′jur) (n.) A surgical technique for the resection of the distal end of the ulna. It can be used for improving the function of the wrist after malunion of a Colles' fracture.

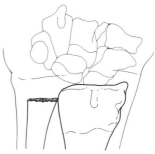

Darrach procedure

Darvon (dar′von) (n.) The proprietary name for a preparation of propoxyphene hydrochloride, an analgesic drug.

Dashboard Fracture (dash′bōrd/frak′chur) (n.) A fracture of the posterior wall of the acetabulum, resulting from a posterior dislocation of the femoral head secondary to forces propagated up the shaft of the femur after striking the flexed knee against the dashboard in a collision. A dislocation without an acetabular fracture is known as a dashboard dislocation. Patellar fractures can also result from dashboard impact.

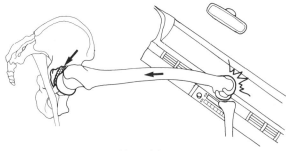

Dashboard fracture

Davis Law (da′vis/law) (n.) A principal which states that ligaments, or any soft tissue, when put under even a moderate degree of unremitting tension, will elongate by the addition of new material. Conversely, when ligaments or other soft tissues remain constantly in a loose or lax state, they will gradually shorten.

Dawbarn's Sign (daw′-barnz sīn) (n.) A sign for subdeltoid bursitis. Tenderness present when the bursa is palpated with the patient's arm by his/her side disappears when the arm is abducted to a right angle.

Daypro (da/pro) (n.) A proprietary brand of Oxaprozim, a nonsteroidal antiinflammatory drug.

DCP Abbreviation for **Dynamic Compression Plate.**

DCS Abbreviation for **Dynamic Condylar Screw.**

DEA Abbreviation for **Drug Enforcement Agency.**

Dead-Arm Syndrome (ded-arm/sin′drōm) (n.) A clinical syndrome associated with recurrent transient anterior subluxation of the shoulder in which the patient experiences episodic pain described as "paralyzing." This pain is accompanied by a feeling of "lameness" brought on by abduction and external rotation of the humerus.

Dead Space (ded/spās) (n.) A cavity that remains after the closure of a wound, leaving a potential area in which fluid or blood can collect.

Debridement (da-brēd-ment′) (n.) The cleansing of wounds by surgical removal of devitalized and contaminated tissue and foreign matter, evacuation of hematoma, and the provision of adequate drainage.

Debris (dĕ-bre′) (n.) Contaminated, devitalized tissue, fragments, and/or foreign matter.

Decalcification (de″kal-si-fi-kā′shun) (n.) The loss or process of removal of calcium salts from a bone or tooth.

Declination Angle (dek″li-nā′shun/ang′g′l) (n.) The angle occurring between the plane of the femoral condyles and the axis of the femoral neck. It is also called a **torsion** or **declination angle of the femur.** See **Anteversion** and **Retroversion**.

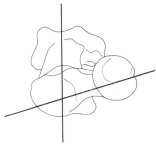

Declination angle

Decompression (de″kom-presh′un) (n.) The reduction of pressure within or exerted on an organ or part of the body by surgical intervention. An example of this is the decompression of a nerve root by discectomy.

Decreased Radiographic Density (dē-krēs′d/rà″de-o-graf′ik/den′si-tē) (n.) A quality of radiographic appearance. Materials with less density or thickness are more easily penetrated by x-ray, which produces, in roentgenography, a darker or grayer area on the film. This may reflect as either increased radiolucency of the photographed structure or increased radiodensity of the surrounding tissues.

Decubitus Position (de-kū′bi-tus/pō-zish′un) (n.) A recumbent or horizontal position or posture. To determine decubitus position, lay a patient down horizontally. Whichever aspect of the body touches the surface is considered decubitus position. For example, left or right lateral decubitus designates lying on the left or right side; dorsal decubitus designates lying on the back (supine); and ventral decubitus designates lying face down (prone).

Decubitus Ulcer (de-kū′bi-tus/ul′ser) (n.) An ulcer that forms in an area where skin tissue has been destroyed and where there is a progressive destruction of the underlying tissue resulting from prolonged, unrelieved pressure in a decubitus position. It is usually caused by local interference with the circulation and typically occurs in regions of bony prominence, such as the sacrum, heel, and trochanters. Also called a **Pressure Sore** or **Bedsore.**

Dedifferentiation (dē-dif″er-en″she-ā′shun) (n.) A process of change toward a more primitive, embryonic, or earlier state. Examples of dedifferentiation include when a highly specialized cell becomes a less specialized cell or when tumor cells differentiate into the highly malignant and aggressive cells seen in chondrosarcoma.

Deep Infrapatellar Bursa See **Infrapatellar Bursa, Deep.**

Deep Palmar Arch (dēp/pal′mar/arch) (n.) In the

palm, the confluence of a branch of the radial artery with the deep palmar branch of the ulnar artery.

Deep Palmar Space (dēp/pal′mar/spās) (n.) A potential space that lies between the fascia covering the matacarpals and their contiguous muscles and the fascia beneath the flexor tendons. Its ulnar border is the fascia of the hypothenar muscles, and its radial border is the fascia of the abductor and other thenar muscles. The deep palmar space is divided into a central compartment, a hypothenar compartment, and a thenar compartment.

Deep Posterior Compartment (dēp/pōs-tēr′e-or/com-part′ment) (n.) One of four fascial compartments of the lower leg, which contains the deep flexor muscles of the leg (flexor digitorum longus, flexor hallucis longus, tibialis posterior), the posterior tibial artery and veins, the tibial nerve, and the peroneal artery and veins. See **Compartment Syndome.**

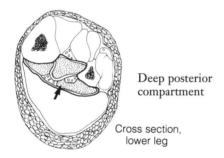

Deep posterior compartment

Cross section, lower leg

Deep Tendon Reflex (dēp/ten′dun/rē′fleks) (n.) See **Muscle-Stretch Reflex.** Abbreviated **DTR.**

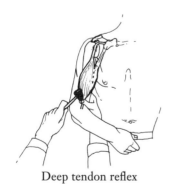

Deep tendon reflex

Deformation (dē′for-ma′shun) (n.) 1. Malformation, abnormality, or alteration that may be congenital or acquired. 2. A term used in biomechanics to define a structural property that is the effect of a load in a known direction placed upon that structure. These measurements are then plotted on a graph, which is known as a **deformation curve**.

Degeneration (dē-jen″er-a′shun) (n.) 1. The deterioration of the cells of a tissue or organ by alteration or chemical change of the tissue. This differs from

infiltration, which is the deposition of abnormal matter in the tissue. 2. A worsening of physical or mental qualities, a deterioration.

Degenerative Arthritis (dē-jen′er-a-tiv/ar-thrī′tis) (n.) See **Osteoarthritis, Degenerative Joint Disease.**

Degenerative Disk Disease (dē-jen′er-a-tiv/disk/dǐ-zēz′) (n.) A condition in which an intervertebral disk loses its normal structural integrity as a result of wear and tear, acute or repeated injuries, or aging. Secondary effects may be disk space narrowing, formation of osteophytes, disk bulging, or herniation. All of these may or may not be associated with clinical signs and symptoms.

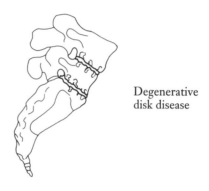

Degenerative disk disease

Degenerative Disease (dē-jen-′er-a-tiv/dǐ-zēz′) (n.) A disease not attributable to an external or internal cause, such as an infection or a metabolic defect. Characterized by the progressive impairment of the function of one or more organs. Examples are Alzheimer's disease or Parkinson's disease.

Degenerative Joint Disease (dē-jen′er-a-tiv/joint/di-zēz′) (n.) A chronic joint disease characterized pathologically by a degeneration of articular cartilage and hypertrophy of bone. It affects predominantly the weight-bearing joints and the distal interphalangeal joints of the fingers. It triggers no systemic symptoms. Synonyms: **Degenerative Arthritis, Hypertrophic Arthritis, Osteoarthritis.**

Degenerative Spondylolisthesis (dē-jen′er-a-tiv/

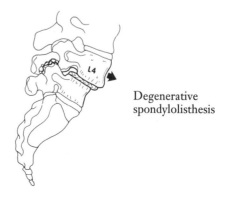

Degenerative spondylolisthesis

spon″di-lō-lis′thē-sis) (n.)   The anterior displacement of a vertebra arising from erosive, degenerative changes in the zygapophyseal joints. Newman first proposed the term to describe a type of spondylolisthesis that occurs as a result of a severe, localized degenerative arthritis and a remolding of the paired zygapophyseal (z-a) joints of the slipped vertebra and its subjacent vertebra. It was originally named pseudospondylolisthesis by Junghanns. Synonyms: **Spondylolisthesis with Intact Neural Arch, Articular Spondylolisthesis.**

Degloving Injury (dē-gluv′ing/in′ju-rē) (n.)   An injury of the hand or foot that characteristically results in avulsion of skin areas. The areas are stripped from their proximal attachment and are subjected to pressure abrasion and a variable amount of heat injury. The combination of interrupted proximal blood supply and tissue trauma in this injury frequently leads to irreparable damage to the soft tissues covering the bones, tendons, and joints of the hand. Treatment is dependent on the extent and location of the skin defect. Injury to a single digit is often the result of a violent avulsion of a ring.

Degrees of Freedom (de-grēz′of/frē-dom) (n.)   In a coordinate system, the number of independent coordinates required to completely specify the position of an object in space. It can be used to describe the motion of a body part—"the knee has 6 degrees of freedom."

Dehiscence (dē-hīs′ens) (n.)   A splitting or bursting open, such as the disruption of opposed surfaces of a surgical wound.

Dehydration (dē′hī-drā′shun) (n.)   The removal or reduction of water from the body or from a substance.

Déjerine's Sign (deh″zher-ēn/sīn) (n.)   A sign of radiculopathy manifested by an aggravation of radicular pain, brought on by sneezing, coughing, straining at stool, or other Valsalva maneuvers.

Déjerine-Sottas Disease (deh″zher-ēn/sot′tahz/di-zēz′) (n.)   A rare congenital, degenerative disease affecting the spine and cerebellum that results in both motor and sensory neuropathies. Biopsy reveals localized swelling of a peripheral nerve in an "onion bulb" pattern. The disease is transmitted as an autosomal recessive trait with an onset in infancy or early childhood. Symptoms include weakness, loss of tendon reflexes, diminished sensation, and distal muscle atrophy. Synonyms: **Familial Interstitial Hypertrophic Neuritis, Progressive Hypertrophic Interstitial Neuropathy.**

Delayed Hypersensitivity (de′lād/hi″per-sen′si-tiv″i-tē) (n.)   The cell-mediated response of a host to an antigen to which it has been previously exposed. The immunologic reaction occurs on exposure to the antigen and results in an inflammatory reaction sometimes apparent in the first few hours but normally appreciable in 24 to 48 hours.

Delayed Muscle Soreness (de′lād/mus′el/sōr′nes) (n.)   A distinct syndrome characterized by discomfort or pain in the skeletal muscles that occurs 24 to 72 hours after heavy exercise. Exercise requiring high intensity and high force production is more likely to result in soreness than low-intensity exercise requiring more endurance. Repetitive muscle stress in the eccentric contraction mode is also associated with a high incidence of soreness. Delayed muscle soreness normally increases in intensity during the first 24 hours after exercise, peaks from 24 to 72 hours, and subsides completely within 5 to 7 days. A transient weakness accompanies delayed muscle soreness, but long-term detrimental effects on performance are not found. Synonym: **Delayed-Onset Muscular Soreness (DOMS).**

Delayed Union (de′lād/ūn′yun) (n.)   A term that indicates it is taking longer than the average time for a given bone injury to heal. The average time for healing of a fracture depends on many variables. See Nonunion for comparison. Contrast with **Nonunion.**

Delbet Walking Cast (del-bā/wok′ing/kast) (n.)   A protective plaster device applied either during traction or at a later point in the fracture healing process. This cast is used in tibia fractures to allow weight-bearing as well as knee and ankle motion. It is made of a series of overlapping plaster splints molded for weight-bearing on the tibial condyles.

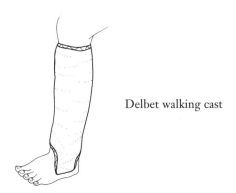

Delbet walking cast

DeLorme Exercises (de-lorm-ā/ek′ser-sīz′es) (n.)   A popular isotonic training program that improves concentric strength. It involves a system of progressive resistance exercises (PRE) in which the load to be lifted is progressively increased during each therapeutic session and over the course of treatment.

Delta Phalanx (del′tah/fā′lanks) (n.)   A triangular or trapezoidal phalanx with an abnormal epiphyseal plate. It results in unequal longitudinal growth and angular deformity.

Deltoid Ligament (del′toid/lig′ah-ment) (n.)   A strong ligament on the medial side of the ankle joint attached proximally to the medial malleolus. It expands distally to attach to the navicular tuberosity, os calcis, and talus.

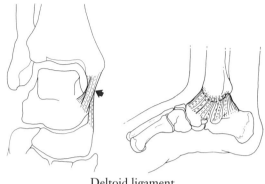

Deltoid ligament

Deltoid Muscle (del'toid/mus'el) (n.) See **Muscle**.

Demarcation Line (de″mar-kā'shun/līn) (n.) 1. A region delineating healthy from diseased tissue. 2. A discrete line separating two structures.

Demerol (dem'er-ol) (n.) The proprietary name for preparations of meperidine, a synthetic narcotic analgesic.

Demianoff's Sign (dem'-yan-offs/sīn) (n.) A sign used in the differentiation of lumbar pain. Place the patient in the dorsal decubitus position and lift extended leg. If "lumbago" is present, this position produces pain in the lumbar region, which is attributed to a stretching of the sacrolumbar muscles. This pain prevents the leg from being raised high enough to form an angle of 10° (or less) with the examining table.

Demineralization (de-min″er-al-i-zā'shun) (n.) The elimination of mineral or organic salts from the tissues of the body.

Demyelination (de-mī″e-li-nā'shun) (n.) 1. The loss of myelin from nerve sheets or tracks. 2. A disorder in which damage to the myelin sheath of a nerve results in impaired function of the nerve fibers normally supported by the myelin. Demyelination may be the primary disorder, as in multiple sclerosis, or it may occur after head injury or cerebral vascular accidents.

Denaturation (de-na″chur-ā'shun) (n.) An alteration of the physical properties and three-dimensional structure of a protein.

Dendrite (den'drīt) (n.) The filamentous or branching extension of a neuron that conducts nerve impulses from its free end toward the cell body. See **Axon** for comparison.

Denervation (de″ner-vā'shun) (n.) An interruption of a nerve's connection to a muscle or part. (EMG testing will show characteristic fibrillation potentials.)

Denial (de-nī'al) (n.) A defense mechanism used by someone who rejects certain aspects or interpretations of external reality, and who may substitute for that reality unrealistic and wishful feelings or idealizations.

Denis Browne Splint (den'is/brown/splint) (n.) An orthosis used for torsional abnormalities in the lower limbs. The splint consists of two plates or devices that can be securely attached to the soles of an infant's shoes and then connected to a cross bar. The foot-plates may be rotated on the cross bar to obtain the desired position of internal and external rotation. The length of the cross bar determines the degree of abduction. Synonym: **Bilateral Shoe Clamp Spreader Bar.**

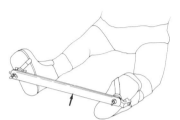

Denis Browne splint

Dens (dens) (n.) 1. The odontoid process of the axis. 2. A toothlike process projecting upward from the body of the second cervical vertebra that articulates with the anterior arch of the atlas. It acts as a pivot around which the atlas rotates.

Density (den'si-te) (n.) A descriptive term related to x-ray films and fluoroscopic screens. Increased density produces a lighter or whiter shadow on the x-ray film or a darker shadow on the fluoroscopic screen. Decreased density allows greater penetration by x-rays and produces a darker or blacker shadow on the x-ray film or a lighter one on the fluoroscopic screen.

Denver Bar (den'ver/bar) (n.) A variant of the metatarsal bar used to relieve pressure on the metatarsal heads. The wedge-shaped bar is usually attached to the outsole of the shoe. The apex of this arc coincides with the posterior edge under the posterior half of the metatarsal shafts. Also called a **Denver Heel**.

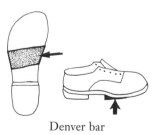

Denver bar

Deossification (dē-os″i-fi-kā'shun) (n.) Loss or removal of the mineral elements or constituents of bone.

Deoxidation (dē-ok″si-dā'shun) (n.) The removal of oxygen from a chemical compound.

Deoxyribonucleic Acid (dē-ok″sē-rī″bō-nū-kle′ik/ as′id) (n.) A macromolecule consisting of a double helix of paired nucleotides, the sequence of which constitutes the genetic code. Abbreviated **DNA**.

Depressed Fracture (de-prest′/frak′chur) (n.) A fracture in which fragments are driven inward, resulting in the depression of one surface of the bone fragment. It is seen frequently in fractures of skull and facial bones. This term also is used to describe intraarticular fractures, such as tibial plateau or skull fractures.

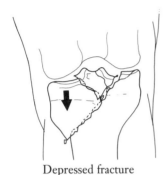

Depressed fracture

Depression (de-presh′un) (n.) A mental state characterized by excessive sadness.

Depressive Neurosis (de-pres′iv/nu-ro′sis) (n.) A psychologic disorder manifested by excessive depression, which is often due to an internal conflict or to an identifiable event, such as the loss of a love object.

Depth Gauge (depth/gāj) (n.) A measuring device used in orthopaedics to determine screw lengths. Insert the end of the gauge into the drilled hole and hook its angled tip over the distal bone cortex. Then advance the sleeve forward. Calibrations on the stem barrel indicate the correct screw length.

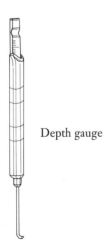

Depth gauge

De Quervain's Disease (de/kār′vanz/di-zēz′) (n.) A stenosing tenosynovitis of the first extensor compartment of the wrist that contains the conjoined tendons of the abductor pollicis longus and extensor pollicis brevis tendons. The disorder is characterized by pain and tenderness in the region of the radial styloid. The most common causes include occupational trauma, repeated hobby use, or use of the wrist in sports such as rowing and tennis. The condition typically occurs between the ages of 30 and 50 years, and women are affected 10 times more frequently than men. The diagnosis is confirmed by the Finkelstein test; pain with resisted thumb extension is also found. The disease is treated most commonly with ice, anti-inflammatory medications, and splinting of the extremity. Occasionally, localized injection of steroids may be required to control the process. A few patients may require surgical release of the first compartment. Synonym: **De Quervain's Stenosing Tenosynovitis**; **De Quervain's Syndrome**. See **Finkelstein Test**.

De Quervain's Fracture (de/kār′vanz/frak′chur) (n.) An eponym for a trans-scaphoid perilunate fracture dislocation.

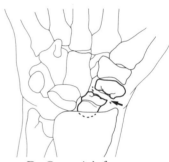

De Quervain's fracture

De Quervain's Stenosing Tenosynovitis (de/kār′vanz/ste-nō′sing/ten″o-sin″ō-vī′tis) (n.) See **De Quervain's Disease**.

Dermal Calcinosis (der′mal/kal″si-nō′sis) (n.) See **Calcinosis**.

Dermatomal Pain (der′ma-tōm′al/pān) (n.) A sharp, sometimes shooting, well-localized pain, arising in the distribution of a specific nerve root. Contrast to **Sclerotomal Pain**.

Dermatome (der′mah-tōm) (n.) 1. A surgical cutting instrument designed to excise split-thickness skin grafts. The thickness of the graft is calibrated by adjusting the depth gauge. The width of the graft is determined by the width of the cutting blade. The two general types are the oscillating blade type and the drum type. 2. The area of skin supplied by the fibers of a single spinal root. 3. An embryo that originates from the somites, giving rise to the dermal layers of the skin.

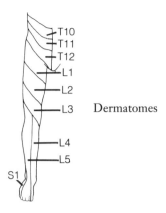

Dermatomes

Dermatomyositis (der″mah-to-mī″o-sī′tis) (n.) An inflammatory disorder of unknown etiology manifested by muscle weakness and often associated with muscle pain and tenderness. These symptoms are preceded or accompanied by a typical rash, in which skin changes usually include periorbital edema and heliotrope, periungual erythema, and scaling erythema over extensor surfaces.

Dermatophytes (der′mah-tō-fīts″) (n.) Fungi that invade and infect superficial skin.

Desault's Dislocations of the Wrist (de-sōz′/dis″lo-kā′shun/of/the/rist) (n.) A volar or palmar dislocation of the distal end of the radius. Volar subluxation is the most common; however, the dislocation or subluxation may be dorsal.

Desiccation (des″i-ka shun) (n.) The removal of water from a material. Commonly association of discs of the lumbar spine.

Desmo (des′mo) The word element for a ligament or fibrous connection.

Desmoid Tumor (des′moid/too′mor) (n.) A slow, progressive fibroblastic proliferation in the striated muscles of any part of the body.

Desmoplastic Fibroma (des″mo-plas′tik/fi-brō′mah) (n.) A rare, intraosseous, collagen-producing fibrous tumor that is characterized clinically by pain. Histologically, it is similar to other fibrous lesions, such as palmar fibromatosis. It is a benign lesion that does not metastasize but does tend to recur locally. The lesion is usually detected in young adults from the 2nd through the 4th decades. There is no significant sex predilection. The tumor occurs generally in a major long bone—the tibia is a common site—or in a flat bone, such as the pelvis. In a limb bone, the metaphyseal end is usually involved. Pathologically, numerous, usually small fibroblasts with oval nuclei are characteristic. Mitotic figures are absent. The cells may be aggregated in whorled bundles with considerable collagen production. Distinguishing desmoplastic fibroma from a low-grade fibrosarcoma is frequently difficult. Radiologic features include a characteristic, expanding lytic area with a wide zone of transition, which indicates an aggressive tumor.

Destot's Sign (des-tōz′/sīn) (n.) A sign seen in conjunction with pelvic fractures. A large hematoma that becomes superficial above the inguinal ligament or in the scrotum.

Detail (dē′tāl) (n.) In a radiograph, a clearness of the finer structures and visibility. Synonym: **Definition**.

Detritus (de-trī′tus) (n.) Particulate matter produced by or remaining after the wearing away or disintegration of a substance or tissue. It is seen pathologically in the synovium of neuropathic joints.

Deutschlander's Disease (doich′len-derz/di-zēz′) (n.) See **March Fracture** or **March Foot**.

Deviation (de″vē-ā′shun) (n.) In orthopaedics, the moving away from a starting position, which frequently denotes abduction or adduction relative to the midline or rotation from a starting point.

Device (de-vīs′) (n.) An instrument, apparatus, implement, machine, contrivance, implant, in vitro reagent, or other similar or related article, including any component, part, or accessory that is:

1. Recognized in the official National Formulary, the United States Pharmacopeia, or any supplements to these;

2. Intended for use in the diagnosis of disease or other conditions or in the cure, mitigation, treatment, or prevention of disease in humans or other animals; or

3. Intended to affect the structure of any function of the body of humans or other animals, without achieving any of its principal goals through chemical action or a dependence on metabolism.

Dextran (dek′stran) (n.) A polysaccharide (glucose polymer) formed outside the cell by the enzymatic action of certain microorganisms. Low-molecular weight dextran is used as a colloid solution, which effectively expands plasma volume, decreases blood viscosity, and increases microcirculatory flow.

Deyerle's Maneuver (dī-er-lēz/mah-noo′ver) (n.) A technique for the reduction of femoral neck fractures. With the patient on a fracture table, exert a strong downward pull on the lower extremity. The foot should be in a slight external rotation to achieve overreduction with respect to length. The foot is internally rotated until the femoral neck is parallel with the floor on the lateral x-ray. Reduction is then achieved in the anteroposterior and mediolateral planes. Apply direct pressure against the greater trochanter, holding the medial side of the knee with one hand while placing the other hand over the lateral side of the greater trochanter. This maneuver levers the neck underneath the head into a slight valgus deformity. Then place both hands just anterior to the greater trochanter and push directly backward toward the floor to move the head in an anatomic or slightly overreduced position in a lateral plane. Hold the pelvis firmly on the opposite side to prevent rotation. (The neck must be parallel with the floor in the lateral projection. If it is not, internally or externally rotate the foot far enough so that it is.) X-rays are then obtained to evaluate the reduction in AP and lateral projections.

Deyerle's Nail (dī-er-lēz/nāl) (n.)   A technique of multiple pin fixation for femoral neck fractures. A metal template is used; this holds the pins securely to the lateral femoral cortex and simultaneously allows the pins to slide.

Deyerle Sciatic Tension Test (dī-er-lē/sī-at'ik/ten'shun/test) (n.)   In sciatica, a test to differentiate the root compression syndrome from other causes of back and leg pain. Several types of test may be used:

1. With the patient seated, holding the back as straight as possible and sitting directly in line with no twist, passively extend the affected leg at the knee until the patient states that the leg pain or a portion of the pain is reproduced. Then lower the leg just below the point of pain. With the leg held clasped between your knees, press with the second and third fingers of both hands on the sciatic nerve in the popliteal space that has been "bowstringed" by this procedure. This maneuver may cause local discomfort, which should be overshadowed by the severe reproduction of the patient's sciatic pain.

2. With the patient seated on the side of the table in a normal position with the head straight, extend the leg slowly to a point at which the pain is reproduced or resistance is met. Then, dorsiflex the foot slightly and lock it between your legs. With both hands clasping the knee, exert firm pressure over the bowstringed popliteal nerve. Usually, this will either cause the patient to rock backward from the sitting position or reproduce his discomfort or pain. The test may be repeated with the patient's back arched and the chin on the chest to reproduce the discomfort. To reproduce the pressure on the stretched popliteal nerve, repeat with the patient flexed forward as far as possible, with the neck also flexed forward to a point of discomfort or tightness. Any test that causes backward motion tends to make the patient straighten up or complain of discomfort; this indicates nerve-root pressure in the lumbar spine region.

Diabetes Mellitus (dī''ah-bē'tēz/me-lī'tus) (n.)   A metabolic disease in which carbohydrate use is reduced. It is caused by a relative or absolute deficiency of insulin and is characterized by hyperglycemia. Chronic diabetes results in complications of neuropathy, retinopathy, nephropathy, and generalized small and large blood vessel disease.

Diagnosis (dī''ag-nō'sis) (n.)   1. A word or phrase used by a physician to identify a disease from which an individual patient suffers; 2. A condition for which the patient needs, seeks, or receives medical care; 3. The art and science of determining the nature and cause of a disease. 4. The identification of a disease process.

Diagnosis-Related Groups (dī''ag-nō'sis/rē-lā'ted/grōōps) (n.)   A classification system of patient illness in terms of expected lengths of hospital stays per group. A process in which direct cost data are grouped by the patient's diagnosis, treatment, and age. Commonly referred to as **DRG**.

Dial Osteotomy (dī-al/os''te-ot'ō-mē) (n.)   An acetabular osteotomy for a dysplastic hip in which the entire acetabulum is freed by osteotomy and redirected as a single segment of bone to cover the femoral head. It is indicated for the truly dysplastic hip in which the head is concentrically located but the CE angle is less than 15 to 20°.

Dialysis (di-al'i-sis) (n.)   The separation of solute molecules by differing rates of diffusion through a semipermeable membrane.

Diaphyseal Fracture (dī''ah-fiz'ē-al/frak'chur) (n.)   A fracture that involves the central shaft of a tubular long bone, such as the femur.

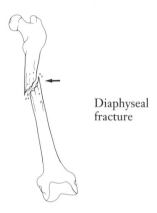

Diaphyseal fracture

Diaphyseal Aclasia (dī''ah-fiz'ē-al/ah-klā'ze-ah) (n.)   A hereditary abnormality of cartilage and bone growth, resulting in many osteocartilaginous outgrowths (exostoses) from the bones formed by endochondrial ossification. Bone growth may also be retarded, causing stunting and deformity. Synonyms: **Multiple Osteochondromatosis**, **Multiple Exostoses**, **Hereditary Multiple Exostoses**.

Diaphysis (dī-af'i-sis) (n.)   The central part of the shaft of a long, tubular bone; embryologically, it represents the primary ossification center. It is bounded by a metaphysis at either end.

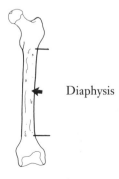

Diaphysis

Diarthrodial Cartilage (dī″ar-thrō′di-al/kar′ti-lij) (n.) Articular cartilage.

Diarthrodial Joint (dī″ar-thrō′di-al/joint) (n.) 1. A type of synovial joint characterized by hyaline cartilage covering the articular ends and synovial membrane lining the interior; 2. Synovial joint.

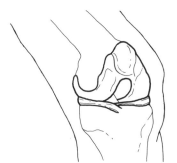

Diarthrodial joint

Diarthrosis (dī″ar-thrō′sis) (n.) 1. Synovial joint; 2. A freely movable joint. The ends of the adjoining bone are covered with a thin cartilaginous sheet, and the bones are linked by a ligament (capsule). This ligament is lined with synovial membrane that secretes synovial fluid. Such joints are classified according to the type of connection between the bones and the type of movement allowed. Example: knee joint.

Diastasis (dī-as′tah′sis) (n.) The dislocation or separation of two normally attached bones, between which there is no true joint. An example is diastasis of the pubic symphysis.

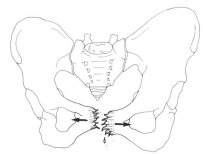

Diastasis pubic symphysis

Diastematomyelia (dī″ah-stem″ah-to-mī-ē′le-ah) (n.) An embryologic spinal defect in which the spinal cord or the cauda equina is divided by a cartilaginous or bony mass located in the midsagittal region of the spinal canal.

Diathesis (dī-ath′e-sis) (n.) An unusual constitutional susceptibility or predisposition to a particular disease.

Diastrophic Dwarfism (dī″ah-strof′ik/dwarf′izm) (n.) A variety of short-limbed dwarfism, characterized by

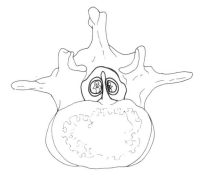

Diastematomyelia

a complex of ear, hand, and foot abnormalities, kyphoscoliosis, joint contractures, and, occasionally, cleft palate. The disorder is inherited as an autosomal recessive condition and may be diagnosed at birth. Lamy and Maroteaux first distinguished this syndrome from other varieties of short stature in 1960, creating the term "diastrophic dwarfism."

Diathermy (dī′ah-ther″mē) (n.) An oscillating, high-frequency electric current which, when used in surgery, generates enough heat to coagulate and destroy body tissues. Heat is generated by the resistance of tissues to the passage of alternating electric current. A short-wave diathermy machine produces a very high frequency of 10 to 100 million cycles per second. It is useful in stopping bleeding from small blood vessels. See **Electrocoagulation**.

Diaz Osteonecrosis (dē′az/os″tē-ō-ne-krōs′sis) (n.) A focal, aseptic necrosis of the talus.

Diazepam (di-āz′e-pam) (n.) A tranquilizer and skeletal muscle relaxant that is marketed under the trade name Valium.

DIC Abbreviation for **Disseminated Intravascular Coagulation**.

Dickens UC Sign (dik-enz/sin) (n.) A radiographic sign in Perthes disease used to measure how much of the femoral head is not covered by the acetabulum. Draw one vertical line from the outer lip of the acetabulum and a second vertical line parallel to it, through the lateral edge of the femoral capital epiphysis. Measure the horizontal distance between these two lines in millimeters. Measure both the affected and unaffected hips. If the acetabulum extends farther laterally than the outer edge of the femoral capital epiphysis in the affected hip, record the measurement as a negative figure. A negative figure signifies coverage of the femoral head by the acetabulum.

Dicloxacillin (dī-kloks″ah-sil′in) (n.) A semisynthetic isoxazolyl penicillin used for oral therapy of infections.

Didiée View (did-yā′/vu) (n.) A radiographic technique useful in identifying posterolateral defects in the humeral head after anterior shoulder dislocation,

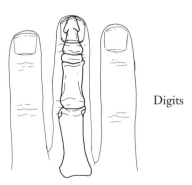

Digits

especially after recurrent dislocation. The patient is prone with the cassette under the shoulder. With the forearm behind the trunk, the shoulder is internally rotated so that the dorsum of the hand is on the iliac crest and the arm is parallel to the table. The x-ray tube is directed laterally to the shoulder joint, with the beam angled 45°. Compare **West Point View**.

Differentiation (dif″er-en″shē-ā′shun) (n.) The structural and functional modification of an unspecialized cell into a specialized one.

Diffuse Idiopathic Skeletal Hyperostosis (di-fūs′/ id″e-ō-path′ik/skel′e-tal/hi″per-ōs-tō′sis) (n.) See **DISH**.

Diffusion (di-fū′zhun) (n.) The migration of molecules or ions from a region of higher to a region of lower concentration. Random movement causes the migration.

Digastric Triangle (dī-gas′trik/trī′ang′g′l) (n.) An anatomic area in the front of the neck, useful in surgical approaches. Its borders are: cephalically, the body of the mandible; ventrally and below, anterior belly of digastric muscle; dorsally and below, posterior belly of and stylohyoid muscles. Also called the **Submandibular Triangle**.

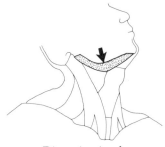

Digastric triangle

Digital Formula (dij′i-tal/for′mū-lah) (n.) A description of the feet according to the length of the toes. The terms were first used by early authors of anatomic atlases, and the names are based on classical works of sculpture and painting. They are:

Greek foot: The big toe is shorter than the second toe (found in 22 percent of patients);

Egyptian foot: The big toe is longer than the second toe (69 percent);

Squared foot: The big toe is the same length as the second toe. See **Metatarsal Formula**.

Digits (dij′its) (n.) Fingers and toes. The names of the digits in the hand are the thumb, index, middle (long), ring, and little fingers. In the foot there are the big, second, third (middle), fourth, and little toes.

Digitus Minimus Varus (dij′i-tus/min′i-mus/var′us) (n.) A clawing of the fifth toe, in which, because of external rotation and adduction, it overlays the dorsum of the fourth toe. Pressure on the toes from footwear may induce symptoms. Synonyms: **Overlap-** ping fifth toe, Congenital dorsal adduction of the little toe.

Dimon and Hughston Osteotomy (dī-mon/and/hū-ston/os″tē-ot′ō-mē) (n.) A surgical technique used to fix unstable intertrochanteric fractures. Osteotomy in the trochanteric area is employed, along with valgus angulation and medial displacement.

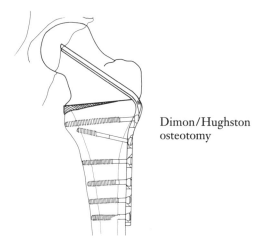

Dimon/Hughston osteotomy

Dinner Pad (din′er/pad) (n.) A pad or roll of material placed over the abdomen before a plaster jacket or body spica is applied. The pad is then removed to leave space under the jacket for expansion of the stomach after eating.

DIP Abbreviation for **Distal Interphalangeal Joint**.

Diplococci (dip″lō-kok′sī) (n.) Cocci occurring in pairs.

Diploid (dip′loid) (adj.) Identically paired representation of each type of chromosome except for the sex chromosomes. Contrast with **Haploid**.

Direct Current Electrical Stimulation (di-rekt′/ kur′ent/ē-lek′trik-el/stim″u-lā′shun) (n.) A type of electric stimulation used in cases of nonunion of fractures. Electrical stimulation occurs through cathodes placed on the skin directly at the site of a fracture nonunion. The cathode pins are then connected to an externally placed power supply that has four cathode lead wires, each delivering 20 microamperes of constant direct current. This constant current to the bone promotes healing.

Disability (dis″ah-bil′i-tē) (n.)   1. An alteration, limiting, loss, or absence of an individual's capacity to meet personal, social, or occupational demands, or to meet statutory or regulatory requirements of physical or psychologic constitution. The disability may be caused by medical impairments or nonmedical factors, but the evaluation or rating of disability is a nonmedical assessment. Permanent disability is a static or stabilized degree of capacity not likely to increase or decrease, in spite of continuing medical or rehabilitative measures. Disability is assessed by nonmedical means. Contrast to **Temporary Disability**. 2. Any physical or medical impairment that substantially limits a major life activity (eg, walking, hearing, working); having a record of such impairment; or being regarded by others as having such an impairment. Physical and mental impairments include, but are not limited to, diseases and conditions, such as tuberculosis, human immunodeficiency virus (HIV) infection and cancer, and such impairments as orthopedic, visual, speech, and hearing.

Disappearing Bone Disease (dis a-pēr-ing/bōn/di-zēz′) (n.)   See **Gorham's Syndrome**.

Disarticulation (dis″ar-tik″u-lā′shun) (n.)   An amputation or separation through the level of a joint.

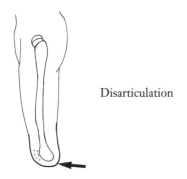

Disarticulation

Disc (disk) (n.)   See **Disk**.

Discectomy (dis-kek′tō-mē) (n.)   An excision of all or part of an intervertebral disk.

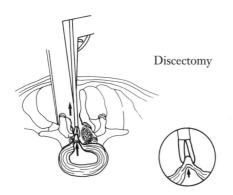

Discectomy

Discharge Diagnosis (dis-charj′/di″ag-nō′sis) (n.)   The complete set or list of diagnoses applicable at discharge to a single patient experience, e.g., an inpatient hospitalization.

Discharge Planning (dis-charj′/plan′ing) (n.)   A coordinated program developed by a hospital to ensure that each patient receives a program for necessary continuing or follow-up care.

Discharge Summary (dis-charj′/sum-ma′rē) (n.)   A clinical resume prepared by the physician at the conclusion of a patient's hospital stay. It summarizes the chief complaint, diagnostic findings, therapy, response to treatment; and recommendations on discharge.

Discharge Transfer (dis-charj′/trans′fer) (n.)   The transfer of an inpatient to another health care institution at the time of discharge.

Discitis (dis-kī′tis) (n.)   An inflammatory disorder of the intervertebral disk.

Discogenic (dis″ko-jen′ik) (n.)   Syndromes characterized by local and radicular pain due to nerve root or spinal cord compression, caused by herniation of the nucleus pulposus.

Discograms (dis′ko-grams) (n.)   Radiographic studies of disk configurations after injection of contrast material. Common readings show that:

1. A normal disc with an intact nucleus pulposus accepts approximately 1/2 cc. of contrast medium. A radiograph made immediately following injection shows that radio-opaque material remains within the area of the nucleus pulposus.

2. A degenerated disc accepts more than 1/2 cc. of contrast medium. The radiograph shows that the fluid extends through cracks or crevices within the disc; if the annulus fibrosus is torn or ruptured, the radio-opaque material may escape through the opening or openings.

Discography (dis-kog′rah-fe) (n.)   The introduction of radio-opaque fluid into the nucleus pulposus for purposes of identifying disc configuration. The resulting studies are known as discograms.

Discometry (dis′ko-me-trē) (n.)   A technique of measuring the pressure within an intervertebral disk.

Discoid Meniscus (dis′koid/mĕ-nis′kus) (n.)   An abnormality in which the cartilaginous meniscus of the

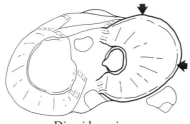

Discoid meniscus

knee joint is discoid in shape rather than semilunar. The lateral meniscus is most frequently affected.

Disease (di-zēz') (n.)   1. Illness or sickness that results from a disturbance of body functions, organs, or systems. 2. A specific disease is a defined morbid process characterized by a known etiology, identifiable signs and symptoms, or a consistent pathology. Disease may be congenital or acquired.

Disfigurement (dis-fig'yer-ment) (n.)   A changed or abnormal appearance, which may be an alteration of color, shape, structure, or a combination of these. Disfigurement may be a residue of an injury or disease, or it may accompany a recurrent or chronic disorder. Prominent bodily disfigurement may have negative psychologic and social consequences that may result in impaired self-image, self-imposed isolation, an alteration of life-style, or other behavioral changes.

DISH (dish) (n.)   Abbreviation for **Diffuse Idiopathic Skeletal Hyperostosis**. A form of osteoarthritis characterized by marked bony proliferation and osteophyte formation effecting the spine as well as the peripheral bones. It usually occurs along the anterolateral aspect and in the posterior longitudinal ligament of vertebral bodies, but also can be seen around major joints. This is a disease of middle-aged and elderly persons, and is more frequently seen in men. While some patients may be asymptomatic, the majority appear to have mild symptoms and signs. The most common complaints are mild stiffness and pain in the middle and lower back regions, which lasts for many years. The radiographic criteria for diagnosis include: a) the presence of flowing calcification and ossification along the anterolateral aspect of at least four contiguous vertebral bodies; b) the relative preservation of intervertebral disc height; and c) an absence of intra-articular bony ankylosis of the sacroiliac and apophyseal joints. The vertically oriented syndesmophytes are in contrast to the horizontal osteophytes of degenerative joint disease of the spine. Synonyms: **Senile Ankylosing Hyperostosis of the Spine**; **Forestier's Disease**; **Ankylosing Vertebral Hyperostosis**.

DISI   The abbreviation for **Dorsal Intercalated Segmental Instability** or **Dorsiflexed Intercalated Segmental Instability Pattern**. This is a carpal instability pattern characterized by a zig-zag collapse of the proximal carpal row. It results in dorsiflexion of the lunate and an increase of the scapholunate angle on a lateral radiograph to greater than 60°. This instability is often the result of scapholunate dissociation.

Disinfectant (dis"in-fek'tant) (n.)   A substance used to destroy pathogens.

Disinfection (dis"in-fek'shun) (n.)   A process by which pathogens, but not spores, are destroyed.

Disk (disk) (n.)   1. A circular or rounded flat plate; 2. Commonly used to refer to the intervertebral disk, which is composed of a nucleus pulposis and an annular fibrosis. Synonym: **Disc**.

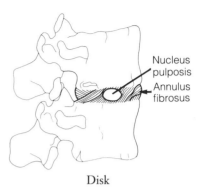

Disk

Disk Degeneration (disk/dē-jen"er-ā'shun) (n.)   The loss of structural and functional integrity of the intervertebral disk. See **Degenerative Disk Disease**.

Disk Space Infection (disk'spās/in-fek'shun) (n.)   An infectious process involving the intervertebral disk space. A needle biopsy of the disk spaces identifies the causative organism.

Dislocation (dis"lo-ka'shun) (n.)   1. A complete loss of contact between the articular surfaces of a joint; 2. A condition occurring when a bone is no longer in normal contact with the bone with which it articulates. Colloq: "out of joint."

Displaced Fat Pad Sign (dis-plāst'/fat/pad/sīn) (n.)   A radiographic sign useful in the diagnosis of occult fractures at the elbow. The sign is produced by any process that may cause a synovial or hemorrhagic effusion within the elbow joint, thus displacing intracapsular or extrasynovial fat pads. The pads appear as radiolucent areas anterior and posterior to the distal end of the humerus and are known as an anterior sail sign and posterior fat pad sign, respectively.

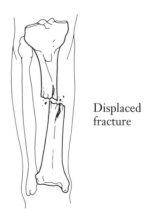

Displaced fracture

Displaced Fracture (dis-plāst'/frak'chur) (n.)   A fracture in which two ends of a fractured bone are separated from each other.

Displacement (dis-plās'ment) (n.)   Positioning in an

abnormal location or placement; the degree of displacement is used to describe the relative position of fracture fragments.

Dissect (di-sekt′) (v.) To cut apart or separate, especially in order to expose structures for anatomic or microscopic study.

Disseminated Intravascular Coagulation (dissem′i-nāt″ed / in″trah-vas′ku-lar / ko-ag″u-lā′shun) (n.) An acquired coagulopathy characterized by intravascular fibrin deposition, principally within arterioles and capillaries. There is a resultant bleeding diathesis with thrombocytopenia, clotting factor deficiencies, and secondary fibrinolysis. The diagnosis is confirmed by the presence of increased fibrin split products and decreased fibrinogen in the serum, in addition to prolonged bleeding time, PT, and PTT. Abbreviated **DIC**. Synonyms: **Consumption Coagulopathy**, **Defibrination Syndrome**.

Dissociation Symptom (dis-so″she-ā′shun/simp′tum) (n.) An inability to feel pain, heat, or cold, although tactile sensibility remains intact.

Distal (dis′tal) (adj.) Situated away from the place or point of reference, origin, or attachment. Contrast with **Proximal**.

Distal Interphalangeal Joints (dis′tal/in″ter-fah-lan′je-al/joints) (n.) Diarthrodial joints between the middle and distal phalanges of the fingers and toes. Abbreviated **DIP**. Compare **Proximal Interphalangeal Joints**.

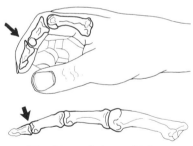

Distal interphalangeal joints

Distal Muscular Dystrophy (dis′tal/mus′ku-lar/dis′tro-fē) (n.) A rare type of progressive muscular dystrophy that initially affects distal, as opposed to proximal, muscles. As the disease progresses, weakness slowly spreads proximally. It is transmitted as an autosomal dominant trait. The age of onset varies, with a mean of 47 years. The disease was first described by Gowers in 1902. Synonyms: **Gower's Muscular Dystrophy**, **Distal Dystrophy**.

Distortion (dis-tor′shun) (n.) Perversion of shape; often used to describe radiographic projections.

Distraction (di-strak′shun) (n.) 1. Refers to a separation or pulling apart of fragments that leaves a gap between them; it can be caused by excessive trac-

tion. 2. Distraction is also often used to refer to the relationship between fracture fragments.

Distraction Epiphysiolysis (di-strak′shun/ep″i-fiz″ē-ol′i-sis) (n.) A method of limb lengthening in which the epiphysis and the metaphysis are transfixed by pins, and a distraction device is then used to produce a fracture at the metaphyseal side of the epiphyseal plate. Subsequent gradual distraction achieves the desired lengthening.

Disuse Osteoporosis (dis-yoos′/os″tē-ō-po-rō′sis) (n.) A type of osteoporosis that occurs in the absence of normal bone stresses. It may be the result of immobilization, weightlessness, or paralysis. The early radiographic signs of disuse osteoporosis are spotty, mottled areas of decreased bone density and some cortical thinning, followed by rather marked periarticular demineralization. The process then continues with a generalized uniform loss of bone density, cortical thinning (due to enlargement of the marrow cavity), and loss of trabeculae. Synonym: **Osteoporosis of Disease**.

Diver's Disease (dī′verz′/di-zēz′) (n.) See **Caissons Disease**.

DJD Abbreviation for Degenerative Joint Disease.

DMS Abbreviation for Delayed Muscle Soreness.

DMSO Abbreviation for Dimethylsulfoxide.

DNA Abbreviation for Deoxyribonucleic Acid.

DNR Abbreviation for Do Not Resuscitate.

Dolichostenomelia (dol″i-kō-ste″nō-mē′le-ah) (n.) Synonym for **Arachnodactyly**.

Dolor (do′lor) (n.) 1. Pain. 2. Used to describe one of the classic signs of inflammation (as in "rubor, tumor, calor, and dolor").

Dome Fracture (dōm/frak′chur) (n.) A fracture involving the weight-bearing surface of the acetabulum.

Dominant (dom′i-nant) (adj.) 1. Controlling or prevailing over all others. 2. In genetics, a gene that exerts its full phenotypic effect to the exclusion of other, or recessive, genes. 3. Used to describe sidedness, such as "right-hand or left-hand dominant."

Doorframe Exercise (dōr-frām/ek′ser-sīz) (n.) A shoulder exercise consisting of moving the hand up along a doorframe to increase the range of motion of the upper limb. It is often described as "climbing a wall like a spider."

Doppler Principle, Phenomenon, or Effect (dop′ler/prin′si-p′l/fe-nom′e-non/or/e-fekt′) (n.) During the rapid movement of a sound or light source, the wave length appears to decrease as the object approaches.

Dorrance Hand (daw′-renz/hand) (n.) The proprietary name of an artificial hand. See also **Dorrance Hook**.

Dorrance Hook (daw′-renz/huk) (n.) The proprietary name of a prosthetic hook with a voluntary opening.

Dorsal (dor'sal) (adj.) Relative to or situated on the posterior or back surface; opposite of ventral.

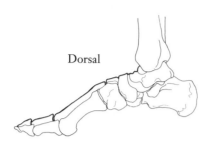

Dorsal

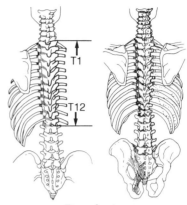

Dorsal spine

Dorsal Bunion (dor'sal/bun'yun) (n.) A pathologic condition of the big toe, consisting of plantar-flexion contracture at the metatarsophalangeal joint and dorsiflexion contracture at the interphalangeal joint and dorsiflexion of the first metatarsal at the cuneiform joint. This condition results in an exostosis over the dorsum of the first metatarsal head, the dorsal bunion. It is often seen in certain muscle imbalances and is less commonly associated with a rocker bottom foot or hallux rigidus.

Dorsal Column (dor'sal/kol'um) (n.) In the three-column theory of spinal stability as described by Francis Denis, the dorsal or posterior column is formed by the posterior bony complex alternating with the posterior ligamentous complex. The posterior column includes the supraspinous and interspinous ligaments, the ligamentum flavum, posterior joint capsules, and the bony arch.

Dorsal Intercalary Segment Instability (dor'sal/inter'ka-ler-ē/seg'ment/stah-bil'i-tē) (n.) See **DISI**.

Dorsal Finger Splints (dor'sal/fing'ger/splintz) (n.) Used for immobilization of the proximal or distal interphalangeal joints or the metacarpophalangeal joints of the hand. The splints are usually fashioned from commercially available metallic splints that have a spongy padding on one side. They are then cut to the proper size and shaped as desired. These are placed on the dorsal or extensor surface of the digit and may be used as extension block splints.

Dorsal Rim Fracture (dor'sal/rim/frak'chur) (n.) See **Barton's Fracture**.

Dorsal Spine (n.) See **Thoracic Spine**.

Dorsal Wrist Angle (dor'sal/rist/ang'g'l) (n.) An angle used to evaluate postreduction radiographs of distal radius fractures. On a lateral radiograph of the wrist, the angle between a line perpendicular to the long axis of the radius and the articular surface of the distal radius. Normal 15°.

Dorsiflexion (dor"si-flek'shun) (n.) A flexing or bending of a body part. For example, dorsiflexion of the ankle implies moving the foot toward the leg so that the angle between the dorsum of the foot and the lower leg is decreased.

Dorsiflexor (dor"si-flek'sor) (n.) A muscle causing backward flexion of a part of the body. For example, contraction of extensors of the foot or hand result in dorsiflexion.

Dorsum (dor'sum) (n.) 1. The back. 2. The upper or posterior surface of a part of the body.

Dorsum Rotundum (dor'sum/rō-tun'dum) (n.) The clinical appearance of increased thoracic kyphosis.

Dosage (dō'sij) (n.) The determination and regulation of the size, frequency, and number of doses of an agent to be administered.

Dose (dōs) (n.) 1. The specified quantity of an agent to be administered at one time. 2. A given quantity of radiation administered or absorbed.

Dosimeter (do-sim'e-ter) (n.) A device to detect and measure accumulated radiation exposure, such as a film badge or ionization chamber that measures radiation dose.

Double Curve (dub'l/kurv) (n.) Two lateral structural curves, scoliosis, in the same spine. See **Double Major Curve**.

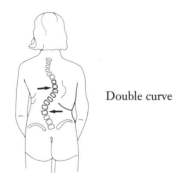

Double curve

Double Fracture (dub'l/frak'chur) (n.) A condition in which a bone is broken at two places or levels without communicating lines of fracture. Synonym: **Segmental Fracture**.

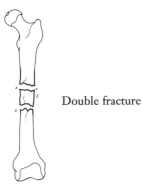

Double fracture

Double Major Curve (dub'l/mā'jer/skō"lē-ō'sis) (n.) Describes a scoliosis where there are two structural curves, usually of equal size.

Double Thoracic Curve (dub'l/tho-ras'ik/kurv) (n.) A scoliosis with a structural upper thoracic curve, a larger more deforming lower thoracic curve, and a relatively nonstructural lumbar curve.

Dowager's Hump (dow ah gerz/hump') (n.) A colloquial term for a high thoracic kyphosis that appears in an elderly female.

Down Syndrome (down/sin'drōm) (n.) A chromosomal abnormality, generally due to trisomy 21. The orthopaedic abnormalities result from generalized ligamentous laxity, and commonly include atlanto-axial instability, recurrent patella dislocation, pes planus, and voluntary, painless hip dislocation. Older term was mongolism.

DPM Abbreviation for a Doctor of Podiatric Medicine. Podiatrist.

Drain (drān) (n.) A device or substance that provides a channel of exit for discharge from a wound.

Drainage (drān'ij) (n.) The removal of fluid from a cavity or wound; also used to describe the fluid removed.

Draping (drāp'ing) (n.) The process of placing drapes over a patient before an operative procedure so as to leave only a minimal area of skin exposed around the site of the incision. This provides a sterile operative field and prevents exposure of unprepared skin areas during surgery.

Drawer Test (drawr/test) (n.) A clinical examination for ligamentous stability. The joint being tested, as well as the direction being tested, must be specified. In general, the test consists of "drawing" the distal part of the joint in the direction of the instability being examined while stabilizing the proximal part of the joint. If instability is present, the examiner will be able to displace the distal aspect of the joint in the direction of the instability, thus implying discontinuity of the normally restraining ligaments. For example, the anterior drawer test of the ankle will evaluate the intactness of the anterior talotibial

ligament. Also see **Anterior Drawer Test, Posterior Drawer Test**.

Dressing (dres'ing) (n.) A material and/or medication applied to cover a wound. Types include occlusive, compressive, and sterile.

DRG Abbreviation for **Diagnosis-Related Groups**.

Drill (dril) (n.) An instrument with a pointed drill bit that revolves to create channels in hard substances, such as bone. It is used to create drill holes for screw placement in bones.

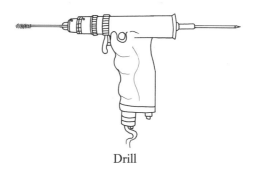

Drill

Drill Guide (dril/gīd) (n.) An instrument used to simultaneously direct the placement of a drill hole and protect the surrounding soft tissues. Synonym: **Drill Sleeve**.

Driller's Disease (dril-lerz/di-zēz') (n.) A post-traumatic disorder characterized by subchondral bone cysts.

Drop Arm Test (drop/arm/test) (n.) A test used during physical examination to detect rotator cuff tears. Instruct the patient to hold the arm at 90 degrees of shoulder abduction, with the elbow bent. Tap the elbow. If there are tears in the rotator cuff, the patient will not be able to lower the arm smoothly or slowly; it will drop to the side from the abducted position.

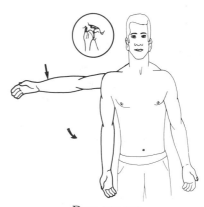

Drop arm test

Drop Foot Gait (drop/foot/gat) (n.)   See **Steppage Gait**.

Drop Foot Splint (drop-foot/splint) (n.)   Splint applied to maintain the ankle joint in a neutral position. Used when there is insufficient voluntary ankle dorsiflexion. Also called **Drop Foot Brace**.

Dropped Foot (dropt/foot) (n.)   See **Foot Drop**.

DTR   Abbreviation for **Deep Tendon Reflex**.

Dual Energy Photon Absorptiometry (du'al/en'er-jē/fō'ton/ab-sorp"shē-om'e-trē) (n.)   A noninvasive technique for the measurement of bone mass that uses two monoenergetic radionuclides. The vertebral body is the anatomic site for measurement.

Dual Onlay Graft (du'al/on-lā'/graft) (n.)   Cortical grafts used to treat nonunions and to bridge bony defects. The grafts consist of two cortical struts placed across each side of the defect and fixed with internal or external fixation devices.

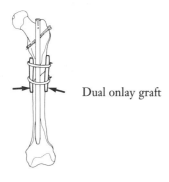

Dual onlay graft

Duchenne's Muscular Dystrophy (du-shenz' mus'kū-lar/dis'tro-fē) (n.)   A progressive muscular dystrophy inherited as a sex-linked recessive trait. It usually appears clinically at about 3 to 5 years as clumsiness and difficulty climbing stairs and rising up from a sitting position (Gower's sign). The proximal lower extremity weakness progresses distally in a fairly constant pattern. Pseudohypertrophy can also be seen in the calf muscles. Affected patients have significantly elevated CPK levels.

Duck Gait (duk/gat) (n.)   A waddling gait.

Duck Waddling Test (duk/wahd'l-ing/test) (n.)   See **Childress' Test**.

Ductility (duk'til-i-tē) (n.)   The ability of a material to absorb relatively large amounts of plastic deformation before failing. Contrast to **Brittleness**.

Dunlops Traction (dun-lopz/trak'shun) (n.)   A side arm skin traction with the elbow held in mild flexion. Countertraction is applied vertically in a downward position by a sling across the distal arm. The traction used to align supracondylar fractures of the humerus.

Dupuytren's Contracture (du-pwē-trahnz'/kon-trak'chur) (n.)   A proliferative fibroplasia of the sub-

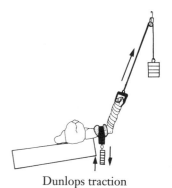

Dunlops traction

cutaneous palmar tissue that occurs as nodules and cords and results in secondary contractures of the finger joints. It is more common in men, epileptics, and alcoholics and is seen most often after 40 years of age. May also show thinning of the subcutaneous tissue with adherence of the dermis to the underlying fibrotic fascia, pitting of the skin, and dorsal "knuckle pads." Pathologically, it is a fibromatosis of the palmer fascia characterized by fibroblastic and myofibroblastic proliferation with little or no inflammatory response.

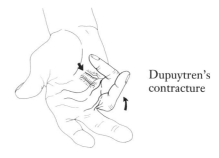

Dupuytren's contracture

Dupuytren's Disease (du-pwē-trahnz'/di-zēz') (n.)   See **Dupuytren's Contracture**.

Dupuytren's Fracture (du-pwē-trahnz'/frak'chur) (n.)   An eponym for a bimalleolar ankle fracture accompanied by a rupture of the tibiofibular ligaments and talar subluxation or dislocation that may follow diastasis. Compare **Bimalleolar Ankle Fracture**.

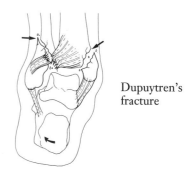

Dupuytren's fracture

Dura (du′rah) (n.)   The outermost of the three membranes covering the spinal cord and brain. It is the toughest and most fibrous of the membranes. Also called **Dura Mater**.

Dutoit Staple (doo-twah′/stāp′l) (n.)   A long, slender staple used to anchor ligaments or tendons to bone, for recurrent anterior shoulder dislocation. In staple capsulorraphy, used for recurrent anterior shoulder dislocation as described by Dutoit and Roux.

Dutoit staple

DuVerney Fracture (duverny/frak′chur) (n.)   A fracture of the ilium just below the anterosuperior spine.

DVT   Abbreviation for **Deep Venous Thrombosis**.

Dwarf (dwarf) (n.)   An abnormally small, short, or disproportioned person.

Dwarfism (dwarf′izm) (n.)   A condition of being undersized, or a dwarf. See also specific dwarfisms.

Dwyer Instrumentation (dwi-er/in″stroo-men-ta′shun) (n.)   An anterior surgical approach to the spine for correction of a scoliotic deformity. Consists of vertebral body screws and staples and a cable that is passed through the screw heads, applying tension between them to gain correction.

Dwyer Osteotomy (dwī-er/os″te-ot′ō-mē) (n.)   A wedge osteotomy of the calcaneus or tarsal bones that is used to correct cavus deformity of the foot.

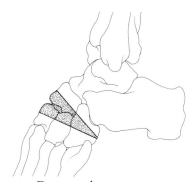

Dwyer wedge osteotomy

DXA (n.)   Abbreviation for dual x-ray absortiometry.

Dynamic Compression Plate (di-nam′ik/kompresh′un/plāt) (n.)   An internal fixation device designed to use the spherical gliding principle in conjunction with the inclined contour of the screw hole and the slope on the underside of the screw head. This design permits oblique insertion of screws through the plate for lag screw placement and the possibility of obtaining compression between any adjacent screw holes. It can produce 2 to 3 mm of impaction at the fracture site. The DCP can be used alone as a compression device, in conjunction with the removable tension device, or as a neutralization plate. Abbreviated **DCP**. See **Hirschhorn Compression Plate**.

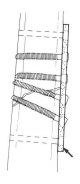

Dynamic compression plate

Dynamic Condylar Screw (di-nam′ik/kon′dī-lar/skru) (n.)   A screw and plate device designed for the internal fixation of distal femoral fractures. It incorporates a lag screw and a compression screw with a 95° DCS plate, which allows for the placing of cancellous screws for interfragmentary compression through the distal screw holes. It is also used in the fixation of subtrochanteric and pertrochanteric femur fractures in the reversed direction. Abbreviated **DCS**.

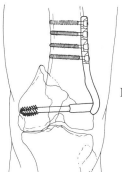

Dynamic condylar screw

Dynamic Hip Screw (di-nam′ik/hip/skru) (n.)   Part of an implant system for the fixation of intertrochan-

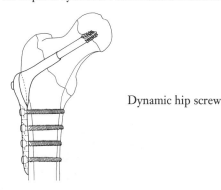

Dynamic hip screw

teric and pertrochanteric femur fractures. It is a sliding device that allows gliding of the lag screw through the barrel of the side-plate as the fracture impacts. Contrast to fixed nail-plate devices.

Dynamic Locking (di-nam'ik/lok'ing) (n.) The placement of a locking intramedullary nail with only proximal or distal interlocking screws. This results in neutralization of translateral movements but permits compression at the fracture site.

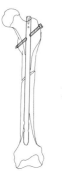

Dynamic locking

Dynamic Splint (di-nam'ik/splint) (n.) A device that aids in the initiation and performance of motion. Example: **Dynamic Hand Splint**.

Dynamics (dī-nam'iks) (n.) 1. The biomechanical study of forces that, when acting on a body, do not add up to zero. 2. A body not in equilibrium. Contrast to **Statics.**

Dynamization (di"nam-i-zā'shun) (n.) The process of converting a statically interlocked, intramedullary nail into a dynamically locked nail by removing the proximal or distal interlocking screw and leaving the nail locked at one end only.

Dynamometer (di"nah'mo-meter) (n.) An instrument for measuring muscular strength.

Dyne (dīn) (n.) The metric unit of force that, if applied to a 1-g mass, will give it an acceleration of 1 cm/sec.

Dysautonomia (dis"aw-tō-nō'mē-ah) (n.) A rare familial condition in which sensory deficits are accompanied by defective lacrimation, salivation, and other autonomic functions. A major orthopaedic complication is the development of neuropathic joints. See **Familial Dysautonomia**, and **Scoliosis**.

Dyschondroplasia (dis"kon-dro-pla'ze-ah) (n.) See **Enchondromatosis** and **Ollier's Disease**.

Dyscrasic Fracture (dis-kre'sik/frak'chur) (n.) A fracture caused by the weakening of a bone owing to a debilitating disease.

Dysesthesia (dis"es-thē'ze-ah) (n.) An unpleasant, abnormal sensation.

Dysostosis (dis"os-to'sis) (n.) A disorder characterized by defective ossification.

Dysplasia (dis-pla'se-ah) (n.) An abnormality or alteration in tissue structure. See **Skeletal Dysplasia** for orthopaedic application.

Dysplasia Epiphysalis Multiplex (dis-pla'se-ah/ep"i-fiz'e alis/mul'ti p'lx) (n.) An abnormal or faulty development of multiple epiphyses. They are flattened, hypoplastic, fragmented, and mottled. Patient has short stature. Syndrome appears late.

Dysplasia Epiphysalis Punctata (dis-pla'se-ah/ep"i-fiz'e-alis/punk'tah-tah) (n.) An abnormal or faulty growth and ossification of the epiphysis. There are radiographic findings of stippling of the epiphysis and short stature. Appears early in infancy.

Dysplastic (dis-plas'tik) (adj.) Referring to dysplasia.

Dysraphism (dis'rah-fizm) (n.) 1. A defective fusion; spinal dysraphism implies the failure of formation of midline spinal elements posteriorly. 2. Any failure of closure of the primary neural tube.

Dysreflexia (dis"re-fleks'e-ah) (n.) An abnormal neuromuscular condition that is characterized by an abnormal motor response to stimuli that normally produce a reflex.

Dystaxia (dis-tak'se-ah) (n.) A mild form of ataxia.

Dystrophic Calcification (dis-trof'ik/kal"si-fi ka'shun) (n.) See **Pathological Calcification**.

Dystrophy (dis-tro-fe) (n.) 1. A disturbance of nutrition either of mineral salts or organic components. 2. A disorder of organ or tissue, usually muscle, due to impaired nourishment of the affected part. Example: **Muscular Dystrophy**.

E

Earth Shoe (erth/shoo) (n.) The proprietary name of a shoe with a large toe box and a heel that is lower than the sole. It was invented in 1957 by Anna Kalso in Denmark and has been marketed in the USA since April 22, 1970—Earth Day (hence its name).

Eburnation (e″bur′na′shun) (n.) 1. Bone sclerosis. 2. The degeneration of the cartilage at the articulating surface of a bone. This exposes the underlying subchondral bone, which then converts into a dense, smooth, ivory-like substance.

Eccentric Contraction (ek-sen′trik/kon-trak′shun) (n.) A muscular contraction in which overall muscle length increases during a tensing of the contractile elements, for example, the hamstring muscles during the deceleration portion of swing phase.

Ecchymosis (ek″i-mō′sis) (n.) A blue-black, purplish, greenish brown, or yellow discoloration caused by extravasation of blood into the skin or mucous membrane. Larger than a petechiae, it is seen in association with bruising or contusion of soft tissue.

ECF Abbreviation for **Extended Care Facility**.

Ecto (ek′to) Prefix denoting outer or outside.

Ectoderm (ek′to-derm) (n.) The embryonic germ cell layer from which will be derived the central and peripheral nervous systems, the sensory epithelia, the epidermis, mammary, pituitary, and subcutaneous glands, and the enamel of the teeth.

Ectomy (ek′to-mē) A suffix used to denote the removal or excision of an anatomic structure.

Ectopic Ossification (ek-top′-ik/os-i-fi-cā-shun) (n.) The formation of bone outside its usual location. See **Heterotopic Ossification.**

Edema (e-dē′mah) (n.) The accumulation of abnormal or excessive amounts of fluid in intercellular tissue spaces or body cavities. Collections of edema fluid may be designated according to site, etiology, and specific characteristics.

Eden-Hybbinette Procedure (e-den-/hib-in-et/pro-sē′jur) (n.) A surgical repair of recurrent anterior dislocation of the shoulder using a bone graft placed against the anterior rim of the glenoid cavity and the scapular neck. See **Bone Block.**

EEG Abbreviation for **Electroencephalogram.**

Efferent (ef′er-ent) (adj.) The conduction or conveying away from a specific site of reference, as in an efferent nerve.

Efferent Nerve (ef′er-ent/nerv) (n.) Any nerve that conveys impulses from the central nervous system to muscles and other effectors. All motor nerves are efferent nerves. Compare **Afferent Nerve Fiber.**

Effusion (e-fū′zhun) (n.) Accumulation of abnormal or excessive amounts of fluid in a joint space, resulting in local swelling. Effusions may be described by the type of fluid contained in the joint; for example, they may be called "bloody," "serous," or "purulent." See **Hemarthrosis** and **Synovial fluid**.

Eggers Plate (eg-erz/plāt) (n.) An early slotted plate used for the internal fixation of fractures.

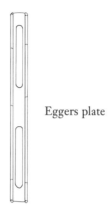

Eggers plate

Eggers Procedure (eg-erz/pro-se′jur) (n.) A surgical technique to correct the spastic cerebral palsy flexed-knee gait. It uses a hamstring–tendon transfer to the most proximal portion of the femoral condyles, capsular releases, and a soleus neurectomy.

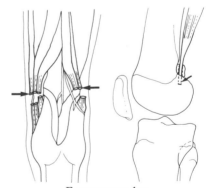

Eggers procedure

Eggshell Gait (eg′shel/gāt) (n.) A type of walk characterized by small steps and reduced motion in the joints of the feet; the patient appears to be actually walking on eggshells. This gait is characteristic of metatarsalgia.

Eggshell Procedure (eg′shel/pro-se′jur) (n.) The thinning of the interior of a vertebra through the pedicle; the fracture of the vertebra so that it can be collapsed. Described by Charles Henig.

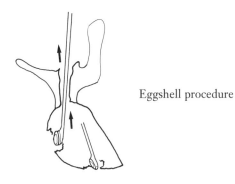

Eggshell procedure

Egyptian Foot (ē-jip'shen/foot) (n.)   A foot in which the big toe is longer than the second toe. Compare with **Square Foot** and **Greek Foot**. See **Digital Formula.**

EHL   Abbreviation for **Extensor Hallucis Longus.**

Ehlers-Danlos Syndrome (a'lerz-dan'los/sin-drōm) (n.)   An inherited connective tissue disorder characterized by skin that is soft, fragile, hyperelastic, and bruises easily. This syndrome is associated with a hyperextensibility of joints, visceral malformation, pseudotumors, and calcified subcutaneous cysts. Wounds heal with delicate "tissue paper" scars. The syndrome has multiple clinical forms. Synonym: **Cutis Hyperelastica.**

Eikenella Corrodens (i"ken-el'ah/ko-rō'denz) (n.)   A gram-negative rod-shaped bacterium that is part of the normal oral flora. An infecting organism in human bite injuries.

Elastic Bandage (e-las'tik/ban'dij) (n.)   A bandage of woven stretchable, elastic material used to exert continuous pressure or support. See **Ace Bandage.**

Elastic Behavior (e-las'tik/be-hāv'yor) (n.)   A biomechanical term that describes a structure that will return to its original shape if a load is applied and then removed; in other words, no permanent deformation occurs.

Elastic Cartilage (e-las'tik/kar'ti-lij) (n.)   A type of nonhyaline cartilage in which the matrix contains a high proportion of elastic tissue. It is found in the

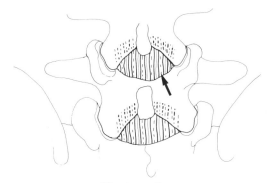

Elastic cartilage

epiglottis, the external ear, and the ligamentum flavum.

Elastic Limit (e-las'tik/lim'it) (n.)   The maximum load to which a structure can be subjected; it will bend or deflect, but it will resume its original shape when the load is released. Synonym: **Yield Point.**

Elastic Modulus (e-las'tik/mod"u-lus) (n.)   See **Modulus of Elasticity.**

Elastic Range (e-las'tik/ranj) (n.)   The range of loading within which a specimen or a structure retains elastic behavior.

Elasticity (e"las-tis'i-tē) (n.)   1. The property of a material or a structure to return to its original form after a deforming load is removed. 2. The ratio of stress to strain for a material. Synonym: **Young's Modulus.**

Elastin (e-las'tin) (n.)   A structural protein that is a major constituent of elastic connective tissues; if present in abundance, it may impart a yellow color.

Elbow (el'bo) (n.)   A joint of the upper extremity that consists of the ulnohumeral and radiocapitellar articulations. Motion takes place in two independent planes—flexion–extension occurs at the ulnohumeral articulation, while forearm rotation occurs through the radiocapitellar articulation. See **Ginglymus Joint.**

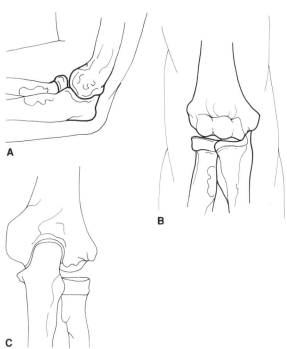

Elbow: A, Lateral view B, Anterior view;
C, Posterior view.

Electric Cast Cutter (e-lek"trik/kast/kut-er) (n.)   An oscillating saw that cuts a cast but not the stockinette or the padding under it. The padding and stockinette remain uncut because they move with the oscillations. Certain models come equipped with vacuums that clean away the dust created by the saw.

Electrical Monitoring of Spinal Cord Function (e-lek″trik′l/mon′i-tor-ing/of spī′nal/kord/funk′shun) (n.) A technique for the detection of intraoperative neurologic complications during spinal surgery. This technique uses electrical stimulation of a peripheral nerve to generate an evoked response more proximally in either the spinal cord or cerebral cortex. Transmission of these potentials, known as somatosensory evoked potentials, is believed to reflect dorsal column function. See **Somatosensory Evoked Potentials (SSEP)**.

Electrical Stimulation of Bone (e-lek″trik′l/stim″u-la′shun/of/bōn) (n.) The application of an electrical current to stimulate osteogenesis. It is used in the treatment of nonunions and may be administered as a constant or pulsed current.

Electrocoagulation (e-lek″tro-ko-ag″u-lā′shun) (n.) The use of a high-frequency electric current to induce the coagulation of tissues. The current is concentrated at one point as it passes through the tissues. Electrocoagulation using a diathermy knife permits bloodless incisions to be made during surgery. See **Diathermy**.

Electroencephalogram (e-lek″tro-en-sef′ah-lo-gram″) (n.) The record obtained by electroencephalography. It refers to the registration of electric potentials of the brain obtained from leads placed on the scalp. Abbreviated **EEG**.

Electrolyte (e-lek′trō-līt) (n.) A substance that breaks apart into electrically charged ions, a solution that conducts electricity via the presence of ions. The positively charged ions are called cations; those in the blood include Na^+, K^+, Ca^{++}, and Mg^{++}. The negatively charged ions in the blood, known as anions, include Cl, PO_4, HCO_3, organic acids, and proteins.

Electromotive Series (e-lek″trō-mōtiv/ser′ēz) (n.) The ranking of metals by their relative tendency to corrode in the presence of other metals.

Electromyogram (e-lek″trō-mī′ō-gram) (n.) The record of intrinsic electrical activity in a skeletal muscle. To obtain this record, electrodes are applied to the surface of the muscle or a needle electrode is inserted into the muscle. The electrical activity is observed with an oscilloscope. Abbreviated **EMG**.

Electromyograph (e-lek″trō-mī′ō-graf) (n.) The instrument used to record and study the intrinsic electric activity of skeletal muscle. The basic components of the electromyograph include an electrode system, a preamplifier, an audioamplifier and loudspeaker, a cathode-ray oscilloscope, and a physiologic stimulator.

Electromyography (e-lek″trō-mī-og′rah-fe) (n.) An expression of the physiologic or pathophysiologic state of muscles. It is determined by inserting a needle electrode into the skeletal muscle, which allows for the detection and recording of variations of electrical activity or voltage. This electric activity is displayed on a cathode-ray oscilloscope and played over a loudspeaker for simultaneous visual and auditory analysis. The technique is used to diagnose nerve and muscle disorders and to assess progress of recovery from some forms of paralysis.

To perform the test, the needle electrode is first inserted. The scope is first observed while the patient is at rest and then engaged in voluntary effort, and finally, when performing at maximum effort. On electrode insertion, a short burst of involuntary potentials, called the insertional potentials, occurs. At rest, there is usually electrical silence. At partial voluntary effort, one can observe individual motor unit potentials. With full voluntary effort, the screen is often obliterated by vertical deflections arranged in what is known as an "interference pattern." In this way it is possible to determine the presence of a disorder, localize the site, and identify the specific nerve or muscle disorder.

Electron (e-lek′tron) (n.) A high-velocity elementary particle that is negatively charged and present outside the nucleus of an atom. It has a specific charge, mass, and spin.

Electron Beam (e-lek′-tron/bēm) (n.) The stream of electrons that emanates from the heated filament of an x-ray tube. It produces x-rays by striking the focal spot on an anode.

Electron Microscope (e-lek′tron/mī′krō-skōp) (n.) A microscope that uses an electron beam, instead of light rays, to produce an image. This image may be viewed firsthand on a fluorescent screen or photographed and then viewed. Electron microscopes are capable of much higher magnification than are light microscopes.

Electron Microscopy (e-lek′tron/mi-kros′ko-pe) (n.) The use of electrons to irradiate clear images of objects within a field. The light source is a beam of electrons; the focusing and magnifying system uses electromagnets.

Electron Volt (e-lek′tron/vōlt) (n.) The energy of motion acquired by an electron accelerated through a potential difference of 1 volt.

Electrophoresis (e-lek″tro-fo-re′sis) (n.) In an electric field, the migration of a substance, such as a protein or a cell, to either the anode or cathode. This technique is used to separate proteins from each other.

Electrospinal Orthosis (e-lek″tro-spi′nal/or-thō′sis) (n.) A treatment modality for scoliosis that uses an intermittent transcutaneous electrical current. This current is applied to the paraspinous or flank musculature, which produces an involuntary contraction of those muscles. Clinical results have been questioned.

Electrosurgery (e-lek″tro-sur′jer-ē) (n.) A technique that uses a high-frequency alternating electric current for the cutting and coagulation of tissue. The current flows between two electrodes as it passes through the tissues; the concentration and flow of this current generates heat as it meets resistance in its passage. This procedure was initiated by Dr. W.T. Bovie, a physicist who developed the first spark-gap tube generator in the 1920s. Also called **Radio-Knife, Surgical Diathermy**, and **Bovie**.

Element (el-e-ment) (n.) Any of more than 100 substances that consist of only one kind of atom and cannot be decomposed into simpler substances.

Elevation (el″e-vā′shun) (n.) The raising or lifting of a body part. Used therapeutically to decrease swelling and edema.

Elevator (el′e-vā″tor) (n.) An instrument used to lift or pry up a body part, e.g., a depressed fracture or soft tissue. See **Periosteal Elevator**.

ELISA Abbreviation for enzyme-linked immunosorbent assay.

Elixir (e-lik′ser) (n.) A liquid containing water, alcohol, and flavoring substances; used as a medium for the administration of medicinal agents.

Ellison Procedure (el′ĭ-son/pro-se′jur) (n.) A lateral extra-articular procedure for the reconstruction of the anterior cruciate ligament in the knee. This technique reroutes a strip of the iliotibial band beneath the fibular collateral ligament.

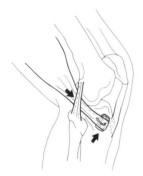

Ellison procedure

Ellis-van Creveld Syndrome (el′is-van-kre-vld/sin′ drōm) (n.) A type of osteochondrodysplasia disorder. It manifests itself at birth and results in short-limbed disproportionate dwarfism. It is transmitted by autosomal recessive inheritance. See **Chondroectodermal Dysplasia**.

Ellsworth-Howard Test (ells wort/how-ard/test) (n.) A method used to determine renal tubular response to parathormone. Normally, injection of parathormone will result in decreased tubular resorption of phosphate. Also, 3 hours after this injection, the output of phosphate in the urine will rise to two to four times the preinjection value. Serum inorganic phosphate may fall by 0.5 to 1 mg/100 mL. In idiopathic and surgical hypoparathyroidism, however, the rise in urinary phosphate may be five to ten times preinjection values, and serum phosphate may fall by 1 to 2 mg/100 mL. In pseudohypoparathyroidism, the urinary phosphate output may rise either not at all, or, at the most, to twice the preinjection value. Interpretation of borderline values and assessment of the potency of the extract may be difficult; the best way to guard against this is to perform a parallel test on a normal control subject.

Elmslie Procedure (elmz-lē/pro-se′jur) (n.) Surgical correction of chronic lateral collateral ligament instability of the ankle by rerouting the peroneus brevis tendon. See **Chrisman-Snook Procedure**.

Elmslie-Trillat Procedure (elmz-le/trē-yah/pro-se′ jur) (n.) Surgical treatment for recurrent patella dislocation. It consists of medial transplantation of the tibial tuberosity, in addition to lateral retinacular release and medial retinacular imbrication.

Elongation (e″long-gā′shun) (n.) A structural property that describes an increase in length as a result of an applied force.

ELPS Abbreviation for **Excessive Lateral Pressure Syndrome**.

Ely's Sign (e′lēz/sīn) (n.) A test to diagnose contracture of the rectus femoris muscle. Place the patient in a prone position and passively flex the knee toward the buttock. In a positive test, the pelvis rises from the table during knee flexion. In a negative test, it does not. Also known as the **Prone Rectus Test**.

E-M Angle (e-m/ang′g′l) (n.) The epiphyseal metaphyseal angle. A simple, quantitative measurement for grading the severity of Blount's disease. On an AP radiograph of the knee, the E-M angle is the inferomedial angle formed by the intersection of the proximal tibial epiphyseal and metaphyseal lines. This angle is a measure of the extent of epiphyseal-metaphyseal depression, and can be used to evaluate the progression and resolution of the tibial bowing caused by Blount's disease.

E/M Codes (ē/em/cōds) (n.) Abbreviation for evaluation and management coding. Effective January, 1992. Medicare mandated the use of these codes for billing and identification of services rendered.

Embolectomy (em-bō-lek′tō-mē) (n.) Surgical removal of a lodged arterial embolus by making an incision into the artery.

Embolism (em′bō-lizm) (n.) The occlusion of a blood vessel by an embolus.

Embolus (em′bō-lus) (n.) Solid or other undissolved foreign matter carried by circulation to a point away from its origin, where it blocks the lumen of a vessel. The obstructing material is usually a blood clot, but may be fat globules, gas bubbles, a piece of tissue, or clumps of bacteria.

Emergency (e-mer′jen-sē) (n.) 1. A situation that involves a potentially disabling or life-threatening condition, thus requiring immediate preventive or treatment intervention. 2. An unforeseen occurrence; a sudden and urgent occasion for action.

EMG Abbreviation for **Electromyelogram**.

Eminence (em'i-nens) (n.) A projection or prominent elevation on the surface of a bone. It is often rounded. Example: tibial eminence.

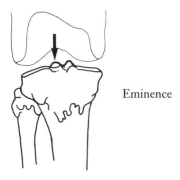

Eminence

Empty Glenoid Sign (emp'te/gle'noid/sīn) An x-ray finding indicating a shoulder dislocation of the glenohumeral joint.

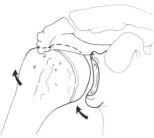

Empty glenoid sign

Emulsion (e-mul'shun) (n.) A mixture consisting of two immissible liquids in which one, in the form of small globules, is dispersed and suspended throughout the other.

EMT Abbreviation for **Emergency Medical Technician.**

Enarthrosis (en'ar-thrō'sis) (n.) 1. A ball-and-socket joint. 2. A multiaxial joint in which the rounded convex head of one bone is received into a socket concavity in another. Examples are the shoulder or hip joint.

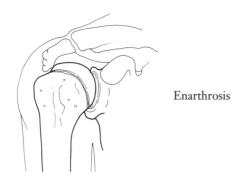

Enarthrosis

Enchondral Ossification (en"kon'dral/os"i-fi-kā'shun) (n.) A series of cellular events that begins with the production of new cartilage cells and eventually results in the formation of new bone. The bone is preformed in cartilage. See **Endochondral Ossification.**

Enchondroma (en"kon-drō'mah) (n.) A benign intramedullary neoplasm of cartilaginous origin. The tumor arises in bone preformed in cartilage; it usually is discovered in the third through the fifth decades of life. Males and females are affected equally. Enchondromas most commonly arise in the short tubular bones of the hands and feet but also occur in the long and flat bones. Frequently, no symptoms or signs are present unless a pathologic fracture supervenes. The lesion is composed of sheets of cartilage cells that generally are uniformly small and mononuclear. The matrix material in the tumor may become calcified; on occasion, lobules of calcium can be observed. The cartilage cells in an enchondroma of a long bone or flat bone tend to resemble the cell pattern of a malignant lesion more closely than do enchondromas in the hand or foot, but the lesion they comprise is still benign. Characteristically, a well-defined, solitary, radiolucent defect is observed in the affected bone; it is also frequently seen in a centric or eccentric ovoid shape. The defect is accompanied by a typically thin zone of transition, and the cortex may be secondarily thinned. The lesion is usually metaphyseal, but often involves the entire shaft of a small tubular bone. It frequently contains lobules of calcific material that look like punctate stippling, and may appear trabeculated. Considerable calcification may be present within the contour of the lesion, in which case, differentiation from a bone infarct may be difficult.

Enchondromatosis (en-kon"dro-mah-tō'sis) (n.) A rare, nonhereditary disorder in which multiple cartilaginous tumors appear throughout the skeleton. Histologically, these lesions resemble solitary enchondromas. Often, the tumors are distributed unilaterally and may result in growth deformities such as shorter limb length. Malignant transformation may occur. Also known as **Ollier's Disease** or **Dyschondroplasia.**

End Artery (end'ar-ter-e) (n.) The terminal branch of an artery. It has no communication or anastomosis with other branches.

End Corn (end/korn) (n.) A hyperkeratotic area seen on the tip of a toe just plantar to the end of the nail. It occurs secondary to rigid hammering of the toe at either the proximal interphalangeal or the distal interphalangeal level. The weight-bearing is concentrated under the tip of the toe rather than under the plantar, "well-upholstered" pulp of the distal phalanx.

End Organ (end/or'gan) (n.) A specialized structure that acts as a terminal for a specific neural pathway.

These peripheral tissues include muscle, skin, and glands.

End Plate (end/plāt) (n.) 1. The bony cortex on the superior and inferior surfaces of each vertebra. 2. The cartilage that defines the disk from above and below, separating it from the adjacent vertebral bone. 3. At a neuromuscular junction, the structure in which motor nerves terminate in skeletal muscle.

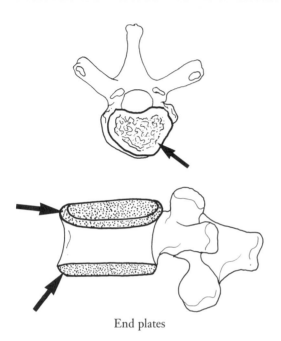

End plates

End Plate Potential (end/plāt/po-ten′shal) (n.) The partial depolarization created in a muscle fiber when it is in the region of an activated neuromuscular junction. Abbreviated **EPP**.

End Point (end/point) (n.) In the clinical examination of ligaments for disruption, this refers to the sensation of stopping when an intact ligament prevents further separation of the joint surfaces. Depending on the examiner, an end point is described as either hard (firm) or soft (mushy).

End Vertebra (end/ver′tĕ-brah) (n.) In the radiographic measurement of a scoliotic curve, a designation applied to the curves of the most cephalad or caudad vertebra, whose superior surface or transverse axis tilts maximally toward the concavity of the curve.

Endemic (en-dem′ik) (adj.) 1. Peculiar to or continuously present in a community; used to characterize diseases or infectious agents. 2. The usual incidence or extent of a particular disease.

Ender's Nail (en′derz/nāl) (n.) Nonreamed, intramedullary nails that are small, flexible, and designed for the fixation of long bone shaft fractures. These nails are pre-bent and rely on the three-point principle to provide adequate fixation. They may be in-

serted retrograde or orthograde, depending on the configuration of the fracture. They are also usually inserted as multiple, stacked nails. Nails 4.5 mm in diameter are used for femoral and larger tibial fractures, whereas 4.0-mm diameter nails are used for small tibial and humeral fractures. Synonym: **Condylocephalic Nail.**

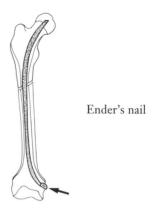

Ender's nail

Endo (en″dō) A prefix used to designate an innermost structure, as in "endoderm" and "endocrine." It is often contrasted with "meso," meaning in the middle, and "ecto," meaning on the outside.

Endochondral Ossification (en″do-kon′dral/os″i-fi-kā′shun) (n.) 1. The process by which bone is formed from cartilage. 2. Ossification that occurs within cartilage and replaces it. 3. The primary ossification process of the axial and appendicular skeletal components. It may recur in selected areas of established bone as part of fracture repair, as in the formation and maturation of callus. This type of bone formation is the synchronous replacement of preexisting cartilaginous tissue by osseous tissue. The overall process is a continuum; it may be arbitrarily divided into a number of steps:

1. The formation of a mesenchymal condensation known as the base anlage.

2. Increased extracellular matrix formation, which creates the precartilaginous model.

3. Extensive ground substance elaboration, which forms the distinct chondral anlage. Hypertrophy of the central chondrocytes begins to occur.

4. Further intercellular and extracellular enlargement of the entire chrondral anlage, with increasing hypertrophy of the central chondrocytes. A trabeculated primary bone collar forms, with an associated periosteum and rudimentary vascular supply at the presumptive diaphysis. There is also increased intracellular and extracellular biochemical activity, especially in the hypertrophied central chondrocytes. This leads to the calcification of the cartilage.

5. The penetration of the primary osseous collar by the fibrovascular tissue, part of which will become the nutrient artery.

6. and 7. The progressive central replacement of cartilage by bone, initially around the area of vascular invasion. This process then extends longitudinally, first to include the collar bone and then toward each end of the anlage. This movement forms the primary ossification center, which will eventually become the diaphysis and metaphyses. An orderly arrangement of the growth mechanism (or physis) is then established along with an actively remodelling metaphysis.

8. and 9. The progressive vascularization of the chondroepiphysis by the cartilage canal system.

10. The appearance of secondary ossification centers within the chondroepiphyses, which is seen primarily as a postnatal process.

Endocrine Gland (en′dō-krin/gland) (n.)   A gland that secretes hormonal substances directly into the blood stream (a ductless gland). Examples: parathyroid, adrenal, and thryoid glands.

Endoderm (en′do-derm) (n.)   The embryonic germ cell layer derived from a number of sources: the epithelial lining of the respiratory tract; the gastrointestinal tract; the bladder and urethra; the tympanic cavity and the eustachian tubes; and the parenchyma of the tonsil, liver, parathyroid, thymus, liver, and pancreas.

Endogenous Infection (en-doj′e-nus/in-fek′shun) (n.)   An infection caused by microbes from the host's own flora.

Endomysium (en″do-mis′ē-um) (n.)   The interstitial connective tissue within muscle fascicles that separates each individual muscle fiber. Compare with **Epimysium.**

Endoneurium (en″do-nu′re-um) (n.)   The interstitial connective tissue in a peripheral nerve that fills the funiculus. By gathering fibers into small bundles, it provides the packing between individual nerve fibers. It contains capillaries that are fed by arterioles and drained by venules in the perineurium. See **Peripheral Nerve.** Compare **Epineurium.**

Endoplasmic Reticulum (en″do-plas′mik/re-tik′ū-lum) (n.)   A cellular organelle that is a complex network of channels extending throughout the cytoplasm. It is known as "rough" endoplasmic reticulum when it is found in association with abundant ribosomes. It is important for cellular transport and, by its ribosome association, has a role in protein synthesis.

Endoprosthesis (en″do-pros-thē′sis) (n.)   An artificial internal body part that is surgically implanted. Also called **Internal Prosthesis.**

Endorphin (en-dor′fin) (n.)   Any of a group of neurotransmitter peptides that occurs naturally in the brain and has potent analgesic properties. The name is an abbreviation for the term endogenous morphine. Also known as **Opioid Peptides.**

Endoscope (en′dō-skōp) (n.)   An illuminated optical instrument that allows the interior of a body cavity or organ to be examined.

Endoscopic Carpal Tunnel Release   A technique for transecting the tranverse carpal ligament using an endoscopic device. Abbreviated **ECTR.**

Endosteal (en′dos′tē-al) (adj.)   Pertaining to the lining of the marrow cavity of a bone. Endosteal cells have osteogenic capacity that is expressed during fracture healing. Compare **Periosteal.**

Endosteal Scalloping (en-dos′tē-al/skal′ō-ping) (n.)   The radiographic finding of an undulating internal cortical edge, usually seen in low-grade malignant intraosseous lesions and represents an internal Codman's triangle.

Endosteum (en-dos′tē-um) (n.)   The membranous layer of connective tissue that lines the medullary cavity of a bone. It is vascular and areolar.

Endothelium (en″do-thē′lē-um) (n.)   The simple squamous epithelium that forms the inner lining of blood and lymphatic vessels, the heart, and the serous cavities of the body.

Endothermic Reaction (en″do-ther′mik/rē-ak′shun) (n.)   A chemical reaction that absorbs heat. Contrast **Exothermic Reaction.**

Endotoxin (en″do-tok′sin) (n.)   1. A toxin released by bacterial cell walls as they disintegrate. 2. The polysaccharide-protein-liquid complex that constitutes an integral part of the cell wall of gram-negative bacteria. It is released on autolysis of the dead cells.

Endotracheal Anesthesia (en″do-trā′kē-al/an-es-thē′zya) (n.)   A form of general anesthesia produced by introducing gases into the trachea by way of a tube.

End-To-End Anastomosis (end/to/end/ah-nas″to-mō′sis) (n.)   A procedure by which the diseased portion of an artery or a severed artery is repaired. Direct anastomosis of the two remaining segments of the artery is used.

Endurance (en-door′ens) (n.)   1. The time limit of a person's ability to maintain either a specific isometric force or a specific power level that involves combinations of concentric or eccentric muscular contractions. 2. The ability of muscles to go on working at high efficiency over a prolonged period. Physiologically, endurance is the expression of circulatory and respiratory efficiency in both the central mechanism and the localized muscles. This efficiency is the result of an ability to eliminate waste products rapidly enough to prevent the onset of fatigue.

Endurance Limit (en-door′ens/lim′it) (n.)   The stress level below which a material can be cyclically stressed indefinitely (psi, dynes/cm^2).

Energy (en′er-jē) (n.)   1. The capacity to do work. 2. The amount of work done by a load on a body. It is measured in units of newton meters or joules.

Energy Absorption Capacity (en′er-jē/ab-sorp′shun/kah-pas′i-tē) (n.)   The mechanical energy absorbed by a loaded structure until it fails.

Engelmann's Disease (eng′el-mahnz/di′zēz) (n.)   A rare familial bone dysplasia of unknown etiology that is marked by a homogeneous fusiform enlargement and thickening of the cortical layers of both the long bones and, occasionally, the short tubular bones. In this disease, there is a striking predilection for symmetric involvement of the extremities, although the epiphysis and the metaphysis are spared. The incidence of skull, spine, and rib involvement is low. The disorder is characterized by retardation of growth, muscle wasting, pain and weakness of the extremities, and a waddling gait. In childhood, the lesion may progress with the involved bones. In adulthood, however, the lesions become static or progress minimally. In general, the severity of the symptoms is proportionate to the extent of skeletal involvement. Radiographically, sclerosis and fusiform enlargement of the diaphyseal cortices of the long bones is characteristic. Synonyms: **Diaphyseal Sclerosis, Progressive Diaphyseal Dysplasia, Camurati-Engelmann Disease.**

English Cane (eng-lish/kān) (n.) A single upright that has a handpiece and a hinged open cuff at the upper end of the forearm extension. Also called a **Forearm Crutch**.

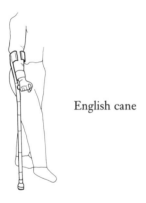

English cane

Enkephalin (en-kef'ah-lin) (n.) Two endogenous pentapeptides with opioid activity. See related term **Endorphin.**

Enlargement Roentgenography (en-larj'ment/rent"gen-og'rah-fē) (n.) The magnification of a roentgenogram to clarify the image and improve detail. This technique also is used as an aid in the evaluation of small and poorly defined lesions.

Enneking's Staging (en-e-kingz/stā'jing (n.) A commonly used system for staging malignant musculoskeletal lesions.

Stage	Grade	Site	Metastasis
IA	Low (G1)	Intracompartmental (T1)	None (Mo)
B	Low (G1)	Extracompartmental (T2)	None (Mo)
IIA	High (G2)	Intracompartmental (T1)	None (Mo)
B	High (G2)	Extracompartmental (T2)	None (Mo)
III	Low (G1)	Intracompartmental (T1)	Yes (M1)
	or	or	
	High (G2)	Extracompartmental (T2)	Yes (M1)

Enostosis (en"os-tō'sis) (n.) A dense bony focus inside a bone that is composed of mature lamellar bone. Also known as a **Bone Island.**

Enteric Coating (en-ter'ik/kō-ting) (n.) A method of coating tablets or capsules to prevent release and absorption of their contents before they reach the intestine. The tablets merely pass through the stomach but dissolve in the intestines.

Enteric Isolation (en-ter'ik/ī"so-lā'shun) (n.) The segregation of people or things to prevent transmission of pathogens caused by contact with fecal matter. This technique is used when diseases can be transmitted by the fecal-oral route, i.e., when pathogens are introduced into the mouth by direct or indirect contact with either feces or articles heavily contaminated with feces.

Enterobacter (en"ter-o-bak'ter) (n.) The genus of gram-negative rods from the family *Enterobacteriaceae*. Present in soil, water, dairy products, and the human intestinal tract, the organisms tend to be less invasive than the *Enterobacteriaceae* in the closely related Klebsiella group. Most infections are associated with alteration in a host's resistance and are acquired during a hospital stay.

Enthesis (en'thē-sis) (n.) 1. The site of attachment of a tendon or ligament into the periosteum of bone. 2. The insertion of synthetic material to replace or repair lost tissue.

Entrapment Neuropathy (en-trap'ment/nu-rop'ah-thē) (n.) A subgroup of compression neuropathies due to:
1. The gradual constriction of anatomic structures around a nerve;
2. The chronic compression of a nerve against an unyielding adjacent fibrous or skeletal structure.

The site of compression is often far removed from the site of symptoms or signs. In addition, the insidious and mild nature of the compression phenomenon is out of proportion to its annoying and often disabling symptoms; it produces sensory and motor changes and is usually quite painful. This pain is referred to the distribution of the involved nerve.

Entropy (en'tro-pē) (n.) A measure of the degree of disorder in any system. A perfectly ordered system has zero entropy; increasing disorder is measured as positive entropy. Spontaneous reactions in a closed system are always accompanied by an increase in disorder and entropy. Designated by the symbol **S.**

Entry Portal (en-trē'/por'tal) (n.) The entry route for microorganisms into a new host.

Enzyme (en'zīm) (n.) A catalyst substance that alters the rate of a chemical reaction but remains unchanged at the end of that reaction.

Eosin (e'o-sin) (n.) An acidic dye used as a counterstain in histology. It will stain acidophilic material pink.

Eosinophilic Granuloma (e"o-sin"o-fil'ik/gran"u-lō'mah) (n.) A benign, self-limiting bone lesion seen classically in males in the first decade. A proliferative disorder of the reticuloendothelial cells. It usually manifests itself with local pain and tenderness. Almost any bone may be affected, but it is most commonly seen in the skull, spine, ribs, pelvis, and proximal skeleton. Radiographically, the lesions are lytic and well-circumscribed. Those that grow most rapidly may produce a premature, destructive appearance, even in the periosteum of new bone. Histologically, the lesions contain a mixture of histiocytes, eosinophils, and chronic inflammatory cells. When electron microscopy is used, rod-shaped inclusion bodies known as Birbeck granules are seen. Synonym: **Eosinophilic Xanthomatous Granuloma.**

Epi (ep″ĭ) A prefix used to designate a structure that is located on top of or over another.

Epicondylar Fracture (ep″i-kon′di-lar/frak′chur) (n.) A fracture that involves an epicondyle of one of the long bones.

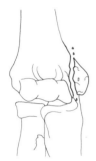

Epicondylar fracture

Epicondyle (ep″i-kon′dīl) (n.) An eminence found on a bone above its condyle. It is usually roughened for attachment with muscles or tendons. Examples are the medial and lateral prominent bony eminences at the distal end of the humerus and just above the elbow joint.

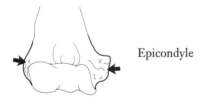

Epicondyle

Epicondylitis (ep″i-kon″di-lī′tis) (n.) Inflammation of the distal, nonarticular medial or lateral bony prominence of the humerus. Inflammation of the lateral humeral epicondyle is commonly referred to as "tennis elbow." Inflammation of the medial humeral epicondyle is commonly referred to as "golfer's elbow."

Epidemic (ep″i-dem′ik) (n.) A temporary and significant increase in the incidence of a disease that sur-

passes what is normally expected over a given time in a community or area.

Epidemiology (ep″i-dēm-ē-ol′-oje) (n.) 1. The dynamic study of health and disease in a population, including its causes, frequency, distribution, and control. 2. The study of the relationship between disease (or health) and the population at risk.

Epidermis (ep″i-der′mis) (n.) The outermost surface tissue of the skin.

Epidermoid Inclusion Cyst (ep″i-der′moid/in-klū′zhun/sist) (n.) A rare, benign, intraosseous lesion most often found in the distal phalanx or calvarium. Radiographically, it appears as a sharply demarcated, lytic area; histologically, it is lined with stratified squamous epithelium and filled with keratin debris.

Epidural (ep″i-du′ral) (n.) The outermost of the three spaces covering the brain and the spinal cord. It is located on or over the dura mater. May be referred to as the **Epidural Space.**

Epidural Anesthesia (ep″i-du′ral/an″es-thē′zē-ah) (n.) A type of regional anesthesia produced by the injection of a local anesthetic agent into the epidural space.

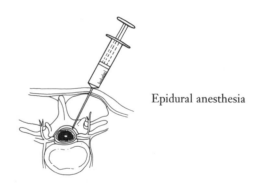

Epidural anesthesia

Epidural Blood Patch (ep″i-du′ral/blud/pach) (n.) A treatment for a refractory postlumbar puncture headache. A patch is used to repair the puncture tear or hole in the dura mater around the spinal cord. If 2 to 10 mL of autologous blood is injected epidurally at the site of the puncture, a gelatinous tampon forms that seals the dural opening.

Epidural Catheter (ep″i-du-ral/kath′e-ter) (n.) A flexible tube that is placed in the epidural space for the administration of prolonged regional anesthesia. It also may be used intraoperatively and postoperatively for continuous analgesia.

Epidural Space (ep″i-du-ral/spās) (n.) The epidural space that surrounds the spinal meninges and extends from the foramen magnum to the sacral hiatus. This space is bounded anteriorly by the posterior longitudinal ligament, laterally by the pedicles of the vertebrae and the intervertebral foramina, and posteriorly by the ligamentum flavum and the anterior surface of the laminae. The epidural space is widest posteriorly, its width varying with the vertebral level—it is narrowest in the cervical region and widest in the lumbar region. In addition to nerve roots, the epidural space contains fat, areolar tissue, lymphatics, arteries, and the vertebral venous plexus of Batson.

Epidural Steroid Injection (n.) A treatment for spinal disorders by the injection of a corticosteroid agent into the epidural space.

Epimysium (ep″i-mis′ē-um) (n.) The sheath of connective tissue that surrounds an entire muscle.

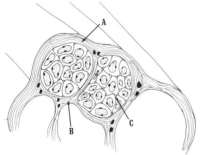

A, Epimysium; B, perimysium; C, endomysium.

Epinephrine (ep″i-nef′rin) (n.) A hormone secreted principally by the medulla of the adrenal gland situated on the kidney. Fear or excitement can stimulate the secretion of epinephrine, producing effects on the circulatory system, glucose mobilization, and so on. Also called **Adrenaline**.

Epineural (ep″i-nu′ral) (adj.) 1. Pertaining to the epineurium. 2. Attached to a neural arch.

Epineural Fibrosis (ep″i-nu′ral/fi-bro′sis) (n.) Scar tissue surrounding a spinal nerve root in the spinal canal or neural foramen. Synonym: **Root Sleeve Fibrosis**.

Epineurium (ep″i-nu′rē-um) (n.) The outer sheath of connective tissue that surrounds the funiculus and the perineural sheaths of a nerve trunk. See **Peripheral Nerve**.

Epiphyseal Cartilage (ep″i-fiz′ē-al/kar′ti-lij) (n.) The temporarily unossified, peripheral region of the epiphyis.

Epiphyseal Disk (ep″ĭ-fiz′e-al/disk) (n.) See **Epiphyseal Plate**.

Epiphyseal Extrusion (ep″i-fiz′ē-al/eks-troo′zhun) (n.) A prognostic sign in Legg-Calvé-Perthes disease that refers to the sighting of a lateral extrusion of the femoral head. It is quantified as the percentage of the width of the femoral head lateral to Perkins′ line; on an AP roentgenogram of the pelvis this can be seen when the hips are in neutral rotation and neutral abduction-adduction. To compute the extrusion, divide the amount of the involved femoral head that is uncovered (A-B) by the width at the epiphyseal

plate of the opposite normal femoral head, (C-D): E = AB/CD × 100.

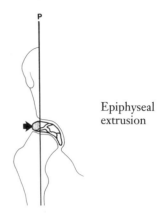

Epiphyseal extrusion

Epiphyseal Fracture (ep″i-fiz′ē-al/frak′chur) (n.) A fracture or separation occurring along or through the epiphyseal plate of a growing bone. These injuries are usually caused by a shearing force that separates the epiphysis from the metaphysis by disrupting the cartilage of the epiphyseal plate. The damage done to this structure may arrest or alter the growth of the

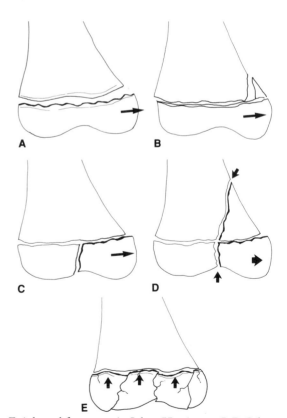

Epiphyseal fractures. A, Salter-Harris type I; B, Salter-Harris type II; C, Salter-Harris type III; D, Salter-Harris type IV; E, Salter-Harris type V.

§ Also: Rang′s 6th type = injury to the perichondrial ring

bone. See also **Salter-Harris Classification of Epiphyseal Fractures**.

Epiphyseal Height (ep″i-fiz′ē-al/hīt) (n.) A radiographic measurement of the distance from the epiphyseal line to the highest point of the epiphysis.

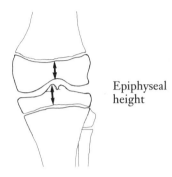

Epiphyseal height

Epiphyseal Index of Cramer (ep″i-fiz′ē-al/in′deks/of/krah′mer) (n.) A radiographic measurement used in the evaluation of a capital femoral epiphysis. An angle formed on an AP radiograph that uses the epiphyseal plate and the femoral head as guides. On the AP radiograph, draw a line demarcating the epiphyseal plate. Then draw a line from the lateral position of the articular surface of the femoral head to the epiphyseal plate line. The angle formed is the epiphyseal index of Cramer. It is normally about 16°.

Epiphyseal Index of Eyre-Brook (n.) See **Eyre-Brook's Epiphyseal Index**.

Epiphyseal Line (ep″i-fiz′ē-al/līn) (n.) A line that represents the junction of the epiphysis and diaphysis of a long bone where longitudinal growth is occurring. 1. The area left at the site of the epiphyseal plate after the fusion of an epiphysis with the diaphysis of a long bone. The site is commonly marked by a cribiform bony plate seen fairly easily in histologic sections. 2. In radiology, a strip of decreased density seen between the metaphysis and the ossified portion of the epiphysis.

Epiphyseal Ossification Center (ep″i-fiz′ē-al/os″i-fi-kā′shun/sen′ter) (n.) The central, ossified portion of an epiphysis.

Epiphyseal Plate (ep″i-fiz′e-al/plāt) (n.) A layer of

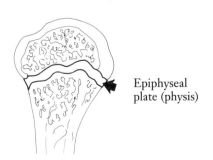

Epiphyseal plate (physis)

hyaline cartilage that separates the epiphysis from the metaphysis. This is the site where most of the longitudinal growth of bones occurs. When growth ceases, the epiphyseal plate is obliterated by ossification. Synonym: **Epiphyseal Disk**, **Physis**, **Growth Plate**.

Epiphyseal Quotient (ep″i-fiz′ē-al/kwō′shent) (n.) See **Sjovall Epiphyseal Quotient**.

Epiphyseal Scar (ep″i-fiz′ē-al/skahr) (n.) A radiodense line present at the ends of mature long bone. It represents a closed epiphyseal plate.

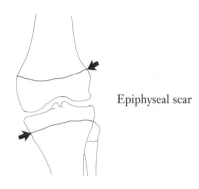

Epiphyseal scar

Epiphyseal Separation (ep″i-fiz′ē-al/sep″ah-rā′shun) (n.) The displacement of an epiphysis that signifies an injury along the epiphyseal plate.

Epiphyseal Stapling (ep″i-fiz′ē-al/stā′pling) (n.) A surgical technique for the correction of a limb length discrepancy. This procedure retards the longitudinal growth of a limb by inserting rigid staples across the epiphyseal plate.

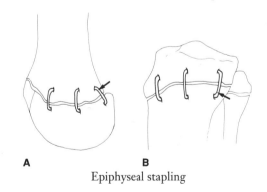

A   **B**
Epiphyseal stapling

Epiphysiodesis (ep″i-fiz″ē-od′e-sis) (n.) A surgical technique that completely arrests longitudinal growth at the epiphysis. It is used for limb equalization in patients whose leg lengths are anticipated to be 2 to 5 cm different.

Epiphyseolysis (ep″i-fiz″ē-ol′ī-sis) (n.) A method of limb lengthening that involves distraction of the epiphyseal plate. See **Distraction Epiphyseolysis**.

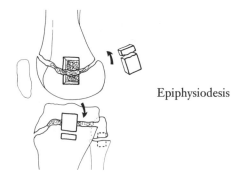

Epiphysiodesis

Epiphysis (e-pif′i-sis) (n.) 1. The end of a bone that lies between the joint surface on one side and the epiphyseal plate on the other. After growth stops, it becomes part of the metaphysis. 2. The portion of a long bone that is developed from the secondary center of ossification. It is separated from the primary center of ossification by the **epiphyseal plate** or **physis**.

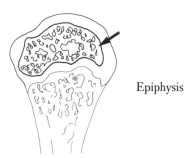

Epiphysis

Epiphysitis (e-pif‴i-sī′tis) (n.) The inflammation of an epiphysis or of the cartilage joining the epiphysis to a bone shaft.

Epithelial Tissues (ep″i-thē′le-al/tish′ūz) (n.) The cellular layers that cover and line outer body surfaces, the interior of hollow organs, and body cavities, acting in these places as absorptive and secretory tissues. Generally, they contain nervous structures, called receptors, that receive stimuli. Many glands are derivatives of epithelial tissues, and these glands secrete a variety of products.

Epitrochlea (ep″i-trōk′le-ah) (n.) The medial epicondyle of the humerus.

Eponym (ep′o-nim) (n.) A commonly used term, phrase, or name describing a disease, structure, syndrome, or theory. It is usually derived from the name of the discoverer or describer; for example, the McMurray test, Apley test, and Dupuytren's contracture are common eponyms.

Epsom Salts (ep′som/sawltz) (n.) A bitter, colorless or white crystalline salt that consists of magnesium sulfate. Popularly used in solution to soak injured body parts.

Equilibrium (ė″kwi-lib′rē-um) (n.) A state of being at rest in which the sum of all forces and all moments acting on an object is zero.

Equine Gait (e′kwīn/gāt) (n.) A gait that results from paralysis of the pretibial and peroneal muscles. To walk, the leg must be lifted abnormally high (as by hip flexion) to clear the foot from the ground. Also known as **drop foot** or **steppage gait**.

Equinovalgus (e-kwī″no-val′gus) (n.) A foot deformity in which the heel is in valgus and plantar flexion and the forefoot is abducted. It is usually seen as an acquired disorder secondary to muscular imbalance. Also known as **talipes equinovalgus**.

Equinovarus (e-kwī″no-vā′rus) (n.) A foot deformity in which the heel is in varus and plantar flexion and the forefoot is adducted. The congenital form is commonly referred to as clubfoot. Also known as **talipes equinovarus**.

Equinus (e-kwī′nus) (n.) A foot deformity in which the heel is in plantar flexion.

Equinus Measurement of Bleck (e-kwī′nus/mezh′er-ment/of/blek) (n.) A radiographic measurement of forefoot alignment. The amount of forefoot equinus, with respect to the horizontal weight-bearing surface of the heel, is measured on a standing lateral radiograph of the foot. The acute angle formed between the first metatarsal shaft and the horizontal plane that is parallel to the plantar aspect of the heel is measured with a goniometer. The normal range is 20° to 30°.

ERB Palsy (erb/pawl′ze) (n.) See **Erb-Duchenne Paralysis**.

Erb-Duchenne Paralysis (erb/du-shen′/pah-ral′i-sis) (n.) A type of brachial plexus injury that causes paralysis of the upper roots of the brachial plexus, commonly from birth injury. This paralysis is due to injury to the fifth and sixth cervical roots, but it does not involve the small muscles of the hand. The lesion that causes the paralysis may result from a closed process (e.g., birth trauma) or a traction injury or fracture. It may be secondary to an open process (e.g., a penetrating injury) or it may result from an

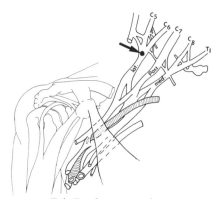

Erb-Duchenne paralysis

infiltrative local process. In the classic form of birth palsy, the arm and forearm are adducted and internally rotated while the forearm is extended and pronated (waiters' tip position). Flaccid paralysis and a wasting of the arm and shoulder muscles are evident. There is no loss of sensation, except perhaps in a small area on the lower border of the deltoid. The paralysis may be transient or permanent, depending on the amount of injury. Synonyms: **Brachial Plexus Paralysis, Duchenne-Erb, Erb's I, Upper Brachial Plexus Paralysis, Erb's Palsy.**

Erb Phenomenon (erb/fe-nom′e-non) (n.)   The finding of increased electric irritability of motor nerves in tetany.

Erg   A unit of work that represents the effort exerted when a body is moved against the force of 1 dyne through a distance of 1 cm.

Ergometry (er″go-me-trē) (n.)   The measurement of work as performed by muscular activity.

Ergonomics (er″go-nom′iks) (n.)   The field of knowledge that looks at the anatomic, physiologic, and psychologic aspects of human work, as well as its laws of mechanics and efficiency. It is considered a branch of ecology.

Ergosterol (er-gos′te-rol) (n.)   The ingestible form of provitamin D_2. At ultraviolet range, sunlight on the skin activates the provitamin, turning it into vitamin D_2 (calciferol).

Erichsen's Sign (er′ik-senz/sīn) (n.)   A maneuver used to diagnose sacroiliac joint disease. In this maneuver, pain occurs when the iliac bones are sharply pressed toward each other. By contrast, in hip joint disease there is no pain when pressure is similarly exerted.

Erlenmeyer Flask Deformity (er′len-mī″er/flask/de-for′mi-tē) (n.)   A deformity caused by failed tubulation. The name is derived from a radiographically appearance of flaring of the metaphyseal end of the distal femur. Examples of this deformity are found in the bony overgrowth due to Gaucher's disease or the failure of osteoclasis in osteopetrosis.

Erysipelas (er″i-sip′e-las) (n.)   An acute infection of the skin and subcutaneous tissues caused by Group A, beta-hemolytic streptococci. The lesion is characteristically hot and red, with a distinct and advancing elevated margin. Central clearing may or may not be evident. The process evolves rapidly and spreads peripherally. Generalized toxic symptoms develop in affected individuals. Also known as **Saint Anthony's Disease.**

Erythema Marginatum (er″i-thē′mah/mar′ji-nā′tum) (n.)   The characteristic maculopapular exanthem of rheumatic fever. The erythematous lesions often have clear centers and round margins; the border of their enlarging ring may be raised or flat. They generally occur on the trunk and proximal extremities; they are rarely seen on the face. The erythema is transient and migratory and may be exacerbated by a hot bath or shower. The lesions are generally nonpruritic, and occur in approximately 10 percent of patients with acute rheumatic fever.

Erythema Multiforme (er″i-thē′mah/mul′ti-for′mah) (n.)   A variety of dermal erythema characterized by acute, self-limited, but often recurrent eruptions, along with secondary epidermal changes. It usually involves both mucous membranes and skin. A symptom complex, it is associated with a wide variety of disorders, the most common being drug reactions, herpes simplex, mycoplasma, histoplasma, and adenovirus infections. Erythema multiforme includes a spectrum of clinical patterns that range from a few trivial lesions on the skin or mucous membranes to a severe, sometimes fatal multisystem illness.

Erythema Nodosum (er″i-thē′mah/no′dōs-um) (n.)   A skin lesion characterized by acute, inflammatory, red cutaneous nodules that are slightly elevated. They are 1 to 5 cm in diameter and heal spontaneously without ulceration or scarring. They principally occur on the anterior surfaces of the lower legs, although occasionally, they are seen on the thighs, arms, and face. Considered a form of hypersensitivity response, the nodules are extremely tender. They evolve from deep red to black and blue; finally, as the subcutaneous hemorrhage resolves, they have a yellowish green tint. Prodromal symptoms such as fever, arthralgia, leg pain, and gastrointestinal disturbances sometimes precede the nodules. Pathologically, one typically sees a perivascular chronic inflammatory cellular reaction, which may involve associated arthralgias or frank arthritis. This is frequently seen in joints adjacent to the nodular lesions.

Erythema nodosum is not a specific disease entity, but a pattern of allergic skin reactions to various blood-borne antigens. It is seen in association with sarcoidosis, inflammatory bowel disease, and Behcet's syndrome, as well as in fungal, viral, mycobacterial, and bacterial (such as streptococcal and yersinial) infections. It is also associated with the use of many drugs, such as oral contraceptives, sulfonamides, and penicillin. Many cases, however, are unassociated with a specific precipitating cause. When no causative factor can be found, the erythema nodosum is termed "idiopathic." Synonyms: **Nodular Vasculitis, Dermatitis Contusiformis, Nodules of the Leg Syndrome.**

Erythrocyte Sedimentation Rate (e-rith′ro-sīt/sed″i-men-tā′shun/rāt) (n.)   The rate at which red blood cells (erythrocytes) settle out of their suspension in blood plasma, measured under standardized conditions and expressed in millimeters per hour. See **Westergreen, Wintrobe,** and **Zeta** sedimentation rates. Abbreviated **ESR.**

Erythrocyte (e-rith′ri-sīt) (n.)   A non-nucleated cell of complex, disklike structure whose primary function is the transport of oxygen. Synonym: **Red Blood Cell.**

Eschar (es′kar) (n.)   A thickened slough of tissue,

usually skin, that is the result of thermal, chemical, or mechanical burning.

Escherichia (esh″er-i′kē-ah) (n.) Genus of gram-negative rods of the family *Enterobacteriacease*, widely distributed in both nature and the human intestinal tract.

Esherich's Sign (esh′er-iks/sīn) (n.) In tetany, a muscular contraction of the lips that resembles a goat's snout.

Esmarch's Bandage (es′marks/ban′dij) (n.) A rolled latex bandage used to squeeze the blood out of an extremity by compressing the superficial vessels. It is used to exsanguinate a limb prior to inflating a pneumatic tourniquet. Alternatively, it can function alone as an elastic tourniquet. The German military surgeon Friedrich von Esmarch introduced the elastic bandage in 1869 for the control of hemorrhage on the battlefield.

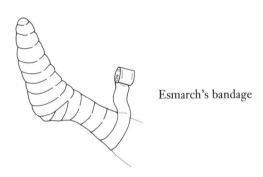

Esmarch's bandage

ESO Abbreviation for Electrospinal Orthosis.

ESR Abbreviation for Erythrocyte Sedimentation Rate.

Essex-Lopresti Fracture (es-ex/lō-prā-stē/frak′chur) (n.) A fracture of the head of the radius that includes an associated dislocation of the distal radioulnar joint. First described by P. Essex-Lopresti in 1951.

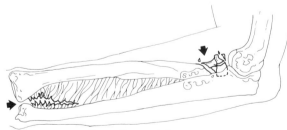

Essex-Lopresti fracture

Essex-Lopresti Technique (es-ex/lō-prā-stē/tek-nēk) (n.) A surgical reduction and fixation of displaced calcaneal fractures. This technique uses an axial pin to manipulate and then fix the fracture fragments.

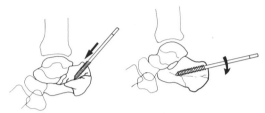

Essex-Lopresti technique

Estrogen Replacement Therapy (es′tro-jen/rē-plās′ment/ther′ah-pē) (n.) A regimen followed to prevent postmenopausal osteoporosis in which estrogens are administered. The estrogen is usually prescribed with cyclic progesterone to avoid complications.

Eu A prefix meaning normal, well, or good.

Eukaryote (u-kar′e-ōt) (n.) An organism whose cells contain a nucleus bounded by a membrane. Often spelled eucaryote.

EULAR Abbreviation for **European League Against Rheumatism**.

Evans Procedure (ev-unz/pro-sē′jur) (n.) Surgical correction of chronic lateral ankle instability that uses the peroneus brevis tendon to reconstruct the calcaneofibular ligament. Compare **Chrisman-Snook Procedure**.

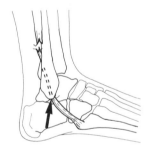

Evans procedure

Everett Crutch (ev-ret/kruch) (n.) An aluminum Canadian crutch. This crutch was first made for its namesake, Charles E. Everett, a patient at the Georgia Warm Springs Foundation. Also called a **Warm Springs Crutch**.

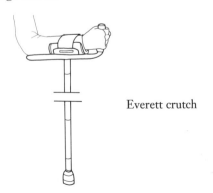

Everett crutch

Eversion (e-ver'shun) (n.) 1. A turning outward. 2. A movement in the foot and ankle that combines pronation, abduction, and dorsiflexion; this turns the sole of the foot so that it tends to face laterally. Requires lateral rotation of the calcaneus on a longitudinal oblique axis through the calcaneus and talus. Also requires motion in the subtalar joint. Compare with **Inversion**.

Eversion Stress Test (e-ver'shun/stres/test) (n.) A clinical assessment of medial ankle instability in which the tibiotalar joint is stressed with eversion. In a positive test, the talus will tilt laterally. Contrast to **Inversion Stress Test**.

Ewing's Sarcoma (u'ings/sar-kō'mah) (n.) A highly malignant, small round-cell neoplasm of bone. The resulting lesion arises in the diaphysis or the metaphysis of long and flat bones. The neoplasm is more common in males than females; it is typically seen in the second decade. Symptoms include pain localized to the area of the tumor, weight loss, fever, and anemia. Leukocytosis with an elevated sedimentation rate is also a symptom, and this may cause the clinical picture of osteomyelitis.

Radiographic studies reveal mottled bone destruction along with extensive involvement of the shaft of the long bones. Growth of the sarcoma within the long bone shaft stimulates the reactive formation of multiple new laminae of bone. This presents a layered, onion-like roentgen appearance.

Grossly, the tumor is gray-white, glistening, and in many instances, soft to almost liquid in consistency. Microscopically, it is composed of small, round, uniform cells that are densely packed. The lack of stroma is conspicuous. With silver stains, groups of cells surrounded by reticulin fibers can be demonstrated. When PAS staining is used, glycogen is evident. Electron microscopy usually offers views of glycogen granules. Current treatment includes the use of adjuvant chemotherapy with radiation and surgical resection.

Exacerbation (eg-zas"er-bā'shun) (n.) An increase in the severity of symptoms or signs of a disorder.

Excessive Lateral Pressure Syndrome (ek-ses'iv/lat'er-al/presh'ur/sin'drōm) (n.) A term originated by Ficat and Hungerford to describe a clinical syndrome that results from extreme pressure on the lateral aspect of the patella. It is characterized by retropatellar pain. Radiologically, there is a tilting of the patella to the lateral side, which is seen on the axial patellofemoral view. In this syndrome, the patella is stable and well-centered in the trochlear sulcus, but there is functional lateralization onto a physiologically and often anatomically prominent lateral facet. Also known as **ELPS**.

Excision (ek-sizh'un) (n.) The operative removal of part or all of a body component.

Excisional Biopsy (ek-sizh'un-al/bī'op-se) (n.) The total excision of tissue for examination in such a manner that the entire lesion is removed.

Excoriation (eks-ko"re-ā'shun) (n.) A superficial abrasion or ulceration of the skin caused by scratching. It is usually linear in appearance. Synonym: **Abrasion**.

Excrescence (eks-kres'ens) (n.) The abnormal outgrowth of a structure.

Excursion of a Tendon (eks-kur'zhun/of/a/ten'dun) (n.) The distance that a tendon must move to facilitate a given movement of a joint.

Exercise (ek'ser-sīz) (n.) 1. Any and all activity involving a generation of force by activated muscle(s) that disrupts a homeostatic state.

2. Exertion of the body or mind to train for an activity, improve health, and/or rehabilitate or correct a physical deformity. Exercise is active if the individual exerts himself, passive if motion occurs without effort.

Exercise Intensity (ek'ser-sīz/in-ten'si-tē) (n.) A level of consistent muscular activity that can be quantified in terms of: (1.) power, or the expended or work performed per unit of time; (2.) isometric force sustained over a period of time; and (3.) the velocity of progression.

Exercise Load (ek'ser-sīz/lōd) (n.) The load with or against which muscular activity is performed. Its function may be assistive, as in the case of weaker muscle groups, or resistive, as when conditioning stronger muscle groups. An exercise load does not necessarily refer to the resistance the muscle must overcome during exercise.

Exercise Testing (ek'ser-sīz/test-ing) (n.) A technique for evaluating cardiovascular response to physical stress. Also called **Stress Testing**.

Exo (ek"so) A prefix denoting outside, outward, or external.

Exocrine (ek'so-krin) (n.) A type of gland that releases its secretion through a duct. Contrast **Endocrine**.

Exostosis (ek"sos-tō'sis) (n.) A benign growth projecting from the surface of a bone. It is formed by endochondral ossification, which results in a characteristically cartilage-capped bony projection contiguous with the normal shaft. Their growth stops when the growth plates close. Diagnosed after pain in the exostotic bursa or a mass effect, they are usually present between the ages of 10 and 25. Radiographically, they appear as sessile or stalked projections in the juxtaepiphyseal region; the stalks characteristically point away from the adjacent joint surface. Malignant transformation rarely occurs. Also known as **osteochondroma** or **osteocartilaginous exostosis**. See related **hereditary multiple exostoses**.

Exothermic Reaction (ek"so-ther'mik/re-ak'shun) (n.) A chemical reaction in which energy is released as heat. Contrast with **Endothermic**.

Exotoxin (ek"so-tok'sin) (n.) A toxin excreted by a

microorganism into its surrounding medium. Contrast with **Endotoxin**.

Exsanguinate (eks-sang′gwi-nāt) (v.) 1. To make bloodless. 2. Removal of blood from a limb by gravity or the application of an elastic bandage prior to the inflation of a tourniquet to create a bloodless field for surgical procedures.

Exstrophy of the Bladder (ek′stro-fē/of/the/blad′der) (n.) A congenital anomaly caused by a failure of fusion of the anterior midline body structures. The presence of pubic diastasis, lateral flaring of the innominate bones, or lateral displacement and external rotation of the acetabuli should be of concern. To facilitate reconstruction of the urologic tract, pelvic bony reconstruction is often indicated.

Extension (ek-sten′shun) (n.) 1. The straightening of a joint so that the two adjacent segments are moved apart, thereby decreasing the joint angle. 2. When the straightening of a joint results in a return to the zero starting position.

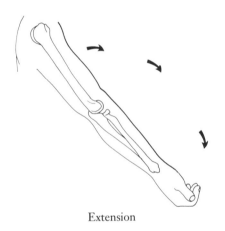

Extension

Extensor (eks-ten′sor) (n.) A muscle whose function it is to extend a joint. See also under **Muscle**.

Extensor Hood (eks-ten′sor/hood) (n.) The dorsal

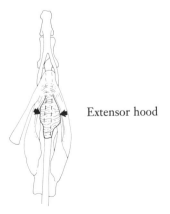

Extensor hood

expansion of the extensor mechanism over the metacarpophalangeal joint.

Extensor Lag (eks-ten′sor/lag) (n.) The inability to actively straighten out a joint into full extension that may result from either a weakness or a disruption of the extensor mechanism of that joint.

Extensor Mechanism of the Finger (eks-ten′sor/mek′ah-nizm/of/the/fing′ger) (n.) A complex anatomic structure responsible for digital extension. It is composed of slips of the digital extensor tendon and requires participation of the adjacent tendons of the lumbrical and interosseous muscles of the hand.

Extensor Tendon Compartments (eks-ten′sor/ten′dun/com-part′ments) (n.) A series of six fibro-osseous canals at the distal end of the forearm through which the extensor tendons gain entrance to the hand. These canals are covered by a substantial retinaculum that keeps the extensor tendons from bowstringing.

1. The first compartment contains the abductor pollicis longus and extensor pollicis brevis.

2. The second compartment contains the radial wrist extensors.

3. The third compartment contains the extensor pollicis longus.

4. The fourth compartment contains the extensor digitorum communis and the extensor indicis proprius.

5. The fifth compartment contains the extensor digiti quinti.

6. The sixth compartment contains the extensor carpi ulnaris.

Extensor Zones of Hand (eks-ten′sor/zonz/of/the/hand) (n.) Zones of the extensor surface of the hand that comply with the different anatomic relationships of the extensor tendons and their attachments.

Zone 1: Extends from the distal insertion of the extensor tendon to the attachment of the central slip at the proximal end of the middle phalanx.

Zone II: Extends from the metacarpal neck to the proximal interphalangeal joint. It includes the extensor mechanism and its contoured surface, the phalanx, and the metacarpal head.

Zone III: Extends proximally from the metacarpal neck to the distal border of the dorsal carpal ligament. The tendons in this area lie freely, without ligamentous attachment, and are covered by paratenon and fascia only.

Zone IV: The area of the wrist under the dorsal carpal ligament. At this level, the tendons have mesotenon. They are held by the dorsal carpal ligament, which acts as a pulley, and are ensheathed in canals similar to the theca on the flexor surface.

Zone V: The zone closest to the proximal margin of the dorsal carpal ligament. Here, many extensor tendons are contained within their respective muscles.

Extent of Lateral Femoral Subluxation Index (ekstent /of/lat′er-al/fem′or-al/sub″luk-sa′shun/in′deks) (n.) A method for quantifying the degree of subluxation of the femoral head from the acetabulum. Lateral subluxation is calculated by first identifying on an AP radiograph of the pelvis the most medial part of the proximal section of the involved femur and then measuring the horizontal distance to the acetabulum. The normal side then is measured at a comparable point and a ratio is formed by dividing the involved side by the normal side.

External Fixation (eks-ter'nal/fik-sa'shun) (n.) A method of fracture management that uses percutaneous transfixing pins in bones. These pins are attached externally to the bone through plaster, metal frames, or other devices (external skeletal fixator).

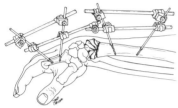

External fixation.

External Rotation (eks-ter'nal/ro-ta'shun) (n.) The movement of a body part away from a central axis.

External Rotation Recurvatum Test (eks-ter'nal/ro-ta'shun/re"kur-va'tum/test) (n.) A test for posterolateral instability of the knee. A way to evaluate abnormal external rotation of the tibia associated with excessive recurvatum at the knee. The test is performed with the patient in a supine position. The knee is moved from approximately 10° of flexion to maximum extension; the tester should observe and palpate the external rotation of the proximal end of the tibia, as well as the amount of recurvatum. In a positive test excessive rotation and a subtle apparent varus deformity in recurvatum occurs. A positive test also signifies the disruption of the posterior cruciate ligament, the posterolateral corner, and the fibular collateral ligament.

External Skeletal Fixator (eks-ter'nal/skel'e-tal/fik-sa'ter) (n.) The frame that holds the percutaneous

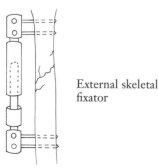

External skeletal fixator

transfixing pins used in external fixation of bone fragments.

Extirpation (ek"ster-pa'shun) (n.) The surgical destruction, eradication, or complete removal of all or part of a tissue from the body.

Extra-Articular (eks"trah-ar-tik'u-lar) (n.) Situated or occurring outside a joint.

Extra-Articular Arthrodesis (eks"trah-ar-tik'u-lar/ar"thro-de'sis) (n.) A surgical technique of obtaining bony fusion across a joint that does not require exposure of the joint surfaces. See **Brittain Arthrodesis**.

Extra-Articular Fracture (eks"trah-ar-tik'u-lar/frak'chur) (n.) A fracture that does not involve a joint surface but is adjacent to the joint.

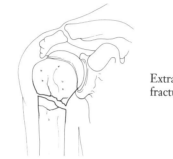

Extra-articular fracture

Extracapsular (eks"trah-kap'su-lar) (adj.) Situated or occurring outside a capsule, usually a joint capsule.

Extracapsular Fracture (eks"trah-kap'su-lar/frak'chur) (n.) A fracture that occurs near or adjacent to, but outside, the capsule of a joint. For example, an intertrochanteric hip fracture is an extracapsular fracture; an intracapsular subcapital hip fracture is not.

Extracellular Fluid (eks"trah-sel'u-lar/floo'id) (n.) The fluid that bathes the cells. Abbreviated **ECF**.

Extrapyramidal System (eks"trah-pi-ram'i-dal/sis'tem) (n.) A complex nervous tract whose function is imperfectly understood. It is believed that the basal ganglia and nuclei of the reticular formation are interconnected and have a diffuse projection system that includes descending and ascending pathways. These pathways significantly influence the upper motor neuron and its function. Diseases of this system involve the movements and the secondary disorders of muscle tone. Commonly seen are the tremor, rigidity, and abnormal posturing of Parkinson's disease. Also seen are athetosis and, less frequently, chorea and hemiballismus, which may be manifestations of cerebral palsy. Further symptoms include diffuse cerebral trauma and anoxia leading to metabolic disorders.

Extravasation (eks-trav"ah-sa'shun) (n.) The exudative leakage or spread of fluid from vessels into surrounding tissues.

Extrusion Index (eks-troo′zhun/in′deks) (n.) On an AP radiograph of the pelvis, it is the width of the portion of the involved femoral epiphysis lateral to a vertical line drawn at the lateral margin of the acetabulum divided by the width of the uninvolved epiphysis.

Exudate (eks′u-dāt) (n.) 1. A fluid with a high content of protein and cells that has passed through the walls of vessels into the adjacent tissues or spaces. Usually the result of inflammation. 2. Any exuded substance. Contrast to **Transudate**.

Eyelet (i′let) (n.) A hole or metal ring on shoes that is used for lacing.

Eyre-Brook Epiphyseal Index (ār-bruk/ep″i-fiz′ē-al/in′deks) (n.) In Legg-Perthes disease, an index used to measure the shape abnormality of the femoral capital epiphysis; also used to express the degree of flattening of the epiphysis. The index is calculated by measuring the height of the epiphysis, which is the distance from the epiphyseal line to the highest point of its outline, and dividing that by its breadth.

Eyre-Brook Head Index (ār-bruk/hed/in′deks) (n.) The percentage relationship of the radius to the diameter of the femoral head. This number is used to express the degree of deformity of the femoral head in Legg-Perthes Disease.

F

Fabella (fah-bel′ah) (n.) A small sesamoid bone often found in the tendon of the lateral head of the gastrocnemius muscle. The bone can be identified in two radiographic views: in the lateral view, the bone is seen at the knee posterior to the distal femur; in the AP view, it is superimposed on the lateral femoral condyle. Degenerative disease of the knee joint may cause the bone to become enlarged and roughened. Fabellae are found in 10 to 18 percent of adults.

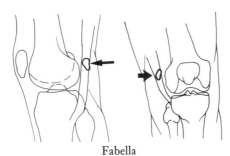

Fabella

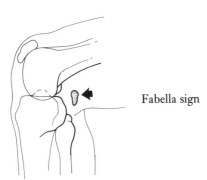

Fabella sign

Fabella Sign (fah-bel′ah/sīn) (n.) In individuals with fabellae, a radiographic sign of effusion and/or intra-

synovial mass. At a normal flexion angle of 120°, the fabella-femoral distance is 9.0 mm and the fabella-tibial distance is 13 mm. With effusion or mass, the fabella is displaced posteriorly, and both distances increase by 1 to 3 mm.

Fabere Test (fā-ber/test) (n.) An acronym derived from the positions of the hip used in the Patrick test: flexion, abduction, external rotation, extension. To carry out the test, have the supine patient place the heel of the affected leg on the opposite knee. Then gently press the thigh downward. If the patient experiences pain in the hip, the test is positive. Also called **Figure of 4 Hip Test**. See **Patrick Test**.

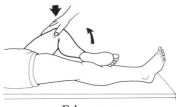

Fabere test

Facet (fas′et) (n.) 1. A small, smooth surface of a bone. 2. In patellae, refers to an articular surface segment. 3. In spine, refers to full articular surface of the ascending and descending articular processes.

Facet Arthrosis (fas′et/ar″thrō-′sis) (n.) See **Degenerative Joint Disease**.

Facet Rhizolysis (fas′et/rī-zō-lī-sis) (n.) See **Facet Rhizotomy**.

Facet Rhizotomy (fas′et/rī-zot′ō-mē) (n.) The denervation of a zygapophyseal joint caused by the destruction of capsular pericapsular tissue and nerve.

Synonyms: **Percutaneous Facet Rhizotomy**, **Facet Rhizolysis**.

Facet Syndrome (fas'et/sin'drōm) (n.) A disorder of the lumbar spine characterized by the sudden onset of low back pain that is positional in nature, relieved in certain postures, and exaggerated in others. The "locking-type" pain usually involves the articular facets of the spinal column.

Facetectomy (fas"e-tek'tō-mē) (n.) The excision of the articular processes that contain the articulations of a zygapophyseal joint.

Facioscapulohumeral Muscular Dystrophy (fa"she-o-skap"ū-lō-hū'mer-al/mus'ku-lar/dis'trō-fē) (n.) A progressive muscular dystrophy transmitted as an autosomal dominant trait. The condition can begin in early childhood, but most often occurs during adolescence.

In the initial stages of the disease, the face and shoulder girdle muscles are affected. In later stages, it spreads to the pelvic girdle. Involvement of the deltoid, scapular rotator, and fixators results in bilateral winging and elevation of the scapula.

Weak facial muscles result in a characteristic appearance: a generally smooth forehead and eye area and a transverse smile. There is an inability to close the eyes properly, whistle, or pout the lips. As muscle weakness progresses, speech becomes indistinct.

Contractural and bony deformities are mild and occur late in the disease. The intelligence level remains normal, and cardiac involvement is rare. Progress of the disease is insidious, with prolonged periods of apparent arrest, and then unusually rapid progression.

FACS Abbreviation for Fellow of the American College of Surgeons.

Factitious (fak-tish'us) (adj.) 1. Artificial and/or contrived; self-induced. 2. An event that is produced artificially or accidentally. Such an event should be discounted when making a diagnosis or when considering the results of an experiment. Example: **Factitious Fever**.

Facultative Anaerobe (fak'ul-tā"tiv/an'er-ōb) (n.) A bacterium that grows under either aerobic or anerobic conditions.

Fadire Test (fā-dīr/test) (n.) An acronym derived from the position used in evaluating disorders of the hip joint: Flexion, Adduction, Internal Rotation, and Extension. Contrast to **Fabere Test** and **Patrick Test**.

Fairbank's Lesions (fār-bankz/le'zhunz) (n.) A range of knee joint changes that are seen on AP radiograph of a knee following a meniscectomy. These include: 1. no abnormality; 2. a squaring or flattening of femoral condyles; 3. marginal osteophyte formation; 4. joint-space narrowing; 5. degenerative osteoarthritis.

Fairbank's Sign of Apprehension (fār-bankz/sīn/of/ap"rē-hen'shun) (n.) A test used in evaluating recurrent dislocation of the patella. With the patient supine and relaxed and the knee straight, attempt a lateral displacement of the affected patella. If the test is positive, the patient becomes apprehensive. Also called **Apprehension Test**.

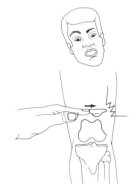

Fairbank's apprehension test

Fajersztajn Test (fa-yer-stān/test) (n.) A variant of the Lasègue test for sciatica. With the patient supine, raise the extended leg to the point of pain. Then dorsiflex the foot to elicit sciatic pain.

False-Negative (fawls'neg'ah-tiv) (adj.) An incorrect report of a test or procedure that falsely indicates the absence of a finding, condition, or disease.

False-Positive (fawls'pos'ĭ-tiv) (adj.) An incorrect result of a test or procedure that falsely indicates the presence of a finding, condition, or disease.

Familial Dysautonomia (fah-mil'e-al/dis"aw-tō-nō'mē-ah) (n.) A rare autosomal recessive disorder of the nervous system characterized by profound, generalized autonomic dysfunction and a diffuse disorder of the central nervous system. Distinctive clinical features include an absence of overflow tears (alacrima) and sweating, a relative indifference to pain, and vasomotor instability, often leading to hyperthermia. The disorder is also frequently characterized by episodic hypertension, postural hypotension, transient blotching of the skin, hyperhidrosis, episodic vomiting, disordered swallowing, dysarthria, and motor incoordination. Familial dysautonomia most often affects Jewish children of Eastern European extraction. They are shorter than normal and may have lower than average intelligence. Most patients die in childhood or early adolescence. Synonym: **Riley-Day Syndrome**.

Familial Metaphyseal Dysplasia (fah-mil'e-al/met"ah-fiz'ē-al/dis-plā'se-ah) (n.) See **Pyle Disease**.

Family (fam"i-lē) (n.) A group of related, similar genera. In taxonomy, family ranks below order and above genus.

Fanconi Syndrome (fahn-kō-nē/sin'drōm) (n.) A group of disorders with characteristic defects of renal tubular function. These include: 1. excessive renal loss of phosphorus, with accompanying hypophosphatemia, vitamin D-resistant rickets, and osteomalacia; 2. renal glycosuria; 3. multiple aminoaciduria; 4. excessive renal loss of uric acid.

Fascia (fash′ē-ah) (n.) A sheet or band of connective tissue that envelops muscles and muscle groups, usually of similar function.

Fascia Graft (fash′e-ah/graft) (n.) A graft of fascial tissue usually taken from the fascia lata, the external investing fascia of the thigh.

Fascia Lata (fash′e-ah/lah′tah) (n.) The external investing fascia of the thigh.

Fascicle (fas′i-k′l) (n.) An arrangement of nerve and muscle fibers resembling a cluster or bundle of rods. Also known as **Fasciculus** or **Funiculus**.

Fasciectomy (fas″e-ek′tō-mē) (n.) An excision of a fascia. For example, this technique is surgically useful in the treatment of Dupuytren's disease.

Fasciitis (fas″ē-ī′tis) (n.) An inflammation of fascia. A common example is plantar fasciitis in the sole of the foot.

Fasciculation (fah-sik″ū-lā′shun) (n.) A brief, spontaneous, and localized involuntary contraction of one or a few motor units in a skeletal muscle. It is grossly detected as a flickering movement under the skin.

Fasciocutaneous Flap (fas″ē-ō-kū-tā′nē-us/flap) (n.) A type of surgical flap that relies on the blood supply from perforating vessels that run up to the superficial surface of the skin in fascial septae located between muscle bellies. With such a flap, there is no need to sacrifice a usable muscle. Many of these flaps contain sensory nerves and thus can be innervated.

Fasciotomy (fash″ē-ot′ō-mē) (n.) A surgical incision in fascia. Used in the treatment of impending compartment syndromes.

Fastidious Organism (fas-tid′ē-us/or′gah-nizm) (n.) An organism difficult to isolate or cultivate on ordinary media.

Fat Embolism (fat/em′bo-lizm) (n.) The sudden blocking of an artery by fat that has been brought by the blood flow to the site where it has lodged. The fat enters the blood circulation usually after fractures of long bones, and it frequently lodges in the lung.

Fat Embolism Syndrome (fat/em″bo-lizm/sin′drōm) (n.) A constellation of symptoms leading to acute respiratory failure after long bone fracture. It is thought to result from deposition of marrow fat or lipids within the pulmonary capillaries. Most commonly encountered in multiple trauma and long bone fractures. Usually presents 12 to 48 hours after injury. Symptoms can range from mild dyspnea to frank coma. Diminished arterial PO_2 is the most consistent laboratory finding. Classic signs, such as fever or petechial rash, may not be present, and diagnosis can require that the physician have a high index of suspicion. The syndrome may present in a subclinical, nonfulminant, or fulminant form. See **Adult Respiratory Distress Syndrome (ARDS)**.

Fat Pad Sign (fat/pad/sīn) (n.) A radiographic sign produced by any process that causes a synovial or hemorrhagic effusion within the elbow joint that displaces the intracapsular or extrasynovial fat pads. A lateral radiograph of the elbow will reveal a "sail-shaped" anterior fat pad or a triangular or elliptical posterior fat pad. This sign is particularly useful in detecting possible obscure fractures around the elbow joint. Anterior fat pad signs can be normal but not posterior signs. See **Displaced Fat Pad Sign**.

Fatigue Failure (fah-tēg′/fāl′yer) (n.) A fracture of bone or implant caused by cyclic loading that may or may not result in permanent deformation. See **Fatigue Fracture**.

Fatigue Fracture (fah-tēg/frak′chur) (n.) A fracture or break in a material caused by repetitive applications of loads that range from the fatigue limit to the yield strength. This fracture results from either low repetitions of high loads or many repetitions of normal loads. See **Stress Fracture** and **Deutschlander's Disease**.

Fatigue Limit (fah-tēg/lim′it) (n.) The load a material can endure indefinitely on subjection to cyclic loading, without bending or breaking.

Fatigue Strength (fah-tēg/strenth) (n.) The maximum load a material can endure without fracturing when subjected to 10 million repetitions or cyclic load. This is probably the most important characteristic in determining a material's functional longevity. Sometimes referred to as the **endurance limit**.

Febrile (feb′ril) (adj.) Pertaining to or marked by fever.

Feedback Inhibition (fēd′bak/in″hi-bish″un) (n.) The down regulation of a given system by the return of output as input, resulting in a signal to decrease that output. Internal regulation within a system allowing maintenance of a range of physiologic levels. This is seen, for example, in hormonal and enzymatic pathways. Also known as negative feedback.

Feiss Line (fīs/līn) (n.) Used for determining the degree of flatfoot, this imaginary line connects the tip of the medial malleolus with the caudal aspect of the head of the first metatarsal. The tubercle of the navicular is normally on this line.

Feldene (fel′dēn) (n.) The proprietary name for Piroxican, a nonsteroidal, anti-inflammatory drug.

Felon (fel′on) (n.) An abscess of the distal finger or toe, where the pulp is divided into many fibrous

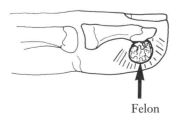

Felon

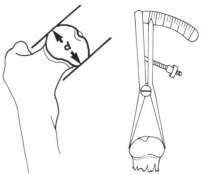

Femoral head size

septa. The abscess may extend into the periosteum of the terminal phalanx, causing osteomyelitis, or it can extend around the nailbed. Also called **Whitlow**.

Felty's Syndrome (fel'tēz/sin'drōme) (n.)   A chronic rheumatoid arthritic disorder associated with splenomegaly, leukopenia, pigmented spots on the skin of the legs, anemia, and thrombocytopenia. See **Still's Disease**.

Femoral (fem'or-al) (adj.)   Pertaining to the femur or the thigh.

Femoral Condyles (fem'or-al/kon'dīlz) (n.)   The distal articular surfaces of the femur that articulate with the tibia and the patella. The medial and lateral condyles are separated by the intercondylar notch and the patellar groove.

Femoral Epicondyles (fem'or-al/ep″-i-kon'dīlz) (n.)   Nonarticular bony lateral or medial projections of the femoral condyles that play a role in ligamentous attachments.

Femoral Head (fem'or-al/hed) (n.)   The nearly spherical extent of the femur that is most proximal and that articulates with the acetabulum.

Femoral Head Width (fem'or-al/hed/width) (n.)   To determine this width, measure the distance from the radiographic "tear drop" to the vertical line tangent to the most lateral portion of the femoral head visible on an AP radiograph of the hip in neutral position.

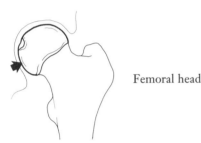

Femoral head

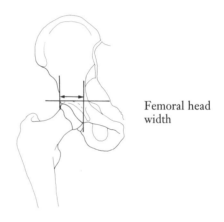

Femoral head width

Femoral Head Coverage (fem'or-al/hed/kov'er-ij) (n.)   A radiographic method of assessing the percent of femoral head articulating within acetabulum in a given position: Calculate the ratio of the depth of the acetabular socket to that of the diameter of the femoral head. This figure expresses the percentage of the femoral head that is uncovered.

Femoral Head Shape (fem'or-al/hed/shāp) (n.)   See **Mose Template**.

Femoral Head Size (fem'or-al/hed/sīz) (n.)   1. The size of the femoral head is measured by drawing a line on the AP radiograph to connect the most medial and lateral points on the femoral head. After measuring the diameter of the normal side, establish the ratio formed by dividing the involved side by the normal side. Coxa magna is present if the involved femoral head has a diameter 10 percent greater than that of the normal side. 2. A measurement obtained directly by putting calipers around an excised femoral head. This measurement is used to determine the replacement size when a hemi- or total hip arthroplasty is performed.

Femoral Neck (fem'or-al/nek) (n.)   The angulated proximal end of the femur that connects the femoral shaft and head.

Femoral Neck Length (fem'or-al/nek/lenth) (n.)   1. The length of the femoral neck is measured by

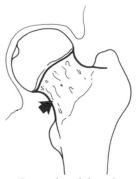

Femoral neck length

using an AP radiograph of the pelvis to determine the relationship of the height of the greater trochanter to the femoral head. The head is divided into four quadrants. If the trochanter reaches the middle of quadrant 2, it has the numerical value of 2.0; if it reaches halfway between quadrants 2 and 3, it has the numerical the value of 2.5, and so on. An imaginary fifth quadrant lies above quadrant 4. Usually lies at the level of the center of the femoral head. 2. Functionally, from the intertrochanteric line to the subcapital region. See **Trochanteric Height**.

Femoral Neck Quotient of Robichon (fem'or-al/nek/kwo'shent/of/raw-bē-shōn') A numerical expression used to evaluate coxa plana. Radiographic measurements of the femoral neck are expressed as the length/width index: the l/w ratio of the affected side divided by the l/w ratio of the normal side multiplied by 100 and then taken to the nearest whole number. Values less than 100 indicate shortening and widening of the affected neck, as seen typically in coxa plana.

Femoral Nerve Traction Test (fem'or-al/nerv/trak'shun/test) (n.) A traction test for midlumbar radiculopathies. With the patient lying on one side, flex the dependent limb at the hip and knee. Also flex the head to increase traction on the cauda equina. Next, extend the relaxed uppermost lower limb maximally at the hip; then flex at the knee. The test is positive when pain radiates down the anterior thigh of that limb. The test is also positive if, on testing the well leg, femoral nerve traction on the pain-free limb produces contralateral anterior thigh pain.

Femoral Shaft (fem'or-al/shaft) (n.) The diaphyseal portion of the femur.

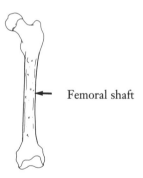

Femoral shaft

Femoral Shaft Line (fem'or-al/shaft/līn) (n.) The line, seen on an AP radiograph of the pelvis and femur, that runs parallel to the long axis of the femur and intersects the tip of the greater trochanter.

Femoral-Tibial Alignment (fem'or-al/tib'ē-al/ah-līn'ment) (n.) The alignment of the femur and tibia as measured on an AP radiograph by the intersection of the vertical axes of the femur and the tibia. On a standing AP view, the tibia is normally at a 7° lateral (valgus) angle to the femoral axis.

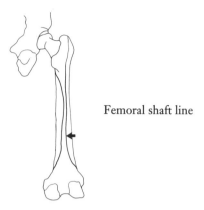

Femoral shaft line

Femoral-Tibial Angle (fem'or-al/tib'ē-al/ang'g'l) (n.) A description of the angular relationship between the femur and tibia at the knee expressed as varus or valgus alignment. It is measured on weight-bearing radiographs of the entire lower extremity or is clinically estimated while the subject is standing.

Femoral Triangle (fem'or-al/trī'ang-g'l) (n.) A triangular subfascial space on the inner side of the upper thigh that is bound laterally by the sartorius muscle, medially by the adductor longus muscle, and superiorly by the inguinal ligament. The space contains the femoral vein, artery, and nerve. See **Scarpa's Triangle**.

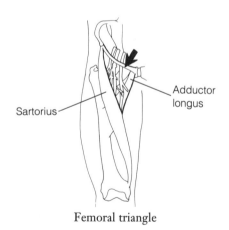

Sartorius

Adductor longus

Femoral triangle

Femorotibial Angle (fem"o-ro-tib'ē-al/ang'g'l) (n.) See **Femoral-Tibial Angle**.

Femur (fe'mur) (n.) The longest and strongest bone of the body, contained in the thigh. It articulates at both the hip and knee joints.

Fenestra (fe-nes'trah) (n.) A windowlike opening or aperture.

Fenestration (fen"es-trā'shun) (n.) A surgical procedure in which a perforation or new opening is formed in bone or other tissue.

Fenoprofen Calcium (fen"o-pro'fen/kal'se-um) (n.)

A nonsteroidal anti-inflammatory drug marketed under the brand name Nalfon.

Ferguson's Angle (fer'gus/unz/ang'g'l) (n.) An angle measured on a lateral radiograph of the lumbosacral spine. It is formed by drawing a horizontal line and its intersection to the plane of the superior margin of the sacrum. The angle is abnormal when it exceeds 34°. Also called the **Lumbosacral Angle**.

Ferguson Method for Scoliosis (fer'gus-un/meth' ud/for/sko"lē-ō-sis) (n.) See **Risser Ferguson Method**.

Festinating Gait (fes"ti-nāt-ing/gāt) (n.) The ambulatory pattern of a patient who involuntarily moves with small, short steps, often on tiptoe, at an accelerating speed. This gait can be seen in Parkinson's disease.

Fever Pattern (fē'ver/pat'ern) (n.) The pattern of elevated body temperature measurement.

Intermittent Fever: High fever interrupted by a return to normal temperature during every 24 hours. Sometimes called hectic, septic, or undulant fever. Pyogenic abscesses often produce this fever pattern.

Relapsing or Recurrent Fever: An elevated temperature, either remittent, intermittent, or sustained for several days, that is followed by several days of normal temperature. This pattern is occasionally referred to as a Pel-Epstein fever.

Remittent Fever: Resembles intermittent fever, except that the temperature does not become normal at any time and the feverish swings are less hectic or severe.

Sustained or Continuous Fever: A low fever with minor diurnal variations and less marked swing in temperature than remittent fever.

Fiberglass Cast (fī"ber-glās/kast) (n.) An immobilizing bandage made of self-curing plastics. These casts are lightweight, long-wearing, water-resistant and radiolucent, as compared with **Plaster-of-Paris Cast**.

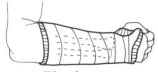

Fiberglass cast

Fibrillation (fi-bri-lā'shun) (n.) 1. A rapid contraction or twitching of muscle fibers. 2. The formation of fibrils or small fibers. 3. A structural defect seen in articular cartilage that is characterized by splitting of the cartilage surface into fibril-like projections.

Fibrillation Potential (fi-bri-lā'shun/po-ten'shal) (n.) An electromyographic representation of individual muscle fiber contractions. These contractions appear as short, spiked waves.

Fibrin (fi'brin) (n.) A coagulated blood protein produced by the action of the enzyme thrombin on a soluble precursor, fibrinogen.

Fibrin Split Products (fi'brin/splint/prod'uktz) (n.) Degradation products of fibrin released into the blood after clot lysis. They may accumulate, resulting in extensive intravascular clotting.

Fibrinogen (fi-brin'o-jen) (n.) A globulin in the blood plasma that, when acted on by the enzyme thrombin, produces the insoluble protein fibrin during the final stage of blood coagulation. Also called **Factor I**.

Fibrinolysin (fi"brĭ-nol'i-sin) (n.) An enzyme produced by hemolytic streptococci that can liquefy clotted blood plasma or fibrin clots. Produced by streptococci (streptokinase). Also called **Plasmin**.

Fibrinolysis (fi"brĭ-nol'ĭ-sis) (n.) Dissolution of fibrin by the enzymatic action of plasmin.

Fibro- (fi"bro) A prefix that denotes the presence or an association of fibrous tissue.

Fibroblast (fi'bro-blast) (n.) The main cell in connective tissue that is involved in the production of fibrous, collagenized stroma. Fibroblasts are derived from mesenchymal cells.

Fibrocartilage (fi"bro-kar'ti-lij) (n.) Cartilage that contains dense, parallel bundles of collagenous fibers in the matrix. The bundles are separated by narrow clefts containing chondrocytes. This type of cartilage is found in the intervertebral disks, the pubic symphysis, at the attachments of tendons and ligaments to bone, and in the menisci of the knee.

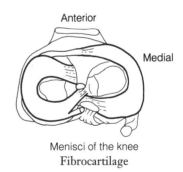

Anterior

Medial

Menisci of the knee
Fibrocartilage

Fibrocyte (fi'brō-sīt) (n.) Used synonymously with fibroblast, although it also can specify the relatively quiescent cell of adult connective tissue.

Fibrodysplasia (fi"bro-dis-plā'sē-ah) (n.) An abnormal development of connective tissue.

Fibrolysis (fib-ro-lī-sis) (n.) The resolution or breakdown of abnormal fibrous tissue, as in the creation of scars.

Fibroma (fĭ-brō'mah) (n.) A benign tumor that consists of fibrous connective tissue. See also specific types.

Fibromatosis (fi"brō-mah-tō'sis) (n.) 1. The presence of multiple fibromas. 2. The formation of a fibrous, tumor-like nodule that arises from the deep fascia, often recurring locally. See **Plantar Fibromatosis** and **Dupuytren's Disease**.

Fibromatosis Colli (fi″bro-mah-to′sis/cō-lī) (n.) See **Congenital Torticollis**.

Fibromyalgia (fi-brō-mī-al-jē-ah) (n.) A nonarticular rheumatism characterized by diffuse musculoskeletal aches and pains and accompanied by exaggerated tenderness at specific areas referred to as **trigger points**. Fibromyalgia is a primary condition of unknown etiology. No laboratory tests are diagnostic. See **Fibrositis**.

Fibromyoma (fi″brō-mī-ō′mah) (n.) A benign tumor consisting of muscular and fibrous materials.

Fibromyositis (fi″brō-mī″ō-sī′tis) (n.) Inflammation of fibromuscular tissue.

Fibronectin (fi″brō-nek′tin) (n.) A group of structural glycoproteins found in the extracellular matrix of connective tissues. It is believed they may play a role in adhesion of fibroblasts and other cell types.

Fibroplasia (fi″brō-plā′se-ah) (n.) The normal production of fibrous tissue that accompanies wound healing.

Fibrosarcoma (fi″brō-sar′kō-mah) (n.) A rare, malignant neoplasm derived from fibrous elements of the medullary cavity of bone. It occurs primarily in soft tissues or in intraosseous areas. Primary fibrosarcoma of the bone usually grows slowly and will manifest itself with pain and/or a mass. The lesions are most commonly found at the ends of long bones. Radiologically, the lesions are radiolucent and without distinct margins. Spindle cells with collagen formation are the histologic findings. There is often a characteristic herring-bone pattern to the cells. Treatment depends on the histologic grading.

Fibrosis (fi″brō′sis) (n.) The formation of fibrous tissues. It may occur de novo, through fibrous degeneration of normal tissue, or by excessive formation, which results in a thickening and scarring of connective tissues.

Fibrositis (fi″brō-sī′tis) (n.) 1. An inflammatory change in the fibrous layers that invest the trunk musculature, producing local pain and tenderness. 2. A generalized musculoskeletal disorder characterized by deep pain and widespread aching, morning stiffness and fatigue, associated sleep disturbance, and specific tender points on physical examination.

Fibrositis is usually divided into two forms: primary fibrositis, in which symptoms occur in the absence of other rheumatic diseases, and secondary fibrositis, in which symptoms arise in the presence of such diseases as rheumatoid arthritis or systemic lupus erythematosus. See **Fibromyalgia**.

Fibrous (fi′brus) (adj.) Containing or composed of fibers.

Fibrous Adhesion (fi′brus/ad-hē′zhun) (n.) A firm attachment of adjacent serous membranes by bands or masses of fibrous connective tissue. Bands may also develop between muscles, tendons, cartilage, and capsules.

Fibrous Ankylosis (fi′brus/ang″ki-lō′sis) (n.) The reduction of joint mobility that results from a proliferation of fibrous tissue.

Fibrous Cartilage (fi′brus/kar′ti-lij) (n.) See **Fibrocartilage**.

Fibrous Connective Tissue (fi′brus/ko-nek′tiv/tish′ū) (n.) Connective tissue in which extracellular fibers are densely packed. The fibers may be interwoven in random or irregular orientation (as in the dermis or in tendon sheaths) or regularly arranged (as in tendons, ligaments, and aponeuroses).

Fibrous Cortical Defect (fi′brus/kor′ti-kal/dē′fekt) (n.) A benign fibrous lesion that appears radiographically as a well-circumscribed, eccentric defect in the metaphyseal region of bones. See **Nonossifying Fibroma**.

Fibrous Dysplasia (fi′brus/dis-plā′se-ah) (n.) A developmental disease of the bone. Abnormal fibrous tissue replaces normal spongiosa and fills the medullary cavity of the affected bones. The tissue contains trabeculae of poorly calcified, primitive bone formed by osseous metaplasia.

The disease may be monostotic or polyostotic. If it is monostotic, it chiefly involves the ribs, facial bones, or long bones. In the long bones, most lesions occur in the femur and tibia. If it is polyostotic (which often occurs when the disease is unilateral) it involves the femur, ilium, tibia, pubis, humerus, fibula, radius, scapula, and clavicle, in that order. The disease is called **Albright Syndrome** when the polyostotic lesions are associated with skin pigmentation and endocrine abnormalities.

Fibrous Proteins (fi′brus/prō′tēnz) (n.) Elongated or filamentous proteins that form the basic structure of connective tissue, muscle (contractile proteins), hair, nails, and the outer skin layer (epidermis). They are relatively insoluble in most dilute solvents.

Fibula (fib′ū-lah) (n.) The long, thin lateral bone of the lower leg. The fibula is smaller than the tibia. Its head joins with the tibia just below the knee. Its

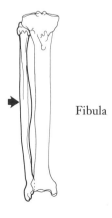

Fibula

lower end projects to the side as the lateral malleolus and articulates with the lateral side of the talus.

Fibular Collateral Ligament (fib'ū-lar/ko-lat-er-al/lig'ah-ment) (n.) The thick ligament that extends from the lateral condylar tubercle of the femur to the lateral surface of the head of the fibula. It runs between the two laminae of the joint capsule.

Fick Angle (fik/ang'g'l) (n.) Angle formed by the axis of the foot and the line of the gait.

Fick Method (fik/meth'ud) (n.) A means of measuring the degree of deformity of hip flexion in stance. On a standing lateral radiograph, draw a line across the superior surface of the first sacral vertebra. Draw another line along the axis of the femoral shaft. The intersection of these lines is the sacrofemoral angle, which is the degree of deformity. Compare to **Milch Method**. Synonym: **Sacrofemoral Angle**.

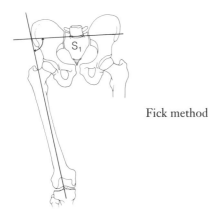

Fick method

Field Block Anesthesia (fēld/blok/an"es-thē'ze-ah) (n.) Regional anesthesia that establishes an anesthetic wall around the operative field by local infiltration around the wound site.

Field Size (fēld/sīz) (n.) The area and shape of a body portion to be irradiated.

Figure-of-8 Bandage (fig'ūr/of/8/ban'dij) (n.) A bandage placed so that the turns criss-cross like a figure 8. Most commonly used for clavicle fractures.

Figure-of-4 Hip Test (fig'ūr/of/4/hip/test) (n.) See **Patrick** or **Fabere Test**.

Filler (fil'er) (n.) In shoe terminology, any cork composition, felt, rubber, or other material placed between the inner sole and the outer sole to level or cushion the foot.

Filleted Graft (fil'e-ted/graft) (n.) A flap of tissue fashioned from nearby skin. This skin is usually taken from a finger or toe from which the bone has been removed but that still retains one or more neurovascular bundles. This graft is appropriate if a damaged finger or toe cannot be salvaged and is to be sacrificed.

Film Badge (film/baj) (n.) A dental-size radiographic film used to estimate amount of radiation to which a person has been exposed. The film is often packaged with an identification badge.

Filum (fī'lum) (n.) A tapered, threadlike or filamentous structure.

Filum Terminale (fī'lum/ter'mi-na-lē) (n.) The tapered, terminal section of the spinal cord.

Finger (fing'ger) (n.) The common name for an upper extremity digit.

Fingernail (n.) The thin, horny plate that covers the dorsum of the distal end of the terminal phalanx of each finger.

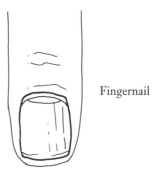

Fingernail

Fingertip (fing'ger-tip) (n.) The portion of the finger distal to the insertions of the flexor and extensor tendons. It includes the terminal portion of the distal phalanx, the nail and nailbed, and the volar pulp. It is highly sensate for function.

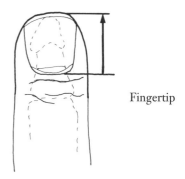

Fingertip

Fingertrap (fing'ger-trap) (n.) A tubular device used to distract fracture fragments in a distal part of the upper extremity. The trap fits on a finger or toe like a glove. It is made of a diagonally woven textile or wire that narrows and tightens when elongated by traction. Also called **Chinese** or **Japanese Finger Traps**.

Finkelstein Test (fink-l-stīn/test) (n.) A diagnostic test for DeQuervain's Disease, a stenosing tenosynovitis of the abductor pollicis longus and the extensor pollicis brevis in the first dorsal extensor com-

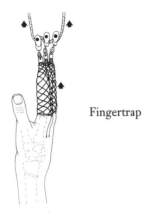

Fingertrap

partment. Have the patient place his or her thumb in the palm of his or her hand and hold it tightly with the other fingers. Then grasp the hand and bend the hand ulnarward. If the test is positive, the patient will feel an intense pain in the region of the radial styloid and first extensor compartment of the wrist. This pain disappears if the thumb is extended, even if the ulnar abduction is maintained.

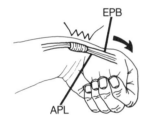

EPB
APL

Finkelstein test

Finsterer's Sign (fin'-ster-erz/sīn) (n.) A diagnostic test for aseptic necrosis of the lunate, known as Kienböck's disease. Have the patient clench his or her hand into a fist. If the test is positive, the base of the third metacarpal is tender when tapped, and its normal prominence is absent.

Fisher's Sign (fish'erz/sīn) (n.) A radiographic sign present in Gaucher's disease that refers to the characteristic Erlenmeyer flask appearance of the distal femur.

Fishmouth Vertebra (fish-mowth/ver'te-brah) (n.)

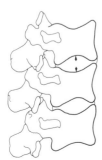

Fishmouth vertebra

A biconcave vertebral body that, on a lateral radiograph of the spine, resembles a fishmouth. Seen in conditions where osteoporosis causes vertebral trabecular collapse.

Fisher Spinal Brace (fish'er/spī'nal/brās) (n.) A thoracolumbar orthrosis used for support and immobilization of the spine. A metal pelvic band with a metal hoop attached to each side is affixed to the spine. Both hoops arch over the iliac crests. Two posterior uprights and two adjustable lateral uprights are joined by a transverse metal bar that is parallel to the inferior angles of the scapulae. The brace ends anteriorly in axillary crutches, which cannot bear weight without causing nerve palsies. All the metal parts, except the lateral uprights, are padded with a thin layer of felt and covered with leather.

A fabric corset provides abdominal support. The corset extends forward from the lateral uprights and fastens at the waist front. Well-padded shoulder straps pass up from the tips of the axillary crutches, go over the shoulders, and cross behind the back. They then swing forward again to buckle on the corset side, parallel with the iliac crests.

The brace limits forward and lateral flexion, rotation of the thoracic spine, and extension of the lower thoracic and upper lumbar spines. The Fisher spinal brace was originally described in 1886.

Fisk Splint (fisk/splint) (n.) A modified Thomas splint that allows for knee flexion.

Fissure (fish'ūr) (n.) A deep, linear groove, ulcer, or crack with sharp edges in the epidermis, organ, or body part.

Fissure Fracture (fish'ūr/frak'chur) (n.) A crack that penetrates the surface but does not go through a long bone.

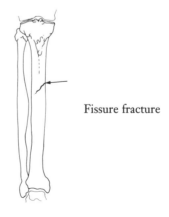

Fissure fracture

Fistula (fis'tu-lah) (n.) 1. An abnormal opening between body tissues. Fistulae usually occur between two hollow organs or between a hollow organ and the skin (eg, the medullary canal to skin). 2. A surgical opening into a hollow organ for drainage.

Five-In-One Procedure (five-in-one/pro-se'jur) (n.) An operative technique for reconstructing the medial compartment of the knee in medial and anteromedial instability. As initially described by J.A. Nicholas, the five parts of the procedure are: (1) total medial meniscectomy, (2) posterior and proximal advancement of the femoral origin of the medial collateral ligament, (3) distal and anterior advancement of the posteromedial part of the posterior capsule, (4) advancement of the posterior part of the vastus medialis, (5) pes anserine transfer. Currently, modifications of this procedure do not require sacrifice of the medial meniscus.

Fixation (fik-sā′shun) (n.) The act, process, or operation of holding, suturing, or fastening something in a fixed position.

Fixed Deformity (fikst/de-for′mi-tē) (n.) An abnormality in joint alignment that is not passively correctible.

Flaccid Paralysis (flak′sid/pah-ral′i-sis) (n.) The loss of muscle tone and tendon reflexes in a paralyzed part resulting from lower motor neuron disorders.

Flail Joint (flāl/joint) (n.) A condition of excess mobility of a joint. It may result from flaccid paralysis or excessive bone and/or soft tissue loss around a joint.

Flanged (flanjd) (adj.) 1. Having a projecting edge. 2. Used in describing the shape of implants and fixation devices.

Flap Tear (flap/tár) (n.) See **Meniscal Flap Tear**

Flat Bone (flat/bōn) (n.) A bone that is in the form of a plate, eg, scapula, ribs, pelvis, and parietal bone.

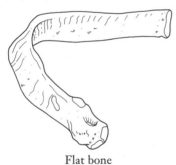

Flat bone

Flat Pelvis (flat/pel′vis) (n.) A pelvis with a short anterior-posterior diameter; **platypelloid**.

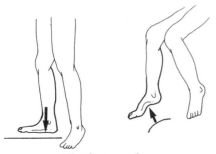

Flat foot, supple

Flatfoot (flat′foot) (n.) A condition in which the loss of height of the medial longitudinal arch of the foot may cause the arch to rest on the ground during stance. This condition may be rigid or flexible, congenital or acquired. See **Pes Planus.**

Flexion (flek′shun) (n.) 1. The act of bending across a joint so that the two adjacent segments approach each other. This results in a decreased joint angle. 2. A motion away from the zero starting position. Contrast to **Extension.**

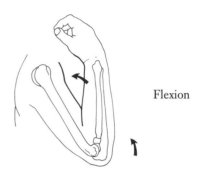

Flexion

Flexion Contracture (flek′shun/kon-trak′tūr) (n.) A fixed deformity in which the joints retain a permanent degree of bending. Terminal extension of that joint cannot be passively achieved.

Flexion-Rotation-Drawer Test (flek′shun/rota′shun/drawr/test) (n.) A diagnostic examination that tests for anterior cruciate ligament insufficiency. Place the patient supine with the knee at 0° of extension. Elevate the leg, allowing the femur to fall into external rotation and permitting the tibia to sublux anterolaterally at the start of the test. As the knee is flexed, the tibia will move backward and the femur will rotate internally, thereby reducing the joint. If this reduction is noted, the test is positive and the anterior cruciate ligament is considered insufficient.

Flexor (flek′sor) (n.) Muscles that flex a joint. See under **Muscle.**

Flexor Pronator Slide (flek′sor/pro-nā′tor/slīd) (n.) A surgical technique used to correct severe flexion deformities of the wrist and hand in patients with cerebral palsy. The origin of the flexor-pronator muscle mass is released and allowed to slide distally; this improves appearance and function.

Flexor Tendon (flek′sor/ten′dun) (n.) The tendinous insertion of a flexor muscle. It is most commonly used in reference to the digital flexor tendons.

Flexor Zones of the Hand (flek′sor/zōnz/of/the/hand) (n.) The five regions of the flexor surface of the hand. These regions are useful because the treatment of flexor tendon injuries may vary with the level of laceration.
Zone I: Extends from just distal to the insertion of the sub-

limis tendon to the site of insertion of the profundus tendon.

Zone II: The critical area of pulleys (No-Man's Land) between the distal palmar crease and the insertion of the sublimis tendon.

Zone III: Comprises the area of the lumbrical origin between the distal margin of the transverse carpal ligament and the first annular pulley.

Zone IV: The zone covered by the transverse carpal ligament.

Zone V: The zone proximal to the transverse carpal ligament, which includes the forearm.

Floating Elbow (flō′ting/el′bō) (n.) A post-traumatic condition in which the elbow joint has no proximal or distal continuity secondary to ipsilateral humeral and forearm fractures.

Floating Knee (flō′ting/nē) (n.) A post-traumatic condition in which the knee joint has no proximal or distal continuity secondary to ipsilateral femoral and tibial fractures.

Fluid Level (floo′id/lev′el) (n.) The horizontal interface between air and fluid. The air is less dense than the fluid below it. See also **Air-fluid Level.**

Fluid Lubrication (floo′id/loo′bri-kā′shun) (n.) A class of mechanisms that completely separates opposite bearing surfaces.

Fluorescence (floo″o-res′ens) (n.) The property of a substance that causes it to turn luminous after exposure to an outside source, such as light or x-rays.

Fluoroscope (floo-o-rō′skōp) (n.) A roentgen device that intensifies internal structures for scanning on a television monitor.

Fluoroscopy (floo″or-os′kō-pē) (n.) An imaging technique for visual diagnostic examination on a screen or monitor; an alternative to conventional x-ray examination.

Flute (flūt) (n.) 1. The longitudinal channels in a screw or a tap that create cutting edges on the thread profile and provide chip spaces. 2. The channel in the outer surface of intramedullary rod designs.

Focal Film Distance (fō′kal/film/dis′tans) (n.) In radiography, the distance between the focal spot, or target, and the film holder. This distance is colinear with the central ray (CR). Known as **FFD.**

Folding Crutch (fōld′ing/kruch) (n.) A single upright metal support for walking. It can be folded at a joint just above the hand-piece for use as a cane or for storage.

Folliculitis (fo-lik″ū-lī′tis) (n.) An infection of the hair follicle.

Foot (fut) (n.) The terminal appendage of the lower

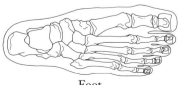

Foot

limb used for support, weight distribution, and locomotion of the body. The foot is composed of the tarsal bones, the metatarsals, and the phalanges.

Foot Slap (foot/slap) (n.) The gait deviation of a person with a dropped foot. Instead of coming down to the surface smoothly, the foot lands flat and briskly, with a loud slap. This occurs immediately after heel strike.

Foot Traction Plate (fut/trak′shun/plāt) (n.) A plate placed at the end of leg traction to which a line and weights are attached.

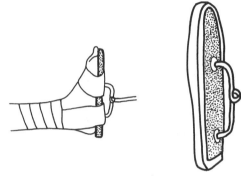

Foot traction plate

Foot Types (foot/tipz) (n.) There are three types of feet based on the relative lengths of the toes: (1) a square pattern, in which the first to the fourth toes are equal in length; (2) the Egyptian type, in which the great toe is the longest and the rays reduce in length progressively from the second to the fifth toe; (3) the Greek type, in which the second toe is longest, followed by the third, first, fourth, and fifth. These types were described by Viladot in 1962.

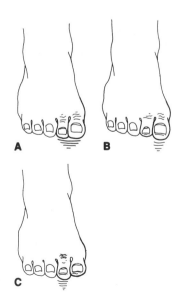

Foot types: **A,** square; **B,** Egyptian; **C,** Greek.

Footboard (fut'bord) (n.) A device used to support the feet in anatomic alignment. It is placed vertically at the foot of a bed to prevent plantar flexion and the development of dropfoot (equinus).

Foot-Dorsiflexion Test (fut-dor'sĭ-flek'shun/test) (n.) A refinement of the straight leg-raising test for sciatica. With the patient supine gently elevate the affected limb to cause sciatic pain. Then apply slow or brisk dorsiflexion of the foot to intensify the pain. See **Fajersztajn Test.**

Footdrop (foot'drop) (n.) An inability to dorsiflex the foot that is caused by paralysis of the anterior muscles of the leg. A flaccid equinus. See **Dropfoot.**

Foot-Flat (foot-flat) (n.) That part of the gait cycle when the forefoot makes initial contact with the walking surface. It immediately follows heel-strike.

Foot Orthosis (fut/or-thō'sis) (n.) A removable appliance placed within a shoe that applies forces to the foot either to relieve pain or to improve balance and function in standing and walking.

Footprint Device (foot'print/de-vīs') (n.) An instrument that measures the pressure distribution between the human foot and the ground. This is known as **foot-to-ground pressure** or **FGP pattern.**

Footprint Slipper Sock (foot'print/slip'er/sok) (n.) A slipper used in the evaluation of pressure areas of the foot. The slipper is made of stretchable polyurethane and contains fragile microcapsules. The capsules break with pressure and spill out a dye, which colors the slipper according to the amount of foot pressure. To test a footprint, the slipper sock is worn either by itself or inside the shoe for a test of about 15 steps.

Foramen (fo-rā'men) (n.) A small opening, orifice, perforation, or passage through which nerves or blood vessels pass; usually found in bones.

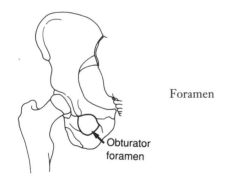

Foramen

Obturator foramen

Foramen Magnum (fo-ra'men/mag'num) (n.) A large opening in the base of the anterior inferior part of the occipital bone that lies between the cranial cavity and spinal canal. The spinal cord passes through the opening.

Foraminotomy (for"am-i-not'o-me) (n.) The surgical removal of a portion of the wall of the intervertebral foramen.

Force (fors) (n.) Any applied action that may change an object's state of rest or motion. The newton is the unit of measure for magnitude of force.

Forearm Cast (for'arm/kast) (n.) A circumferential cast that extends from just below the elbow to the proximal transverse crease of the palm. Used for immobilization of injuries about the radial metaphysis and wrist. Synonym: **Short Arm Cast.**

Forearm Crutch (for'arm/kruch) (n.) A cane with a handpiece pointing forward at a 90° angle. The forearm extension deviates posteriorly at a 15° angle. A hinged open cuff at the upper end reaches two to three fingerbreadths below the elbow. The crutch is usually made of aluminum. It is also called a **Lofstrand Crutch.**

Forearm Splint (for'arm/splint) (n.) A splint that extends from just below the elbow to the proximal transverse crease of the palm.

Forefoot (for'fut) (n.) The front part of the foot, including the metatarsals and the phalanges.

Foreign Body (for'in/bod'e) (n.) A substance or material abnormally present in a body space or tissue.

Foreign-Body Giant Cell (for'in-bod'ē/jī'ant/sel) (n.) A large multinucleated cell derived from a coalescence of macrophages. It is seen in association with chronic granulomatous inflammation surrounding a foreign body. Also known as **Langhans Giant Cell.**

Foreign Body Reaction (for'in/bod'ē/rē-ak'shun) (n.) The inflammation around a foreign body in a tissue or organ.

Forepart (fōr'part) (n.) In a shoe, the portion of the last that extends from the ball break to the toe.

Forestier's Bowstring Sign (fo"res-tē-āz/bō'string/sīn) (n.) The ipsilateral contracture of spine muscles that occurs when a patient with ankylosing spondylitis bends to the side. Normally, the contralateral muscles tighten.

Forestier's Disease (fo"-res-tē-ā/dĭ-zēz') (n.) Eponym for Diffuse Idiopathic Skeletal Hyperostosis (DISH). See **DISH.**

Forme Fruste (fōrm/frūst) (n.) An atypical form of a disease; the usual symptoms fail to appear, and the disease stops sooner than expected.

Fossa (fōs'ah) (n.) In anatomy, a hollow or depressed area in a bone.

Fouchet's Sign (foo-shāz'/sīn) (n.) A clinical test that suggests, if positive, the diagnosis of chondromalacia patella. Have the patient extend the knee fully. The sign is present if the extension produces point tenderness or if compression of the patella against the femur causes pain.

Four-Legged Cane (for/leg-ed'/kān) (n.) A support for walking with four relatively long tips. Also called a **Quad Cane.**

Four-Point Cane (for/point/kān) (n.) A support for walking with four tips.

Four-Point Gait (for/point/gāt) (n.)   A mode of walking that develops when using a pair of crutches or canes. It has the following sequence: left crutch, right foot, right crutch, left foot.

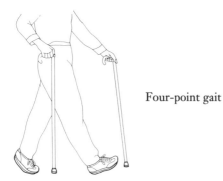

Four-point gait

Four-Poster Collar (for/pos'ter/kol'ler) (n.)   An orthosis that immobilizes or supports the neck. Its construction includes padded mandibular and occipital supports that are attached to the thoracic and chest plates by two rigid adjustable front and back supports. Bilateral flexible leather straps connect the mandibular and occipital supports. Also known as a **Four-Poster Brace** or a **Four-Poster Orthosis**.

Fovea (fō've-ah) (n.)   A small pit or cup-shaped depression.

Fovea Centralis (fō-vea/sen-tra'lis) (n.)   A small pit or central depression near the center of the acetabulum; the ligamentum teres begins here.

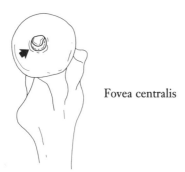

Fovea centralis

Fowler-Phillip Angle   (fow'ler/fil'ip/ang'g'l) (n.)   The radiographic angle formed on the calcaneus between the posterior and the plantar bone surfaces. Described by Fowler and Phillip, the angle uses fixed anatomic landmarks to measure adult calcaneal bones in the dry state, using fixed anatomic landmarks. The angle can also be used to draw lines tangential to these surfaces.

Fowler Position (fow'ler/pō-zish'un) (n.)   A semi-sitting or reclining position, attained when supine by raising the trunk and thighs to a 45° angle while the feet remain flat.

Fowler Procedure (fow'ler/prō'sē'jur) (n.)   A surgical technique of forefoot arthroplasty for the treatment of symptomatic forefoot deformities in patients with rheumatoid arthritis. It involves resection of metatarsal heads via a plantar approach.

Fracture (frak'chur)   1. (v.) To break. 2. (n.) A break or disruption in the continuity of a bone; this usually includes a severed periosteum. The fracture is **complete** if it involves the entire cross-section of the bone; it is **incomplete** if it involves only a portion of the cross-section. Every fracture is either open or closed. In an open type, the wound extends through the skin or mucous membrane. Without such a wound, the fracture is closed (ie, it does not communicate with the outside air). Fractures are classified by anatomic location, direction of the fracture line, presence or absence of overlying skin wounds, associated joint injuries, and other specific characteristics. One classification system is as follows:

Comminuted Fracture (kom'i-nūt″ed)   A bone splintered into multiple fragments.

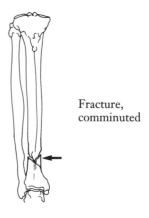

Fracture, comminuted

Compound (open) Fracture (kom-pownd)   When a skin wound communicates with the fracture site.

Depressed Fracture (de-prest)   A fracture with central wedging or displacement, e.g., skull, tibial plateau.

Greenstick Fracture (grēn'stik)   A bone broken and bent, but still securely hinged at one side. A bone in which fracture has occurred in a portion of its circumference under tension.

Impacted Fracture (im-pakt'ed)   The broken bone and a fragment are wedged into another fragment. Implies some stability.

Longitudinal Fracture (lon″ji-tū'di-nal)   When the break runs parallel to the bone.

Oblique Fracture (o-blēk)   A slanting break on the bone.

Pathologic Fracture (path″ō-loj'ik)   The break occurs at the site of preexisting bone disease. It is usually transverse.

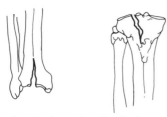

Fracture, longitudinal

Segmental Fracture (seg-men′tal)   More than one complete break in a given bone.

Simple (closed) Fracture (sim′p′l)   When the skin remains intact over the fracture site.

Spiral Fracture (spī-ral)   The break coils around the bone. Caused by rotation, its length is generally 2½ times the diameter at its center.

Stress Fracture (stres)   A fatigue fracture that results from repetitive stresses.

Torus Fracture (to′rus)   A buckling fracture seen in pediatric patients. Fracture under compression.

Transverse Fracture (trans-vers′)   The break runs across bone.

See also **Specific Fractures**.

Fracture Bed (frak′chur/bed) (n.)   A bed with an overhead frame and attachments for traction, suspension, and other procedures. A board under the mattress prevents sagging.

Fracture Board (frak′chur/bord) (n.)   A firm wooden platform placed under the mattress of a bed to prevent sagging.

Fracture Disease (frak′chur/di-zēz) (n.)   When a fracture is treated by prolonged immobilization, chronic edema, soft tissue atrophy, osteoporosis, and joint stiffness may result. Fracture disease prevents early active exercise of joint muscles and causes delayed return of function after bony healing.

Fracture-Dislocation (frak′chur/dis″lo-kā′shun) (n.)   A joint dislocation that is accompanied by a fracture of one or more of the bones that form the joint.

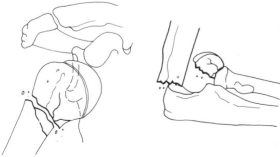

Fracture-dislocation

Fracture Line (frak′chur/līn) (n.)   Any line or x-ray shadow considered to be the result of a fracture.

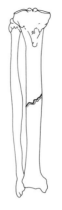

Fracture line

Fracture Strength (frak′chur/strenth) (n.)   The degree of stress at which a material breaks (psi; dynes/cm²).

Fracture Table (frak′chur/ta′b′l) (n.)   A table devised for immobilizing an extremity to help in treatment of fractures.

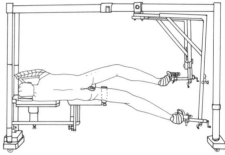

Fracture table

Fracture Terminology (frak′chur/ter″mi-nol′ō-jē) (n.)   The description of fracture components may include displacement, comminution, compounding, angulation, location in bone, and mechanism. The displaced distal fragment is always related to the proximal, or stationary, part. To describe angular deformity, consider the distal fragment of an angle to the proximal. Angulation also may be described by defining the direction of the apex of the angulation.

Frankel's White Line (freng′kelz/wīt/līn) (n.)   A widened layer of calcified cartilage that appears on a radiograph as a characteristic transverse line of density (white) in the juxtaepiphyseal area. It is seen in children with scurvy.

Fragilitas Ossium (frah-jil′i-tas/ōs′ē-um) (n.)   An abnormal fragility of the bones in which minor trauma readily produces fractures. See **Osteogenesis Imperfecta.**

Fragmentation (frag″ment-tā′shun) (n.)   The breakage of a material, such as bone or wire, into multiple pieces.

Frame (frām) (n.) A rigid structure for supporting or immobilizing a part.

FRCS Abbreviation for Fellow of the Royal College of Surgeons.

Free-Body Analysis (frē/bod′ē/ah-nal′i-sis) (n.) A technique used to determine the internal stresses in a structure subjected to external loads.

Free Fibular Graft (fre/fib′u-lar/graft) (n.) A type of vascularized free osseous transfer that uses the fibular.

Free Flap (fre/flap) (n.) A technique for covering defects with soft tissue that uses an arterialized flap that has been completely detached from its donor bed. When sutured into a new site, the principal artery and vein are joined to the recipient vessels by microvascular techniques. Also known as **Vascularized Free Flap.**

Free Graft (frē/graft) (n.) A graft of tissue completely freed from its bed. The tissue is detached from the donor site and transplanted into the recipient site. Its vascular supply can come from the capillary ingrowth of the recipient site, or it may be transplanted as a vascularized graft through microsurgery.

Free Tendon Graft (frē/ten′dun/graft) (n.) A tendon that is detached from a donor site and transplanted into a recipient site.

Freeze-Drying of Bone (frēz-drī′ing/of/bōn) (n.) A technique of preparing bone for preservation (e.g., for deposit in a bone bank) that involves rapidly freezing the bone and then dehydrating it in a high vacuum. Also known as **Lyophilization.**

Freiberg's Infraction (frī-bergz/in-frak′shun) (n.) An idiopathic avascular necrosis of a metatarsal head. It is most commonly seen in the head of the second metatarsal. This infraction was described by Freiberg in 1914 and by Kohler in 1915. Synonym: **Kohler's Second Disease; Juvenile Deforming Metatarsophalangeal Osteochondritis.**

Frejka Pillow (frā-ka/pil′o) (n.) A large, bulky device used to maintain the reduction of congenitally dislocated hips. This bulky pillow is placed over the diaper in the baby's groin; this keeps the thighs abducted. Two long shoulder straps are attached to the upper end of the pad. The pillow must be reapplied with each diaper change so that redislocation cannot occur. Also called: **Frejka Orthosis, Frejka Pillow Splint, Abduction Pillow.**

Friction (frik′shun) (n.) The resistance to motion between two bearing surfaces. This includes: 1. Moving friction—the resistance to continued motion; 2. Starting Friction—the resistance to the beginning of motion between two bearing surfaces; it is a higher resistance than moving friction.

Friedman's Position (frēd′manz/po-zish′un) (n.) A radiographic position for an axiolateral view of the head, neck, trochanter, and upper shaft of the femur.

Friedreich Ataxia (frēd′rīk/ah-tak′sē-ah) (n.) A type of spinal cerebellar degenerative disease, with onset usually in the first decade. Initially, most patients present with a staggering gait and a high plantar arch. Progressive ataxia then occurs. The predominant orthopaedic disorders are cavus feet and scoliosis. It is generally inherited in an autosomal recessive pattern.

Frog Cast (frog/kast) (n.) A plaster cast that holds the hips in a 90° position of abduction/flexion and lateral rotation. It is used in the treatment of congenital hip dislocation and is similar in principle to the Von Rosen, Barlow, and Denis-Browne splints. See **Lorenz Plaster Cast.**

Frog Leg Attitude (frog/leg/at′i-tūd) (n.) A position in which the hips are flexed, abducted, and externally rotated, while the knees are flexed and the feet are in equinovarus posture.

Frog Leg Lateral (frog/leg/lat′er-al) (n.) A lateral radiograph of the hip showing the legs in 90° of flexion, full abduction, and external rotation. A radiograph of the pelvis taken from anterior to posterior in this position will show a lateral projection of each proximal femur.

Frog Position (frog/pō-zish′un) (n.) A position in which a child lies prone with the thighs in external rotation and abducted to about 90°. The knees are also at right angles. This is often seen in the newborn. Known also as **Spread-eagle Position.**

Frog Splint (frog/splint) (n.) A malleable device for the treatment of a mallet finger. When open, it gives the appearance of a frog.

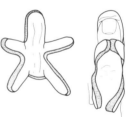

Frog splint

Froment's Paper Sign (fro-mahz′/pā′per/sīn) (n.) A diagnostic test of ulnar nerve palsy. When the patient attempts to pinch a piece of paper forcefully between the thumb and index finger, increased flexion of the interphalangeal joint of the thumb occurs. The sign is caused by the loss of adduction power in the thumb and abduction of the index finger.

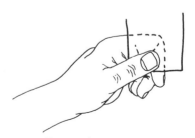

Froment's paper sign

Frontal Plane (frun'tal/plān) (n.) Any vertical plane parallel to the long axis of the body and perpendicular to the sagittal plane. It divides the body into ventral and dorsal segments.

Frozen Section (frō'zen/sek'shun) (n.) A histologic section that has been quick-frozen by microtome and immediately stained for rapid microscopic study and diagnosis. It is the method of pathologic study used intraoperatively, but not as accurate as permanent sectioning.

Frozen Shoulder (frō'/zen/shōl'der) (n.) A clinical entity of unclear origin whose hallmark is a painful shoulder with a markedly limited range of motion. This syndrome may be associated with inflammation of the rotator cuff. An arthrogram characteristically shows diminished capsular volume with obliteration of the normal capsular recesses. Also known as **Adhesive Capsulitis.**

Frykman Classification (frīk-man/klas"si-fi-ka' shun) (n.) A classification of distal radius (Colles) fractures made according to the presence or absence of a distal ulnar fracture and the involvement of the articular surface.

Fulguration (ful"gu-rā'shun) (n.) A destruction of tissue by electric sparks generated by a high-frequency current.

Full-Length Crutch (ful-lenth/kruch) (n.) An axillary crutch.

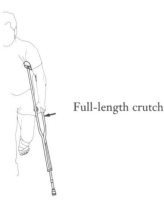

Full-length crutch

Full-Thickness Skin Graft (ful-thik'nes/skin/graft) (n.) 1. A graft that consists of a full thickness of skin with little or no subcutaneous tissue. 2. The removal or elevation of the epidermis, corium, and subcutaneous fat at a depth greater than 0.035 in (1 mm). These grafts inhibit wound contraction better than split-thickness grafts, and they are preferred on the face, neck, hands, elbows, axillae, knees, and feet.

Full Weight-Bearing (ful/wāt/bār'ing) (adj.) A prescription for ambulation that permits unrestricted and unprotected loading on the extremity. Contrast to weight-bearing as tolerated. Abbreviated **FWB.**

Fulminant (ful'mi-nant) (n.) See **Fulminating.**

Fulminating (ful'mi-nāt'ing) (adj.) A severe condition or symptom with a very sudden onset and short duration. Also known as **Fulminant,** or **Fulgurant.**

Function (funk'shun) (n.) 1. The specific action or property of an organ or body part. 2. The performance by an organ or body part of its special action.

Functional Assessment (funk'shun-al/a-ses'ment) (n.) A way to measure an individual's coping skills. This includes describing abilities and limitations in performing daily tasks needed for living, leisure activities, vocational pursuits, social interactions, and other required behaviors.

Functional Curve (funk'shun-al/kurv) (n.) See **Nonstructural Curve.**

Functional Disease (funk'shun-al/diz-ēz) (n.) An ailment or problem involving body functions not caused by a structural defect or organic lesion.

Fungal Infection (fung'gal/in-fek'shun) (n.) A septic process initiated by a fungus; it may occur locally or systemically.

Fungicide (fung-i-sīd) (n.) A substance or agent that kills fungi.

Fungus (fung'gus) (n.) Any member of the kingdom fungi, comprising single cell or multinucleated organisms. Most fungi are multicellular and have spores (reproductive elements), hyphae (tubular branching filaments), mycelia (mass of hyphae), and, sometimes, organized tissue layers. As mycelia branch and come in contact with organic material, they secrete enzymes that hydrolyze proteins, carbohydrates, and fats. They then absorb the split products.

Funiculus (fū-nik'ū-lus) (n.) 1. A bundle of nerves surrounded and bound by the perineurium (a thin sheath of connective tissue). Each funiculus may contain motor, sensory, or sympathetic fibers in various numbers. The number and size of the funiculi may vary in any given nerve and along the course of the nerve. Funiculi, along with their perineural sheaths, may branch, divide, or anastomose with the nerve trunk. See **Peripheral Nerve.** 2. Any of the three main columns of white matter found in each lateral half of the spinal cord.

FUO Abbreviation for Fever of Unknown Origin.

Furuncle (fu'rung-k'l) (n.) A focal suppurative inflammation or infection of the skin and subcutaneous tissues that usually originates in or about a hair follicle. It encloses a central slough or "core." Also called **Boil.**

Fusiform (fū'zi-form) (n.) Tapered at both ends, spindle-shaped.

Fusion (fū'zhun) The surgical formation of a bony ankylosis. Synonym: **Arthrodesis.** See specific fusions.

FWB Abbreviation for Full Weight Bearing.

Fx Abbreviation for Fractures.

G

G-Suit (g̅-so̅o̅t) (n.)   See **Antigravity Suit.**

Gaenslen Test (genz'len/test) (n.)   A technique used in the evaluation of the sacroiliac joint. Ask the patient to lie supine and draw both knees to the chest. Shift the patient to the side of the examining table so that one buttock extends over the edge. Allow the unsupported leg to drop gently over the edge while the patient pulls the other leg into the knee-chest position. Increased pain suggests pathology of the sacroiliac joint.

Gage's Sign (gājz/sīn) (n.)   A radiologic variation seen in Legg-Calvé-Perthes disease. A V-shaped radiolucent area is seen at the lateral epiphyseal-metaphyseal junction of the femoral head. Catterall describes this as one of the "head at risk" signs. This represents a dense, collapsed segment of the epiphysis, embraced laterally by a "V" of viable epiphysis.

Gait (gāt) (n.)   A manner or style of walking, stepping, or running. A normal gait is smooth, coordinated, and rhythmic, although gaits vary from person to person. Many factors, such as pain, joint motion, paralysis, and any deformity of the lower extremities, may alter gait.

The gait cycle may be divided into two phases: the stance phase (60 percent of the cycle) and the swing phase (40 percent of the cycle). The stance phase occurs during the weight-bearing portion of walking. Each stance phase is subdivided into heel strike, foot-flat midstance, push-off, and toe-clearance. Toe-clearance initiates the swing phase, with acceleration in the first half and deceleration in the second half. Swing phase terminates with the heel strike. See **Stance Phase** and **Swing Phase.**

Galant's Reflex (gah-lantz/rē'fleks) (n.)   A righting reflex normally present at birth. To elicit the reflex, stimulate the child's flank between the rib cage and the pelvic rim. The normal response is an incurvation of the trunk ipsilateral to the stimulus. Persistence of the reflex beyond the third month suggests diffuse neurologic deficit. Synonym: **Incurvation Reflex.**

Galeazzi Fracture-Dislocation (gal"e-at'zē/frak'chur/dis"lo-kā'shun) (n.)   A fracture of the radial shaft with an associated dislocation of the distal radioulnar joint. It is often called "the fracture of necessity," which refers to the need to treat this fracture by surgical intervention for optimal result. It was first described in 1934 by R. Galeazzi and is also called **Piedmont Fracture, Dupuytren's Fracture,** and **Reverse Monteggia Fracture.**

Galeazzi's Sign # 1 (gal"e-at'zēz/sīn) (n.)   A clinical sign indicative of developmental dysplasia of the hip in an infant. Lay the infant flat on a firm table. Flex the hips and knees to right angles, leaving the feet flat on the table. Apparent shortening of the femur, seen as differing knee levels, indicates a positive test.

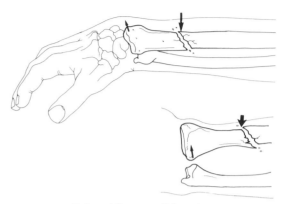

Galeazzi fracture-dislocation

This sign will be positive in any condition that results in unequal femoral lengths and therefore is suggestive but not diagnostic of congenital hip dislocation or developmental hip dysplasia. See **Allis Sign.**

Galeazzi's Sign # 2 (gal"e-at'zēz/sīn) (n.)   A sign of developmental dysplasia of the hip. The standing patient shows curvature of the spine from a shortening of the leg.

Gallie Fusion (gal'ē/fū'zhun) (n.)   A surgical technique of atlantoaxial fusion that uses a posterior approach to the cervical spine followed by passage of a wire around the posterior arch of the atlas and around the spinous process of the axis.

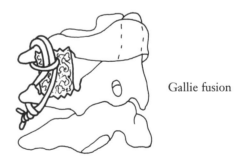

Gallie fusion

Gallium Scan (gal'e-um/skan) (n.)   A nuclear imaging test that uses gallium[67] as the radionuclide tracer. This tracer is preferentially picked up by white blood cells. Imaging is performed 24 to 72 hours after injection. This test is useful in identifying areas of inflammation and abscess formation.

Game-Keeper's Thumb (gām/ke'perz/thum) (n.)   A rupture of the ulnar collateral ligament of the metacarpophalangeal joint of the thumb. Despite its name, it is more commonly caused by falls while skiing. The thumb is forced radially by the ski pole or strap when the hand hits the ground. Also known as **Skier's Thumb.**

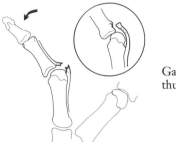

Game-keeper's thumb

Gamma Camera (gam′ah/kam′er-ah) (n.)   A radioactivity detector made of a single large NaI crystal and multiple amplifiers. The camera visualizes an organ by recording the gamma radiation emitted by a scanning agent in that organ. The technique resembles the optical radiation recorded in a camera. Used in nuclear medicine scanning procedures.

Gamma Globulin (gam′ah/glob′u-lin) (n.)   A class of serum proteins identified by a characteristic rate of movement in an electric field. These globulins usually function as antibodies.

Gamma Rays (gam′ah/rāz) (n.)   Electromagnetic radiations spontaneously emitted from radioactive materials. The rays are more penetrating than alpha or beta particles. They are either waves or particles without mass. 2. High energy, short wavelength electromagnetic radiation that originates in the nucleus of an unstable atom. Dense material is the best shield against these highly penetratng rays. Unlike gamma rays, x-rays originate outside the nucleus of an atom and generally have lower energies.

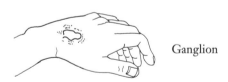

Ganglion

Ganglion (gang′gle-on) (n.)   1. A small mass of nerve tissue with neuron cell bodies, which often have numerous synapses. 2. Swellings in the posterior sensory roots of the spinal nerves that contain cell bodies but no synapses. Chains of ganglia parallel the spinal cord in the sympathetic nervous system. Ganglia are situated in or near the innervated organs in the parasympathetic nervous system. 3. A cystlike swelling arising near a tendon sheath or joint capsule. This occurs most commonly on the back of the hand or wrist. Fibrous sheath tissue proliferates with mucoid degeneration, producing the cystlike swelling. The ganglion contains no true lining.

Gangrene (gan′grēn) (n.)   The death and decay of part of the body caused by a deficiency or failure of the blood supply. Bacterial invasion and putrefaction follow.

Gangrene may be classified as wet or dry. **Wet gangrene** develops where fluid is in the tissue. It occurs in disorders that include an obstruction of the venous return from a tissue or an organ. The tissue is usually infected. **Dry gangrene** results from obstruction of the arterial circulation, which causes the tissue to become dehydrated and shriveled and to appear blackened and mummified. A red zone of granulation tissue marks the demarcation of dead tissue from living tissue. See also **Gas Gangrene.**

Garden's Alignment Index (gar′denz/ah-līn′ment/in′deks) (n.)   A measurement used in determining the adequacy of reduction of fractures of the femoral neck. An angle is constructed on AP and lateral radiographs of the hip by drawing a line parallel to the femoral neck that intersects a line parallel to the primary compressive trabecula of the femoral neck and head. These angles should be 160° to 180°. The index is calculated by dividing the AP angle by the lateral angle. Ideally the index should be 160/180.

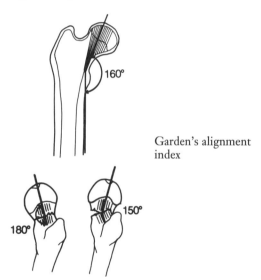

Garden's alignment index

Garden's Femoral Neck Fracture Classification (gar′denz / fem′or-al / nek / frak′chur / klas″sĭ-fĭ-ka′shun) (n.)   A commonly used system for the classification of femoral neck fractures. It has prognostic value.

Stage I: An incomplete fracture with the head tilted in a posterolateral direction; a so-called impacted fracture.

Stage II: Complete but undisplaced fracture.

Stage III: Complete and partially displaced fracture, as judged by the direction of the trabeculae in the head fragment. The two fragments remain in contact with each other.

Stage IV: Completely displaced fracture.

Gardner's Syndrome (gard′nerz/sin′drōm) (n.)   A familial syndrome whose clinical disorders include

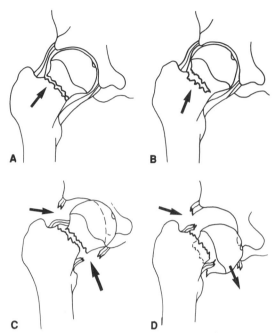

Garden's femoral neck fracture classification.
A, Garden's type 1 intracapsular fracture; **B**, Garden's type 2; **C**, Garden's type 3; **D**, Garden's type 4.

multiple large bowel polyps, multiple osteomas, dental anomalies, fibrous tissue tumors, and cystic lesions of the skin. Some patients also show inadequate response to the action of parathormone, resulting in a clinical picture of pseudohypoparathyroidism.

Gardner-Wells Tongs (gard/ner-welz/tongz) (n.) A rigid device applied to the sides of the skull for skeletal traction that is useful in treating fractures of the cervical spine. These tongs feature a self-contained tension device and are designed to follow the coronal contour of the calvarium. See **Barton Tongs** and **Crutchfield Tongs** for comparison.

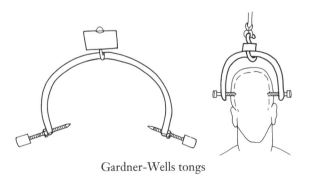

Gardner-Wells tongs

Gargoylism (gar'goil-izm) (n.) A genetically transmitted, autosomal recessive form of osteochondro-

dystrophy manifested by joint changes, congenital corneal opacities, hepatosplenomegaly, and mental deficiency. Facial characteristics include thick lips, a depressed bridge of the nose, low set ears, and widely spaced teeth. The facial appearance has been likened to that of a gargoyle, hence the designation. The disorder results in excessive urinary excretion of dermatin sulfate and heparan sulfate. This is more properly called **Hurler's Syndrome** or **Dysostosis Multiplex.**

Garre's Osteomyelitis (gar-āz'/os"te-ō-mī"e-lī'tis) (n.) A form of chronic, nonsuppurative osteomyelitis characterized by a protracted course of dull and constant pain localized to the site of the lesion. Most commonly seen in the tibia and femur. Radiographically, gradual thickening and increased cortical density are seen; occasionally, small foci of decreased density within the sclerotic area are noted. Also known as **Idiopathic Cortical Sclerosis** and **Garre's Sclerosing Osteomyelitis.**

Gas Gangrene (gas/gang'grēn) (n.) A fulminant, necrotizing infection caused by a gram-positive, anaerobic gas-producing bacillus, most commonly *Clostridium perfringens.*

Successful treatment depends on prompt recognition, emergent thorough debridement and decompression, and intravenous antibiotic therapy. If available, hyperbaric oxygen is a useful adjunctive therapy.

Gas-in-Nucleus Pulposus (gas/in/nu'kle-us/pul'posus) (n.) In the intervertebral cartilage, a radiographic sign indicative of degenerative conditions of the disk. See **Vacuum Sign.**

Gastroc (gas"trok) (n.) A colloquial term for the gastrocnemius and soleus muscles.

Gastrocnemius Muscle (gas"trok-ne'me-us/mus'el) (n.) See **Muscle.**

Gastrografin (gas"tro-graf'in) (n.) A proprietary name for a preparation of meglumine diatrizoate, a diagnostic radiopaque medium.

Gatch Bed (gach/bed) (n.) A bed with a mattress support made of three parts, each of which can be operated separately to achieve various positions of the trunk, thighs, and legs.

Gate Theory (gāt/the'o-rē) (n.) A theory used to explain pain perception and suppression. If noxious stimulation of small-diameter nerve fibers opens the "pain gate" in the brain, another kind of stimulus of the large-diameter nerve fibers closes the gate, shutting out pain. Postulated by Melzack and Wall.

Gaucher's Disease (gō-shāz/di-zēz') (n.) A familial metabolic disorder characterized by the accumulation of kerasin, a glucocerebroside, in the reticuloendothelial cells of the spleen, lymph nodes, bone marrow, and liver. It results from a deficiency of the enzyme glucocerebrocidase. An autosomal recessive disease, it is highly prevalent in the Jewish population. The characteristically large, lipid-filled histio-cytes, Gaucher's cells, are pathognomonic and are best demonstrated by bone marrow biopsy. Three types of Gaucher's disease are described.

Type I: The chronic, non-neuropathic type, also known as the adult or benign form.

Type II: The actual fatal neuropathic type, also known as the infantile or malignant form.

Type III: The rare type, also known as the subacute neuropathic or juvenile form.

Skeletal changes are widespread and variable and include mottling and medullary widening because of replacement by pathologic tissue, pathologic fracture, avascular necrosis, acute periosteal reactions known as Gaucher's sterile periosteal reaction, and late deformity and degenerative changes.

Gauntlet Bandage (gawnt'let/ban'dij) (n.)   A covering that fits the hand and fingers like a glove.

Gauntlet Cast (gawnt'let/kast) (n.)   A rigid cover extending from below the elbow to the proximal palmar crease, including the thumb. Also known as a **Thumb Spica Cast**.

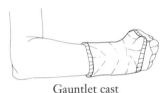
Gauntlet cast

Gauvain's Sign (gō-vānz/sīn) (n.)   A diagnostic marker found in tuberculosis of the hip joint. To perform the test, grasp the femoral condyles of the affected side with one hand. Place the palm of the other hand on the abdomen between the iliac spines. The sign is positive if rotation of the femur provokes a reflex spasm of the abdominal muscles due to irritation of the psoas muscle.

Gauze (gawz) (n.)   A thin, woven, open-meshed material used in surgical dressings.

Gel (jel) (n.)   A colloid substance that is firm in consistency but contains a large proportion of liquid.

Gelatin Sponge (jel'ah-tin/spunj) (n.)   A sterile, gelatin-based material that is absorbable and water-insoluble; it is available in either powder, film, or compressed-pad form. The pad comes in many sizes and can be cut without crumbling. The sponge is a hemostatic agent. To use it, place it on an area of capillary bleeding. Fibrin is deposited in the interstices of the sponge, which then swells, forming a substantial clot.

Gelfoam (gel'fōm) (n.)   The trademark for an absorbable gelatin sponge material. It is used as a local hemostatic agent. See **Gelatin Sponge**.

Gene (jēn) (n.)   1. The basic unit of heredity defined by the functions it controls. The gene is a small section of the chromosome. Each gene specifies a protein and controls the development of a particular trait that is determined by the interaction of the gene product with its total environment. Genes are capable of self-replication and transmission as a part of the chromosome. 2. A linear sequence of nucleotides along a segment of DNA that provides the code instructions for synthesis of RNA.

General Anesthesia (jen'er-al/an"es-thē'ze-ah) (n.)   The administration of a drug, usually in liquid or gaseous form, that produces a state of unconsciousness.

Generic (jě-ner'ik) (adj.)   Nonproprietary. It denotes a product or drug name not protected by patent.

Genetic Code (je-net'ik/kōd) (n.)   The four-symboled system of base-plan sequences in DNA. It is called a code because it determines both the amino acid sequence in the enzymes and other protein components synthesized by the organism.

Geniculate Arteries (jě-nik'u-lāt/ar'te-rēs) (n.)   Branches of the popliteal artery around the knee. These include: the lateral superior geniculate artery, the medial superior geniculate artery, the middle geniculate artery, the lateral inferior geniculate artery, and the medial inferior geniculate artery.

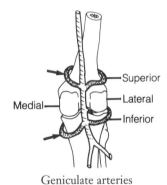
Geniculate arteries

Genitofemoral Nerve (jen"i-to-fem'or-al/nerv) (n.)   A branch of the lumbar plexus formed by branches of the anterior portions of L1 and L2. This nerve gives off a genital branch to supply the cremaster muscle and sensory twigs to the scrotum and adjacent thigh. The femoral branch supplies sensation to the skin of the femoral triangle.

Genotype (jēn'o-tīp) (n.)   The particular set of genes present in an organism and its cells; a person's entire genetic constitution. Compare **Phenotype**.

Gentamicin (jen"tah-mī-sin) (n.)   An aminoglycoside antibiotic.

Genu (je'nu) (n.)   1. The knee. 2. Any bent anatomic structure resembling the knee.

Genu Articularis Muscle (je'nu/ar-tik'u-lar-is/mus'el) (n.)   See **Muscle**.

Genu Recurvatum (je′nu/re″kur-va′tum) (n.) Hyperextension of the knee, commonly known as **back knee**. It is measured on a standing lateral radiograph of the knee.

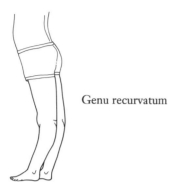

Genu recurvatum

Genu Valgum (je′nu/val′gum) (n.) An angular deformity of the knee in which the lower leg deviates outward in relationship to the upper leg. It results in separated feet when the knees touch; also referred to as **knock knee**. Normal adult stance is approximately 6° to 7° of genu valgum.

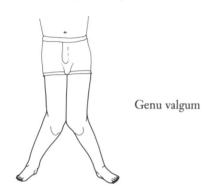

Genu valgum

Genu Varum (je′nu/va′rum) (n.) An angular deformity of the knee in which the lower leg deviates inward in relationship to the upper leg. It results in separation of the knees when the feet are placed together. Commonly known as **bow legs**.

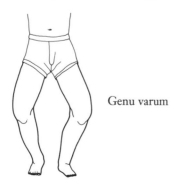

Genu varum

Genus (jē′nus) (n.) In taxonomy, the level between the ranking of species and family. A group of related species constitutes a genus.

Gerdy's Tubercle (gher-dēz/too′ber-k′l) (n.) The anterior lateral tubercle of the tibia. It is the site of insertion of the iliotibial band onto the proximal tibia.

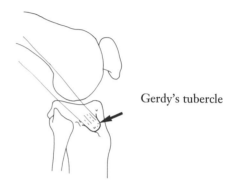

Gerdy's tubercle

Geriatrics (jer″ē-at′riks) (n.) The branch of medicine dealing with the problems of disease, disabilities, and care of the elderly.

Germ Layer (jerm/lā-yer) (n.) One of the three basic embryonic tissue layers—ectoderm, endoderm, mesoderm—that give rise to all body tissues and organs.

German Crutch (jer′man/kruch) (n.) See **Forearm Crutch.**

Germicide (jer′mi-sīd) (n.) An agent capable of killing germs or microbes. Synonym: **Bactericide.**

Gerontology (jer″on-tol′o-jē) (n.) The study of the phenomena, processes, and problems of aging.

Geyser Sign (gī′ser/sīn) (n.) A radiographic sign seen in tears of the rotator cuff. On a shoulder arthrogram, leakage of dye from the glenohumeral joint into the subdeltoid bursa outlines the acromioclavicular joint. The sign is indicative of a full-thickness rotator cuff tear.

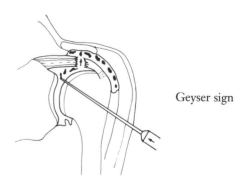

Geyser sign

Ghillie (gil-ē) (n.) In shoe terminology, a shoe open from throat to instep.

Giant Cell (jī′ant/sel) (n.)   A large, multinucleated cell.

Giant-Cell Arteritis (jī′ant-sel/ar″te-rī′tis) (n.)   An inflammatory disease of arteries in the elderly characterized by multinucleated giant cells. It can affect any large or medium-sized artery, but is commonly seen in the superficial temporal artery, carotid artery, vertebral artery, and aorta. This condition is accompanied by fever, headache, and a variety of neurologic disturbances, including blindness. It is often associated with the polymyalgia rheumatica syndrome and is also known as **cranial arteritis** or **temporal arteritis**.

Giant-Cell Reparative Granuloma (ji′ant/sel/re-par′ah-tiv/gran″u-lō′mah) (n.)   A benign, intraosseous lesion most commonly seen in the mandible and maxilla, but also in the small bones of the hands and feet. It appears radiographically as an expansile, lucent defect. Histologically, spindle-shaped fibroblasts with scattered giant cells predominate, especially in areas of hemorrhage.

Giant-Cell Tumor of Bone (ji′ant-sel/too′mor/of/bōn) (n.)   A locally aggressive bone tumor that usually involves the epiphyseal region of a long bone. It occurs in early adult life, generally after the age of 20, and can affect either sex. It most frequently occurs around the knee or distal radius. Radiographically, the lesion appears as a well-defined lytic, multilocular cystic or bubble-like defect in the metaphysis and epiphyseal end of the bone. It is usually eccentric and extends to the region of the subchondral bone. The microscopic appearance of the tumor varies with the degree of hemorrhage and degeneration. In unaffected areas, the tumor is made up of spindle-shaped stromal cells that are moderately vascularized with multinucleated giant cells and collagen fibrils interspersed throughout the tumor cells. In areas of degeneration, osteoid trabeculae and new bone may be found. The more cellular and atypical the stromal cell type, the more likely that the tumor will recur or metastasize. Conventional giant cell tumors are locally aggressive. Full malignant tumors that metastasize also occur.

Giant-Cell Tumor of Tendon Sheath (ji′ant-sel/too′mor/of/ten′dun/sheeth) (n.)   A benign neoplasm of synovial cell origin. It may include the tendon sheath, joint, or bursa. Two clinical types exist—the nodular form and the villous form. The nodular form presents as a solitary, well-circumscribed lesion; the villous form consists of multiple nodules associated with hyperplastic synovium. The latter lesions are more commonly known as **pigmented villonodular synovitis**. The former are the giant-cell tumors of the tendon sheath most often seen in the hand.

The tumor usually appears as a solitary, often lobulated nodule that is slow-growing, painless, tan-colored, and smooth-surfaced. Histologically, it consists of a pleomorphic cell population, which includes lipid-laden foam cells, multinucleated giant cells, and round or polygonal stromal cells. The cells often have hemosiderin deposits in a collagenous stroma. Synonyms: **Xanthogranuloma, Myeloplaxoma, Nodular Tenosynovitis, Benign Synovioma, Fibrous Xanthoma of Synovium, Pigmented Nodular Synovitis, Villous Synovitis, Giant Cell Fibrohemangioma, Myeloid Giant Cell Tumor of Tendon Sheath**.

Gibbus Angle (gib′us/ang′g'l) (n.)   The degree of angular deformity that results from acute, kyphotic curvature of the spine. This angle is measured on a lateral radiograph by determining the angle between the upper end-plate of the normal vertebrae above the affected vertebrae and the lower end-plate of the normal vertebrae below the affected vertebrae.

Gibbus Deformity (gib′us/dē-for′-mi-tē) (n.)   A sharply angular kyphosis or posterior curvature of the vertebral column. Clinically, this is seen as a hump or posterior protuberance in the midline of the spine.

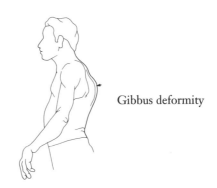

Gibbus deformity

Gibney Boot (gib′-nē/būt) (n.)   An adhesive-tape strapping used for the treatment of ankle sprains. To apply, wrap alternate strips on the foot sole and around the back of the leg. The strips make a herring-bone or basket-weave pattern. Also called **Gibney Strapping** or **Gibney Bandage**.

Gigantism (ji-gan′tizm) (n.)   Excessive stature; the result of oversecretion of growth hormone prior to skeletal maturity, which results in massive growth of the skeleton. Some patients reach huge proportions. See **Acromegaly**.

Gigli Saw (jēl′yē/saw) (n.)   A flexible, saw-toothed wire that has detachable handles at either end. It is used to cut through bone.

Gilchrest Sign (gil′krest/sīn) (n.)   A clinical test of biceps tendon subluxation. Have the patient hold a 5-lb weight in each hand and raise the hands directly overhead, and then lower them slowly with the arms abducted and externally rotated. The test is positive if there is pain or a sharp, painful snap in the region of the origin of the biceps muscle.

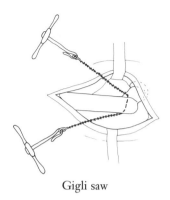

Gigli saw

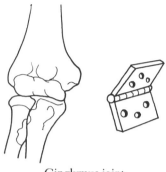

Ginglymus joint

Gill Procedure (gil/pro′se-jur) (n.) A technique for the treatment of painful spondylolisthesis in which no fusion is performed. Through a posterior approach, the loose neural arch and the dense fibrocartilaginous tissue at the defect in the pars interarticularis are excised in order to decompress the fifth lumbar and first sacral nerve roots.

Girdlestone Operation (ger′d′l-stōn/op″er-ā′shun) (n.) A resection of the femoral head and neck, intended to create a painless pseudoarthrosis. Originally described for treatment of persistent tuberculous and pyogenic hip infections.

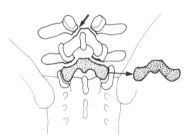

Gill procedure

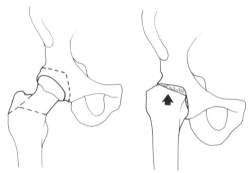

Girdlestone operation

Gill's Sign (gilz/sīn) (n.) A clinical sign of hip joint effusion. To feel the swelling, place your thumb over the femoral artery at the point where it crosses the inguinal ligament and the other four fingers on the buttock opposite the thumb. Grasp the joint with its soft tissues between the thumb and fingers. The affected hip feels thicker than normal.

Gilliat Tourniquet Test (jēl-yah/toor′ni-ket/test) (n.) A technique used to diagnose carpal tunnel syndrome. Place a blood pressure cuff around the upper arm of the affected extremity. Inflate the cuff above the systolic pressure to 220 mm Hg. Normally, the patient feels a tingling in the entire hand and fingers in two or three minutes. In carpal tunnel syndrome, the patient feels a tingling in the sensory distribution of the median nerve in 30 to 60 seconds.

Ginglymus Joint (jin′gli-mus/joint) (n.) A hinge joint. In these joints, a broad, transversely cylindrical convexity of one bone fits into a corresponding concavity on the other. This is a uniaxial joint, which allows angular movement in only one plane. The elbow is an example of a ginglymus joint.

Girth (gerth) (n.) In shoe terminology, the dimension around the last.

Gissane's Angle (gīs-ānz′/ang′g′l) (n.) In the calcaneus, a cortical strut extends along the side of the posterior facet of the subtalar joint. Anteriorly, this strut forms an acute angle known as the crucial angle, or Gissane's angle. Just superior to this angle is the apex of the wedge-shaped, lateral process of the talus.

Giving-Way Sensation (giv′ing/wā/sen-sā′shun) (n.) A nonspecific, subjective symptom noted by patients with knee disorders. This may be a complaint in patients with ligamentous instability, quadriceps weakness, meniscal tears, loose bodies, or chondromalacia.

Gland (gland) (n.) A cell or organ that produces one or more secretions.

Glasgow Coma Scale (glas′gō/kō′mah/skāl) (n.) A practical, standardized system to assess neurologic function and degree of consciousness impairment after a head injury. The system involves three determinants: eye opening, verbal response, and motor response. Each function is assessed numerically by the best response according to the following scale.

Eye Opening:

spontaneous	4
to voice	3
to pain	2
none	1

Verbal Response:

oriented	5
confused	4
inappropriate	3
incomprehensible	2
none	1

Motor Response:

obeys command	6
localizes pain	5
withdraws (pain)	4
flexion	3
extension (pain)	2
none	1

Total Score: 3–15

Glenohumeral (glē″nō-hū′mer-al) (adj.)   Relating to the glenoid cavity and the humerus.

Glenohumeral Joint (glē″nō-hū′mer-al/joint) (n.)   The articulation between the glenoid and the proximal end of the humerus. Commonly called the **Shoulder**.

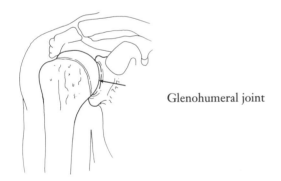

Glenohumeral joint

Glenohumeral Ligaments (glē″nō-hū′mer-al/lig-ah′ ments) (n.)   Thickenings in the anterior aspect of

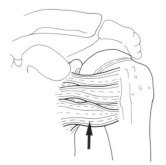

Glenohumeral ligaments

the capsule of the glenohumeral joint that play a significant role in anterior stability of the shoulder joint. These three ligaments are called the superior, the middle, and the inferior glenohumeral ligaments.

Glenoid Cavity (glē′noid/kav′i-tē) (n.)   The depression or cavity in the lateral angle of the scapula. It articulates with the head of the humerus to form the shoulder joint. Also called the **Glenoid Fossa**.

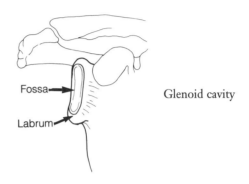

Glenoid cavity

Glenoid Fossa (glē′noid/fos′sah) (n.)   See **Glenoid Cavity**.

Glenoid Labrum (glē′noid/lā′brum) (n.)   The fibrocartilaginous structure formed at the glenoid rim by the conjoined periosteum, articular cartilage, capsule, and synovium. In cross-section, the labrum is triangular and has a sharp, thin, free edge.

Glenoid Rim (glē′noid/rim) (n.)   The edge or lip of the glenoid fossa. The labrum attaches to this.

Glia (gli′ah) (n.)   The special connective tissue of the central nervous system. Also called **Neuroglia**.

Glider Cane (glīd′er/kān) (n.)   A four-legged support for walking. Its two inner legs have wheel tips that glide when the outer legs are raised and tilted. Also called a **Cane Glider**.

Gliding Joint (glīd′ing/joint) (n.)   A synovial joint formed by the apposition of two relatively flat surfaces—one slightly convex, the other slightly concave. This allows gliding movements. Intervertebral facet joints are examples. Also called **Arthrodial Joint** and **Plane Joint**.

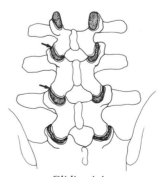

Gliding joint

Gliding Movement (glīd'ing/m$\overline{oo}$v'ment) (n.) The simplest joint movement. One surface glides or moves over another without angular or rotatory motion.

Glioblastoma (glī''ō-blas-tō'mah) (n.) A malignant brain neoplasm derived from non-nervous (glial) tissue.

Glioma (gli-ō'mah) (n.) 1. Any tumor composed of non-nervous cells (glia) in the nervous system. 2. A neoplasm composed of neuroglia in any state of development. It includes all intrinsic neoplasms of the brain and spinal cord, such as astrocytomas and ependymomas.

Globulin (glob'u-lin) (n.) A protein soluble in dilute solutions of neutral salts but insoluble in water. Serum globulins are the major protein components of blood plasma, and have a variety of functions, which include transport, blood clotting, and antibody activity. See also specific globulins.

Glomangioma (glō-man''jē-ō'mah) (n.) See **Glomus Tumor**.

Glomus Tumor (glō'mus/tū'mer) (n.) A vascular hamartoma arising from a normal glomus or other arteriovenous anastomosis. These are rare, painful lesions most commonly found in the subungual region in the fingers. Synonym: **Glomangioma**.

Glucocorticoids (gloo''ko-kor'tĭ-koidz) (n.) Adrenocortical steroids that regulate metabolism.

Gluconeogenesis (gloo''ko-nē-ojen'-esis) (n.) The biosynthesis of glucose from nonglucose metabolic precursors.

Glucose (gloo'kōs) (n.) A simple sugar or monosaccharide. Its formula is $C_6H_{12}O_6$. The basic building block for common polysaccharides, this is a major fuel source for most organisms.

Gluteal Gait (glū'tē-al/gāt) (n.) A gluteal limp. This type of gait is characterized by a tilt of the trunk toward the weak side during the stance phase to compensate for a drop of the pelvis on the normal side. The pelvic drop is usually caused by paralysis or weakness of the gluteus medius muscle, which stabilizes the pelvis in stance phase. Synonyms: **Trendelenburg Gait; Gluteus Medius Gait; Gluteus Medius Lurch**.

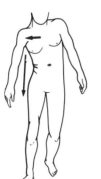

Gluteal gait
Gluteus medius gait

Gluteal Line (glū'tē-al/līn) (n.) One of three rough curved lines on the outer surface of the ilial ala. The posterior line is frequently encountered harvesting a posterior iliac crest graft.

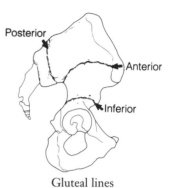

Gluteal lines

Gluteus Maximus Lurch (glū'tē-us/mak'si-mus/lerch) (n.) A type of gait characterized by a tilt of the trunk backward toward the weak gluteus maximus muscle during the stance phase to compensate for the weak muscle. Synonyms: **Gluteus Maximus Gait, Gluteus Maximus Limp**.

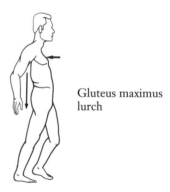

Gluteus maximus lurch

Gluteus Maximus Muscle (glū'tē-us/mak'si-mus/mus'el) (n.) See **Muscle**.

Gluteus Medius Gait (glū'tē-us/mē'dē-us/gāt) (n.) See **Gluteal Gait**.

Gluteus Medius Muscle (glū'tē-us/mē'dē-us/mus'el) (n.) See **Muscle**.

Gluteus Minimus Muscle (glū'tē-us/min'ĭ-mus/mus'el) (n.) See **Muscle**.

Glycogen (glī'kō-jen) (n.) A polysaccharide that is a polymer of glucose. Its formula is $C_6H_0O_5$. It is converted into glucose in times of metabolic need by enzymatic release.

Glycolysis (glī-kol'i-sis) (n.) The anaerobic degradation of glucose by enzymes into lactic acid or pyruvic acid, with release of energy.

Glycosaminoglycans (glī''kos-ah-mē''no-glī'sens) (n.) A group of noncollagenous proteins, including keratan and dermatan sulfate, which are part of the bone matrix. Aggregates of these monomers impart the essential anionic characteristic to proteoglycans, which aids in cross-linking and the stability of the protein structure.

gm   The abbreviation of gram.

Goldthwaits' Sign (gōld'thāwts/sīn) (n.)   A clinical sign seen in sprains of the sacroiliac joint. To elicit the sign, lay the patient supine. Extend the limb on the involved side and then flex the hip and the knee so that the thigh is on the abdomen. Then extend the leg slowly, with one hand under the lower spine. Gradually apply leverage to the side of the pelvis as the hamstrings tighten. Normally, this leg can extend to form a right angle with the table before pain, muscle spasm, or pelvic shift occurs. A lesion—either caused by arthritis or a ligamentous sprain of the sacroiliac joint—is present if pain occurs before the lumbar spine moves. The disease or injury may be located in the sacroiliac, or, more probably, the lumbosacral articulations if pain occurs after the lumbar spine moves. Repeat the test on the other leg. A lumbrosacral lesion is present if pain occurs when both legs are raised to the same height. A sacroiliac lesion is present if no pain occurs when the uninvolved leg is raised higher than the other leg.

Golfer's Fracture of the Ribs (gol'ferz/frak'chur/of the ribs) (n.)   Multiple stress fractures of the upper posterior ribs. These fractures typically occur in beginning golfers.

Golgi Complex (gol'jē/kom'pleks) (n.)   A system of concentrically folded membranes and vesicles found in the cytoplasm of eukaryotic cells. The Golgi complex plays a role in the production and release of secretory materials.

Golgi Tendon Organ (gol'jē/ten'dun/or'gan) (n.)   A subset of mechanoreceptors lying within muscle tendons and ligaments immediately beyond their attachment to the muscle fibers. The tendon organs detect changes in muscle and soft tissue tension. Signals are transmitted through large, rapidly conducting type A alpha nerve fibers to local areas of the spinal cord and to the cerebellum.

Gonarthritis (gōn″ar-thrī'tis) (n.)   An inflammatory, arthritic process in the knee.

Goniometer (gō″nē-om'e-ter) (n.)   A dual-armed instrument for measuring angles. One arm has a pointer, the other a protractor scale. These are joined by a pivot that provides enough friction to stabilize the instrument for easy reading.

Gonococcal Arthritis (gon″o-kok'al/ar-thri'tis) (n.)   An acute infectious arthritis due to *Neisseria gonorrhoeae*. Smears of joint fluid are likely to demonstrate the gram negative diplococci, but it is often difficult to recover gonococci on joint fluid culture. These infections usually respond rapidly to intravenous antibiotics, preferably penicillin.

Gonorrhea (gon″o-rē'ah) (n.)   A sexually transmitted

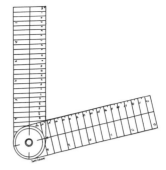

Goniometer

infectious disease caused by *Neisseria gonorrhoeae*. The disease produces a purulent urethral discharge in both males and females, cervicitis and salpingitis in adolescent and older women, vulvovaginitis in children, and ophthalmia in the newborn and occasionally in adults. Synonym: **Clap** (from the French **clapoir**, or brothel). See also **Gonococcal Arthritis**.

Gony Laxometry (gōn'ē/laks-om-et-rē) (n.)   The measurement of knee laxity.

Good Samaritan Statutes (gud/sam-ar-i-tan/stat-ūtz) (n.)   Statutes that exempt physicians from liability for ordinary negligence after giving emergency care to accident victims. These have been enacted in various forms by different state legislatures.

Goodyear Welt Shoe (gud'yēr/welt/shoo) (n.)   A shoe in which the insole, outsole, and upper are stitched together. It includes an 8-mm strip of leather, known as a welt, along the border. This construction eases certain orthotic modifications, notably those between outsole and insole. The Goodyear welt machine was perfected in the 1870s by Charles Goodyear, Jr.

Goose-Neck Deformity (goos-nek/dē-for'mi-tē) (n.)   A marked forward tilt of the cervical vertebral column and skull in relation to the neutral vertical plane of the dorsal and lumbar regions.

Gordon Reflex (gor'don/rē'fleks) (n.)   A type of toe extensor response that appears in corticospinal or pyramidal tract injury. To elicit it, compress the calf muscles; if pathology exists, the toes will extend and spread. See **Babinski Sign**, **Oppenheim Sign**, and **Chaddock Sign** for modifications of this maneuver.

Gorham Syndrome (gor-am/sin'drōm) (n.)   A rare and unusual affectation of the skeletal system. Characterized by massive osteolysis of bony structures. An entire bone or even several bones may disappear from the roentgenogram. The course of this condition is unpredictable. Synonyms: **Disappearing Bone Disease, Massive Osteolysis**, and **Phantom Bone**.

Goring (gor'ing) (n.)   In shoe terminology, a woven elastic fabric inserted in the front or sides of a shoe upper. Its expansion allows a larger opening for the foot.

Gortex Graft (gor′teks/graft) (n.) Any graft made of Gore-Tex, an inert polymer made of polytetrafluoroethylene. In orthopaedic use, a cruciate ligament prosthesis constructed from an expanded polytetrafluoroethylene.

Gouffon Pin (gū-fōnh′/pin) (n.) A trademark of Howmedica; a modified Knowles pin used to fix hip fractures. It has a trocar point, distal cancellous threads, hex collar, and a break-off shank.

Gouge (gowj) (n.) A chisel with a concave-convex cross-section used for cutting and removing bone.

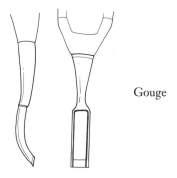

Gouge

Gout (gowt) (n.) A metabolic disorder that results from the deposition of urate crystals in the joints and in the viscera, especially the kidneys.

Two forms of gout exist: primary gout, a metabolic disease based on an inborn error in the intermediary metabolism of purines and related compounds, and secondary gout, which exists when hyperuricemia results from various disorders that increase the production or decrease the excretion of uric acid. Clinically, gout may present as an acute, painful arthritis. Examination of the synovial fluid reveals an inflammatory exudate and the diagnostic, negatively birefringent crystals. The first metatarsophalangeal joint is the most common site of initial involvement. An intermediate stage of intercritical gout is then seen. In the last stage, chronic tophaceous gout may be present in which diffuse deposition of urate crystals occurs.

Gower's Sign (gow′erz/sīn) (n.) A diagnostic marker in muscular dystrophy and congenital myopathies that reflects hip extensors and trunk weakness. If an affected patient (usually a child) is placed prone on the ground, the patient must "climb up his legs" to get up. He first puts his hands on his legs, then he walks his hands proximal to the knee in order to stabilize the quadriceps weakness before being able to extend the back. The patient has a positive sign prior to losing quadriceps strength.

Gracilis Muscle (gras′il-is/mus′el) (n.) See **Muscle**.

Graft (graft) 1. (n.) Any transplanted or implanted

Gowers' is correct ←

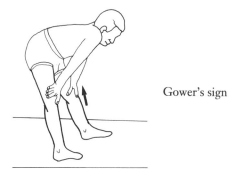

Gower's sign

organ, tissue, or object. 2. (v.) To implant or transplant such tissue. See also specific grafts.

Grain (grān) (n.) A unit of weight equal to 0.0648 gm. One grain is usually considered to be equal to 60 mg for convenience of calculation.

Gram (gram) (n.) A metric unit of mass and weight equal to 1/100 kilogram or 15,432 grains. Abbreviated g. or gr.

Gram Stain (gram/stān) (n.) A differential histologic stain used to classify bacteria. The differentiation depends on whether the bacteria examined retain or lose the primary stain (crystal violet) when treated with a decolorizing agent. An organism is considered gram positive if it retains the stain, and gram negative if it loses the stain.

Granulation (gran″u-lā′shun) (n.) 1. The tiny red flecks visible in a wound during healing, as seen in the base of an ulcer. They consist of loops of newly formed capillaries and fibroblasts. 2. The process of forming tissue in or around an inflammation. 3. The formation of small, rounded outgrowths. These outgrowths consist of small blood vessels and connective tissue. They are present on the healing surface of an ulcer or a wound that does not have tight-fitting edges. Granulation is a normal stage in the healing process.

Granulation Tissue (gran″u-la′shun) (n.) the new tissue formed in the repair of all wounds. It consists of organized hematoma, connective tissue cells, and newly formed capillaries. In soft tissue, it ultimately forms scar or fibrous tissue. In hard tissue, it may progress to bone or fibrous tissue.

Granuloma (gran″ū-lō′mah) (n.) A circumscribed mass or nodule consisting mainly of histiocytes. It occurs in reaction to the presence of a living agent (infectious granuloma) or a nonliving foreign body (foreign body granuloma). It may occur idiopathically.

Grating (grāt′ing) (n.) A subjective sensation of rubbing or rasping that occurs with the motion of a joint. On examination, crepitus will be elicited.

Grattage (grah-tahzh′) (n.) The process of rubbing, brushing, or scraping the surface of a slowly healing ulcer or wound to stimulate healing.

Gravity Method of Stimpson (grav'i-tē/meth'ud/of/ stimpson) (n.) A technique for the closed reduction of hip dislocations. May be applied to both acute posterior and acute anterior dislocation. The patient is placed prone, with the lower extremities hanging from the end of the table. The pelvis is immobilized, and gentle downward pressure is applied to the lower leg with the knee flexed to 90 degrees. Rotary motion of the limb may be needed to effect reduction.

Gravity Stress Test (grav'i-tē/stres/test) (n.) A diagnostic method in medial instability of the elbow, especially useful in acute injuries. With the patient supine, externally rotate the shoulder and place the elbow in 15° to 20° of flexion. In an unstable elbow, just the weight of the forearm and hand will exert sufficient valgus stress to open the medial side. This can be confirmed radiographically during the stress test.

Gray Matter (grā/mat'er) (n.) The regions of the central nervous system (the brain and spinal cord) that contain aggregations of nerve cell bodies. These appear grayish in color in the fresh state, unlike those that are fixed or preserved. In the spinal cord the gray matter is predominantly found in the anterior and posterior horns.

Grayson's Ligament (grā'sonz/lig'ah-ment) (n.) A small digital ligament that runs from the volar aspect of the flexor tendon sheath to insert into the skin. It holds the digital neurovascular bundle in place, preventing bowstringing.

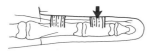

Grayson's Ligament

Grease Gun Injuries (grēs/gun/in'jur-ēs) (n.) A hand disorder that results from penetration of the tissues by grease or diesel fuel under high pressure. The grease will follow the route of least resistance, resulting in ischemia and chemical irritation. These injuries require immediate decompression and debridement.

Greater Multangular (grāt'er/mul-tang'gu-lar) (n.) A carpal bone. Also known as the **Trapezium**.

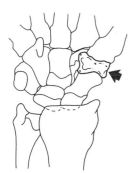

Greater multangular (trapezium)

Greater Trochanter (grāt'er/tro-kan'ter) (n.) The bony, lateral prominence of the hip that marks the proximal end of the femoral shaft. The greater trochanter serves as the insertion site for the tendons of the gluteus medius, gluteus minimus, obturator externus, obturator internus, gemelli and piriformis muscles. The trochanter is covered by a bursa.

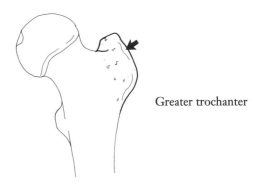

Greater trochanter

Greater Tuberosity (grāt'er/too"be-ros'i-tē) (n.) The most lateral prominence of the proximal humerus. It serves as the insertion site for the supraspinatus, infraspinatus, and teres minor tendons. Also known as the **Greater Tubercle**.

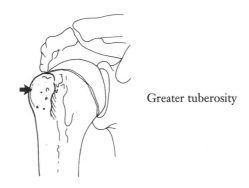

Greater tuberosity

Greek Foot (grēk/fut) (n.) A foot with a big toe shorter than the second toe. Compare with square foot and Egyptian foot. See **Digital Formula**.

Green-Anderson Tables (grēn-an'der-son/tā'b'lz) (n.) Charts that predict the growth remaining in the femur and tibia in skeletally immature patients. These data are used in the evaluation and treatment of leg length discrepancies.

Green Transfer (grēn/trans'fer) (n.) A technique for tendon transfer in the treatment of flexion deformities of the wrist and fingers in patients with cerebral palsy. The flexor carpi ulnaris is transferred dorsally to remove a deforming force and promote forearm supination and wrist extension.

Greenstick Fracture (grēn′stik/frak′chur) (n.) An incomplete break in a long bone in which a portion of the cortex and the periosteum remain intact on the compression side of the injury. The intact cortex is often plastically distorted, which results in an angular deformity if not overcorrected. Seen commonly in children, this fracture results from bending or compression forces.

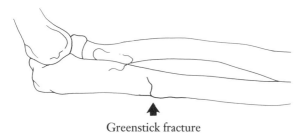

Greenstick fracture

Greulich and Pyle Tables (groy-lik/pīl/tā′b′lz) (n.) An atlas of the left-hand and wrist radiographs of presumably normal children of progressive ages. It is used for the determination of skeletal maturity (bone age). In practice, an AP radiograph of the left hand and wrist is compared to the appearance of the average normal radiographs shown in the atlas. Standards are given for both sexes.

Grice-Green Procedure (grīs/gvēn/prō-se′jur) (n.) An extra-articular bone block arthrodesis of the subtalar joint for correction of paralytic flat feet in children.

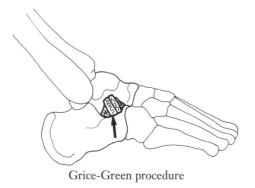

Grice-Green procedure

Grid (grid) (n.) 1. An array of evenly spaced perpendicular lines. 2. A device used in radiography for reducing the amount of scattered radiation reaching the x-ray film. The grid is composed of a stationary arrangement of thin strips of lead. To improve the efficiency of a grid and to eliminate grid lines on the radiograph, a moving grid, known as a Potter Buckey diaphragm, is used.

Grind Test (grīnd/test) (n.) A clinical maneuver used to aid in the diagnosis of a meniscal tear, originally described by Alan Apley. Have the patient lie prone, with the affected knee flexed to 90°. Stabilize the back of the thigh while leaning on the heel to produce compression across the knee. Then rotate the tibia internally and externally on the femur while maintaining compression. In a positive test, this maneuver elicits pain in the medial or lateral compartment of the knee, suggesting meniscal damage on the same side. Also known as **Apley's Grind Test** or **Apley's Compression Test.**

Grip Strength (grip/strength) (n.) A composite measurement of hand, wrist, and forearm strength. It can be used serially to determine improvement or worsening in the function of the distal upper extremity. Strength is measured by having the patient exert maximum grip on a previously calibrated grip dynamometer. The best of three attempts with each hand is noted.

Gristle (gris′l) (n.) The colloquial term for cartilage or cartilagenous.

Gritti-Stokes Amputation (gre′te-stōks/am″putā′shun) (n.) An amputation of the lower limb through the femoral condyles. The patella is retained, and, after removing its articular cartilage, it is applied to the end of the femur. This amputation method is rarely used.

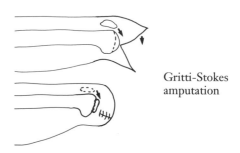

Gritti-Stokes amputation

Groin Flaps (groin/flaps) (n.) A cutaneous flap from the iliofemoral region that may be used as a pedicle flap or as a free flap. It is based on the superficial circumflex iliac vessels. In situations that require a bone graft, the underlying iliac crest may be included with the groin flap.

Groove (grūv) (n.) A narrow channel or depression. Synonym: **Sulcus.**

Grosse-Kempfe Interlocking Nail (grōs-kemf′/in″ter-lok′ing/nāl) (n.) A reamed, intramedullary fixation device that has the potential for screw insertion through both ends of the nail. The curved femoral nail has both a diagonal hole for proximal interlocking that runs from superolateral to inferomedial and two transverse distal holes. The tibial nail uses two proximal and distal screws.

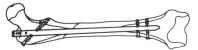

Grosse-Kempfe interlocking nail

Gross Pathology (grōs/pah-thol′o-jē) (n.)   The description of changes in the tissue and organs of the body resulting from disease that are visible to the unaided eye.

Ground-Glass Appearance (grownd-glas/ah-pēr′ans) (n.)   A radiographic finding in which a relatively radiolucent zone in the bone has a hazy appearance on the film owing to diffusely distributed punctiform mineral densities ("ground glass"). These spicules are too small to be seen individually on the roentgenogram. This appearance is often seen in fibrous dysplasia lesions. Also known as **Smoky appearing**.

Ground Substance (grownd/sub′stans) (n.)   The gel-like matrix in which connective tissue cells and fibers are imbedded.

Group Fascicular Nerve Graft (grōōp/fah-sik′u-lar/nerv/graft) (n.)   A technique of peripheral nerve grafting in which groups of fasciculi are bridged with small cutaneous nerves. It is useful when there are gaps of 3 to 7 cm and the nerve cannot be repaired without tension.

Group Fascicular Nerve Repair (grōōp/fah-sik′u-lar/nerv/re-par′) (n.)   A technique for peripheral nerve repair in which bundles of fasciculi are aligned and then apposed by epineurial suturing. Also known as **Bundle Repair**.

Group Practice (grōōp/prak′tis) (n.)   The combined practice of three or more health professionals who share office space, equipment, records, office personnel, expenses, and income.

Growth Factor (grōth/fak′ter) (n.)   A substance that promotes the growth of a specific portion of an organism. These are small proteins in weight. Examples include platelet-derived growth factor, which modulates fibrous tissue, and transforming growth factor-β, which stimulates the growth of cartilage.

Growth Failure (grōth/fāl′yer) (n.)   A term that denotes failure to achieve a height commensurate with the average for a chronologic age.

Growth Hormone (grōth/hor′mōn) (n.)   A small protein molecule produced by the anterior pituitary gland that exerts an effect on nearly all body tissues. It promotes increases in both cell size and number, resulting in growth of all tissues capable of growing. Also known as **Somatomedin**.

Growth Increase (grōth/in′krēs) (n.)   An increase in the size of an organism that results from an increase in number of cells, their size, and the amount of intercellular matrix. Any or all of these factors can cause growth increase.

Growth Plate (grōth/plāt) (n.)   See **Epiphyseal Plate** and **Physis**.

Growth Prediction Chart (grōth/prē-dik′shun/chart) (n.)   See **Green-Anderson Chart**.

Guanine (gwan′īn) (n.)   A purine component of nucleotides and nucleic acids.

Guépar Knee Prosthesis (gā-pahr/nē/pros-thē′sis) (n.)   An early design for total knee arthroplasty. It was a constrained, uniaxial hinged device intended for implantation with methylmethacrylate cement.

Guide Pin (gīd/pin) (n.)   Any wire device placed during surgery in order to direct subsequent reaming, overdrilling, or cannulated screw placement.

Guillain-Barré Syndrome (gē-yan′-bar-rā/sin′drōm) (n.)   An acute lower motor neuron paralysis with areflexia and variable sensory involvement. It is of unknown etiology, and affects people of all ages and both sexes. In approximately 50 percent of cases, a mild upper respiratory or gastrointestinal infection precedes the neuritic symptoms by one to three weeks. The weakness usually presents initially in the lower extremities, with progressive involvement of the trunk, upper extremities, neck, and cranial nerves. Pain is uncommon, but paresthesias are frequent; sensory impairment is usually minimal. In most cases CSF protein levels are elevated several days after infection. A pleocytosis is found in the CSF in only about 10 percent of patients; otherwise, laboratory data are unremarkable. The prognosis for recovery is very good; the speed of recovery is variable. Complete recovery is possible once respiratory failure is overcome. However, many patients show residual muscle weakness. Synonyms: **Guillain-Barré-Stohl Syndrome**, **Glanzmann-Salaud Syndrome**, **Kussmaul-Landry Syndrome**, **Landry Syndrome**, **Ascending paralysis**, **Acute Infective Polyneuritis**, **Postinfectious Radiculoneuropathy**, **Acute Idiopathic Polyneuritis**.

Guillotine Amputation (gil′ō-tēn/am″pu-tā′shun) (n.)   An open amputation in which the entire cross-section of the stump is left open for dressing. It is performed by transection without dissection or flap creation. Also called **Chop Amputation**.

Gull Wing Sign (gul/wing/sīn) (n.)   A sign of fracture-dislocation of the posterior acetabular rim and/or dislocation of the femoral head. Radiographically this is visible in lateral projection as a gull wing–like shadow produced by the intact and fractured portions of the acetabulum.

Gumma (gum′ah) (n.)   A rubbery tumor-like lesion associated with tertiary syphilis.

Gunshot Fracture (gunshot/frak′chur) (n.)   A fracture produced by a bullet or other missile. All gunshot fractures are classified as open fractures.

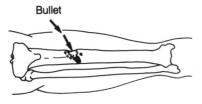

Gunshot fracture

Gunshot Wounds (gunshot/wo͞ondz) (n.) An injury that results from penetration of the skin by a bullet or other missile. This may result in the disruption of skin, underlying soft tissue, neurovascular structures, and bone. The severity of a wound is directly related to the amount of kinetic energy lost by the bullet in the body, because the kinetic energy of a missile is dissipated in bullet deformation and tissue damage. The three recognized mechanisms of bullet injury are: (1) laceration and crushing of tissues forced apart (the principal effect of low velocity missiles); (2) shock waves due to compression of the medium in front of the missile, moving out at approximately the speed of sound in water (4800 ft/sec or 1500 m/sec). These shock waves instantaneously raise pressures up to 100 atmospheres, or 1500 foot pounds per square inch; and (3) temporary cavitation.

Gunstock Deformity (gun'stok/dē-for'mi-tē) (n.) Refers to a cubitus varus deformity. This deformity classically results from supracondylar elbow fractures in children who have residual coronal angulation of the distal fragment postreduction. See **Cubitus Varus Deformity**

Gutter Splints (gut'er/splintz) (n.) A type of splint used for the immobilization of phalangeal and metacarpal fractures. The splint is formed by using plaster slabs cut to the proper size and then applied and molded into a U-shaped splint over either the radial or ulnar half of the forearm and hand. The splint

should extend from the fingertips to just below the elbow, permitting flexion and extension at the elbow joint. The splints are held in place with an elastic bandage.

Guttmann's Test (gut'manz/test) (n.) An examination for interruption of a peripheral nerve that evaluates autonomic function by determining areas of anhydrosis. This is a starch-iodine test using quinizacin powder. With normal sweating, the skin is dyed a deep purple color by the quinizacin powder; the area of anhydrosis remains undyed.

Guyon's Canal (gē-yōnz/kan'al) (n.) The "loge de Guyon," as originally described by Felix Guyon in 1861, is a semirigid canal or tunnel of the wrist. The roof of the canal is formed by the volar carpal ligament, which is blended with the tendinous insertion of the flexor carpi ulnaris into the pisiform bone, and the distal extension of the flexor carpi ulnaris, the pisohamate ligament. The lateral wall is formed by the hook of the hamate and the insertion of the transverse carpal ligament. The medial wall is formed by the fibrous attachments of the pisohamate ligament and the pisiform bone itself. The ulnar nerve and artery traverse Guyon's canal. See **Ulnar Tunnel**.

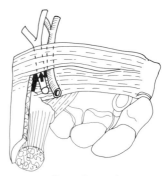

Guyon's canal

H

H-Band (h-band) (n.) See **H-Zone**.

H-Line (h-līn) (n.) See **Hilgenreiner's Line**.

H-Zone (h-zōn) (n.) Part of the organization of striated muscle myofibrils, the H Zone is a region of low density occupied only by myosin filaments; it bisects the A band. It is seen microscopically as a relatively light band; a darker, somewhat indistinct M band is seen in the center of the H Zone. Synonym: **Hensen's disk** or **H-band**.

Habituation (ha-bit-chū-ā'shun) (n.) The process of physiological tolerance or psychological dependence through repeated use or exposure.

Hackenbroch Sign (hah'ken-brok) (n.) In claw foot, a shortened distance between the lateral malleolus and the Achilles tendon.

Hagie Pin (n.) A partially threaded pin designed for use in the fixation of hip fractures. The large screw head has cutting edges on both the proximal and distal portions; this eases insertion and removal. The midportion is smooth, allowing a lag effect. The threaded proximal portion allows compression by a corresponding bolt.

Haglund Disease (hahg'loond/di-zēz') (n.) A painful disorder of the posterior heel characterized clini-

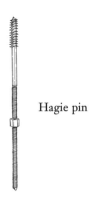

Hagie pin

cally by a painful "pump bump" or thickening of the soft tissues at the point of insertion of the Achilles tendon. Clinically, the disorder is noted by the presence of retrocalcaneal bursitis, Achilles tendinitis, superficial soft-tissue swelling posterior to the tendon insertion, and a prominent posterior superior calcaneal border of bursal projection. The condition is caused by compression of the distal Achilles tendon and the surrounding soft tissue between the os calcis and the posterior shoe counter. Synonym: **Haglund Syndrome**; **Retrocalcaneal Bursitis**.

Hairpin Splint (hār-pin/splint) (n.) A splint used for fractures of the distal phalanx of the fingers. This splint, fashioned out of a thin metal strip or a large hairpin, provides protection from further external injury for fractures that often do not require much immobilization.

Half-Life (half'līf) (n.) 1. The time required for the body's biologic processes to eliminate half of a given amount of an introduced substance. 2. The period of time it takes for half of the atoms of a radioactive element to disintegrate or become stable. The rate of disintegration depends on the element's atomic structure; its half-life cannot be affected by changes in temperatures, pressure, chemical combination, or any other measurable condition. The half-life of different elements varies from a few seconds to several billion years.

Hallux (hāl'uks) (n.) Great toe.

Hallux Rigidus (hāl'uks/rig'idus) (n.) A disorder of

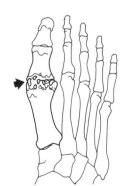

Hallux rigidus

the metatarsophalangeal joint of the great toe, associated with stiffness and limitation of motion.

Hallux Valgus (hāl'uks/val'gus) (n.) 1. A developmental deformity of the great toe and first metatarsophalangeal joint. In this condition, the great toe subluxates or dislocates laterally from its rectus position. Simultaneous but varying degrees of axial rotation also occur. 2. One of the components of the bunion deformity complex. See **Bunion**.

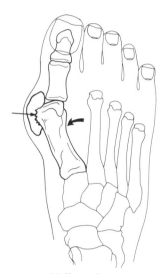

Hallux valgus

Hallux Varus (hāl'uks/vā'rus) (n.) A deformity of the first metatarsophalangeal joint in which the proximal phalanx assumes an adducted position, deviating away from the other toes toward the midline.

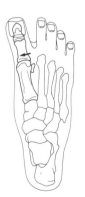

Hallux varus

Halo (hā'lo) (n.) An apparatus for immobilization and/or traction of the cervical spine. Under general or local anesthesia, a metal ring is secured to the skull, just below its maximum diameter, with four pins in diagonally opposed positions. The halo ring then allows for three-dimensional control of the head. It may then be combined with appropriate distal counterforces such as a plaster cast, a plaster vest, femoral pins, or a pelvic hoop, which in combination provide effective immobilization of the spine.

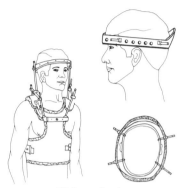

Halo orthosis

Halo-Femoral Traction (hā′lo/fem′or-al/trak′shun) (n.) A technique of spinal distraction that provides correction of spinal deformities by using a halo ring in combination with pins placed in the distal femoral diaphyses.

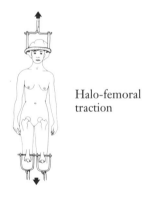

Halo-femoral traction

Halo-Pelvic Traction (hā′lo/pel′vik/trak′shun) (n.) A technique of spinal distraction that provides correction of spinal deformities by using a halo ring in combination with another metal hoop secured through pins into the pelvis. Developed by Ronald DeWald.

Hamartoma (ham-ar-tō-mah) (n.) A local malformation that may appear to be neoplastic but actually results from abnormal development. Histologically, it is characterized by a forced overgrowth of mature, normal cells and tissues in an organ; these cells and tissues are usually composed of elements identical to those of the organ.

Hamate Bone (ham′āt/bōn) (n.) A hook-shaped bone of the wrist that articulates with the pisiform and triquetral bones proximally and the fourth and fifth metacarpal bones distally.

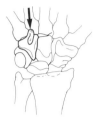

Hamate bone and hook of hamate

Hammer Finger (ham′er/fing′ger) (n.) See **Mallet Finger**.

Hammer Toe (ham′er/tō) (n.) A deformity characterized by flexion contracture of the proximal interphalangeal joint of the toe. The distal interphalangeal joint may be in flexion, in neutral extension, or in slight hyperextension. The proximal phalanx is usually dorsiflexed, which eventually results in hyperextension at the metatarsophalangeal joint. Painful calluses develop at the tip of the toe, over the dorsum of the proximal interphalangeal joint, and occasionally, under the metatarsal head. Compare **Claw Toe**.

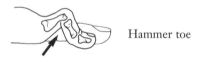

Hammer toe

Hamstring (ham′string) (n.) Any of the tendons at the back of the knee that attach the posterior femoral muscles to their insertions in the lower leg. These muscles include the semitendinosus, semimembranosus, and biceps femoris.

Hamulus (ham′u-lus) (n.) Any hook-shaped process, e.g., those on the hamate and sphenoid bones.

Hand (hand) (n.) The terminal component of the upper extremity. Anatomically, the hand includes the carpus, the metacarpals, the phalanges, and the overlying soft tissue structures.

Hand Orthosis (hand/or-tho′sis) (n.) A mechanical device designed for the upper extremity that uses applied force to improve stability and function or to correct deformity.

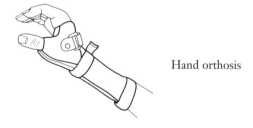

Hand orthosis

Handicap (han′di-kap) (n.) 1. An extra burden that the individual must either overcome or circumvent to avoid significant reduction of a specific functional ability. 2. Partial or total inability to perform an activity. Usually related to an identifiable structural abnormality, a handicap is often determined by the range of two standard deviations from the main observation of a large number of apparently healthy subjects. The widely accepted alternative terms are **impairment** and **disability**. 3. The functional disadvantages and limitations of potential based on a physical or mental impairment.

Handlebar Palsy (han'-dl-bar/pawl'ze) (n.) An overuse injury syndrome associated with bicycling. It is characterized by an ulnar neuropathy caused by excessive and repetitive pressure of the hand against a bicycle handlebar. To prevent this ulnar neuropathy, the cyclist should wear well-padded gloves and pad the handlebars of the bicycle.

Hand-Schüller-Christian Disease (hand-shil'er/kris'chan/di-zēz') (n.) A syndrome that occasionally includes the clinical triad of exophthalmos, diabetes insipidus, and multiple osteolytic bone lesions. It results from a chronic disseminated histiocytosis. This disease is one of a group of disorders known as **Histiocytoses**; other related disorders are **Eosinophilic Granuloma** and **Letterer-Siwe disease**.

Hanging Cast (hang-ing/kast) (n.) A support structure used for certain fractures of the humerus. It is a lightweight cast that extends from the upper arm to the hand. The elbow is flexed to 90°, which leaves the thumb and fingers free. A strap running through a loop proximal to the wrist and around the neck suspends the arm. The arm must remain dependent during treatment to allow the cast to provide a traction force.

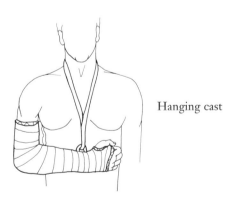

Hanging cast

Hangman's Fracture (hang'manz/frak'chur) (n.) A fracture of the cervical vertebra (axis), usually through the pars interarticularis just posterior to the pedicles, without fracture of the odontoid. The term is derived from pathology caused by judicial hanging in which the noose knot is used submentally.

Hangnail (hang/nāl) (n.) 1. A small piece of partially detached skin at the side or base of the fingernail.

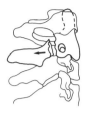

Hangman's fracture

2. A tag of the lateral nail folds that becomes detached and torn.

Hansen-Street Nail (han'sen/strēt/nāl) (n.) A solid intramedullary nail used for fixation of femoral shaft fractures. It has a diamond-shaped cross-section, a blunt point on one end, and a threaded, pointed stud at the other end.

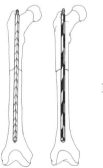

Hansen-Street nail

Haploid (hap'loid) (adj.) Having a single set of unpaired chromosomes in each nucleus. A characteristic of a mature gamete.

Hapten (hap'ten) (n.) An incomplete antigen that requires another substance to become antigenic. It reacts with an antibody but does not stimulate antibody formation by itself.

Hard Corn (hard/korn) (n.) A cone-shaped hyperkeratotic skin lesion that occurs where there is irritation between the skin and an outside source (usually a shoe). A hard corn also may result from prominence of a phalangeal condyle, an unreduced dislocation, or an exostosis. Hard corns are commonly found on the lateral aspect of the fifth toe and the dorsal aspect of the terminal end at the proximal or distal interphalangeal joint level. At the terminal

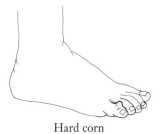

Hard corn

end of the toes, an end-corn may form, especially if there is a flexion or mallet-toe deformity. Synonym: **Heloma Durum**. Compare **Soft Corn**.

Harrington Rod (har'ing-ton/rod) (n.) See **Harrington System**.

Harrington System (har'ing-ton/sis'tem) (n.) A method used for internal instrumentation of the spine. Rods and hooks produce distraction or compression forces that can be applied over a length of the spine. The system was introduced for use in the correction of scoliosis but is also applicable to internal fixation of spine fractures. A spinal fusion that spans the distance from the uppermost to the lowermost hook usually accompanies this form of spinal instrumentation. Invented by Paul Harrington of Houston, Texas.

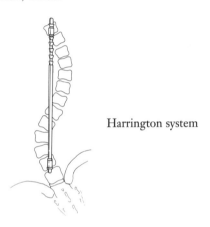

Harrington system

Harris Condylocephalic Nail (har'is/kon"di-lō'-se-fal'ik/nāl) (n.) A long, flexible, solid nail intended for closed intramedullary fixation of pertrochanteric fractures. Technically, these nails are inserted in a retrograde fashion from the femoral condyle into the femoral head.

Harris Footprint Mat (har'is/foot'print/mat) (n.) A rubber mat used to take footprints. Small ridges of varying heights are inked with a roller and covered with a sheet of paper on which the patient stands and walks. Areas of greatest pressure are revealed by the thickness of the ink in the footprint. A thin variety of the Harris mat also can be cut to fit inside a shoe to reveal areas of excessive pressure while walking.

Harris Footprint Test (har'is/foot'print/test) (n.) A test used to evaluate the pressure areas on the sole of the foot. The test is taken on a ridged rubber mat inked with a printer's brayer. Place a piece of plain white paper on the inked mat to record the imprint. Then place the foot on the paper and ask the patient to stand for 10 seconds with his weight evenly distributed on both feet. Increasing pressure is represented by darker inking and more intersections.

Harris Growth Arrest Lines (har'is/grōth/ah-rest/ līnz) (n.) Radiodense transverse striations seen radiographically in the metaphysis. These striations are manifestations of a disturbance in longitudinal growth seen following injury or illness. These lines run parallel to the contour of the provisional zone of calcification in the physis. Also known as the **Transverse Lines of Park**.

Harris HD-2 Total Hip System (har'is/hd-2/to'tal/ hip/sis'tem) (n.) A total hip arthroplasty that is a trademark of Zimmer, Inc.

Harris Hip Rating Scale (har'is/hip/rat'ing/skal) (n.) A numerical scale used in evaluation of the hip. This system evaluates pain, function, absence of deformity, and range of motion. One hundred points is the highest possible total. Also called **Harris Hip Rating System**.

Harrison's Grooves (har'i-sunz/grōovz) (n.) A radiographic sign of rickets characterized by a depression or horizontal groove of the rib cage. This depression or groove is caused by the diaphragm's pull on weakened ribs.

Hart's Sign (hartz/sīn) (n.) A diagnostic marker in congenital dislocation of the hip. In a positive sign, with the patient supine and both hips flexed to right angles, the motion of abduction is limited on the affected side and the adductor muscles are tight or contracted.

Hauser Bar (how'zer/bar) (n.) See **Comma Bar**.

Hauser Procedure (how'zer/pro-se'jur) (n.) A surgical technique for treating recurrent dislocation of the patella in adults. In this procedure, the insertion of the patellar tendon, along with a thick block of tibia, is transferred distally and medially.

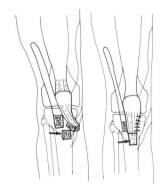

Hauser procedure

Haversian Canal (ha-ver'shan/kah-nal) (n.) The central canal of the osteon that contains the blood and nerve supplies of the bone. In a transverse section of bone, these canals appear as round holes at the center of each Haversian system. The canals run longitudinally for a short distance, then branch and communicate through cross-channels known as **Volkmann's canals**.

Harris Hip Rating Scale

Pain	n	Function	n	Function	n	Deformity	n	Range of Motion	n
Degree		Limp		Stairs		Fixed Adduction		Flexion	
none	44	none	11	normal	4	<10°	1	>90°	1
slight	40	slight	8	without railing	2	>10°	0	<90°	0
moderate	20	moderate	5	any manner	1	Fixed Internal Rotation		Abduction	
marked	10	severe	0	unable	0	<10°	1	>15°	1
disabled	0	Support		Shoes and Socks		>10°	0	<15°	0
		none	11	with ease	4	Flexion Contracture		Adduction	
		cane, long walks	7	with difficulty	2	<15°	1	>15°	1
		cane	5	unable	0	>15°	0	<15°	0
		1 crutch	3	Sitting		Leg-length Discrepancy		External rotation	
		2 canes	2	any chair, 1 hour	4	<3 cm	1	>30°	1
		2 crutches	0	high chair	2	>3 cm	0	<30°	0
		Distance walked		unable to sit	0			Internal Rotation	
		unlimited	11	comfortably				>15°	1
		6 blocks	8	Public Transportation				<15°	0
		3 blocks	5	able to use	1			Trendelenburg	
		indoors	2	unable to use	0			negative	1
		bed and chair	0					positive	0

Harris WM: Traumatic arthritis of the hip after dislocation and acetabular fractures: Treatment by mold arthroplasty. An end-result study using a new method of result evaluation. J Bone Joint Surg 48A:737–755, 1969.

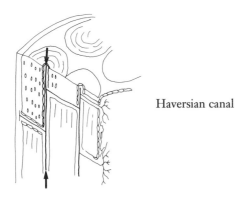

Haversian canal

Haversian System (ha-ver′shan/sis′tem) (n.)   The functional unit of mature cortical bone. Also known as an osteon, a cylindrical structure about 250 μ wide by 1 to 5 cm long composed of concentric layers of bony lamellae surrounding a central haversian canal. Osteocytes in the lacunae line the lamellae and communicate with each other through canaliculi.

Hawkin's Classification   (haw′kinz/klas″sĭ-fĭ-ka′shun) (n.)   In talar neck fractures, a commonly used classification based on the amount of disruption of blood supply to the talus.

Type I: Nondisplaced vertical fracture.

Type II: Displaced fracture with subluxation or dislocation of the subtalar joint.

Type III: Displaced fracture with subluxation or dislocation of the body of the talus from the ankle and subtalar joints.

Some physicians add a *Type IV* that includes any complicated fractures that cannot otherwise be classified.

Hawkin's Sign (haw′kinz/sīn) (n.)   A radiographic means of evaluating the viability of the talar body following fractures of the talar neck. If, in the AP radiograph of the ankle, a zone of translucency appears beneath the subchondral plate of the talus, avascular necrosis is not present. The lucent zone represents bone resorption and requires an intact blood supply to appear. Hawkin's sign usually appears 6 to 8 weeks after an injury.

Haygarth's Nodes (ha′garths/nōdz) (n.)   The fusiform swellings of the proximal interphalangeal joints of the hand in rheumatoid arthritis. These swellings are usually associated with pain and swelling.

Head Acetabular Index of Heyman-Herndon (hed/as″e-tab′u-lar/in′deks/of/hā′man-hern′den) (n.)   A radiographic measurement used to evaluate the congruity of the femoral head epiphysis within the acetabulum. It is measured by dividing the width of the epiphysis by the width of the acetabulum. Normal hips oscillate with an index between 70 and 100.

Head of a Screw (hed/of/a/skru) (n.)   The uppermost part of a screw, designed to hold the tip of a screwdriver.

Head of Femur (hed/of/fē′mur) (n.)   The rounded upper end of the femur that articulates with the acetabulum to form the hip joint.

Head of Radius (hed/of/rā′dē-us) (n.) The proximal end of the radius that articulates with the capitellum at the distal end of the humerus.

Head-Neck Quotient (hed/nek/kwo′shent) (n.) A radiographic measurement of the abnormality of the shape of the femoral head and neck. On an AP radiograph, tracing lines are drawn and measured from the superior border of the femoral head, through the center of the neck to the intertrochanteric line, divided by another line measuring the width of the femoral neck at its narrowest diameter. A quotient of 100 indicates no deformity in this respect.

Head-Shaft Angle (hed-shaft/ang′g′l) (n.) A radiographic measurement used to evaluate the varus-valgus angulation of the femoral neck. On an AP radiograph of the hip, draw a straight line through the widest part of the femoral head parallel to the femoral neck. Intersect this line with another line going through the longitudinal axis of the femoral shaft. The angle this forms is the head-shaft angle. The average angle is 127°.

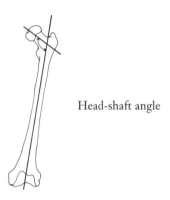

Head-shaft angle

Head-Stem Offset of Femoral Component (hed-stem/off-set/of/fem′or-al/kom-po′nent) (n.) A calculation of a prosthetic femoral component that is measured from the center of the prosthetic head to a line going through the axis of the distal part of the femoral stem.

Healing (hēl′ing) (n.) The restoration of structure and function to injured or diseased tissues.

Healing by First Intention (hēl′ing/by/ferst/in-ten′shun) (n.) The primary union of a wound in which cleanly incised skin edges are reapproximated and repair occurs without granulation.

Healing by Second Intention (hēl′ing/by/sek′und/in-ten′shun) (n.) The process of wound closure in which the wound heals by the formation of granulation tissue. Eventual coverage occurs by spontaneous migration of epithelial cells over the defect.

Health Care (helth/kār) (n.) The provision by professional and paraprofessional personnel of services that maintain health and treat illness or injury.

Health Maintenance Organization (helth/mān′ten-ans/ōr′gan-i-zā′shun) (n.) An organization responsible for providing prepaid, comprehensive health care services to its clients. Abbreviated **HMO**.

Heberden's Node (he′ber-denz/nōd) (n.) A cartilaginous and bony enlargement at the distal interphalangeal joint of a finger, characteristic of osteoarthritis.

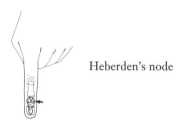

Heberden's node

Heel (hēl) (n.) 1. In common usage, the hindmost part of the foot, the calcaneus. 2. In shoe terminology, a heel consists of two parts: the rigid proximal section that comes in contact with the foot, and the distal section (plantar surface) that comes in contact with the ground.

Heel Base (hēl/bās) (n.) In shoe terminology, the part of the heel next to the sole. It is usually made concave to fit the heel seat.

Heel Bisector Method (hēl/bi-sek′tor/meth′ud) (n.) A radiographic technique for grading the severity of metatarsus adductus. On an AP radiograph of the foot, construct a reference line (referred to as the heel bisector) that bisects the hindfoot. This is the major axis of the elliptical weight-bearing surface of the heel; normally, it crosses between the second and third toes. A deformity is considered mild if the line crosses through the third toe, moderate if it crosses between the third and fourth toes or through the fourth toe, and severe if it crosses between the fourth and fifth toes.

Heel Cord (hēl/kord) (n.) The long tendon of the calf that inserts into the calcaneus. It is composed of the gastrocnemius-soleus and plantaris tendons. Also known as **Triceps Surae** or **Achilles Tendon**.

Heel Breast (hēl/brest) (n.) In shoe terminology, the forward face of the heel, which is often concave toward the shank.

Heel Elevation (hēl/el-e-vā′-shun) (n.) In shoe terminology, the height of the heel measured in a vertical line at the posterior aspect of the heel; the distance is calculated from the plantar surface to the heel point at the heel seat. Also known as **Heel Height**.

Heel Height (hēl/hīt) (n.) See **Heel Elevation**.

Heel Off (hēl/off) (n.) In gait analysis, the event near the end of the stance phase when the heel rises off the floor at the beginning of the push-off interval.

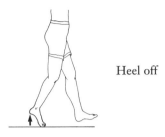

Heel off

Heel strike

Heel Pad (hēl/pad) (n.)   A cushioning or protective material placed in the heel seat of a shoe.

Heel-Pad Thickness Sign (hēl-pad/thik′nes/sīn) (n.) A clinical sign of acromegaly characterized by increased thickness of the heel pad—usually to more than 20 mm.

Heel Pain Syndrome (hēl/pān/sin′drōm) (n.)   A disorder characterized by pain in the plantar aspect of the heel on heel strike and tenderness over the central area of the heel at the calcaneal tuberosity. It is an inflammatory process believed to result from cumulative repetitive loading of the heel during heel strike while walking. Also known as **Calcaneodynia**, **Painful Calcaneal Spur**, **Heel Spur Syndrome**, and **Painful Heel Pad Syndrome**, and **Plantar Fasciitis**.

Heel Pitch (hēl/pich) (n.)   In shoe terminology, inclination of the heel (from the vertical) at the posterior surface.

Heel Point (hēl/point) (n.)   In shoe terminology, the rearmost point of the last at the heel seat.

Heel Seat (hēl/sēt) (n.)   In shoe terminology, the place to which the heel is attached; the area on which the anatomic heel rests.

Heel Spur (hēl/sper) (n.)   An osteophyte that protrudes from the plantar surface of the anterior end of the calcaneus. Also known as **Calcaneal Spur**.

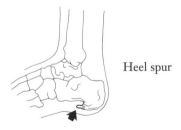

Heel spur

Heel Spur Syndrome (hēl/sper/sin′drom) (n.)   See **Heel Pain Syndrome**.

Heel Strike (hēl/strīk) (n.)   In gait analysis, the initial event of the stance phase; the instant the heel of the reference limb touches the floor. Also known as **Heel Contact**.

Heel-Toe Gait (hēl/tō/gāt) (n.)   Any manner of walking in which the heel strikes the ground first and the toes are the last part of the foot to leave the ground at the end of stance phase.

Heifetz Tong (hī′fets/tong) (n.)   A stainless steel arc with three self-drilling bolt drills used for skeletal traction for the cervical spine. It is applied to the vertex of the skull.

Helbing's Sign (hel′bingz/sīn) (n.)   A diagnostic marker in hyperpronation of the foot. With the patient standing, visualize a plumb line dropped from the middle of the popliteal space; this line should bisect and run parallel to the Achilles tendon. The sign is present if medial or inward deviation of the Achilles tendon is noted, indicating that the foot is in pronation.

Helfet Test (hel′-fet/test) (n.)   A maneuver used to determine proximal tibiofibular joint instability. Instruct the standing patient to flex the involved knee while leaning all of his weight on it. If the proximal tibiofibular joint is unstable, the patient will instinctively attempt to stabilize the involved leg by supporting it with the contralateral foot.

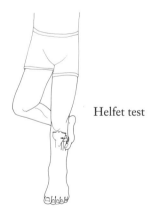

Helfet test

Helping Hand (help′ing/hand) (n.)   A device used to grasp an object otherwise out of reach.

Hemangioma (he-man″je-ō′mah) (n.)   A benign proliferation of vascular endothelium that creates a mass resembling neoplastic tissue. Usually asymptomatic, these lesions can occur in any organ or tissue. Intraosseous lesions usually occur in the skull or vertebral bodies; they are usually solitary. Roentgenographically, these lesions are relatively lytic, with a coarse, trabeculated bone pattern that is often honeycombed in appearance.

Hemarthrosis (hēm″ar-thrō′sis) (n.) An accumulation of blood in a joint.

Hematocrit (hē-mat′o-krit) (n.) The ratio of the volume of packed red blood cells to the volume of whole blood as measured in marked tubes. The ratio is expressed as a percentage. To calculate, multiply the red cell column in millimeters × 100 total height of column in millimeters. Abbreviated **Hct.**

Hematoma (hēm″ah-tō′mah) (n.) A localized accumulation of extravasated blood that clots to form a semisolid swelling within the tissues.

Hematoxylin (hēm″ah-tok′si-lin) (n.) A colorless crystalline compound used in various histologic stains.

Hematuria (hēm″ah-tū′re-ah) (n.) The presence of blood or red blood cells in the urine. Usually microscopic hematuria is differentiated from gross hematuria.

Hemiarthroplasty (hem″ē-ar-thrō′plas-tē) (n.) An arthroplasty that addresses only one side of a joint. Example: **Bipolar Hip Prosthesis.**

Hemihypertrophy (hem″ē-hī-per′trō-fē) (n.) Overgrowth of one side of the body, body part, or organ.

Hemilaminectomy (hem″ē-lam″i-nek′tō-mē) (n.) Removal of half of a lamina of a vertebra.

Hemimelia (hem″ē-mē′lē-ah) (n.) Literally "half a limb," this term refers to the congenital absence of the major portion of a limb. These anomalies are subdivided: **complete hemimelia,** in which the entire distal limb is absent; **incomplete hemimelia,** in which most of the distal limb is absent; and **paraxial hemimelia,** in which the preaxial or postaxial portion of the distal half of the limb is absent. Paraxial hemimelia may be terminal or intercalary.

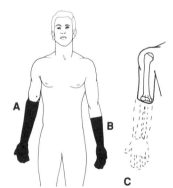

Hemimelia. **A,** Complete hemimelia; **B,** incomplete hemimelia; **C,** transverse hemimelia.

Hemiparaplegia (hem″ē-par″ah-plē′jē-ah) (n.) Paralysis of one side of the lower half of the body.

Hemiparesis (hem″ē-par′ē-sis) (n.) Paresis, or partial paralysis, that affects one side of the body.

Hemiplegia (hem″ē-plē′je-ah) (n.) Paralysis of one side of the body.

Hemiplegic Gait (hem″ē-plē′jik/gāt) (n.) The typical gait of a hemiplegic patient. On the paralyzed side, there is usually a flexed elbow, stiff knee, and an inverted, plantarflexed ankle, with the lower limb swinging forward in a semicircular fashion.

Hemisacralization (hem″ē-sa″kral-i-zā′shun) (n.) Fusion of the fifth lumbar vertebra to the first segment of the sacrum on only one side.

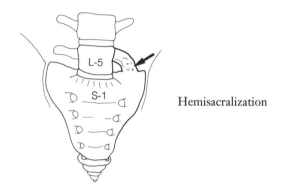

Hemisacralization

Hemivertebra (hem″ē-ver′te-brah) (n.) A congenital anomaly of the spine caused by the incomplete development of one side of a vertebra.

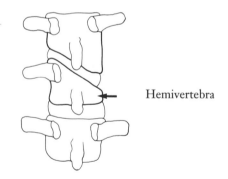

Hemivertebra

Hemochromatosis (hē″mō-krō″mah-tō′sis) (n.) A condition that results from excessive iron accumulation. It may be secondary to excessive iron intake or repeated blood transfusions, or it may be idiopathic. The disease is seen mostly in older men and affects the skin and visceral organs. It may be seen in bones and joints as a noninflammatory arthropathy involving the metacarpophalangeal joints as well as the shoulders and elbows. Radiographically, nonspecific periarticular cysts and erosions may be seen. Grossly, the affected synovial tissue has a brown discoloration, and hemosiderin deposits are seen on histologic examination.

Hemoglobin (hē′mō-glō″bin) (n.) A conjugated protein in red blood cells consisting of heme and globin that transports O_2 and CO_2 in the blood. Abbreviated as **Hb.**

Hemolysis (hē-mol′i-sis) (n.) The process of breaking down or destroying red blood cells so that hemoglobin is released.

Hemophilia A (hē″mō-fil′ē-ah/A) (n.) The classic form of hemophilia. It is characterized by the defective synthesis of thromboplastin, which is caused by deficiency of Factor VIII (antihemophiliac globulin or AHG). Bleeding occurs either after trivial trauma or spontaneously; the skin, the mucous membranes, and the joint cavities are most frequently involved. The disease is transmitted as an X-linked recessive gene and therefore tends to spare females, who carry the abnormal gene. Many carriers show a lower blood level of AHG (Factor VIII), and in some, a mild clotting defect may occur. In 30% of hemophiliacs, no family history can be elicited. Synonyms: **AHG Deficiency: Factor VIII Deficiency.**

Hemophilia B (hē″mō-fil′ē-ah/B) (n.) A variety of hemophilia caused by an inborn deficiency of plasma thromboplastin component (also known as PTC or Factor IX). Transmitted as a sex-linked recessive, it accounts for about 15% of all cases of hemophilia. Clinically, it is indistinguishable from classic Hemophilia A; laboratory findings are also very similar. Synonym: **Christmas Disease.**

Hemophilic Pseudotumor (hē-mō-fil′ik/soo″dō-tū′mor) (n.) A progressive cystic swelling produced by recurrent hemorrhaging into soft tissue. It may be seen after a subperiosteal hemorrhage. Radiographically, this would appear as an erosion into the bone associated with soft tissue that may be calcified.

Hemophilus (hē-mof′i-lus) (n.) The genus of gram-negative rods ascribed by some to the family *Brucellaceae*. Most members are part of the normal flora of the upper respiratory tract mucous membranes.

Hemorrhage (hem′or-ij) (n.) A discharge of blood from the blood vessels. Usually used in reference to profuse bleeding.

Hemosiderin (hē″mō-sid′er-in) (n.) An iron-containing glycoprotein pigment found in most tissues, including the liver, that represents colloidal iron in the form of granules much larger than ferritin molecules. It is insoluble in water and differs from ferritin in electrophoretic mobility. Pathologic accumulations of hemosiderin are known to occur in a number of disease states.

Hemosiderosis (hē″mō-sid″er-ō′sis) (n.) The accumulation of hemosiderin in tissues.

Hemostasis (hē″mō-stā′sis) (n.) The arrest of bleeding.

Hemostat (hē′mō-stat) (n.) An instrument designed for clamping a bleeding blood vessel.

Hemovac (hē′mō-vak) (n.) A proprietary name for a closed-wound, suction-drainage device.

Hennequin's Sign (hen-e-kinz/sīn) (n.) In the clinical examination of a patient with a fracture of the neck of the femur, digital compression below Poupart's ligament and lateral to the major femoral vessels will elicit pain and tenderness.

Henry Approach (hen″rē/ah-prōch) (n.) A system of extensile approaches to the extremities. For example, an anterior surgical approach to the radius. The incision is extended from the lateral side of the biceps tendon insertion along the medial border of the brachioradialis to the radial styloid. Use part or all of this incision as necessary.

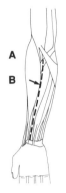

Henry approach.
A, Biceps tendon;
B, brachioradialis muscle.

Heparin (hep′ah-rin) (n.) A mucopolysaccharide that functions as an anticoagulant by inhibiting the enzyme thrombin in the final stage of blood clotting.

Herbert Screw (herbert/skru′) (n.) A double-ended threaded screw with different pitches of the screw threads at either end. This enables compression of the fracture fragments as the screw is advanced without the need for a screw head. Most commonly used in the scaphoid bone.

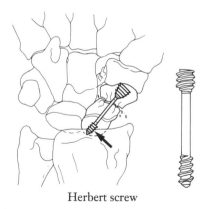

Herbert screw

Hereditary Multiple Exostosis (he-red′i-ter-ē/mul′ti-p′l/ek″sos-tō′sis) (n.) A generally benign, hereditary disorder of enchondral growth of bone. It is marked by the development of multiple exostoses in the extremities near the long bone diaphyses. The disease has an autosomal dominant pattern of inheritance. Radiographically and pathologically, the lesions are analogous to solitary osteochondramata. This disorder is also known as **Multiple Osteocartilaginous Exostosis** or **Diaphyseal Aclasis**.

Herniated Disk (her-ne-āt″ed/disk) (n.) A pathologic condition in which the nucleus pulposus of an intervertebral disk has protruded through the surrounding fibrocartilage or annulus fibrosus. Symptoms may result from pressure on the spinal nerves or the spinal cord. Four degrees of displacement are recognized: 1. **Internal disk disruption.** 2. **Bulging:** The displaced material causes a discrete bulge in the annulus, but no material escapes through the annular fibers. 3. **Extrusion:** The displaced material presents in the spinal canal through disrupted fibers of the annulus but remains connected to material persisting within the disc. 4. **Sequestration:** Nuclear material escapes into the spinal canal as one or more free fragments, which may migrate to other locations. Colloquially called **Ruptured** or **Slipped Disk**.

Herniated Nucleus Pulposus (her′ne-āt″ed/nu′kle-us/pŭl-pō′sŭs) (n.) Abbreviated **HNP**; see **Herniated Disk**.

Herniation (her″ne-a′shun) (n.) A protrusion of an organ or other body structure through a defect or natural opening in a covering wall, membrane, muscle, or bone.

Herpes Zoster (her′pēz/zos′ter) (n.) An acute viral infection of one or more dorsal root ganglia or sensory ganglia of the spinal nerves. It is accompanied by a painful rash of the skin and/or mucous membranes, and is distributed in the corresponding dermatome along the course of the peripheral sensory nerves that arise in the affected ganglia. The rash is a vesiculobullous eruption. The causative varicella virus also produces chickenpox, and it has been proposed that the zoster represents reactivation of a previously acquired, dormant, virus. Synonyms: **zoster, shingles**.

Hesitant Gait (hez′i-tant/gāt) (n.) A gait characterized by initial hesitation; it is characteristic of Parkinson's disease.

Heterograft (het′er-o-graft) (n.) Tissue transplant from one species to another, such as grafting pigskin onto a human. Synonym: **Xenograft**.

Heterotopic Ossification (het″er-o-top′ik/os″ĭ-fi-ka′shun) (n.) See **Myositis Ossificans**.

Hexachlorophene (hek″sah-klō′rō-fēn) (n.) A germicidal compound commonly used in soaps and dermatologic agents.

Hex Screw (heks/skru) (n.) A screw that has a hexagonal head.

Hexcelite Cast (hex-e-līt/kast) (n.) A proprietary brand of fiberglass cast.

Hey's Amputation (hāz/am″pu-tā′shun) (n.) Am-

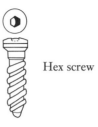
Hex screw

putation of the foot between the tarsus and metatarsus.

Hiatus (hi-ā′tus) (n.) A gap, cleft, or opening.

Hibbs Angle (hibz/ang′g′l) (n.) The radiographic angle between the talus and the first metatarsal, used as a measurement of cavus. On the lateral radiograph of the foot, draw a line through the center of the longitudinal axis of the talus and the longitudinal axis of the first metatarsal. Measure the angle formed by the intersection of these lines. In a normal foot, the longitudinal axis of the talus is parallel with that of the first metatarsal. In a cavus foot, the angle is greater than 15°.

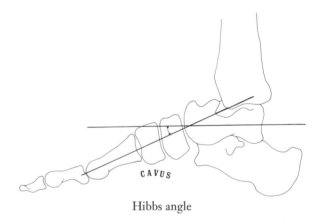
Hibbs angle

Hibbs Arthrodesis (hibz/ar″thrō-dē′sis) (n.) A surgical technique for arthrodesis of the hip characterized by using the greater trochanter as a graft.

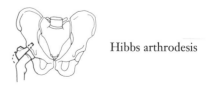
Hibbs arthrodesis

Hibbs Retractor (hibz/re-trak′tor) (n.) A flat, right-angled surgical instrument with a serrated edge used for retraction of soft tissues.

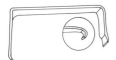

Hibbs retractor

Hibbs Spinal Fusion (hibz/spi′nal/fu′zhun) (n.) A surgical technique for fusion of the lumbar spine characterized by its goal of obtaining fusion at four different points—the laminas and articular processes on each side.

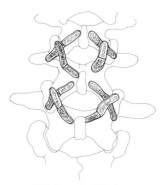

Hibbs spinal fusion

Hibiclens (hi-bi-klenz) (n.) Proprietary name for chlorhexidine gluconate, a skin antiseptic.

High Tibial Osteotomy (hi/tib′ē-al/os″te-ot′ō-mē) (n.) A technique for the treatment of unicompartmental gonarthrosis that uses a wedge-shaped, or dome-shaped osteotomy in the proximal end of the tibia.

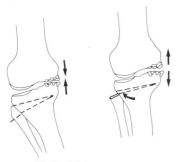

High tibial osteotomy

High-Definition Intensifying Screen (hi/def″i-nish′un/in-ten″si-fī′ing/skrēn) (n.) A radiographic screen composed of extremely small fluorescent crystals that provides the highest quality resolution of the radiographic image.

High-Riding Patella (hi-rīd′ing/pah-tel′ah) (n.) See **Patella Alta**.

High-Riding Scapulae (hi-rīd′ing/skap′yū-lē) (n.) See **Sprengel Deformity**.

High-Speed Intensifying Screen (hi/spēd/in-ten″si-fī′ing/skrēn) (n.) A fluoroscopic screen composed of large fluorescent crystals that requires the shortest composition time to produce satisfactory radiographs.

High-Velocity Missile (hi-ve-los′i-tē/mis-īl) (n.) Any missile whose velocity is greater than 2500 ft/sec.

Highet's Scale (hī′etz/skāl) (n.) A method of grading muscle strength based on a scale of 0 to 5.

0 Zero: Total paralysis, no evidence of contractility

1 Trace: Muscle flicker, no joint motion

2 Poor: Muscle contraction, complete range of joint motion with gravity eliminated

3 Fair: Complete range of joint motion, against gravity

4 Good: Complete range of joint motion against gravity with some resistance

5 Normal: Complete range of joint motion against gravity with full resistance.

Hilgenreiner's D Line (hil-gen-rī-nerz/D-līn) (n.) In the evaluation of developmental dysplasia of the hip, this radiographic measurement is the distance from the lateral edge of the triradiate cartilage to the intersection of Hilgenreiner's H Line with Hilgenreiner's horizontal line. This distance is increased when congenital hip dislocation is present.

Hilgenreiner's Epiphyseal Angle (hil-gen-rīnerz/ep″i-fiz′ē-al/ang′g′l) (n.) An angle useful in predicting the progression of a coxa varus deformity. On an AP radiograph of the pelvis, the angle formed by the intersection of Hilgenreiner's horizontal line with a line drawn parallel to the epiphyseal plate of the proximal femur. If the angle is less than 45°, spontaneous correction occurs. If the angle is greater than 60°, patients usually show progressive varus deformity, which requires surgical intervention.

Hilgenreiner's Fold (kil-gen-rī-nerz/fold) (n.) In the physical examination of an infant with developmental dysplasia of the hip, have the patient lie prone. The lateral fold between the thigh and buttock will become shortened and flattened, or even absent, on the affected side.

Hilgenreiner's H Line (hil-gen-rī-nerz/H-līn) (n.) In the evaluation of developmental dysplasia of the hip, this radiographic measurement is the distance from the most proximal part of the femoral neck to Hilgenreiner's Y line. This distance may be shortened if the hip is dislocated proximally.

Hilgenreiner's Y Line (hil-gen-rī-nerz/y/līn) (n.) A

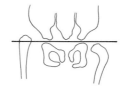

Hilgenreiner's Y line

line used in the evaluation of infants with developmental dysplasia of the hip. On an AP radiograph of the pelvis, a horizontal line drawn through the triradiate cartilages. Also known as **Hilgenreiner's Horizontal Line.**

Hill-Sachs Lesion (hil′-saks/lē′zhun) (n.) A radiographic sign of recurrent anterior dislocation of the shoulder characterized by an osteochondral lesion occurring in the posterolateral aspect of the humeral head. Radiographically, the lesion is seen when the humeral head is internally rotated; it can, however, be completely obscured by external rotation. The defect results from the impingement during an anterior dislocation of the posterolateral aspect of the humeral head against the anteroinferior aspect of the glenoid fossa.

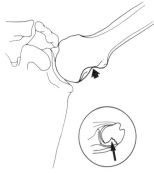

Hill-Sachs lesion

Hilton's Law (hil′tunz/law) (n.) A law of joint innervation stating that the trunks of nerves whose branches supply the groups of muscles moving a joint also provide sensory nerves to both the skin overlying the insertions of these muscles and to the interior of the joint.

Hindfoot (hīnd′foot) (n.) The posterior portion of the foot, which consists of the talus and calcaneus.

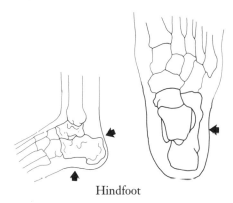

Hindfoot

Hinge Joint (hing/joint) (n.) See **Ginglymus Joint.**

Hip (hip) (n.) The joint at which the proximal femur articulates with the acetabulum of the pelvis.

Hip Arthroplasty (hip/ar′thro-plas″tē) (n.) A general term referring to any of a number of surgical procedures involving the reconstruction of the hip joint.

Hip Fractures (hip/frak′churz) (n.) In common usage, a general term for fractures of the proximal femur near the hip joint.

Hip Joint (hip/joint) (n.) The joint formed at the head of the femur and the acetabulum of the hip bone; commonly called the **hip.**

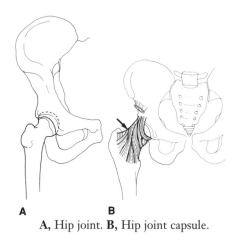

A, Hip joint. **B,** Hip joint capsule.

Hip Pointer (hip/point′er) (n.) A colloquial sports term referring to a very painful inflammation of tissue along the anterior superior iliac crest. It is usually caused by a direct fall or blow.

Hip Spica (hip/spi′kah) (n.) A cast applied to the trunk and one or both legs. It is used for postoperative care and fracture management. The various kinds of hip spicas are:

1. Single hip spica, which extends from the nipple line to include the pelvis and one thigh and leg.

2. Double hip spica, which extends from the nipple line or upper abdomen to include the pelvis, both thighs, and the lower legs.

3. One and a half spica, which extends from the upper abdomen to include one entire leg and the knee of the other leg.

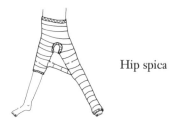

Hip spica

Hip Station of Gage and Winter (hip/sta′shun/of/gāj/and/win′ter) (n.) A radiographic measurement used to evaluate the position of the femoral head in relation to the acetabulum in congenital dislocation of the hip. This is measured while the child is in traction, prior to any attempt at reduction. The station is defined by the position of the medial corner of the femoral neck metaphysis. The various stations are:

Minus-One Station: Superior to Hilgenreiner's horizontal line.

Zero Station: Between Hilgenreiner's line and the reduced position.

Plus One Station: At the same level as the normal hip.

Plus Two Station: Below the opposite normal hip.

Hippocratic Maneuver (hip″o-krat′ik/mah-noo′ver) (n.) A technique for the reduction of shoulder dislocations. Place your shoeless heel into the axilla for countertraction; then apply straight traction at the wrist, with the elbow extended. The pressure of the heel against the humeral head is thought to help ease it back into the joint.

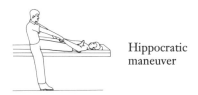

Hippocratic maneuver

Hippocratic oath (hip″o-krat′ik/ōth) (n.) The vow taken by a physician to observe the code of behavior and practice devised and followed by the Greek physician Hippocrates (460 to 370 BC).

Hirschhorn Plate (n.) An original fracture fixation and compression plate used to treat fractures of the long bones. Developed by Ralph Hirschhorn of Long Island, New York.

Histiocytosis X (his″te-o-si-to′sis/X) (n.) A group of syndromes characterized by a proliferation of histiocytes, along with eosinophils and chronic inflammatory cells. This group includes eosinophilic granuloma (solitary or multiple), Hand-Schüller-Christian Disease, and Letterer-Siwe Disease.

Histocompatibility (his″to-kom-pat″ĭ-bil′i-tē) (n.) The genetically determined degree to which cellular antigens are alike in two individuals of the same species.

Histology (his-tol′o-je) (n.) The study of the structure and arrangement of tissues.

HLA Abbreviation for Human Leukocyte Antigens. This refers to the complex of antigens controlled by the major histo-compatibility complex of gene loci for leukocyte antigens in man.

HMO Abbreviation for Health Maintenance Organization.

HNP Abbreviation for Herniated Nucleus Pulposus.

Hodgen Splint (hoj′en/splint) (n.) An apparatus for applying balanced suspension to a fractured extremity. The splint consists of two sturdy wires that are continuous at their lower ends and a padded ischial ring with two loops at both the proximal and distal ends. Ropes leading from these loops to another rope and a pulley allow the limb to be suspended and traction to be applied. This apparatus has been used in the treatment of femur fractures; a similar wire suspension splint was designed for use in forearm fracture treatment.

Hodgkin's Disease (hoj′-kinz/di-zēz′) (n.) A malignant disease of lymphoreticular origin that occurs mostly in young and middle-aged adults. Histologically, the disease is characterized by Reed-Sternberg cells and a variable proliferation of lymphocytes and histiocytes. If bone lesions occur, they are usually osteoblastic. Radiographically, vertebra of ivory color are characteristic. Also known as **Hodgkin's Lymphoma.**

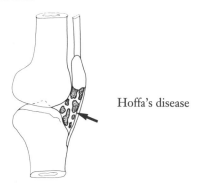

Hoffa's disease

Hoffa's Disease (hof′az/di-zēz′) (n.) Necrosis of the infrapatellar fat pad. On physical examination, one may see swelling caused by the presence of an enlarged fat pad or a mild effusion. Forced extension produces pain, and deep palpation will elicit local tenderness. Radiographically, either small, irregular, calcific flecks or dense, calcific clumps may be seen inferior to the patella. Clinically, patients usually give a long history of exertion-related pain in the anterior compartment of the knee. Synonyms: **Infrapatellar Fat Pad Hypertrophy, Hoffa-Kaster Disease.**

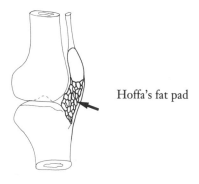

Hoffa's fat pad

Hoffa's Fat Pad (hof′az/fat/pad) (n.) The infrapatellar fat pad of the knee.

Hoffa's Sign (hof′az/sīn) (n.) A clinical finding associated with avulsion fractures of the calcaneal tuberosity. In this finding, when the legs are in comparable positions, the Achilles tendon on the injured side will be less taut than on the contralateral side. A loose fragment may be seen and felt behind the malleolus.

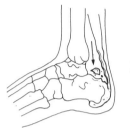

Hoffa's sign

Hoffman External Fixator (hof'man/eks-ter'nal/fiksa'ter) (n.)   A system for external fixation of fractures, using percutaneous transfixing pins in bone, that are attached to a rigid external metal frame. The components include transfixing pins, universal ball joints, adjustable connecting rods, and articulation couplings. Half-pins also can be obtained. The components are made of stainless steel; aluminum alloy hoop frame components are available. The original Hoffman is a trademark of Jaquet Freresand and is manufactured by Howmedica, Inc. Also known as a **Hoffman Frame** or a **Hoffman-Vidal Frame**.

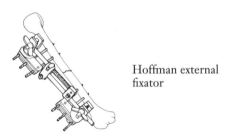

Hoffman external fixator

Hoffman's Sign (hof'manz/sīn) (n.)   An abnormal reflex whose unilateral presence suggests pyramidal tract disease. To elicit the sign, support the patient's hand in a relaxed and pronated position. Extend the long finger and grasp the middle phalanx between your thumb and long fingers. With your opposite thumb, snap and release the nail of the patient's middle finger to flex the distal phalanx and stretch flexor. A positive Hoffman sign is present when the thumb flexes and adducts.

Hohmann Retractors (hō-mahn/re-trak'torz) (n.)   Surgical instruments used for retraction of the soft tissues around bones. They are available in a variety of sizes and tip-shapes that allow subperiosteal retraction after adequate exposure of the bone.

Also known as the **Homan Retractor**, a variation in spelling.

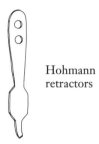

Hohmann retractors

Hoke Corset (hōk/kor'set) (n.)   A thoracolumbosacral canvas corset with front opening and multiple stays. The corset was developed about 1930 by surgeon Michael Hoke of Warm Springs, Georgia; he developed it primarily as a support for scoliosis due to poliomyelitis. It is also called the **Warm Springs Corset**.

Holding Power (hold'ing/pow'er) (n.)   The ability of a screw to provide functional resistance to loads that tend to pull the screw directly out of bone.

Hole Zones (hōl/zōnz) (n.)   The spaces that occur within the substance of collagen fibrils due to the internal organization of collagen fibrils in mineralized tissues. Mineralization seems to occur in these hole zones.

Holmgren's Sign (holm'grenz/sīn) (n.)   A radiographic sign of intra-articular fractures of the knee. On a cross-table lateral view of the knee, a lipohemarthrosis will appear as a layering in the suprapatellar pouch (the bone marrow fat floats on top of the blood).

Holt Nail-Plate (holt/nāl-plāt) (n.)   A type of fixed-nail-plate device designed for fixation of hip fractures. The nail-plate angle is 130°.

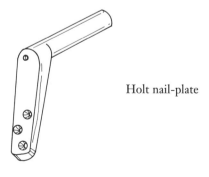

Holt nail-plate

Holt-Oram Syndrome (hōlt-orem/sin'drōm) (n.)   A congenital malformation that presents with atrial septal defects or other cardiovascular manifestations, along with upper limb deficiencies, usually radial club hand and hypoplasia of the clavicles.

Homans' Sign (hō-mahnz/sīn) (n.) A clinical sign of deep vein thrombophlebitis in the calf. With the patient supine and the knee extended, dorsiflexion of the ankle elicits pain at the back of the calf or knee.

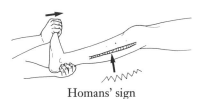

Homans' sign

Home Health Agency (hōm/helth/a′jen-sē) (n.) A public or private organization that provides health services in the patient's home, either directly or through other organizations.

Home Health Aide (hōm/helth/ād) (n.) A person who, under the supervision of a home health or welfare agency, assists elderly, ill, or disabled persons with household chores, bathing, and other daily needs. Also called **Homemaker**.

Home Health Care (hōm/helth/care) (n.) The provision of such services as nursing, therapy, and health-related homemaker or social services in the patient's home, for the purpose of restoring and maintaining the patient's maximal level of comfort, function, and health.

Home Health Institution (hōm/helth/in′sti-tū′shun) (n.) An establishment with permanent facilities and medical, nursing, and other professional and technical services that provides treatment for patients at home.

Home Traction (hōm/trak′shun) (n.) A general term for any type of traction used by a patient and his family outside the hospital setting. Examples are cervical halter traction or intermittent skin traction for the lower extremity in Legg-Calvé-Perthes disease.

Homecare (hōm′kār) (n.) The provision of equipment and services to the patient in the home for the purpose of restoring and maintaining his or her maximal level of comfort, function, and health.

Homocystinuria (hō″mō-sis″tin-ū′rē-ah) (n.) An inheritable disorder of amino acid catabolism characterized by an increased concentration of homocystine in the blood and urine. There are three distinct forms of the disease, the most common of which is due to a deficiency of cystathione β-synthase. This results in an accumulation of methionine and homocystine, the latter of which interferes with the normal cross-linking of collagen. This causes skeletal complications, among other problems. Some skeletal findings are fragility of bones, scoliosis, excessive length of long bones, and enlarged ossification centers.

Homogentisic Acid (hō″mō-jen-tis′ik/as′id) (n.) 2, 5-dihydroxyphenylacetic acid, an intermediate product in the metabolism of tyrosine and phenylalanine. It is excreted in the urine in alkaptonuria, an inborn error of metabolism.

Homograft (hō′mō-graft) (n.) A tissue transplant from one individual to a genetically nonidentical individual of the same species. Synonyms: **Allograft**; **Homologous Graft**; **Homogenous Graft**.

Hook (hook) (n.) 1. A substitute for a missing hand, it is the most frequently used terminal device of an upper-limb prosthesis. Resembling two neighboring fingers in a slightly flexed position, it comprises a double hook of metal that can open to grasp objects of various sizes. Only one hook finger is moveable. It is operated via a steel cable by the wearer's shoulder muscles or by pneumatic mechanisms. 2. A surgical instrument with a bent or curved tip used to hold, lift, or retract tissue.

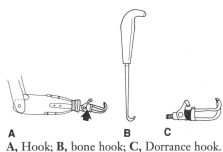

A, Hook; **B,** bone hook; **C,** Dorrance hook.

Hoover Cane (hoo′ver/kān) (n.) A long, light aluminum cane used by the blind in walking. See **Long Cane**.

Hoover Test (hoo′ver/test) (n.) A test used to differentiate true inability to raise a leg from malingering in a patient with back pain who states that he or she cannot raise his or her legs. With the patient supine, place your palms beneath the heels. Ask the patient to raise one leg. The truly disabled person involuntarily offers counterpressure with the heel of the other leg. This sign is absent in hysteria or malingering. When the normal leg is lifted, the hysterically "paralyzed" leg will press down normally. When the patient attempts to lift the hysterically or fallaciously "paralyzed" leg, however, the down-pressing movement of the normal leg will be absent or trifling commensurate with the absence or paucity

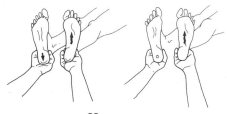

Hoover test

of effort made. The downward pressure in the opposite heel may be quantified with a manometer. Synonym: **Phenomenon of Complementary Opposition.**

Hoppenfeld's Ankle Clonus Test (hopen-feldz/ang′kl/klo′nus/test) (n.) See **Ankle Clonus Test.**

Hoppenfeld's Law (hopen-feldz/law) (n.) A principle that states that wherever a nerve touches a bone, it grooves that bone. Examples: the radial nerve in the spiral groove, the ulnar nerve at the medial epicondyle of the elbow, and the spinal nerves at the base of the pedicles.

Horizontal Cleavage Tear (hor″i-zon-tal/klēv′ij/tār) (n.) A tear that occurs in the horizontal plane of a meniscus, thereby dividing its superior and inferior surfaces. See **Meniscal Tears** and **Interstitial Tear.**

Horizontal Plane (hor″i-zon-tal/plān) (n.) Any plane through the body that lies parallel to the horizon. Also known as **Transverse Plane.**

Hormone (hor′mōn) (n.) An organic compound produced in one part of a body that is carried in the blood to exert an effect on the activities of cells in another organ or part.

Horner's Syndrome (hor′nerz/sin′drōm) (n.) The result of an injury to the superior cervical sympathetic ganglion. Characteristics are ipsilateral ptosis, miosis, and anhidrosis.

Horseback Rider's Knee (hors-bak/rī′derz/nē) (n.) A common term for posterior dislocation of the fibular head in the proximal tibiofibular joint.

Hospital (hos′pit′l) (n) An institution that provides medical and surgical treatment for sick and injured persons.

Hospital, Affiliated (hos′pit′l/a-fil-ē-ā-ted) (n.) A hospital allied with another institution or program, such as a medical school, shared services organization, multi-hospital system, or religious organization.

Hospital, Certified (hos′pit′l/ser″ti-fīd′) (n.) A hospital recognized by the United States Department of Health and Human Services as meeting its standards as a provider in the Medicare program.

Hospital Cane (hos′pit′l/kān) (n.) A standard wooden cane. Also known as a **C Cane.**

Host (host) (n.) An animal, plant, or person on or within which microorganisms live.

Hot Isostatic Pressing (hot/i′so-stat′ik/pres′ing) (n.) A procedure in the manufacturing of metals that simultaneously applies heat and pressure for the consolidation of a part. It increases the strength of a casted component and is abbreviated as HIP.

Hot Pack (hot/pak) (n.) Any device used to provide superficial heat therapy to a body part.

House Staff (hows/staf) (n.) Physicians and other health care professionals still in training who participate in an accredited, hospital-sponsored program of graduate medical education.

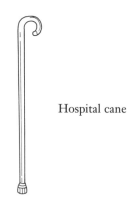

Hospital cane

Housemaid's Knee (hows′mādz/nē) (n.) A common term for a prepatellar bursitis thought to result from chronic, recurrent, minor trauma to the prepatellar bursa. Radiographically, one may see an enlarged bursa anterior to the patella. Patients complain of anterior knee pain, especially on kneeling. Prepatellar swelling with local tenderness is also found.

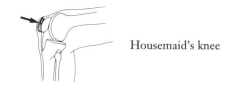

Housemaid's knee

Houston A-Frame Brace (hu′ston/A-frām/brās) (n.) An ambulatory abduction orthosis used in Legg-Calvé-Perthes Disease.

Howships Lacunae (how′ships/lah-kū′nē) (n.) Microscopic cavities along bone surfaces that contain osteoclasts. These osteoclasts are resorbing bone.

Hoyne's Sign (hoynz/sīn) (n.) A way of confirming the meningeal irritation seen in acute poliomyelitis. Bring the head and neck of the supine patient over the edge of the bed. Support the patient's shoulders as he or she attempts to elevate his or her trunk; normally, the head follows the plane of the trunk. In polio, the head will fall back limply.

Hubbard Tank (hub-ard/tank) (n.) A large, keyhole-shaped water tank in which a patient may be immersed for therapeutic exercise. Also called a **Full Body Tank.**

Hueter's Line (hē′terz/līn) (n.) A straight line connecting the epicondyles of the humerus with the tip of the olecranon when the elbow is extended.

Hueter's Sign (hē′terz/sīn) (n.) 1. In the evaluation of fracture healing by osteophony. When a bone is tapped distal to the fracture line, soft tissue remains between the fracture fragments if vibration is not heard proximally. 2. In patients with rupture of the biceps tendon, pain is elicited in the shoulder when the supinated forearm is flexed against resistance.

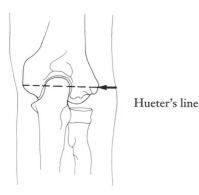

Hueter's line

Hueter-Volkmann Law (he'ter/folk-man/law) (n.) The rate of epiphyseal growth is affected by pressures applied to its axes: increased pressure inhibits growth; decreased pressure accelerates growth. Also referred to as the **Inverse Pressure Epiphyseal Rule**.

Hughston Jerk Test (hū-ston/jerk/test) (n.) A clinical examination of the knee that elicits a pivot shift indicative of anterior cruciate ligament insufficiency. See **Jerk Test** for details of this maneuver.

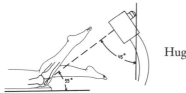

Hughston view

Hughston View (hū-ston/vū) (n.) A radiographic technique for obtaining a tangential view of the patella. The view is taken with the knee in 50° to 60° of flexion and with the x-ray tube angled 45° from the vertical position.

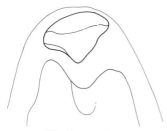

Hughston view

Human Position (hū'man/po-zish'un) (n.) A description of the positioning of the lower extremities for cast application in the treatment of congenital dislocation of the hip. This position, in contrast to the frog leg position, avoids extreme abduction and flexion of the hips that may contribute to the development of aseptic necrosis of the femoral head.

Humeral Head (hū'mer-al/hed) (n.) The termination of the humerus proximal to the anatomic neck; it articulates with the glenoid cavity of the scapula.

Humeral Triangular Space (hū'mer-al/tri-ang'gu-lar/spās) (n.) A triangular anatomic space in the upper posterior arm through which the radial nerve and the brachial artery leave the axilla. The space is bounded by the teres major muscle, the long head of the triceps brachii muscle, and the proximal humerus.

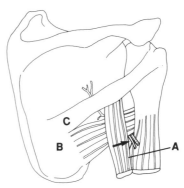

Humeral triangular space. **A,** Triceps long head; **B,** Teres major; **C,** Teres minor.

Humerotangential Angle (hū″mer-o-tan'jen'shul/ ang'g'l) (n.) An angle measured on a tangential x-ray view of the distal humerus used to assess the reduction of distal humerus fractures, especially supracondylar fractures. Measure the angle formed by the longitudinal axis of the humerus and the line that joins both epicondyles. Compare that angle with the angle in the normal elbow.

Humerus (hū'mer-us) (n.) The long bone of the upper arm. It is composed of a shaft and two articular surfaces that form a part of the shoulder and the elbow joints.

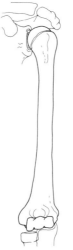

Humerus

Humoral (hū'mor-al) (adj.) Pertaining to body fluids; it especially refers to biologically active chemical agents carried in body fluids.

Humphrey's Ligament (hum'frēz/lig'ah-ment) (n.) The lateral meniscofemoral ligament that courses anterior to the posterior cruciate ligament in the knee.

Hunchback (hunch'bak) (n.) 1. A rounded deformity, or hump, of the back. 2. A person with such a deformity. This condition is often the result of excessive thoracic kyphosis. It may be secondary to severe scoliosis, causing a large posterior thoracic rib-hump.

Hunter's Canal (hunt'erz/kah-nal') (n.) A triangular fascial tunnel located in the anterior middle third of the thigh. This canal extends from the apex of the femoral triangle to the opening in the adductor magnus. It is bounded anteriorly by the sartorius muscle, laterally by the vastus medialis, and posteriorly by the adductor longus and adductor magnus. It contains the femoral artery, the femoral vein, and the saphenous nerve. Also called the **Adductor** or **Subsartorial Canal**.

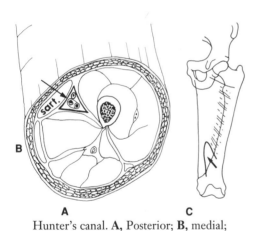

Hunter's canal. **A,** Posterior; **B,** medial; **C,** adductor hiatus.

Hunter Rod (hunt'er/rod) (n.) A Dacron-impregnated silicone rod used in a two-stage procedure for flexor tendon repair in the hand. In the first stage, the rod is inserted in the area of the excised tendon to maintain the tunnel until passive motion is restored to the digit. In the second stage, the rod is removed, and a tendon graft is inserted.

Hunter's Syndrome (hun'terz/sin'drōm) (n.) An inheritable disorder of mucopolysaccharide metabolism transmitted as an X-linked recessive trait. It is characterized chemically by excessive dermatan sulfate and heparan sulfate in tissues and urine. Clinical findings are similar to those found in Hurler's syndrome, but milder in severity; for example, mental deterioration progresses more slowly, and cornea clouding does not occur. Dwarfing, deafness, and heart defects are common. Also known as **Mucopolysaccharidosis II**.

Hurler's Syndrome (hoor'lerz/sin'drōm) (n.) An inheritable disorder of mucopolysaccharide metabolism transmitted as an autosomal recessive trait. It is characterized chemically by excessive dermatan and heparan sulfate in tissues and urine. Clinically, the generalized connective tissue disturbance is manifested early in life. Owing to the progressive involvement of many organs and organ systems (including the skin, brain, liver, eyes, and skeletal system), these children rarely survive past adolescence. Also known as **Mucopolysaccharidosis I-H**, or **Gargoylism**.

Hutchinson's Fracture (huch'in-sunz/frak'chur) (n.) A fracture of the radial styloid. Also known as **Chauffeur's Fracture**.

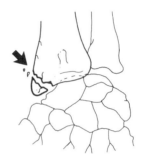

Hutchinson's fracture

Hyaline Cartilage (hi"ah-līn/kar'ti-lij) (n.) A type of elastic cartilage that grossly appears smooth and semitransparent with a bluish-white tint. It forms most of the fetal skeleton. Found on the articular surfaces of the skeleton and in the respiratory passages of adults.

Hyaluronic Acid (hī"ah-lu-ron'ik/as'id) (n.) An acid mucopolysaccharide that occurs in the synovial fluid and in the extracellular ground substance of vertebate connective tissues. It is a straight-chain polymer that consists of a repeating unity of a disaccharide composed of N-acetyl glucosamine and glucuronic acid. It forms the backbone of the aggregated proteoglycan molecule.

Hyaluronidase (hi"ah-lu-ron'i-dās) (n.) An enzyme that catalyzes the hydrolysis of hyaluronic acid.

Hydroarthrosis (hy"dro-arthrō'sis) (n.) The accumulation of excessive synovial fluid in a joint.

Hydrocephalus (hi"drō-sef'ah-lus) (n.) A condition in which an excessive amount of cerebrospinal fluid accumulates in the cerebral ventricles.

Hydrocollator (hi"dro-kol'la-ter) (n.) The proprietary name of a small stainless-steel tank used for either hot or cold packs. The hot pack is a cotton bag filled with bentonite, a silicate gel that absorbs hot water (about 70°C) to form a soft, heat-retaining mass. The cold pack (under the name of ColPac) is a similar bag, filled with bentonite and a glycol solution. It is maintained at 6°C in a dry unit resembling the deep-freeze compartment of a refrigerator.

Hydrocortisone (hī″drō-kor′ti-sōn) (n.) The principle glucocorticoid secreted by the adrenal gland. Synonym: **Cortisol**.

Hydrodynamic Lubrication (hī″drō-dī-nam′ik/lū-bri-kā-shun) (n.) In engineering terms, a type of fluid film lubrication that occurs when bearing surfaces are moving tangentially to each other and their shape is such that a converging wedge of fluid is formed. A lifting pressure is then generated because the viscosity of the fluid causes it to be dragged into the gap between the surfaces. It has been proposed that this mechanism is one type of lubrication that occurs at joint surfaces.

Hydrolysis (hī-drol′i-sis) (n.) The decomposition of a substance by the insertion of water molecules between some of its bonds.

Hydrostatic Bed (hī″drō-stat′ik/bed) (n.) See **Water Bed**.

Hydrostatic Lubrication (hī″drō-stat′ik/lū-bri-kā-shun) (n.) In engineering terms, a type of fluid film lubrication that occurs where there is no relative sliding motion of the bearing surfaces and the pressure in the fluid is generated externally.

Hydrotherapy (hī″drō-ther′ah-pē) (n.) The external application of water in the treatment of disease and injury. Because water absorbs and gives up heat slowly, it is an effective tool in all its states—liquid, solid and gaseous—for heating and cooling the body. Sprays and whirlpools also can be used for stimulation and wound care.

Water also is used therapeutically by invoking the Archimedes Principle, which states that weight-bearing joints thrust upward under water undergo minimal stress. Buoyancy can therefore be used to assist or resist activity.

Hydroxyapatite (hī-drok″sē-ap′ah-tīt) (n.) 1. An inorganic constituent of bone matrix and teeth. It is a crystal with a specific lattice configuration; it contains calcium, phosphate, and hydroxyl ions. 2. A bioactive calcium phosphate ceramic. It can form a chemical bond with bone. Abbreviated **HA**.

Hydroxyproline (hī-drok″sē-pro′lēn) (n.) An amino acid that occurs naturally as a constituent of collagen.

Hypalgesia (hī″pal-jē′ze-ah) (n.) Elevation of the threshold for tolerating pain and other noxious stimuli.

Hyper (hī′per) Prefix for greater than normal, above, or beyond.

Hyperabduction Maneuver (hī″per-ab-duk′shun/mah-nōō′ver) (n.) A diagnostic procedure involving compression of the neurovascular bundle as it passes beneath the pectoralis minor; this maneuver is used to evaluate thoracic outlet syndrome. With the patient sitting in a comfortable position, determine the amplitude of the radial pulse. Then, hyperabduct the arm and determine the change in amplitude, if any, of the pulse. Note the degree of hyperabduction that produces obliteration of the pulse as well as whether it is diminished or obliterated in more than one position within the hyperabduction arc. A positive test, along with a compatible history, is highly suggestive of thoracic outlet syndrome. See **Wright** and **Adson Test**.

Hyperalgesia (hī″per-al-jē′ze-ah) (n.) Increased sensitivity to noxious stimulation.

Hyperbaric Oxygen (hī″per-bār′ik/ok′si-jen) (n.) Oxygen that is delivered at pressures above those of the atmosphere. Delivered in a hyperbaric chamber, this type of oxygen therapy is an effective adjunctive treatment of clostridial myonecrosis. It has other applications.

Hypercalcemia (hī″per-kal-sē′me-ah) (n.) The presence of high concentration of calcium compounds or ions in the blood. A variety of symptoms may present, including malaise, muscular weakness, polyuria, polydipsia, constipation, dehydration, nausea, vomiting, anorexia, and mental derangement. Increased serum and urine calcium levels are diagnostic. Electrocardiographic changes, especially a shortened Q-T interval, also may occur. The etiology varies widely, but the underlying disorder is usually diagnosed on the basis of history, physical examination, and other laboratory tests.

Hypercalciuria (hī″per-kal″si-u′re-ah) (n.) The presence of high calcium levels in urine.

Hypercapnia (hī″per-kap′ne-ah) (n.) The presence of excessive carbon dioxide in blood.

Hyperesthesia (hī″per-es-thē′ze-ah) (n.) The depression of the threshold for touch stimulation; it is usually measured in comparison with normal areas of the same patient's body.

Hyperextension (hī″per-ek-sten′shun) (n.) The extension of a limb or joint beyond its normal limit.

Hyperextension Orthosis (hī″per-ek-sten′shun/or-thō′sis) (n.) A thoracolumbosacral orthosis that places the spine in extension and prevents flexion. Also known as a **Flexion Control Orthosis**.

Hyperflexia (hī″per-flek′shē-ah) (n.) An abnormally increased or exaggerated action of the reflexes.

Hyperflexion (hī″per-flek′shun) (n.) Flexion of a limb or joint beyond its normal limit.

Hyperkalemia (hī″per-kah-lē′mē-ah) (n.) The presence of excessive potassium in blood.

Hyperkyphosis (hī″per-kī-fō′sis) (n.) A kyphosis of greater than normal range. Usually used in reference to the thoracic spine.

Hyperlordosis (hī″per-lor-dō′sis) (n.) A lordosis of greater than normal range. Frequently used in reference to the lumbar spine.

Hypermobile Flatfoot Deformity (hī″per-mō-bīl/flat′foot/de-for′mi-tē) (n.) A condition in which the medial arch of the foot appears normal, but when weight *is* borne, the height of the arch decreases significantly.

Hypermobility Syndrome (hī″per-mō-bil′i-tē/sin′drōm) (n.) A benign syndrome in an otherwise healthy individual that consists of musculoskeletal pain and dysfunction along with joint laxity in three or more paired joint areas. Often provoked by strenuous effort after a period of sedentary or inactive living, the condition may present at any age and in either sex. There can be generalized pain or local joint pain and dysfunction. The areas most commonly involved include the knees, the feet, the hands, and the lower back.

Hypernatremia (hī″per-nah-trē′mē-ah) (n.) The presence of excessive sodium in blood.

Hyperostosis (hī″per-os-tō′sis) (n.) The presence of excessive growth or enlargement of bony tissue.

Hyperparathyroidism (hī″per-par″ah-thī′roid-izm) (n.) A pathologic state in which there is an excessive amount of parathyroid hormone in the blood. Clinical manifestations result from either the *direct* action of increased PTH on bone, the gut and the kidney, or *indirectly* from the resultant hypercalcemia. Diagnosis is based on finding increased PTH in the blood. Other laboratory tests are necessary to distinguish primary and secondary hyperparathyroidism.

  Primary Hyperparathyroidism (prī′mer-ē/hī″per-par″ah-thi′roid-izm) (n.) A condition resulting from the excessive production of PTH owing to parathyroid gland hyperplasia, adenoma, or carcinoma.

  Secondary Hyperparathyroidism (sek′un-der″ē/hī″per-par″ah-thī′roid-izm) (n.) A condition caused by excessive secretion of PTH as a result of other disease states in which there is resistance to the metabolic actions of PTH. For example, it is seen in chronic renal disease and in some forms of osteomalacia.

Hyperpathia (hī″per-path′e-ah) (n.) A painful syndrome characterized by overreaction and after-sensation to a stimulus.

Hyperplasia (hī″per-plā′zē-ah) (n.) An absolute increase in the number of cells in a tissue or organ.

Hyperpyrexia (hī″per-pi-rek′se-ah) (n.) See **Malignant Hyperthermia**.

Hypersensitivity (hī″per-sen′si-tiv″i-tē) (n.) A condition in which the response to a stimulus is excessive. A state of induced hypersensitivity is commonly known as an **Allergy**.

Hypertonia (hī″per-tō-′nē-ah) (n.) A state of increased muscle tension, rigidity, or spasm.

Hypertonic (hī″per-ton′ik) (adj.) A solution with a higher osmotic pressure than a comparable solution.

Hypertrophic Arthritis (hī″per-trōf′ik/ar-thrī′tis) (n.) See **Osteoarthritis**.

Hypertrophic Pulmonary Osteoarthropathy (hī″per-trōf′ik / pul′mo-ner″ē / os″tē-ō-ar-throp′ah-thē) (n.) A clinical syndrome characterized radiographically by the formation of symmetric periosteal new bone in the diaphysis. Patients present with aching bone pain and/or arthralgias. In addition to periostitis, they may have synovial hypertrophy, which results in large effusions and clubbing of the fingers and toes. This syndrome is seen in association with neoplastic and chronic diseases of the lung, and, less commonly, with other organ system diseases. Also known as **Marie-Bamberger Syndrome** or **Osteopulmonary Arthropathy**.

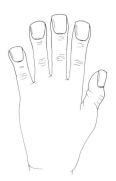

Hypertrophic pulmonary osteoarthropathy

Hypertrophic Scar (hī″per-trof′ik/skar) (n.) Bulky scars that stay within the boundaries of a wound. Hypertrophic scars tend to regress over a period of months or years; *keloids*, in contrast, may continue to enlarge over time.

Hypertrophy (hī″per-trō-fē) (n.) An increase in size or volume of a part or organ produced by enlargement of existing cells, not by an increasing number of cells.

Hyperuricemia (hī″per-ū″ri-sē′mē-ah) (n.) The presence of high blood uric acid levels.

Hypesthesia (hīp″es-thē′zē-ah) (n.) An elevation of the threshold for touch stimulation; usually noted in comparison with normal areas on the same patient's body. The opposite of this is **Hypoesthesia**.

Hypnosis (hip-nō′sis) (n.) An artificially induced trance-like state, characterized by heightened susceptibility to suggestion.

Hypnotic (hip-not′ik) (n.) An agent or drug that produces sleep or depression of the senses.

Hypo (hī′po) A prefix meaning less than normal, under, below, or down.

Hypoalgesia (hī″po-al-jē′sē-ah) (n.) Diminished sensitivity to noxious stimulation.

Hypocalcemia (hī″pō-kal-sē′me-ah) (n.) The presence of a decreased amount of calcium in the blood. This state produces increased neuromuscular excitability, which results in tetany and seizures. Clinically, one also may see lethargy, impaired cognitive function, and heart failure in patients with heart disease. An electrocardiogram shows a prolonged Q-T interval.

Hypochondriasis (hī″pō-kon-drī′ah-sis) (n.) A disorder characterized by an excessive preoccupation and concern with one's own physical health or the unfounded belief that one is suffering from a serious disease. The predominant disturbance is an unrealistic and persistent interpretation of physical signs or sensations as abnormal when professional physical evaluation does not support the existence of any physical disorder that can account for this interpretation. The unrealistic fear or belief persists despite medical reassurance, causing impairment in social or occupational functioning. The condition is not due to any other medical disorder, such as affective or somatization disorders or schizophrenia.

Hypoesthesia (hī″pō-es-thē′zē-ah) (n.) Decreased sensitivity to stimulation; this excludes the special senses. The opposite is **Hypesthesia**.

Hypokalemia (hī″pō-ka-lē′mē-ah) (n.) The presence of decreased potassium in blood.

Hypokyphosis (hī″pō-kī-fō′sis) (n.) A kyphosis of the thoracic spine less than the normal range.

Hypolordosis (hī″pō-lor-dō′sis) (n.) A curvature of the cervical and lumbar spine less than the normal range.

Hypoparathyroidism (hī″pō-par″ah-thī′roid-izm) (n.) The clinical state that results from an insufficient blood level of parathyroid hormone. This disease is characterized biochemically by a low level of serum calcium and a high level of serum phosphate. Various clinical signs and symptoms result from these chemical abnormalities. Hypoparathyroidism is most commonly seen postsurgically after thyroid or parathyroid surgery, and less often as an idiopathic condition. A transient hypoparathyroidism with mild hypocalcemia may occur in the neonatal period.

Hypophosphatasia (hī″pō-fos″fah-tā′zē-ah) (n.) An inborn error in alkaline phosphatase metabolism where either the synthesis of that enzyme is decreased or its destruction is increased. It is characterized by a low serum alkaline phosphatase level, increased urine and blood levels of phosphoethanolamine, and defective bone mineralization, which results in an excessive unmineralized bone matrix. This disorder occurs in three different forms: infantile, childhood, or adult. The infantile form is the most severe, with a rapid clinical course. The childhood form produces rachitic defects; the adult form results in osteomalacia.

Hypopituitarism (hī″pō-pi-tū′i-tah-rizm) (n.) An endocrine disturbance resulting from deficient secretion of one or more of the trophic hormones—growth hormone, gonadotropic, thyrotropic, or adrenocorticotropic hormone—by the anterior lobe of the pituitary gland. The clinical findings in hypopituitarism vary with the age of onset, the severity of the lesion, and the hormones involved.

Hypoplasia (hī″pō-plā′zē-ah) (n.) A condition of arrested development in which a part of the body remains in an immature state or below normal size.

Hyporeflexia (hī″pō-rē-flek′sē-ah) (n.) Diminished function or weakening of the reflexes.

Hypothenar Hammer Syndrome (hī-poth′e-nar/ham′mer/sin′drōm) (n.) A disorder that results from the occlusion of the ulnar artery or its digital branches in the region of the hypothenar space. It is thought to result from repetitive blunt trauma to the hand. Patients present with cool, pale, and ulcerated ulnar digits, and possibly with a thickening and tenderness of the hypothenar eminence. Angiography is usually diagnostic.

Hypothenar Muscles (hī-poth′e-nar/mus′elz) (n.) The abductor digiti minimis, flexor digiti minimi, and opponens digiti minimi muscles. See **Muscle**.

Hypothenar Space (hī-poth′e-nar/spās) (n.) The anatomic compartment on the ulnar side of the palm that contains the hypothenar muscles.

Hypothesis (hī-poth′e-sis) (n.) A tentative assumption or proposed solution for a scientific problem. It must be tested by experimentation, and if not validated, discarded.

Hypothyroidism (hī″po-thī′roid-izm) (n.) The clinical expressions of a deficient supply of thyroid hormone.

Hypotonia (hī″pō-tō′nē-ah) (n.) A state of reduced muscle tension.

Hypotonic (hī-pō-ton′ik) (adj.) Having a lower concentration of solute, and therefore a lower osmotic pressure than a reference solution.

Hypovolemic Shock (hī″pō-vō-lē′mik/shok) (n.) Shock that results from inadequate intravascular volume; it is usually secondary to hemorrhage. This is the most common type of shock seen in the multiply traumatized patient.

Hypoxia (hī-pok′sē-ah) (n.) Decreased amounts of oxygen in the blood delivered to the tissues. Synonym: **Hypoxemia**.

Hysteria (his-tēr′e-ah) (n.) A pyschoneurosis in which the individual converts anxiety created by emotional conflict into physical symptoms that have no organic basis. Also called **Conversion Reaction** or **Conversion Hysteria**.

Hysterical Scoliosis (his-ter′i-kal/skō″le-ō′sis) (n.) A nonstructural deformity of the spine that develops as a manifestation of a conversion reaction.

I

I & D (n.) Abbreviation for 1. Incision and drainage. 2. Irrigation and debridement.

I-Band (I-band) (n.) The single refracting, or isotropic, band of a sarcomere. It appears light on microscopy and is composed only of actin filament. Also known as **I-Disc**.

ICD Abbreviation for International Classification of Diseases (World Health Organization Classification).

ICDA International Classification of Diseases. (World Health Organization Classification, adapted for use in the United States.)

ICD-9-CM Abbreviation for International Classification of diseases, 9th revision, clinical modification. A reference for reporting diagnoses codes. Refer to CPT for current procedure codes.

I-Disc (I-Disk) (n.) See **I-Band**.

I Fibrinogen Scan (I/fi-brin'ō-jen/skan) (n.) A nuclear scanning technique for the detection of an acute thrombotic process. It uses fibrinogen labeled with intravenously injected radioactive iodine. The accumulation of label is evaluated with a scintillation counter along the affected area.

Iatrogenic (ī-at"ro-jen'ik) (adj.) 1. Resulting from the professional activities of a physician or surgeon. 2. A term used to describe adverse responses or complications of prescribed therapy.

Ibuprofen (i-bu'prō-fen) (n.) A nonsteroidal anti-inflammatory drug marketed under various brand names (e.g., Advil, Nuprin, Rufen, and Motrin).

Ice Rub (īs/rub) (n.) The rubbing of a body area with a piece of ice. The technique may be used to decrease extravasation of blood in acute injuries, as therapy in low back pain and similar acute conditions, or as an agent in facilitation techniques. Sometimes incorrectly called an **ice massage**.

Ideal Foot (ī-de'l/foot) (n.) The configuration of a foot that best adapts to modern footwear—one would have a Greek-type forefoot and an "index plus" or "index plus-minus" type of metatarsal formula. See **Metatarsal Formula**, **Digital Formula**, **Index Plus**, and **Index Plus Minus**.

Idiopathic (id"ē-ō-path'ik) (adj.) A condition or disorder having an unknown or obscure cause.

Idiopathic Scoliosis (id'ē-o-path-ik/sko"le-o'sis) (n.) A structural spinal curvature for which a cause has not been established.

IDK Abbreviation for internal derangement of the knee.

Ig Abbreviation for Immunoglobulin. See **Immunoglobulin**.

Ilfeld Splint (īl-feld/splint) (n.) An abduction splint used for infants with congenital hip dislocation or developmental dysplasia of the hip. It consists of a transverse adjustable metal bar with two universal joints that can be adjusted and locked. These joints are attached to two padded, trough-shaped devices designed to encircle the thighs; similar to a Craig splint.

Iliac Crest (il'ē-ak/krest) (n.) The thickened and expanded superior border of the ilium. A commonly used site of autogenous bone graft because of its superficial location and large quantity of bone available.

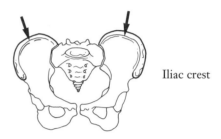

Iliac crest

Iliac Crest Height Test (il'ē-ak/krest/hīt/test) (n.) A clinical maneuver used to evaluate any obliquity of the pelvis. The examiner sits on a stool or kneels behind the subject, placing the palmar surfaces of his or her index fingers on the patient's iliac crests and noting their relative heights. The examiner then records whether the pelvis is level (=), low on the left side (L), or low on the right side (R).

Iliac Epiphysis (il'ē-ak/e-pif'i-sis) (n.) The epiphysis along the crest of the ilium. Also known as the **Iliac Apophysis**.

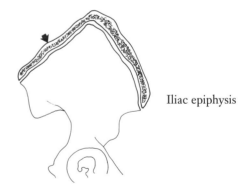

Iliac epiphysis

Iliac Epiphysis Sign (il'ē-ak/e-pif'i-sis/sīn) (n.) The state of ossification of the iliac epiphysis as noted on the AP roentgenogram of the pelvis. This sign reflects the degree of skeletal maturity and is graded I to V: I, 25% excursion; II, 50% excursion; III, 75% excursion; IV, 100% excursion; V, Fusion of the epiphysis to the iliac crest. Also called the **Apophysis Sign** or **Risser's Sign**.

Iliac Fossa (il′ē-ak/fos′sah) (n.) The concave interior aspect of the wing of the ilium. The iliacus muscle arises from it.

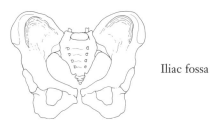

Iliac fossa

Iliac Spine (il′ē-ak/spīn) (n.) A small but prominent bony projection along the surface of the iliac crest. There are four of these prominences: the anterior superior iliac spine, the anterior inferior iliac spine, and the posterior inferior and superior iliac spines. These are useful anatomic and radiographic landmarks.

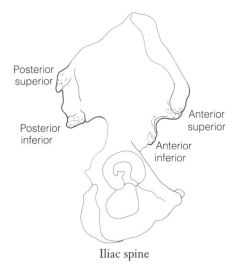

Iliac spine

Iliac Tuberosity (il′ē-ak/too″be-ros′i-tē) (n.) A large rough area on the posterior superior aspect of the ilium that serves as an attachment for the posterior sacroiliac ligaments.

Iliacus Muscle (il′iakus/mus′el) (n.) See **Muscle**.

Iliofemoral Ligament (il″e-o-fem′or-al/lig′ah-ment) (n.) See **Ligament**.

Iliolumbar Ligament (il″ē-o-lum′bar/lig′ah-ment) (n.) A strong band of connective tissue that radiates from the fifth lumbar transverse process to the iliac crest.

Iliopectineal Line (il″ē-o-pek-tin′ē-al/līn) (n.) The bony ridge that divides the pelvis into two areas: the one above, known as the greater or false pelvis, and the one below, the true or lesser pelvis. The ridge is formed by the pecten of the pubic bone, along with

its lateral extension to the iliopubic eminence (which is actually a ridge, not a line).

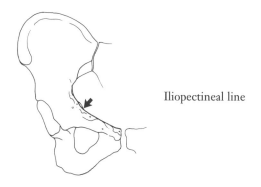

Iliopectineal line

Iliopsoas Muscle (ilē-o-sō′as/mus′el) (n.) See **Muscle**.

Iliopsoas Sign (il″ē-o-sō′as/sīn) (n.) A radiographic diagnostic aid in which the iliopsoas fat plane is displaced, reflecting intra-articular or periarticular disease of the hip. This plane is medial and parallel to the iliopsoas muscle as it inserts into the lesser trochanter.

Iliopubic Column (il″ē-o-pū′bik/kol′um) (n.) The anterior bony column of the acetabulum, composed of contributions from the ilium and the pubis. To visualize the iliopubic column in profile, obtain an internal oblique radiographic view of the pelvis.

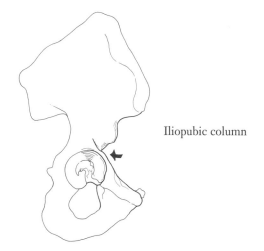

Iliopubic column

Iliopubic Eminence (il″ē-o-pū′bik/em′i-nens) (n.) A bony ridge on the pelvis that marks the site of fusion of the ilium and pubis.

Iliotibial Band (il″ē-o-tib′ē-al/band) (n.) A thickened strip of fascia that runs laterally in the thigh from the iliac crest to the lateral tibial tubercle. It receives part of the insertion of the tensor fascia lata

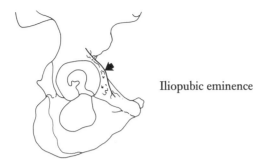

Iliopubic eminence

and gluteus maximus muscles. Also known as the **iliotibial tract**.

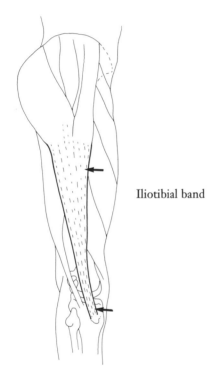

Iliotibial band

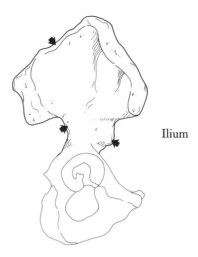

Ilium

day) sliding a bone fragment internally to fill a bone defect. Slow bone distraction stimulates neogenesis, producing new bone growth behind the distracted bone fragment.

Illness (il′nes) (n.) An acute or chronic medical or mental condition, exclusive of an injury.

IM An abbreviation for 1. Intramuscular. 2. Intramedullary.

Image Intensification (im′ij/in-ten″sif-i-cā′shun) (n.) Electronic amplification of the x-ray beam. The final light image is significantly brighter than that seen on a conventional fluorescent screen. The image can be recorded, televised, filmed, or photographed.

Imbrication (im″bri-kā′shun) (n.) The surgical technique of suturing tissues in overlapping layers.

Immediate Postoperative Prosthesis (i-mē′de-it/pōst-op′er-ah-tiv/pros′thē-sis) (n.) A technique for fitting a lower-limb prosthesis. The socket is applied to the stump immediately after amputation by applying a rigid dressing that allows for the attachment of a pylon and an ankle-foot assembly. Commonly referred to by the abbreviation **IPOP**.

Immersion Foot (i-mer′shun/fut) (n.) A circulatory disturbance similar to *trench foot*. It results from prolonged exposure to dampness and cold or, less commonly, warmth. The feet are discolored, swollen, and blistered. It may seem that massive gangrene from the ankle down is imminent, but in the absence of infection and with proper treatment, the prognosis is good, although recovery is usually slow.

Immobilization (im-mo″bil-i-zā′shun) (n.) The process of rendering a structure or body part fixed, or immovable.

Immune Response (i-mūn′/re-spons′) (n.) The complex reaction of the immunologic mechanism to an antigen that leads to the induction of sensitivity as a primary response or the production of antibodies that tend to resist the antigen as a secondary response.

Immunity (i-mu′ni-tē) (n.) The state of being able to

Iliotibial Band Syndrome (il″ē-o-tib′ē-al/band/sin′drōm) (n.) An inflammatory condition characterized by localized pain over the lateral femoral condyle. It is believed to result from friction between it and the overlying iliotibial band or by the development of bursal tissue with secondary inflammation between these two structures. Also called **Iliotibial Band Friction Syndrome**.

Ilium (il′ē-im) (n.) The fan-shaped bone that forms the superior aspect of the innominate bone.

Ilizarov Procedure (ilizarov/pro-se′jur) (n.) 1. A method of immobilization of fractures using percutaneous transfixing wires in bone, that are attached to a rigid external circular metal frame. 2. A bone lengthening method that consists of slowly (1 mm/

resist and/or overcome harmful agents or influences. Immunity may be active, passive, specific, or adaptive.

Immunodeficiency (im″u-nō-de-fish′en-sē) (n.)   A condition that results from inadequate or ineffective functioning of the body's immunologic mechanisms.

Immunoelectrophoresis (im″u no-e-lek″tro-fo-rē′sis) (n.)   A technique for identifying antigenic fractions in a serum. The components of the serum are separated by electrophoresis and allowed to diffuse through agar gel toward a particular antiserum. Where the antibody meets its antigen, a band of precipitation occurs.

Immunofluorescence (im″u-no-floo″o-res′ens) (n.)   A technique for observing the amount and/or distribution of antigen by using fluorescein-labeled antibodies specific to that antigen. The binding of these antibodies is determined microscopically by using ultraviolet rays for observation.

Immunogens (im′ū-nō-jens) (n.)   Substances that induce antibody production in a host. Also known as **Antigens**.

Immunoglobulin (im″ū-no-glob′ū-lin) (n.)   A class of structurally related proteins that contain two pairs of polypeptide chains all linked by disulfide bonds. They are classified as immunoglobulin IgG, IgA, IgM, IgD, and IgE, depending on their structural and antigenic properties. See **Ig**.

Immunosuppression (im″ū-no-su-presh′un) (n.)   The use of a drug or other agent, such as an x-ray, to inhibit the immune response.

Impacted Fracture (im-pakt′ed/frak′chur) (n.)   A compression injury in which the broken bone ends are driven together and rendered immovable by the force producing the fracture. This occurs most often near the metaphysis. See **Torus Fracture**.

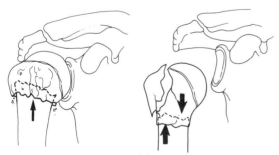

Impacted fracture

Impairment (im-pār′ment) (n.)   The loss of, the loss of use of, or the derangement of any body part, system, or function. An objective, quantifiable pathophysiologic condition that does not always result in secondary disability. See **Permanent Impairment**. Contrast to **Disability**.

Impingement (im-pinj′ment) (n.)   Encroachment or infringement upon.

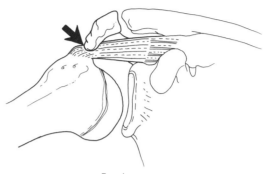

Impingement

Impingement Sign (im-pinj′ment/sīn) (n.)   A diagnostic test in evaluating shoulder pain. Stand behind the seated patient; prevent scapular rotation with one hand while raising the arm in forced forward elevation with your other. This forces the greater tuberosity with the insertion of the supraspinatus tendon, to impinge against the acromion. It will cause pain in patients with impingement lesions of all stages and with many other shoulder conditions. If the pain is from an impingement lesion, it can be eliminated or reduced by the injection of 10 mL of 1.0% xylocaine beneath the anterior acromion (positive impingement test). Pain due to other causes, with the possible exception of calcific bursitis is not relieved. This helps distinguish impingement lesions from other causes of shoulder pain, such as cervical radiculopathy.

Impingement Syndrome (im-pinj′ment/sin′drōm) (n.)   A painful inflammatory condition of the shoulder characterized by the occurrence of pain during abduction or elevation of the arm. The underlying pathophysiology involves entrapment of the supraspinatus and biceps tendons against the anterior and inferior aspects of the acromion, the coracoacromial ligament, and the acromioclavicular joint. With time, rotator cuff tendonitis develops, which may progress to fibrosis and rupture. Also known as **Supraspinatus** or **Rotator Cuff Syndrome**.

Implant (im′plant) (n.)   A tissue, device, or substance that is transferred, grafted, or inserted into the living body.

Implant Arthroplasty (im′plant/ar′thro-plas″tē) (n.)   A technique in which the resected joint is replaced by a manufactured prosthesis.

Inactivate (in-ak′ti-vāt) (n.)   To destroy the activity of a substance.

Incision (in-sizh′un) (n.)   The surgical cutting of tissues.

Incisional Biopsy (in-sizh′un-al/bi′op-se) (n.)   A biopsy in which only part of a lesion is removed.

Inclination Angle (in″klī-na′shun/ang′g′l) (n.) The radiographic angle formed by the incident of the longitudinal axis of the neck with that of the shaft of the femur in neutral rotation. Also called the **Angle of Inclination** and the **Neck-Shaft Angle**. Compare **Declination Angle**.

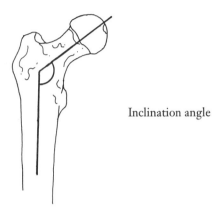

Inclination angle

Inclinometer (in″kli-nom′e-ter) (n.) An instrument used to measure the angle of thoracic inclination or rib hump. Developed by Dr. William Bunnell.

Inclusion Cyst (in′klu′zhun/sist) (n.) See **Epidermal Inclusion Cyst**.

Incomplete Fracture (in-kom′plēt/frak′chur) (n.) A fracture involving only a portion of the cross-section of bone; some trabeculae are disrupted completely, but others only buckle, bend, or remain intact. An angular deformity may occur, but there can be little or no displacement.

Incubation Period (in″kū-bā′shun/pe′rē-od) (n.) 1. Elapsed time between exposure to infection and the appearance of disease symptoms. 2. The period during which microorganisms inoculated into a medium are allowed to grow.

Index Finger (in′deks/fing′ger) (n.) The second digit of the hand, next to the thumb. Synonym: **Forefinger**.

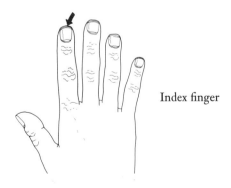

Index finger

Index Plus-Minus Type (in′deks/plus-mī′nus/tīp) (n.) A measurement of the foot in which the first metatarsal is equal in length to the second while the other three metatarsals progressively diminish in length.

Index Plus Type (in′deks/plus/tīp) (n.) A measurement of the foot in which the first metatarsal is longer than the second while the others decrease progressively in length.

Indication (in″di-kā′shun) (n.) A strong reason for believing that a particular remedy or course of treatment is appropriate.

Indium Scan (in′de-um/skan) (n.) A nuclear medicine scanning technique useful in the diagnosis of bone and joint infections using a radiopharmaceutical. This scan requires intravenous injection of indium-labeled autologous white blood cells. Images are taken at 4 and 24 hours after injection.

Indocin (in′dō-sin) (n.) Proprietary name for Indomethacin, a nonsteroidal, anti-inflammatory drug.

Indolent (in′dō-lent) (adj.) A characterization of disease processes that persist or fail to heal.

Indomethacin (in″dō-meth′ah-sin) (n.) A nonsteroidal, anti-inflammatory drug marketed under the brand name Indocin.

Induction (in-duk′shun) (n.) In anesthesiology, the period from the beginning of the administration of an agent until the patient loses consciousness.

Induration (in″du-rā′shun) (n.) Hardening of a tissue or structure.

Indwelling Catheter (in′dwel-ing/kath′e-ter) (n.) A catheter designed to remain stable as it runs through the urethra into the bladder to continuously drain urine. Example: **Foley Catheter**.

Inertia (in-er′shē-ah) (n.) The property of all bodies to resist change in a state of rest or motion when under the action of applied loads.

Infantile Cortical Hyperostosis (in′fan-tīl/kor′ti-kal/hi″per-os-tō′sis) (n.) A disease usually occurring in the first 3 months of life characterized by a classic triad of hyperirritability, soft tissue swelling, and palpable hard masses over multiple bones. Radiographically, there is diffuse, dense periosteal thickening, hyperostosis of the compact portions of bone, and sclerosis of spongy partitions of the diaphysis. The clinical course may include several exacerbations and remissions, but spontaneous recovery usually occurs. Synonym: **Caffey's Disease**.

Infantile Paralysis (in′fan-tīl/pah-ral′i-sis) (n.) The major form of **poliomyelitis**.

Infantile Scoliosis (in′fan-tīl/sko″lē-ō′sis) (n.) A curvature of the spine that develops during the first 3 years of life.

Infantile Spinal Muscular Atrophy (in′fan-tīl/spi′nal/mus′ku-lar/at′ro-fē) (n.) See **Werdnig-Hoffman Disease**.

Infantile Tibia Vara (in′fan-tīl/tib′ē-ah/vā′-ra) (n.) A torsional and varus angulation of the proximal end of the tibia caused by a disturbance of the growth of the proximal medial epiphysis and its cartilage. See **Blount's Disease**.

Infarction (in-fark′shun) (n.) A localized area of ischemic necrosis within a tissue or organ; it is produced by occlusion of arterial supply or venous drainage.

Infection (in-fek′shun) (n.) The entry into and multiplication of microorganisms in the body of a human or animal. This is not synonymous with infectious disease, and its result may or may not be manifest.

Infectious (in-fek′shus) (adj.) Capable of producing disease in a susceptible host.

Infectious Arthritis (in-fek′shus/ar-thrī′tis) (n.) See **Septic Arthritis**.

Infectious Disease (in-fek′shus/di-zēz′) (n.) A disease caused by pathogenic organisms, e.g., bacteria, viruses, protozoa, or fungi. It may or may not be contagious.

Inferior (in-fēr′ē-or) (adj.) Lower in place or position.

Inferior Pubic Ramus (in-fēr′ē-or/pū′bic/rā′mus) (n.) The lower and shorter arm of the pubis that bounds the obturator foramen inferiorly and joins the ischial ramus laterally.

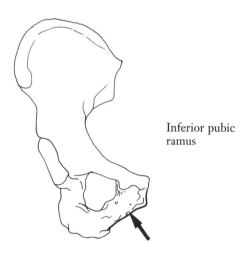

Inferior pubic ramus

Infiltration Anesthesia (in″fil-tra′shun/an″es-the′ze-ah) (n.) Injection of an anesthetic solution directly into a local area of terminal nerve endings.

Inflammation (in″flah-mā′shun) (n.) The reaction of living tissues to all forms of injury; it involves vascular, neurologic, humoral, and cellular responses at the injury site. This response is characterized by pain, heat, redness, swelling, and loss of function.

Inflammatory Joint Disease (in-flam′ah-to″rē/joint/di-zēz) (n.) A general term for any of the arthridites resulting from an inflammatory process. An inflammatory process is suggested by examination of a synovial effusion that is yellow, translucent, and low in viscosity. It has an elevated white blood cell (WBC)

count of 2000 to 75,000 WBC/mm^3, an increased percentage of polymorphonuclear leukocytes, a friable mucin clot, and a negative culture.

Inflatable Splint (in-fla′ta-b′l/splint) (n.) A first-aid device used in the emergency immobilization of an injured limb. Also called an **air-splint** because its relative rigidity is a result of infusing air into the plastic splint.

Informed Consent (in-form′d/kon′sent) (n.) In law, the requirement that a patient or the patient's guardian be advised of and understand the risks attending a proposed procedure or treatment. The patient should understand the nature of his or her condition; the nature of the proposed treatment and possible alternative treatments; and the risks, consequences, and chances of failure of any treatment. This understanding is usually indicated by a signed statement.

Infra (in′frah) Prefix meaning below or beneath.

Infraction (in-frak′shun) (n.) A minor, localized break in the cortex of a bone. This causes only slight local deformity.

Infraglenoid Tubercle (in″frah-gle′noid/too′ber-k′l) (n.) A small bony prominence immediately below the glenoid cavity.

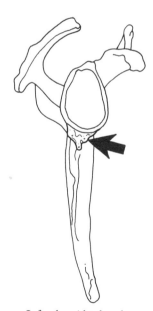

Infraglenoid tubercle

Infrapatellar Bursa, Deep (in-fra-pah-tel′-ar/ber′sah/dēp) (n.) The bursa between the tibia and the patellar tendon.

Infrapatellar Bursa, Superficial (in-fra-pah-tel′-ar/ber′-sah/soo″-per-fish-al) (n.) The bursa between the patellar tendon and the skin.

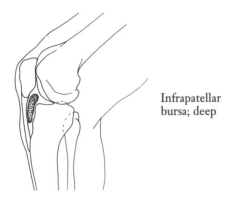

Infrapatellar
bursa; deep

Infrapatellar Ligament (in″frah-pah-tel′ar/lig′ah-ment) (n.) The ligament that connects the inferior pole of the patella to the tibial tubercle.

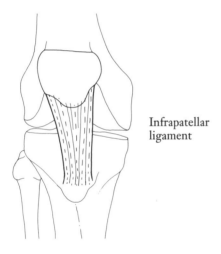

Infrapatellar
ligament

Infrapatellar Tendon (in″fra-pah-tel′ar/ten′dun) (n.) The tendinous portion of the extensor mechanism of the knee. It runs from the inferior pole of the patellar to insert into the tibial tuberosity.

Infraspinatus Muscle (in″frah-spī′na-tus/mus′el) (n.) See **Muscle**.

Infraspinous (in″frah-spī′nous) (adj.) Commonly used to denote "beneath the spine of the scapula."

Infusion (in-fu′zhun) (n.) The introduction of a solution into a vessel.

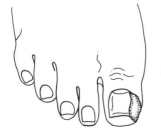

Ingrown toenail

Ingrown Toenail (in′grōn/tō′nāl) (n.) The aberrant growth of a toenail, with one or both lateral margins pushing deep into adjacent soft tissue. This causes pain, inflammation, and possibly infection.

Inguinal (ing′gwi-nal) (adj.) Pertaining to, or situated in, the groin.

Inguinal Ligament (ing′gwi-nal) (n.) The groin ligament that extends from the anterior superior iliac spine to the pubic tubercle and the pectineal line. It is part of the aponeurosis of the external oblique muscle of the abdomen. Synonym: **Poupart's Ligament**.

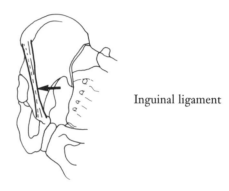

Inguinal ligament

Inguinal Triangle (ing′gwi-nal/trī′ang′g′l) (n.) A triangular anatomic area bounded laterally by the inferior epigastric artery, medially by the rectus abdominis, and inferiorly by the medial half of the inguinal ligament.

Injection (in-jek′shun) (n.) The introduction of a substance into a vessel, passage, tube, cavity, or tissue, usually through a needle puncture.

Injury (in′ju-rē) (n.) Damage or impairment resulting from an accidental or intentionally inflicted trauma.

Inlay (in′lā) (n.) In shoe terminology, any type of arch support or foot mold inserted into a shoe.

Inlet of Pelvis (in′let/of/pel′vis) (n.) The space within the brim of the pelvis. Synonym: **Superior Pelvic Strait**.

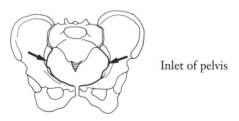

Inlet of pelvis

Inlet View (in′let/vū) (n.) A radiographic view of the pelvis taken with the patient supine and the x-ray beam directed 25° caudad in the sagittal plane. This view is useful in evaluating rotational deformity or medial displacement in pelvic fractures.

Innersole (in′er-sōl) (n.) In shoe terminology, a sole of leather, cork, or other material that is cut to fit the exact size and shape of the last bottom. Synonym: **Insole**.

Innervation (in″er-vā′shun) (n.) The distribution of nerves to a particular body part.

Innervation Ratio (in″er-vā′shun/ra′shē-ō) (n.) The number of muscle fibers per motor nerve fiber.

Innominate Bone (i-nom′i-nāt/bōn) (n.) The so-called unnamed bone of the pelvis, composed of the ilium, the ischium, and the pubis. Also known as the **Hip Bone or Os Coxae**.

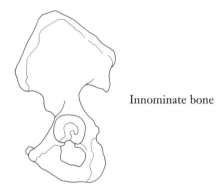

Innominate bone

Innominate Osteotomy (i-nom′i-nāt/os″tē-ot′ō-mē) (n.) See **Salter Osteotomy**.

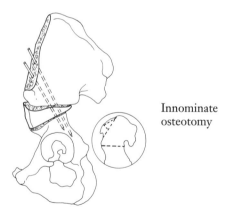

Innominate osteotomy

Inorganic (in″or-gan′ik) (adj.) A characterization of all compounds that do not contain carbon as well as a few simple carbon-containing substances, such as carbon dioxide and the carbonates.

Insall-Burstein Knee Prosthesis (in-sall/ber-stīn/nē/pros-thē′sis) (n.) A total knee arthroplasty system manufactured by Zimmer, Inc.

Insall and Salvati Patellar Position (in-sall/and/salvati/pah-tel′ar/po-zish′un) (n.) A radiographic method of diagnosing patella alta. On the lateral radiograph of the knee at 50° of flexion, a measurement of the length of the patella (LP) to the length of the patella tendon (LT). In a normal knee, the ratio of LP to LT is 1.0. A variation of more than 20% indicates abnormal position of the patella.

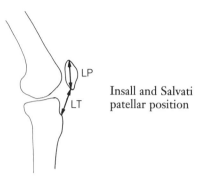

Insall and Salvati patellar position

Insertion (in-ser′shun) (n.) The anatomic point of attachment of a muscle, tendon, or ligament onto a bone. With few exceptions, the more distal end of the structure is described as the insertion.

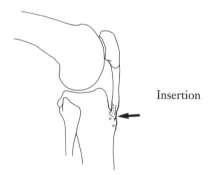

Insertion

In Situ (in/sī′tu) (n.) In its original or normal place or natural position.

Insole (in′sōl) (n.) In shoe terminology, the area between the sole of the foot and other segments of the shoe. See also **Innersole**.

Instability (in″sta-bil′i-tē) (n.) The loss of stability. This term is used in the description of joints after ligament injury.

Instability Index (in″sta-bil′i-tē/in′deks) (n.) In congenital dislocation of the hip, a measurement of the inherent tendency to dislocate. To determine, add the amount of femoral anteversion to the amount of acetabular anteversion. A total value of 60 represents the upper level of normal.

Instant Center of Rotation (in′stant/sen′ter/of/ro-tā′shun) (n.) In analysis of surface joint motion in the sagittal and frontal but not the transverse plane, a description of the relative uniplanar motion of two adjacent segments of a body and the direction of displacement of the contact points between the segments is given. There is an instant during rotation when a point has zero velocity; this constitutes the instant center.

Instep (in'step) (n.)   The arched middle portion of the foot.

Insufficiency Fractures (in"su-fish'en-sē/frak'churs) (n.)   Fractures occurring in bones affected with nontumorous disease. See **Stress Fracture**.

Insulin (in'su-lin) (n.)   A hormone synthesized in islet cells of the pancreas that promotes the conversion of glucose to the storage material glycogen.

Integument (in-teg'u-ment) (n.)   The outer covering of the body. Synonym: **Skin**.

Interbody Fusion (in"ter-bod'ē/fū'zhun) (n.)   A surgical technique for obtaining bony fusion between intervertebral bodies. Most interbody fusions are performed through anterior approaches to the spine, but posterolateral interbody fusions also may be performed.

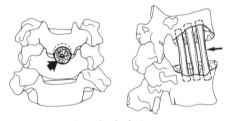

Interbody fusion

Intercalary (in-ter'kah-ler"ē) (adj.)   Inserted or occurring between two others. Used in certain classifications of congenital failure of formation of parts to describe segmental deficiencies of an extremity.

Intercondylar (in"ter-kon'di-lar) (adj.)   Between the condyles. Used in reference to humeral or femoral condyles.

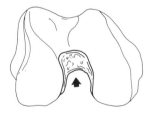

Intercondylar, femoral

Intercondylar Line (in"ter-kon'di-lar/līn) (n.)   A transverse ridge separating the floor of the intercondylar fossa from the popliteal surface of the femur. It affords attachment to the posterior portion of the articular capsule of the knee. Also known as the **Intercondylar ridge**.

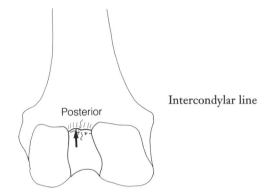

Posterior

Intercondylar line

Intercondylar Notch (in"ter-kon'di-lar/noch) (n.)   A fossa present at the distal end of the femur; it separates the femoral condyles.

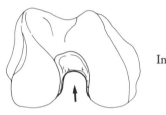

Intercondylar notch

Intercostal (in"ter-kos'tal) (adj.)   Between the ribs.

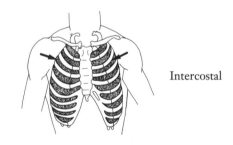

Intercostal

Intercostal Muscles (in"ter-kos'tal/mus'elz) (n.)   The muscles occupying the spaces between the ribs that are responsible for controlling some rib movements.

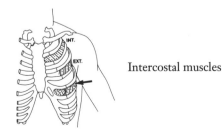

Intercostal muscles

Intercurrent Disease (in″ter-kur′ent/di-zēz′) (n.) A health problem occurring during the course of another disease with which it has no connection.

Interdigital Neuroma (in″ter-dij′i-tal/nu′rōma) (n.) A painful affection of a digital nerve in the foot, usually in the third web space. Pathologically, the nerve is greatly thickened by perineural fibrosis. Also known as **Morton's neuroma**.

Intermediate Care Facility (in″ter-mē′de-it/kār/fah-sil′i-tē) (n.) A provider of health services to patients who do not need the degree of care provided by a hospital or nursing facility but who do require institutional care. Also known as an **intermediate care institution**.

Intermediate Disk (in″ter-me′de-it/disk) (n.) In a striated muscle fiber, a thin, dark, doubly refractive disk in the middle of the isotropic disk. Synonyms: **Krause's Membrane, Z Disk**.

Intermuscular Septum (in″ter-mus′kū-lar/sep′tum) (n.) A fascial attachment found in upper both and lower extremities that gives regional organization to muscle groups and may provide the fibrous origin for certain muscles.

Internal Derangement of the Knee (in-ter′nal/de-rānj′ment/of/the/nē) (n.) A general term describing a mechanical derangement of knee structure or function. The term is often used when the examiner is not sure of the exact diagnosis but suspects that something is functionally incorrect. Abbreviated **IDK**.

Internal Fixation (in-ter′nal/fik-sa′shun) (n.) In the surgical management of orthopaedic disorders and fractures, the use of metallic or other devices to obtain firm attachment either between bones or between soft tissue and bone.

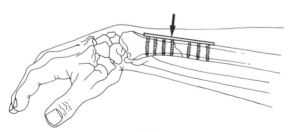

Internal fixation

Internal Fixation Devices (in-ter′nal/fik-sa′shun/dē-vī-sez) (n.) Nails, screws, plates, wires, sutures, and intramedullary rods used within the body to restrict movements.

Internal Oblique View of Pelvis (in-ter′nal/o-blēk/vū) (n.) A radiographic projection of the pelvis taken with the pelvis rotated approximately 45° away from the affected side with the beam centered on the affected hemipelvis. It is useful in the evaluation of acetabulum fractures by providing a profile of the anterior column, visualization of the posterior lip of the acetabulum, and an on-edge view of the iliac wing. Also known as an **obturator oblique**.

Internal Tibial Torsion (in-ter′nal/tib′ē-al/tor′shun) (n.) A rotational deformity of the lower leg that results in a toeing-in appearance. The angle between the transmalleolar and transcondylar axes of the tibia is used to measure torsion. Also known as **Medial Tibial Torsion**. Abbreviated **I.T.T.**

International System of Units (in″ter-na′shun-al/sis′tem/of/ū′nits) (n.) An extension of the metric system approved by the General Conference on Weights and Measures in 1960. Expanded for the health professions, it has been adopted by most European countries and Canada. The abbreviation, **SI**, comes from the French le Système International d'Unités.

Interneuron (in″ter-nu′ron) (n.) In a chain of neurons, any one that is intermediary. Synonyms: **Internuncial Neuron, Intercalated Neuron**.

Interosseous (in″ter-os′ē-us) (adj.) Between two parallel bones in the same extremity.

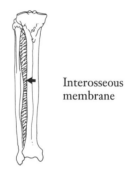

Interosseous membrane

Interosseous Membrane (in″ter-os′ē-us/mem′brān) (n.) The fascia that interconnects two parallel long bones in a given extremity, such as that between the radius and ulna. The membranes provide stability and add to the regional organization of the muscle groups of that extremity.

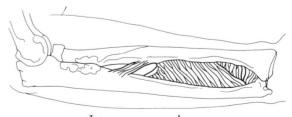

Interosseous membrane

Interosseous Muscles (in″ter-os′ē-us/mus′els) (n.) See **Muscle**.

Interpedicular Distance (in″ter-pe-dik′ū-lar/dis′tans) (n.) A gradually varying distance between the inner margins of the pedicles as shown on AP radiographs of the thoracic and lumbar vertebrae. It is measured in millimeters.

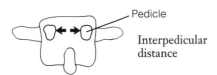

Interphalangeal Joint (in″ter-fah-lan′jē-al/joint) (n.) An articulation between two phalanges.

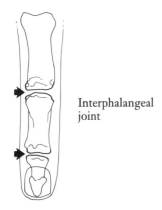

Interpositional Arthroplasty (in″ter-po-zish′un-al/ar′thrō-plas″tē) (n.) A technique of arthroplasty in which the joint is resected and soft tissues, usually fascia, are placed between the former articular surfaces. These arthroplasties are intended to provide improved stability over simple resection arthroplasties.

Interscalene Space (in-ter-skā-lēn/spās) (n.) The enclosed space formed when the prevertebral fascia splits to envelop the scalene muscles and then fuses again at their lateral margins. This is a continuous enclosure in which the neural, perineural, and vascular structures extend from the cervical transverse processes to several centimeters beyond the axilla. It can be divided into an axillary perivascular space, a subclavian perivascular space, and an interscalene space.

Interscapular (in″ter-skap′u-lar) (adj.) Between the scapulae.

Interspinal (in-ter-spi′nal) (adj.) Between or connecting spinous processes. Synonym: **Interspinous**.

Interspinous (in″ter-spi′nus) (adj.) Between or connecting spines or spinous processes. Synonym: **Interspinal**.

Interspinous Ligament (in″ter-spi′nus/lig′ah-ment) (n.) Membrane structures that extend between the roots and apices of the vertebral spines.

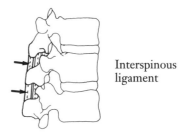

Interspinous Pseudarthrosis (in″ter-spi′nus/soo″dar-thrō′sis) (n.) The development of a false joint between two spinous processes.

Interstitial (in″ter-stish′al) (adj.) Describing the area between and around cells.

Interstitial Calcinosis (in″ter-stish′al/kal″sĭ-no′sis) (n.) A disease process in which deposits of calcium lie in subcutaneous fatty tissues.

Interstitial Fibrosis (in″ter-stish′al/fī-brō′sis) (n.) The laying down of fibrous tissue in the interstitial tissues between normal structures.

Interstitial Fluid (in″ter-stish′al/flōō′id) (n.) Extracellular fluid that circulates between and around the cells. It is composed of water and electrolytes.

Interstitial Tear (n.) See **Meniscal Interstitial Tear**.

Intertransverse Ligaments (in″ter-trans-vers′/lig′ah-ments) (n.) Ligaments that connect adjacent vertebral transverse processes.

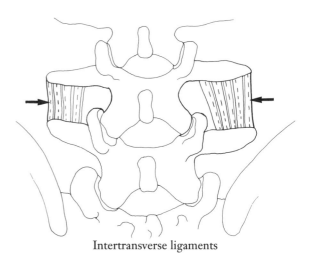

Intertransverse ligaments

Intertrochanteric (in″ter-tro″kan-ter′ik) (n.) The portion of the femur between the greater and the lesser trochanters.

Intertrochanteric Crest (in″ter-tro″kan-ter′ik/krest) (n.) A ridge on the posterior surface of the femur connecting the greater and lesser trochanters.

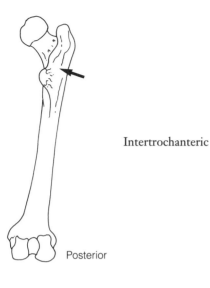

Intertrochanteric

Posterior

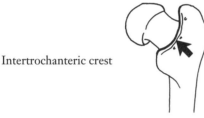

Intertrochanteric crest

Intertrochanteric Fracture (in″ter-tro″kan-ter′ik/
hip/frak′chur) (n.)   A fracture extending between
the trochanters of the upper end of the femur.

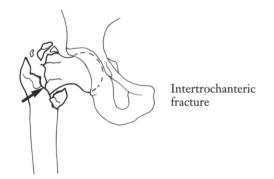

Intertrochanteric
fracture

Intertrochanteric Line (in″ter-tro″kan-ter′ik/līn) (n.)
A roughened line that separates posteriorly the neck
and shaft of the femur. It passes downward and medially from the greater trochanter and continues into
the medial lip of the linea aspera.

Intertrochanteric Osteotomy (in″ter-tro″kan-ter′ik/
os″te-ot′ome) (n.)   A surgical procedure designed to
change the neck-shaft angle of the hip.

Intervertebral (in″ter-ver′te-bral) (adj.)   Situated between two adjacent vertebrae. Example: between
L_1-L_2.

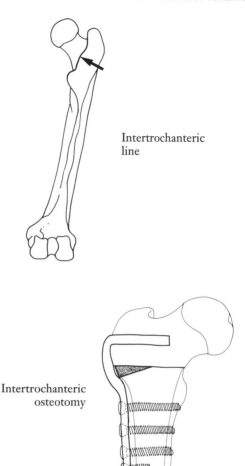

Intertrochanteric
line

Intertrochanteric
osteotomy

Intervertebral Disc Rupture (in″ter-ver′te-bral/disk/
rup′chur) (n.)   See **Herniated Nucleus Pulposus**.

Intervertebral Disc (in″ter-ver′te-bral/disk) (n.)
The layer of fibrocartilage interposed between the
bodies of adjoining vertebrae. Each consists of three
intimately related and interacting parts: the nucleus
pulposus, the annulus fibrosus, and the cartilage
endplates.

Intervertebral Foramen (in″ter-ver′te-bral/for-ā′
men) (n.)   The aperture formed by the opposing
notches in the laminae of the adjacent vertebrae
through which spinal nerves and vessels pass. It has
the shape of an inverted tear drop. The superior
boundary is the pedicle of the vertebrae above. The
anterior wall is formed by the posterior aspect of the
vertebral body, the disk, and the body below. The
inferior boundary is the pedicle situated caudal to
the nerve root. The posterior wall or roof is formed
by the pars interarticularis, the ligamentum flavum
attached to it, and the apex of the superior articular
process of the vertebra, which is situated at the inferior aspect of the foramen.

181

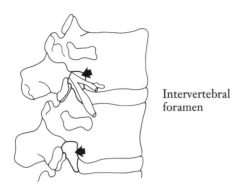

Intervertebral
foramen

of a joint. An example of this is a subcapital fracture of the femoral head.

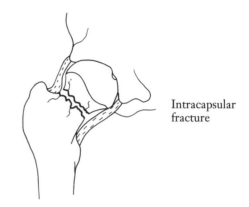

Intracapsular
fracture

Intervertebral Joints of Luschka (in″ter-ver′te-bral/joints/of/lush′kah) (n.)   The synovia-lined joints found between the bodies of the cervical vertebrae, beginning with C2 and ending with C6-7, that are lateral to the intervertebral disks. These joints are independent of the disk cartilage and the lateral articulations. Also known as **Uncovertebral Joints**. See **Luschka, joints.**

Intervertebral Space (in″ter-ver′te-bral/spās) (n.) The space between the vertebral bodies occupied by the intervertebral disk.

Intima (in′ti-mah) (n.)   The inner layer of the wall of an artery or vein. It is composed of a lining of endothelial cells and an elastic membrane. Also called **Tunica Intima.**

Intoeing (in′tō-ing) (n.)   A gait or stance in which the feet point inward or medially. Commonly called **Pigeon-toe.**

In Toto (in/tō′tō) (n.)   In the whole.

Intra (in′trah) (n.)   Prefix meaning within.

Intra-arterial (in″trah-ar-te′re-al) (adj.)   Within or directly into an artery.

Intra-articular (in″trah-ar-tik′u-lar) (adj.)   Within a joint.

Intra-articular Fracture (in″trah-ar-tik′u-lar/frak′chur) (n.)   A fracture within a joint and/or involving the articular surface.

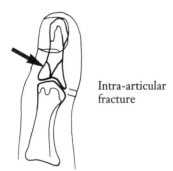

Intra-articular
fracture

Intracapsular Fracture (in″trah″kap′su-lar/frak′chur) (n.)   A fracture occurring within the capsule

Intracapsular Volar Wrist Ligaments (in″trah-kap′su-lar/vo′lar/rist/lig′ah-menz) (n.)   A complex of ligaments that connect the osseous structures of the wrist.

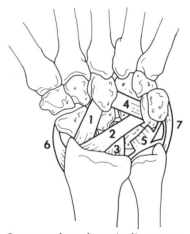

Intracapsular volar wrist ligaments:
1, radioscaphocapitate; *2*, radiolunotriquetral;
3, radioscaphoid; *4*, triquetrocapitate; *5*, ulnolunate;
6, radiocollateral; *7*, ulnocollateral.

Intracellular (in″trah-sel′u-lar) (adj.)   Within cells.

Intractable Pain (in″trak′tah-b′l/pān) (n.)   Pain that causes incapacitation of function and cannot be relieved satisfactorily by drugs short of drug addiction or large doses of sedatives.

Intradermal (in″trah-der′mal) (adj.)   Within the skin.

Intramedullary (in″trah-med′u-lār″e) (adj.)   Within the central portion or medullar cavity of a bone.

Intramedullary Nail (in″trah-med′u-lār″e/nāl) (n.) A metal rod or nail inserted into the medullary canal of a tubular bone to provide internal fixation and stabilization of diaphyseal fractures. The nail may be rigid or flexible, straight or curved, hollow or solid, and may have various shapes, including diamond-shaped, clover-leaf, cylindrical, fluted, or double I-beam. See **Küntscher Hansen, Enders**, and **Lottes Nail**.

Intramembranous Ossification (in″trah-mem′brah-nus/os″i-fi-kā′shun) (n.) The process by which bone is formed directly from membrane without a cartilaginous stage. This includes periosteal and endosteal new bone formation.

Intramuscular (in″trah-mus′ku-lar) (adj.) Within a muscle.

Intraneural (in″trah-nū′ral) (adj.) Within a nerve.

Intraneural Fibrosis (in″trah-nū′ral/fi-bro′sis) (n.) The formation of scar tissue within the substance of a nerve.

Intraspinal (in″trah-spī′nal) (adj.) Within the spinal canal.

Intrathecal (in″trah-thē′kal) (adj.) 1. Within a sheath. 2. In orthopaedics, something that runs through the theca of the spinal cord into the subarachnoid space.

Intrauterine Fracture (in″trah-u′ter-in/frak′chur) (n.) A fracture of a fetal bone in utero.

Intravascular (in″trah-vas′ku-lar) (adj.) Within the blood vessels.

Intravenous (in″trah-ve′nus) (adj.) Within or into a vein.

Intrinsic-Minus Deformity (in-trin′sik/mī′nus/dē-for′mi-tē) (n.) A position of the hand characterized by the extension of the metacarpophalangeal joints and flexion of the interphalangeal joints. This results from interruption of intrinsic muscle function. Contrast with **Intrinsic-Plus Deformity**.

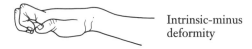

Intrinsic-minus deformity

Intrinsic Muscles (in-trin′sik/mus′elz) (n.) Muscles whose origins and insertions both lie within the hand. These include the thenar group, the hypothenar group, the adductor pollicis, the lumbricals, and the interosseous muscles.

Intrinsic-Plus Deformity (in-trin′sik/plus/de-for′mi-tē) (n.) A position of the hand characterized by flexion of the metacarpophalangeal joints and extension of the proximal interphalangeal joints. This is caused by intrinsic muscle tightness. Contrast with **Intrinsic-Minus Deformity**.

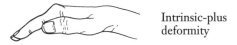

Intrinsic-plus deformity

Intrinsic Tightness Test (in-trin′sik/tīt/nes/test) (n.) A test of the degree of resistance of the intrinsic muscles of the hand. The test is performed in two stages: 1. With the hand and wrist in neutral position, the examiner applies passive flexion to all three digital joints of a finger to exclude pathologic conditions of the extrinsic extensor tendon or the digital joints. 2. The intrinsic muscles are tensed by holding the metacarpophalangeal joint in full extension and applying dorsal pressure to the tip of the finger in an attempt to produce passive flexion. In the normal hand, passive flexion is still possible in this position. If disease is affecting the intrinsic muscles, the degree of resistance to passive flexion is directly proportional to the severity of the disease.

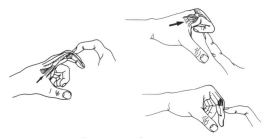

Intrinsic tightness test

Intubation (in″tū-bā′shun) (n.) The introduction of a tube into part of the body for the purpose of diagnosis or treatment. The term is most commonly used in reference to placing a tube into the trachea to provide an airway.

Inunction (in-ungk′shun) (n.) The rubbing in of an ointment or liniment.

Invasive Technique (in-vā′siv/tek′nēk) (n.) A method, procedure, or treatment in which equipment and/or substances are introduced into the body.

Inversion (in-ver′zhun) (n.) The turning inward of a body part, such as the foot or sole, so that it tends to face medially. Compare to **Eversion**.

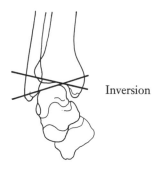

Inversion

Investigational Drug (in-ves-ti-gā′-shun-l/drug) (n.) An agent intended solely for investigational use by qualified experts to study its safety and effectiveness.

In Vitro (in/vē′trō) (adj.) Literally, "in glass." Used to describe biologic experiments performed in test tubes, glassware, or any laboratory, or nonclinical setting. Contrast to **In Vivo**.

In Vivo (in/vē′vō) (adj.) Within the living organism. Used to describe laboratory testing of agents within living organisms. Contrast to **In Vitro**.

Involucrum (in″vo-lū′krum) (n.) A growth of new bone formed from the periosteum in response to osteomyelitis. It tends to surround a mass of infected and/or necrotic bone known as the **Sequestrum**.

Involuntary Muscle (in-vol′un-ter″ē/mus′el) (n.) 1. Muscle not under conscious control, e.g., the muscles of the stomach, blood vessels, and heart. 2. A nonstriated muscle.

Iodoform Dressing (ī-o′do-form/dres′ing) (n.) A proprietary brand of gauze wound-dressing impregnated with an iodine compound.

Ion (ī′on) (n.) An atom or group of atoms characterized by an electrical charge arising from the gain or loss of electrons. Ions are positive (cation) or negative (anion).

Ionic Bond (i-on′ik/bond) (n.) The chemical bond formed between ions of opposite charge.

Ionizing Radiation (i′on-īz″ing/rā-dē-ā′shun) (n.) Radiation capable of causing ionization, i.e., the physical force whose characteristic ability is transfer of its energy to matter by separating orbital electrons from their atoms, thus forming physical ion pairs.

Iontophoresis (ī-on″to-fō-rē′sis) (n.) The introduction of drugs and/or chemicals into the body by means of a galvanic current.

Iowa Hip Rating Scale (ī′ow-ah/hip/rāt′ing/skāl) (n.) A standardized method for the evaluation and comparison of the degree of impairment of the hip joint.

IP Abbreviation for Interphalangeal.

Ipsilateral (ip″si-lat′er-al) (adj.) On the same side. The opposite of **contralateral**.

Iridocyclitis (ir″i-do-sī-klī′tis) (n.) An inflammatory condition of the anterior uveal tract often seen in association with rheumatoid diseases, especially juvenile rheumatoid arthritis. Diagnosis is made on slit lamp examination.

Iron (ī′ern) (n.) In shoe terminology, a measure of sole thickness—1/48 inch equals 1 iron.

Irradiation (i-rā″dē-ā′shun) (n.) Exposure to any type of rays (ultraviolet, radium, or roentgenographic) for diagnostic or therapeutic purposes.

Irreducible (ir″re-dūs′i-b′l) (adj.) In orthopaedics, not capable of being replaced in a normal position. Used in reference to displaced fractures or joint dislocations that cannot be aligned (reduced) by nonoperative treatment and frequently require open reduction.

Irrigation (ir″i-gā′shun) (n.) The process of washing out a body cavity or wound with a continuous flow of water or medicated solution.

Irritability (ir″i-tah-bil′i-tē) (n.) The ability to respond to stimuli or changes in environment. This is a general property of all living organisms.

Ischemia (is-kē′mē-ah) (n.) A deficient flow of blood to a part of the body that is caused by obstruction, constriction, or blockage of the blood vessels supplying it.

Ischemic Contracture (is-kem′ik/kon″trak′chur) (n.) See **Volkmann's Ischemia**.

Ischial Epiphysis (is′ke-al/ĕ-pif′i-sis) (n.) A growth center of the ischial bone.

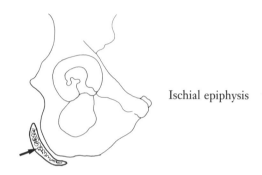

Ischial epiphysis

Ischial Ramus (is′kē-al/ra′mus) (n.) The arm of the ischium that extends forward from the tuberosity to join the inferior ramus of the pubis.

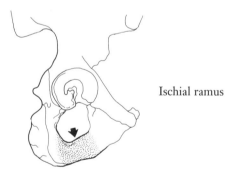

Ischial ramus

Ischial Spine (is′ke-al/spīn) (n.) A pointed projection of the ischium directed medially at the pelvic outlet. It separates the lesser and greater sciatic notches.

Ischial Tuberosity (is′kē-al/too″be-ros′i-tē) (n.) The blunt, inferior aspect of the ischium on which the body rests in the sitting position.

Ischial Weight-Bearing (is′kē-al/wāt/bār′ing) (n.) Any prostheses, orthoses, or cast that transfers weight from the lower extremity onto the ischial tuberosity.

Ischiopubic Column (is″kē-ō-pū′bik/kol′um) (n.) The posterior bony column of the acetabulum that is formed by contribution of the ischium, the pubis, and the ischiopubic ramus. To visualize this column

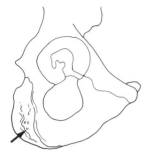

Ischial tuberosity

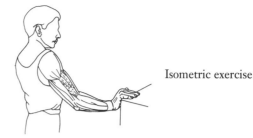

Isometric exercise

radiographically, obtain an extended oblique x-ray view of the pelvis.

Ischium (is'kē-um) (n.)   The heavy posterior, inferior portion of the innominate bone.

Iselin's Osteonecrosis (i-ze-linz/os″te-ō-ne-krō′sis) (n.)   A focal aseptic, necrosis of the fifth metatarsal.

Isoenzyme (ī″so-en′zīm) (n.)   Any of the electrophoretically distinct forms of an enzyme that share the same function. Synonym: **Isozyme.**

Isograft (ī′so-graft) (n.)   A tissue transplant from one individual to another genetically identical.

Isokinetic (ī″so-kin′et-ik) (adj.)   1. A dynamic contraction that causes a shortening of muscle length in which resistance accommodates to the force applied and the speed is held constant by a special device. 2. A contraction in which the limbs move at a constant velocity but the shortening speed of the contracting muscle(s) is not constant.

Isokinetic Exercise (ī″so-kin′et-ik/ek′ser-sīz) (n.)   Exercise requiring the use of an apparatus that holds joint motion to a constant speed by offering resistance to muscle activity that matches the degree of that activity.

Isolation Techniques (ī″so-la′shun/tek-nēks′) (n.)   Practices used to prevent the transfer of microorganisms. Also called **Communicable Disease Techniques.**

Isomer (ī′so-mer) (n.)   One of a group of compounds identical in atomic composition but different in structural arrangement.

Isometric (ī″so-met′rik) (adj.)   A muscle contraction in which the length of the total muscle remains unchanged during the exercise; resistance is equal to the force applied, and velocity is zero.

Isometric Exercise (ī″so-met′rik/ek′ser-sīz) (n.)   An active exercise performed against stable resistance in which there is change in the length of the muscle. Therefore, in isometric or "muscle-setting" exercises, muscles contract without producing any motion of the joint. Synonym: **Static Exercise.**

Isotonic (ī″so-ton′ik) (adj.)   1. The contraction of a muscle that is allowed to shorten as it exerts a steady force. 2. A contraction that causes a change in the length of the muscle, which in turn causes a movement of the part(s) to which it is attached. Resis-

tance is constant and velocity is inversely proportional to the load applied. There are two types of isotonic contractions: In a **concentric** or **shortening** contraction, the joint motion occurs in the direction of pull, decreasing the joint angle. This is known as **positive work.** An **eccentric** or **lengthening** contraction occurs during the lengthening of a muscle to resist the lengthening. This is known as **negative work.** Isotonics are the easiest and most common method of resistive exercise, and various apparatuses are available—the Universal Gym, Nautilus, and free weights are examples. 3. A solution having the same osmotic pressure as another solution.

Isotonic Exercise (ī″so-ton′ik/ek′ser-sīz) (n.)   An active exercise in which there is muscle contraction and movement of the joint through an arc of motion against a constant resistance.

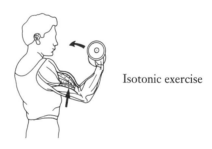

Isotonic exercise

Isotope (ī′so-tōp) (n.)   One of several possible forms of a chemical element that differ from other forms in the number of neutrons in the atomic nucleus but not in chemical properties.

Isotropic Material (ī′so-trop′ik/mah-te′re-al) (n.)   A material whose mechanical properties are the same in all directions.

Isthmus (is′mus) (n.)   A narrow or constricted structure connecting two other structures.

-itis   Suffix: inflammation of.

ITB   Abbreviation for Iliotibial band.

ITT   Abbreviation for Internal tibial torsion.

IV   Intravenous.

Ivory Bones (ī′vo-re/bōnz) (n.)   Very dense bones that appear ivorylike on radiograph. They are seen, for example, in osteopetrosis and osteoblastic lesions.

Ivory Phalanx (ī-vo-re/fa'lanks) (n.) A radiologic sign of psoriatic arthritis characterized by an increased density of the terminal phalanges, with or without bony spiculation and with minimal bony resorption of the tuft.

I/Y Ratio (ra'shē-o) (n.) A radiologic measurement used in the evaluation of congenital dislocation of the hip. On the AP radiograph of the pelvis, I is the horizontal distance between the lateral wall of the ilium just above the edge of the acetabulum and the inner wall of the ilium. Y is the distance between the inner wall of both iliums just above the triradiate cartilage. In patients with unilateral dislocation, compare the ratio of I/Y on the dislocated side with that on the normal side. In normal hips, the ratio of I/Y is equal on both sides. In unilateral dislocations, the ratio before reduction is higher on the normal side than on the dislocated side.

J

Jaccoud's Arthritis (zhah-kōoz'/ar-thrī'tis) (n.) A rare syndrome seen after repeated attacks of rheumatic fever. The arthropathy results in hand and foot deformities that may be mistaken for rheumatoid arthritis: ulnar deviation and subluxation at the metacarpophalangeal and metatarsophalangeal joints. Radiographically, a notch or hook may be seen on the ulnar side of each metacarpal head. Also known as **Jaccoud's Syndrome, Chronic Postrheumatic Fever Arthropathy, Chronic Fibrous Rheumatism**.

Jack-knife Position (jak'nīf/po-zish'un) (n.) A prone position with the patient's hips positioned over a central break on the operating table. The table is flexed at a sharp angle of 90°, raising the hips and lowering the head and feet. Also called **Kraske Position**.

Jack Toe-Raising Test (jak/to-rās'ing/test) (n.) A means of evaluating an anatomic site where the foot sags in pes planus. With the patient standing, the great toe is passively dorsiflexed. This maneuver elevates the longitudinal arch of the foot in all cases of naviculocuneiform sag and in most cases of combined (naviculocuneiform and talonavicular) breaks; this maneuver, however, does not restore the arch when the talus is plantar-flexed and the sag is at only the talonavicular joint.

Jacob's Chuck (jā'kubz/chuk) (n.) An adapter for a hand- or power-drill for attachment of drill bits, wires, etc. Sometimes cannulated at its attachment to the drill. See **Chuck**.

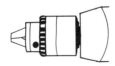

Jacob's chuck

Jammed Finger (jam'd/fing'ger) (n.) A diffusely painful and swollen proximal interphalangeal joint of a digit, resulting from a sudden, longitudinal directed force on the extended proximal interphalangeal joint. Diagnosis is made by excluding other injuries, including fracture and/or disruption of the volar plate, collateral ligaments, or extensor mechanism of the finger. X-ray findings, with the exception of soft tissue swelling, are negative. This condition is associated with prolonged morbidity (6 to 12 months) and often causes permanent residual thickening about the joint.

Jansen's Disease (jan-zenz/dǐ-zēz') (n.) A rare type of metaphyseal chondrodysplasia, a condition, transmitted by autosomal dominant inheritance. A short-limbed type of dwarfism manifested in late infancy and associated with mental and physical retardation. Radiographically, there is generalized demineralization and the metaphyses show characteristic cupping, flaring, and vacuolated areas. Also known as **Metaphyseal Dysostosis, Murk-Jansen's Syndrome**.

Jansen's Test (yan'senz/test) (n.) A clinical test for evaluation of osteoarthritis of the hip. Instruct the patient to cross his or her legs with a point just above the ankle resting on the opposite knee. This motion is impossible when osteoarthritis of the hip is present.

Japanese Finger Traps (jap-e-nēz/fin-ger/trapz) (n.) See **Fingertraps**.

Jaundice (jawn'dis) (n.) A condition characterized by yellowish discoloration of the plasma, skin, and mucous membranes, resulting from an abnormal accumulation of bilirubin in the serum. It may be recognized on careful examination when the serum bilirubin concentration reaches approximately 2 mg/100 mL.

JBJS Abbreviation for the *Journal of Bone and Joint Surgery*.

JCAH Abbreviation for Joint Commission on Accreditation of Hospitals.

Jeanne's Sign (jēnz/sīn) (n.) A diagnostic test used in the evaluation of ulnar nerve palsy. The patient is asked to hold a piece of paper tight between the thumb and index finger. In ulnar nerve palsy, the classic posture is characterized by flexion of the interphalangeal joint and hyperextension of the metacarpophalangeal joint of the thumb due to paralysis of the adductor pollicis, the extensor pollicis brevis, and the first dorsal interosseous muscles. See **Froment's Sign.**

Jefferson Fracture (jef′er-son/frak′chur) (n.) A fracture of the ring of C1 (atlas). The mechanism of an injury on top of the head that forces the occipital condyles of the skull against the lateral masses, causing a burst fracture of C1. An AP radiograph generally shows widening of the distance between the odontoid and the lateral masses of C1, and the lateral film frequently shows cracks or frank disruption of the ring posteriorly. Described by Sir Godfrey Jefferson in 1919.

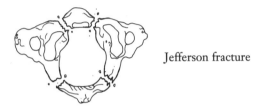

Jefferson fracture

Jendrassik's Maneuver (jen-drah′siks/mah-noo′ver) (n.) A technique to distract the patient during testing of a peripheral reflex, in order to elicit a latent reflex or increase the amplitude of a reflex. Ask the patient to interlink his or her flexed fingers, placing the palmar surfaces of the fingers of one hand against the palmar surfaces of the other; then pull them apart at the time of the test. Also called **Reinforcement Maneuver.**

Jerk (jerk) (n.) 1. The sudden contraction of a muscle in response to a nerve impulse. 2. A sudden reflex or involuntary movement.

Jerk Test (jerk/test) (n.) A maneuver used to evaluate anterolateral instability of the knee joint. The test is similar to the **pivot shift test** but begins with the knee flexed and the tibia reduced. Using valgus stress and internal rotation of the tibia, the knee is gradually extended. In a positive test, subluxation occurs maximally at about 30° of flexion; then spontaneous relocation, in the form of a sudden jerk, will occur near full extension.

Jeune's Syndrome (zh-unz/sin′drōm) (n.) A very rare type osteochondrodysplasia manifested at birth. The most striking deformity is a diminished thorax, resulting in significant pulmonary problems. Also known as **Asphyxiating Thoracic Dysplasia.**

Jeweler's Forceps (jool-erz′/fōr′seps) (n.) A type of forceps used in microsurgery.

Jewett Brace (joo′et/brās) (n.) A framelike thoracolumbosacral orthosis, based on the three-point pressure principle and designed to maintain an erect posture. It consists of two anterior pressure pads, one over the upper part of the sternum, the other over the pubis, and one posterior pad in the thora-columbar area for counterpressure. Thus it restricts, in particular, flexion of the vertebral column. Also called **Hyperextension Brace.**

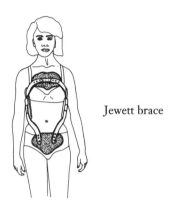

Jewett brace

Jewett Nail-Plate (joo′et/nāl/plāt) (n.) A fixed plate with a tri-flanged nail, used in the fixation of femoral neck and intertrochanteric hip fractures.

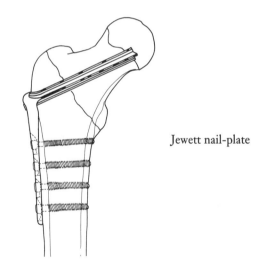

Jewett nail-plate

Jimmy (jim′ē) (n.) In shoe terminology, a piece of material of felt, cork, or leather shaped as the forepart of an insole and inserted to tighten a shoe.

Jobst Boot (jōb-st/boot) (n.) An inflatable compression unit combined with an electric timing device for rhythmic inflation and deflation; used to reduce edema in a limb. Synonym: **Jobst Sleeve.**

Jobst Stocking (jōb-st/stok′ing) (n.) A compressive elastic stocking used to control edematous conditions, such as post-phlebitic edema or burns.

Jogger's Heel (jog-erz′/hēl) (n.) A condition seen in runners and athletes, characterized by discomfort and pain about the heel caused by repetitive and forceful strikes of the heel on a hard surface.

Jogger's Toe (jog-erz′/tō) (n.) 1. A subungal hematoma of the great toe. The patient frequently presents 3 to 4 weeks after jarring the toe while jogging with an asymptomatic bluish discoloration of the nail. 2. Involvement of any of the toes; frequently bilateral, involving the toe that is most forward in the toe-box. There is a characteristic petechial eruption of the fat pad of the toe tip. It is caused by repeated trauma to the nail of the hallux by sudden deceleration against the toe-box of a tight-fitting running shoe. Also known as **turf toe** among football players or **tennis toe** among tennis players.

John Wayne Procedure (jon/wān/pro-se′jur) (n.) A facetious statement referring to the surgical axiom: "Go in and do what's right."

Johnson's Position (john′sonz/po-zish′un) (n.) A position used to obtain an axiolateral radiographic projection of the femoral head, neck, and trochanter region.

Joint Capsule (joint/kap′sūl) (n.) The articular capsule. A connective tissue housing of a joint. It adds to joint stability. Synovium lines its inner surface.

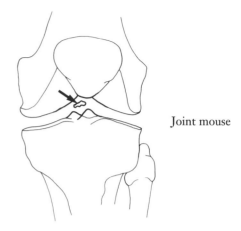

Joint mouse

Joint Space (joint/spās) (n.) 1. The space between two or more articulating bones or articulating prosthetic components. 2. On radiographic evaluation of articulations, the radiolucent space between the subchondral bone edges. This should reflect the overall height of the articular cartilage and will be diminished or narrowed in arthritic conditions.

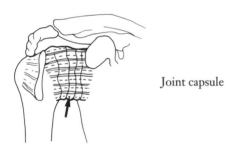

Joint capsule

Joint Commission on Accreditation of Hospitals (joint/kom′ish-un/on/ak″red-i-tā′shun/of/hospitals) (n.) A private accrediting agency that inspects hospitals and accredits those that meet its criteria. It has published standards for the various services and departments in hospitals. Abbreviation **JCAH**.

Joint Manipulation (joint/mah-nip″u-lā′shun) (n.) A skilled passive movement of a joint, either within or beyond its active range of motion.

Joint Mobilization (joint/mo″bi-li-zā′shun) (n.) A very general term that may be applied to any active or passive attempt to increase movement at a joint.

Joint Mouse (joint/mows) (n.) A small, loose body or osteochondral fragment within a synovial joint. Synonyms: **Joint Body, Loose Body, Arthrophytes, Corpora Mobile, Arthroliths**.

Joint Reaction Force (joint/re-ak′shun/fōrs) (n.) The internal reaction force when a joint is subjected to external loads and/or muscle forces. The unit of measure is newtons (poundforce).

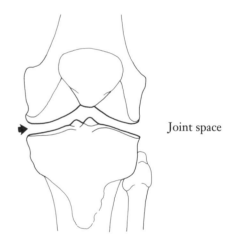

Joint space

Joints of Luschka (joints/of/lush′kah) (n.) Diarthrodial synovial joints lying between the uncus on the superior and lateral articulating margins of an inferior cervical vertebra, articulating with the inferior and lateral surface of the superior vertebra. Also referred to as the **uncovertebral joints**. See also **Luschka Joints**.

Joker (jō′ker) (n.) A blunt, flat surgical instrument. May be useful in levering small fracture fragments.

Jones Abduction Frame (jōnz/ab-duk′shun/frām) (n.) A special apparatus used on hospital beds to assist in gaining hip abduction in various diseases of the hip.

Jones Bandage (jōnz/ban′dij) (n.) See **Jones Compression Dressing**.

Jones Bar (jōnz/bar) (n.) In shoe terminology, a metatarsal bar placed between the innersole and the outersole.

Jones Compression Dressing (jōnz/kom-presh′un/dres′ing) (n.) A bulky, nonocclusive compression dressing commonly used for soft-tissue injuries. It provides relative immobilization of the joint and uniform compression for reducing swelling. The dressing is applied in layers of cotton bandage alternating with elastic bandages. Also known as **Jones Bandage**.

Jones Criteria (jōnz/kri-te′re-ah) (n.) A standardized list of clinical findings of major and minor importance for making the diagnosis of acute rheumatic fever.

Jones Fracture (jōnz/frak′chur) (n.) A fracture of the proximal diaphyseal portion of the fifth metatarsal. Described by Robert Jones in 1902. It is to be distinguished from an avulsion fracture through the styloid process of the base of the metatarsal.

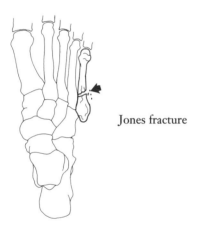

Jones fracture

Jones Procedure (jōnz/pro-sē′jur) (n.) A technique for reconstruction of the anterior cruciate ligament using the central one-third of the bone–patellar tendon–bone complex leaving the graft attached distally to the tibia and routing it through a femoral tunnel proximally.

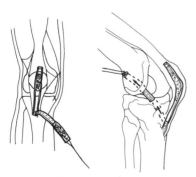

Jones procedure

The Journal of Bone and Joint Surgery Official publication of the American Academy of Orthopaedic Surgeons, the British and Canadian Orthopaedic Associations, and many other national and international orthopaedic societies. Abbreviated **JBJS**.

JRA Abbreviation for Juvenile rheumatoid arthritis.

Judet Prosthesis (zhú-dā/pros-thē′sis) (n.) An early total hip design intended for press fit instead of cement fixation.

Jugular Compression Test (jug′u-lar/kom-presh′un/test) (n.) A maneuver to increase the intraspinal pressure; it causes exaggeration of radicular pain in patients with space-occupying lesions that press on the nerve roots. The test may be performed with the patient either supine or upright. Apply simultaneous compression to the internal and external jugular veins for a period of 2 minutes or more. If the patient, without prompting, complains of increased pain in the back, in the hip and the thigh, and finally, in the leg down to the ankle—and possibly says that a toe feels numb and is tingling—the test is positive. A positive test is pathognomonic of an intraspinal lesion, although not necessarily of a ruptured disc; it may point to a neoplasm involving the spinal roots. Synonym: **Viet's test**.

Jugular Fossa (jug′u-lar/fos′ah) (n.) An area of pronounced depression in the temporal bone.

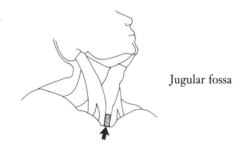

Jugular fossa

Jump Position (jump/pō-zish′un) (n.) The posture of a spastic child who stands with knees and hips flexed and ankles in the equinus position.

Jump Sign (jump/sīn) (n.) An involuntary reaction by the patient to stimulation of a tender area or trigger point. This may take the form of wincing or sudden jerking of the part being examined, of adjacent areas, or even of the entire body. The sign must be distinguished from reactions not elicited from specific, consistent topographic sites, that are more prolonged, or that take the form of pushing the examiner away. Contrast to **Trigger Point**.

Jumper's Fractures (jump′erz/frak′churz) (n.) A term applied to one or more thoracolumbar fractures caused by a vertical plunge. The vertebral pedicles, lamina, articulating facets, or vertebral body may be involved.

Jumper's Knee (jump′erz/nē) (n.) 1. An overuse syndrome seen in athletes who subject their knee extensor mechanisms to intense and repeated stress. It results in tendinitis of the patellar, or less commonly, of the quadriceps tendon. Clinically, there is point tenderness at the site of involvement at the superior or inferior pole of the patella or the insertion of the patellar tendon into the tibial tuberosity. 2. A condition of partial avulsion of the fibers of the patellar tendon from the lower pole of the patella. Also called **Patellar** or **Quadriceps Tendonitis.**

Junctura Cartilagenae (junk-tur-a/kar-til-adj-en-ā) (n.) See **Amphiarthrosis.**

Juvenile Aponeurotic Fibroma (joo′ve-nīl/ap″ō-nū-rot′ik/fi-brō′mah) (n.) A distinctive, benign, soft-tissue tumor of young children. It usually occurs in the palms and soles. Synonym: **Cartilage Analogue of Fibromatosis.**

Juvenile Osteochondroses (joo′ve-nīl/os″te-ō-kon-drō′sēs) (n.) A group of regional clinical entities, each designated by its own eponym. These conditions occur mostly in children, have similar roentgenographic appearances, and mostly affect the epiphyseal or apophyseal centers. The two basic groups of these conditions are:

 1. Those due to localized osteonecrosis of an apophysis or an epiphysis. Examples include Legg-Calvé-Perthes disease and Freiberg Disease.

 2. Those related to abnormalities of endochondral ossification either congenitally or post-traumatic. Examples include Osgood-Schlatter disease and Schuermann disease.

Juvenile Rheumatoid Arthritis (joo′ve-nīl/rōō″mah-toid/ar-thrī′tis) (n.) Chronic synovitis in children, probably including several distinct disease processes. Recognizable subgroups are: systemic-onset disease (20%), rheumatoid factor-negative polyarthritis (25%), rheumatoid factor-positive polyarthritis (5%), pauciarthritis associated with antinuclear antibodies and chronic iridocyclitis (30%–35%), pauciarthritis associated with sacroiliitis and HLA-B27 (10%–15%). Rheumatoid factor-positive polyarthritis appears to be the childhood equivalent of classic adult rheumatoid arthritis. The pauciarthritis type associated with HLA-B27 appears to be closely related to the spondyloarthropic diseases. Although there are no diagnostic laboratory tests, various subgroups differ in immunogenetic findings as well as in clinical appearance and prognosis. Also called **Still's Disease.**

Juvenile Scoliosis (joo′ve-nīl/skō″le-ō′sis) (n.) Scoliosis developing between the ages of 3 and 7 years. Occurs equally in boys and girls.

Juvenile Spinal Muscular Atrophy (joo′ve-nīl/spī′nal/mus′kū-lar/at′rō-fē) (n.) See **Kugelberg-Welander Syndrome.**

Juxta (juks′tah) Prefix: near, beside, or close to.

Juxtacortical Chondroma (juks″tah-kor′ti-kal/kon-drō′mah) (n.) A benign cartilaginous tumor of bone usually found in the metaphyseal cortex of long bones and short tubular bones. Characteristically, a radiograph shows a well-defined saucer-like cortical defect surrounded by sclerotic bone, often with an overhanging edge. Calcification may be seen.

Juxtacortical Osteosarcoma (juks″tah-kor′ti-kal/os″te-ō-sar-kō′mah) (n.) A type of malignant bone tumor that is usually slow-growing and histologically low-grade. Most commonly, it occurs on the posterior aspect of the distal femur. Radiographically, the lesion is usually a large, well-circumscribed, dense, juxtacortical mass. A radiolucent line or space is usually apparent between the tumor and the underlying cortex. Also known as **Parosteal Osteogenic Sarcoma.**

K

K 1. The symbol for potassium. 2. The symbol for the Kelvin temperature scale.

K-Rod Abbreviation for Küntscher Rod.

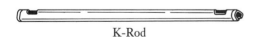

K-Rod

KAFO Abbreviation for Knee-Ankle-Foot Orthosis.

Kanavel's Sign (kan-a′velz/sīn) (n.) The four cardinal signs of flexor tendon sheath infection: (1) posture of slight finger flexion, (2) fusiform swelling of the digit, (3) pain on passive extension, (4) tenderness along the flexor tendon sheath.

Kanavel's Triangle (kan-a′velz/tri′ang-ġ′l) (n.) An area in the middle of the palm beneath which lies the common tendon sheath of the digital flexor tendons.

Kaplan's Cardinal Line (kap′lanz/kar′di-nal/līn) (n.) A topographic guide to the deep structures of the hand. To locate it, lie the hand flat and supinated. Draw a line from the apex of the interdigital fold between the thumb and the index finger toward the ulnar side of the hand that is parallel to the middle crease of the palm of the hand. It passes near the pisiform bone, touching its distal pole.

Kaposi's Sarcoma (kah′po-shēz/sar-kō′mah) (n.) A slowly evolving endothelial neoplasm of reticuloendothelial cells. Multifocal and proliferative, it pri-

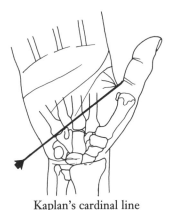

Kaplan's cardinal line

marily affects the skin but can occur in other organs. Characteristically, the lesion presents as a nodule or plaque of violaceous hue. It typically occurs in the lower extremity. Its etiology is unclear.

Kaposi's sarcoma generally affects 40- to 70-year-old males of Eastern Europe, Ashkenazy Jewish, and Equatorial South African heritage. A resurgence of Kaposi's sarcoma is found as a side-effect of acquired immunodeficiency syndrome (AIDS). Approximately 10% of diagnosed patients may exhibit visceral involvement. Synonyms: **Multiple Idiopathic Hemorrhagic Sarcoma, Angioendothelioma Cutaneum, Acrosarcoma; Sarcoma Cutaneum Telangiectaticum Multiplex, Angioreticulomatosis, Multiple Angiosarcoma.**

Karyotype (kar′ē-ō-tīp) (n.) The total chromosomal complement of a cell.

Keflex (kef′leks) (n.) A proprietary brand of cephalexin, an orally administered first-generation cephalosporin antibiotic.

Keflin (kef′lin) (n.) A proprietary brand of cephalothin, an intravenously administered first-generation cephalosporin antibiotic.

Kefzol (kef′zōl) (n.) A proprietary brand of cefazolin, a first-generation cephalosporin antibiotic.

Kehr's Sign (kārz/sīn) (n.) A symptom of pain referred to the shoulder. It comes from an acute or subacute inflammation of the undersurface of the diaphragm, as in a rupture of the spleen.

Keith's Law (Kēths/law) (n.) A principle that states that ligaments are never used for the continuous support of any joint or part.

Keller Procedure (kel′er/pro-se′jur) (n.) A surgical technique for correction of hallux valgus. It includes resection of the proximal end of the first proximal phalanx, release of the adductor tendon, and resection of the bony medial eminence of the first metatarsal. Keller was an army physician. The hospital at the U.S. Military Academy at West Point is named for him. Also known as **Keller's Resection Arthroplasty.**

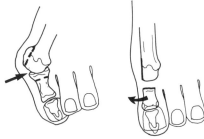

Keller procedure

Kelly Clamp (kel′ē/klamp) (n.) A surgical clamp.

Keloid (ke′loid) (n.) A large, firm mass of scarlike tissue. It is usually the result of trauma but sometimes occurs spontaneously. Hypertrophied scars are similar but often have a less dense connective tissue with skin appendages. Keloid scarring occurs in people with a predisposing genetic factor, most commonly in the Negroid race.

Kempf Nail (kemf′/nāl) (n.) The Grosse-Kempf intramedullary nail system for fixation of femoral and tibial shaft fractures. See **Grosse-Kempf Interlocking Nail.**

Kennedy Ligament Augmenting Device (ken′e-dē/ lig′ah-ment/awg-men′ting/de-vīs′) (n.) A type of synthetic stent used to augment or lengthen autogenous tissues in the repair or reconstruction of the anterior cruciate ligament. The **Kennedy LAD** is made of braided polypropylene yarn.

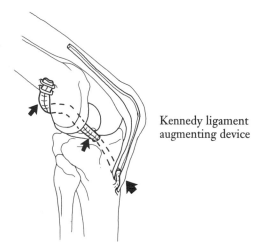

Kennedy ligament augmenting device

Kenny Crutch (ken′e/cruch) (n.) A double-upright forearm crutch with a leather cuff at the upper end. This device was named for the Australian nurse, Elizabeth Kenny, also known as Sister Kenny.

Kenny–Howard Splint (ken′ē/how-ard/splint) (n.) A device used in the treatment of acromioclavicular joint disruption. Designed to exert downward pressure on the superiorly displaced clavicle and upward pressure on the arm.

Kenny Treatment (ken′ē/trēt′ment) (n.) A form of physical therapy used in poliomyelitis. It consists of the application of hot moist packs to the affected muscles followed by passive and then active exercises with muscle reeducation. Synonym: **Sister Kenny Treatment**.

Keratin (ker′ah-tin) (n.) One of a group of tough, fibrous proteins; a horny tissue formed by certain epidermal tissues. It is especially abundant in skin, claws, and hair.

Keratin Sulfate (ker′ah-tin/sul′fāt) (n.) One of the connective tissue proteoglycans.

Kerlix Dressing (ker′-lix/dres′ing) (n.) A proprietary brand of gauze bandage packaged in rolls.

Kernig's Sign (ker′nigz/sīn) (n.) A sign of meningeal irritation. To perform the test, lay the patient supine. Then flex the hip and extend the knee. Normal knee extension may reach 135°. The test is positive when knee extension is limited and painful.

Kerrison Rongeur (ker′-i-son/rawn-ghur′) (n.) A type of biting forceps especially useful in spinal surgery.

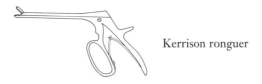

Kerrison ronguer

Ketoprofen (kē′tō′prō′fen) (n.) A type of nonsteroidal, anti-inflammatory drug derived from proprionic acid. Brand name Orudis and Oravil.

Key Pinch (kē/pinch) (n.) Grasping strength, as in holding a coin between the thumb and index fingers.

Kg Abbreviation for Kilogram.

Kidner Procedure (kid′ner/pro-sē′jur) (n.) A surgical technique for the correction of the symptomatic pes planus associated with an accessory navicular. In this procedure, the accessory navicular is excised, and the tibialis posterior tendon is rerouted into a more plantar position.

Kidney Rests (kid′nē/rests) (n.) A kidney-bean–shaped device attached to an operating room table that helps maintain the position of a patient during a surgical procedure. The device is a covered concave metal piece with grooved notches at the base that attach to the table.

Kienböck's Disease (kēn′beks/dĭ-zēz′) (n.) An osteochondrosis or aseptic necrosis of the carpal lunate bone.

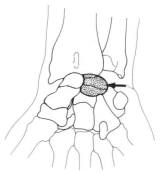

Kienböck's disease

Kilian's Line (kel′e-anz/līn) (n.) A prominent ridge on the promontory of the sacrum.

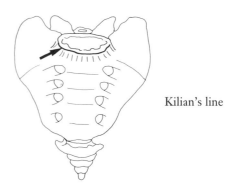

Kilian's line

Kilian's Pelvis (kil′e-anz/pel′vis) (n.) A deformed osteomalacic pelvis. Synonyms: **Osteomalacic Pelvis, Pelvis Obtecta**.

Kilogram (kil′ō-gram) (n.) A metric weight measure equaling 1000 g or 2.2 lbs.

Kinematics (kin″e-mat′iks) (n.) The division of mechanics that examines the geometry of the motion of bodies. It includes displacement, velocity, and acceleration but does not deal with motion-producing forces.

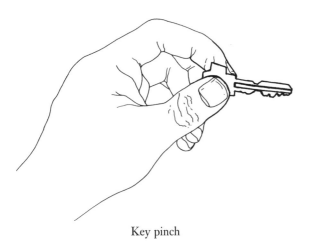

Key pinch

Kineplasty (kin′e-plas″tē) (n.) A type of amputation involving the arrangement of muscles and tendons in the stump so that they can be used to move parts of a prosthetic appliance. The types of kineplastic amputations include the club, the loop, the tendon, and the muscle tunnel.

Kinesthesia (kin′es-thē′ze-ah) (n.) The brain's constant awareness of muscle position and movement throughout the body. It is achieved by means of proprioceptors, which send impulses from muscles, joints, and tendons back to the brain.

Kinetic Energy (ki-net′ik/en′er-jē) (n.) The energy that a body possesses due to its velocity. The unit of measure is newton-meters or joules.

Kinetics (ki-net′iks) (n.) A branch of mechanics that studies the relation between the force system acting on a body and the change it produces in the body motion.

Kinin (ki′nin) (n.) One of a group of polypeptides produced in the blood or tissues. Kinin dilates blood vessels and produces the pain associated with inflammation.

Kirner's Deformity (ker′nerz/de-for′mi-tē) (n.) A deformity of the little finger in which an abnormal angle of the distal phalanx is the result of the angular fusion of the epiphysis with the shaft. It is usually bilateral and symmetric. Synonym: **Dystelephalangy.**

Kirschner's Traction Bow (kērsh′nerz/trak′shun/bo) (n.) A clamplike device used with fine wires for skeletal traction. It is based on the use of tension applied to wires and pins to obtain increased resistance to angulation, which therefore permits the use of small-diameter wires or pins for traction.

Kirschner Wire (kērsh′ner/wīr) (n.) A threaded or smooth metallic wire with a small diameter and a trochar or diamond-pointed ends. It has multiple uses, including skeletal traction, internal fixation of fractures, and percutaneous pin fixation of fractures.

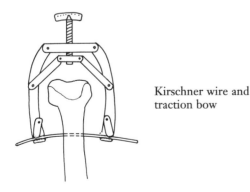

Kirschner wire and traction bow

Kite's Angle (kītz/ang′g′l) (n.) A measurement of the relationship between the talus and calcaneus as seen on an AP radiograph of the foot. It is the angle between a line drawn parallel to the anterolateral border of the calcaneus and another line drawn parallel to the medial border of the talus.

Kite's Rotation Test (kītz/ro-tā′shun/test) (n.) A maneuver used to distinguish between congenital and acquired medial leg torsion. Have the patient lay supine. Grasp the ankles and rotate the limbs medially and laterally at the hip joints. In the congenital form of medial leg torsion, the patellae can be turned medially and laterally to the same degree as in a normal child. In the acquired form, the patellae can be turned medially 90° or more, but they cannot be rotated laterally.

Klebsiella (kleb″sē-el′lah) (n.) A genus of short, gram-negative rods found in the family Enterobacteriaceae. The rods have been isolated from several animals and inanimate objects. They may be either pathogenic or part of the normal flora.

Klein's Line (klīnz/līn) (n.) A line drawn on an AP radiograph of the pelvis to detect medial slippage of the capital femoral epiphysis. Draw a line along the superior surface of the femoral neck toward the acetabulum. This line should intersect the femoral head. In a slipped capital femoral epiphysis, the femoral head will remain medial to this line.

Klenzak Ankle Joint (klen-zak′/ank′k′l/joint) (n.) A type of spring-loaded ankle dorsiflexion-assisting device used in braces. It has a spring adjustment and a plantar flexion stop.

Klenzak Brace (klen-zak′/brās) (n.) A double-bar ankle foot orthosis used with a Klenzak joint for footdrop. The spring assist provides dorsiflexion of the ankle. The Klenzak joint and double stirrup attach to a steel plate located between the sole and the heel of the shoe.

Kling Dressing (kling/dres′ing) (n.) A proprietary brand of gauze wound dressing material.

Klippel-Feil Sign (kli-pel′fīl/sīn) (n.) A diagnostic sign in pyramidal tract disorders. To elicit the sign, support the patient's wrist; then have him or her flex and quickly extend the fingers. The sign is positive if flexion and adduction of the thumb occur.

Klippel-Feil Syndrome (kli-pel′fīl/sin′drōm) (n.) A congenital malformation of the cervical spine characterized by the fusion of two or more cervical vertebrae. This may result in restricted neck motion, low hairline, and occasionally, neurologic involvement. It is also called **Congenital Short Neck Syndrome,** or **Brevicollis.**

Klumpke Paralysis (kloom′kē/pah-ral′i-sis) (n.) A type of brachial plexus injury involving the lower plexus. The sensory and motor deficits involve C8 and T1, with or without C7 dysfunction. The primary functional deficits result from paralysis of the intrinsic hand muscles and the wrist and finger flexors. Compare to **Erb's Palsy.**

Knee (ne) (n.) The articulation between the femur, the patella, and the tibia.

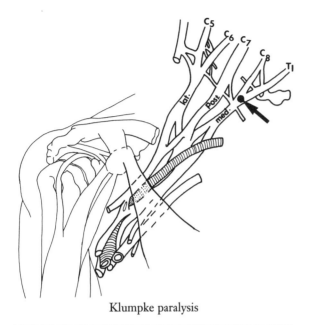

Klumpke paralysis

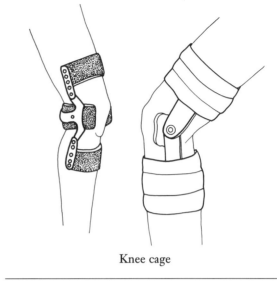

Knee cage

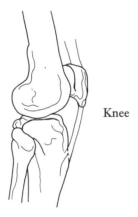

Knee

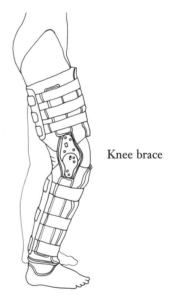

Knee brace

Knee Brace (nē/brās) (n.)   An orthosis used to provide support for the knee. It extends from mid-thigh to about mid-leg. The support may or may not have a joint. See **Lenox-Hill Orthosis**.

Knee Cage (nē/kāj) (n.)   Device used for stabilizing, supporting, protecting, or splinting the knee. Knee cages consist of steel bars or stays that extend from the mid-thigh to the upper third of the calf. They have a mechanical joint in juxtaposition to the knee. This joint may have stops arranged to restrict flexion and extension to a prescribed degree.

Knee-Chest Position (nē-chest/pō-zish′un) (n.)   An anatomic position in which the head, shoulder, and chest rest on the table with the knees bent placed under the abdomen, and the hips and buttocks elevated.

Knee-Elbow Position (nē-el′bō/pō-zish′un) (n.)   An anatomic position in which the patient is prone, resting on his or her knees and elbows with the chest elevated.

Knee Immobilizer (nē/im-mō′bilīzer) (n.)   See **Knee Splint**.

Knee Jerk (nē/jerk) (n.)   See **Quadriceps Reflex**.

Knee Pad (nē/pad) (n.)   In orthotics, a pad placed in front of the knee and attached to an orthosis. The pad is usually made of leather. It restricts the forward displacement of the knee inside the orthosis.

Knee Splint (nē/splint) (n.)   A device used for immobilizing, supporting, or stabilizing the knee.

Kniest Syndrome (nēst/sin′drōm) (n.)   A type of short-limbed, short-trunked, disproportionate dwarfism recognizable at birth. Also known as **pseudo-metatropic dwarfism**.

Knight Brace (nīt/brās) (n.)   A thoracolumbosacral orthosis. It consists of two lateral and two posterior rigid uprights and a full-front abdominal flexible support. This brace limits flexion and extension of the lumbar spine, decreases the lumbar lordosis, restricts lateral flexion, and assists the abdominal musculature in increasing intra-abdominal pressure. It is often called a **Chair Back** or **Lumbosacral A-P and L Orthosis**.

Knight-Taylor Brace (nīt-tā'ler/brās) (n.)   A thoracolumbar orthosis. This brace combines the features of the Knight brace and the Taylor brace. It consists of a metal frame (that has paraspinal and lateral uprights and pelvic and thoracic bands), shoulder straps, and an abdominal support. This brace particularly restricts flexion and extension in the thoracolumbar and upper lumbar joints.

Knock-Knee (nok-nē) (n.)   The colloquial name for an abnormal incurving of the legs that results in a gap between the feet when the knees touch. See **Genu Valgum**.

Knowles Pin (nōlz/pin) (n.)   A threaded pin with a trocar point, a distal thread, a hex collar, and a break-off shank. It is used mostly for fixation across the femoral neck, as with hip fractures or the treatment of a slipped capital femoral epiphysis.

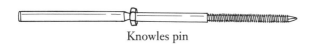

Knowles pin

Knuckle (nuk'l) (n.)   A colloquial term referring to the dorsum of the metacarpophalangeal joints prominent when the hand is clenched into a fist.

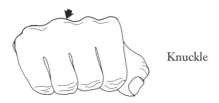

Knuckle

Knuckle Pad (nuk'l/pad) (n.)   A well-defined dermal and epidermal thickening over the articular areas that occurs on the dorsal surface of one or more fingers or toes. It was described in 1893 by Garrod.

Koch Functional Hand Splints (kōk/funk'shun-al/hand/splintz) (n.)   Aluminum and leather glove splints for hand injuries and deformities.

Kocher Clamp (kōk'er/klamp) (n.)   A surgical clamp.

Kocher Fracture (kōk'er/frak'chur) (n.)   A fracture of the capitellum of the distal end of the humerus. A

fragment of the articular surface and bone may be displaced into the elbow joint.

Kocher-Langenbeck Incision (kōk'er/lahng'en-bek/in-sizh'un) (n.)   Posterior approach to the hip joint. It extends from a point distal to the posterior superior spine of the ilium obliquely to the greater trochanter and then distally down the femoral shaft.

Kocher Maneuver (kōk'er/mah'noo-ver) (n.)   A technique for the reduction of the anterior dislocated humeral head into the glenoid. There are four steps to this maneuver: 1. With the elbow flexed 90°, traction is applied in line with the humeral shaft. 2. The arm is slowly brought into external rotation. 3. The humerus is adducted across the front of the chest, approximately to the midline. 4. The arm is rotated internally until the hand rests on the opposite shoulder. During this maneuver, the humeral head is levered on the anterior glenoid, and the shaft is levered against the anterior thoracic wall until the reduction is complete.

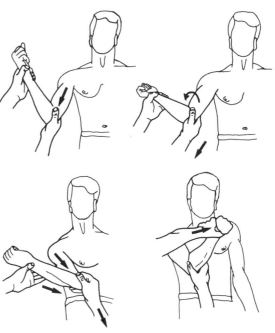

Kocher maneuver

Koebner Phenomenon (keb'ner/fe-nom'e-non) (n.)   The rash associated with systemic juvenile rheumatoid arthritis. It is composed of discrete, faint pink macules or maculopapules. If the rash is absent during the examination, it can be elicited by scratching or rubbing a susceptible area.

Köhler's Disease (kā'lerz/di-zēz') (n.)   An avascular necrosis or osteochondrosis of the tarsal navicular bone.

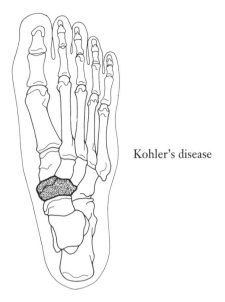

Kohler's disease

Köhler's Line (kā′lerz/līn) (n.) A radiographic line used in measuring protrusio acetabuli. On the AP radiograph of the pelvis, draw a line from the pelvic border of the ilium to the medial border of the body of the ischium. If the outline of the acetabular dome passes medial to this line, a protrusion exists. Kohler's line is useful with serial radiographs of an individual patient, but is not suitable for comparing patients. As protrusio acetabuli progresses, the femoral head projects medial to Kohler's line.

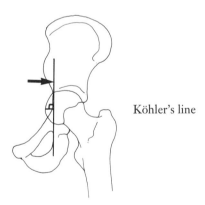

Köhler's line

Köhler's Second Disease (kā′lerz/sek′und/di-zēz′) (n.) An avascular necrosis of the second metatarsal head. Synonyms: **Freiberg's Infarction, Juvenile Deforming Metatarsophalangeal Osteochondritis.**

Köhler's Teardrop Sign (kā′lerz/tēr′drop/sīn) (n.) An anatomic radiographic landmark. On an AP roentgenogram of the pelvis, a normal radiodense projection that resembles a teardrop. Laterally, it is formed by the most inferior and anterior portion of the acetabular fossa. Medially, it is formed by the

anterior flat part of the quadrilateral surface of the iliac bone. The ilioischial line intersects or is tangential to the teardrop. Also known as the **Radiographic "U."**

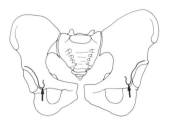

Kohler's teardrop sign

König Disease (kōn′iġ/di′zēz′) (n.) 1. Osteochondritis dissecans of the knee. 2. Osteochondritis of the tubular bones in adult males. It is associated with subchondral inflammatory processes and necrotic dissection of cartilaginous fragments. It results in loose bodies in the bone and joint cavities. Synonyms: **Paget's Quiet Necrosis of Bone, Osteochondritis Dissecans, Osteochondrolysis.**

Kopitz Parallelogram (kō′-pits/par″ah-lel′-o-gram) (n.) In congenital dislocation of the hip, a parallelogram made up of four lines passing from the medial and lateral edges of the acetabular roof to the medial and lateral edges of the proximal femoral epiphysis. On the AP radiograph, draw a line from the most lateral ossified margin of the roof of the acetabulum to the most medial ossified margin of the acetabulum. Draw another line along the superior surface of the ossified femoral neck. Then draw two additional lines—one from the lateral edge of the superior line to the lateral edge of the medial protruding tip of the ossified femoral neck, and the other from the medial edge of the inferior line. Normally, the four lines form a parallelogram or rectangle, with the femur lying close to the center. In congenital dislocation of the hip, the figure takes on a rhomboidal or trapezoidal shape, and the femoral head has an eccentric position.

Kosovicz Carpal Angle (kō-sō-vits/kar′pal/ang′ġ′l) (n.) A radiographic measurement useful in the evaluation of carpal instability. It is the angle formed be-

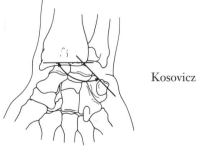

Kosovicz carpal angle

tween a line tangential to the proximal edge of the lunate and the scaphoid, and a line tangential to the lunate and triquetrium. This angle depends on race, sex, age, and wrist position. Normal values: 123° to 133° for males; 127° to 131° for females.

Krebs Cycle (krebz/sī'kl) (n.) An enzyme system that converts pyruvic acid to carbon dioxide in the presence of oxygen. The energy released by the process is captured in the form of ATP molecules. This is also referred to as the **Citric Acid Cycle** or the **Tricarboxylic Acid (TCA) Cycle**.

Krukenberg Operation (kroo'ken-berg/op''er-ā'shun) (n.) A surgical reconstructive procedure that converts the forearm to forceps after the amputation of a hand. The radial ray acts against the stabilizer ulnar ray in function so that the two bones act as a claw.

KUB (kub) (n.) An abbreviation for a plain AP roentgenogram of the abdomen that includes the areas of the kidney, ureters, and bladder.

Kugelberg-Welander Disease (kū'gl-berg-vā-lander/diz-ēz) (n.) A type of spinal muscular atrophy whose onset is between the ages 2 and 15 years. Also known as **Juvenile Spinal Muscular Atrophy**.

Kummel's Disease (kim'elz/di-zēz') (n.) A syndrome that follows a compression fracture of a vertebral body. It is actually a post-traumatic spondylitis characterized by the formation of a gibbus and kyphosis. It may have neurologic symptoms that include pain, paralysis, and sphincter disturbances. Synonym: **Spondylitis Traumatic Tarda**.

Küntscher Nail (kint'sher/nāl) (n.) A clover leaf–shaped intramedullary nail used for fixation of femoral shaft fractures. Also called a **K-Rod**. Named for Gerhardt Küntscher.

Kutler V-Y Advancement Flap (kut'ler/V-Y/advans'ment/flap) (n.) A surgical technique for the coverage of fingertip amputations that involves use of the injured finger alone. In this technique, two lateral triangular flaps are developed, each with its apex pointing proximally. The flaps are then mobilized toward the tip of the finger to cover the defect.

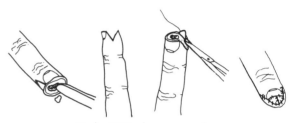

Kutler V-Y advancement flap

K-Wire (K-wir) (n.) See **Kirschner Wire**.

Kyphoscoliosis (kī''fō-skō''lē-ō'sis) (n.) A structural scoliosis associated with a kyphosis. The kyphosis appearance is caused by the rib fullness. The spine is usually lordotic at the apex of the scoliosis deformity.

Kyphosis (kī-fō'sis) (n.) A posterior convex angulation of the spine as evaluated on a lateral view of the spine. Contrast **Lordosis**.

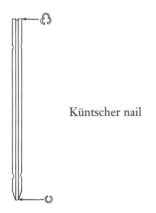

Küntscher nail

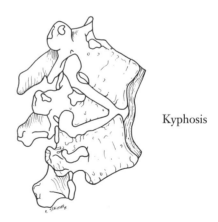

Kyphosis

L

L 1. Lumbar, as in lumbar spine. 2. Left, when written with a circle drawn around the letter.

L1 The first lumbar vertebra or nerve root.

L1-2 The intervertebral space between the first lumbar vertebra and the second lumbar vertebra.

L2 The second lumbar vertebra or nerve root.

L2-3 The intervertebral space between the second lumbar vertebra and the third lumbar vertebra.

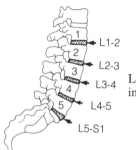

Lumbar vertebrae and intervertebral disk spaces

L3 The third lumbar vertebra or nerve root.

L3-4 The intervertebral space between the third lumbar vertebra and the fourth lumbar vertebra.

L4 The fourth lumbar vertebra or nerve root.

L4-5 The intervertebral space between the fourth lumbar vertebra and the fifth lumbar vertebra.

L5 The fifth lumbar vertebra or nerve root.

L5-S1 The intervertebral space between the fifth lumbar vertebra and the first sacral vertebra.

L Chain (L-chān) (n.)   See **Light Chain**.

Laboratory Medicine (lab′o-rah-to″rē/med′i-sin) (n.) The field of medical study encompassing the use and interpretation of certain tests and observations significant to the diagnosis, prognosis, and treatment of disease. Also known as **Clinical Pathology**.

Labrum (lā′brum) (n.)   A fibrocartilaginous rim attached to the margin of the glenoid cavity that effectively deepens and enlarges the glenoid fossa. This labrum is triangular in cross-section, with a sharp, thin free edge. Also known as **Glenoid Labrum**.

Labyrinthine Reflex (lab″i-rin′thīn/rē′fleks) (n.)   A normal infantile reflex that should disappear by 6 months of age. In this reflex, when a child is prone, tone is reduced and the arms and legs flex. Conversely, if the child is supine, tone is increased and the arms and legs extend.

LAC   Abbreviation for Long Arm Cast.

Lace Stay (lās/stā) (n.)   In shoe terminology, a portion of the upper containing eyelets for lacing.

Laceration (las″er-ā′shun) (n.)   A tear of any body tissue producing a wound with jagged or irregular edges. If the tissue is the skin, the laceration is further described as superficial or full-thickness, depending on the depth of the wound.

Lacertus (lah-ser′tus) (adj.)   Certain fibrous attachments of muscles.

Lacertus Fibrosus (lah-ser′tus/fi-brō-sis) (n.)   The commonly used term for the **bicipital aponeurosis**, which is a band of fibrous tissue running from the distal tendon of the biceps brachii muscle medially across the forearm to insert into the subcutaneous border of the proximal ulna. It forms part of the roof of the cubital fossa and this overlies the median nerve and the brachial artery.

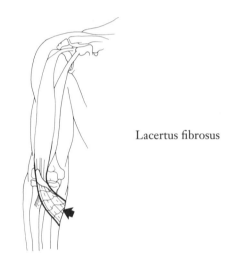

Lacertus fibrosus

Lachman Test (lahk′-man/test) (n.)   An extremely reliable clinical test used in the evaluation of anterior cruciate ligament (ACL) integrity. Place the patient supine on the examining table and stand next to the table on the side of the involved extremity. Hold the distal end of the femur proximal to the patella with one hand and the proximal portion of the tibia, just distal to the tibial tubercle, with the other hand. Hold the knee in approximately 15° to 20° of

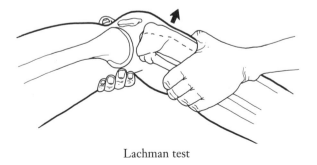

Lachman test

flexion and apply an anteriorly directed force to the back of the proximal tibia while holding the femur posteriorly displaced. If the ACL is intact, a firm endpoint will be present. If the ACL is incompetent, increased anterior translation of the tibia will be present. This should be compared with the uninvolved extremity.

Lackum Jacket (lak′-um/jak′et) (n.) A plaster jacket formerly used in the treatment of scoliosis. Also called **Surcingle Cast**.

Lactated Ringer's (lak′tāt-ed/ring′erz) (n.) See **Ringer's Lactate Solution**.

Lacuna (lah-kū′nah) (n.) A small space, cavity, or depression; pl. lacunae. See **Howship's Lacunae**.

LAD Abbreviation for Ligament Augmentation Device.

Lag Screw (lag/skru) (n.) A screw used to compress (or lag) two bony fragments together by providing purchase in one fragment, while being able to turn freely in the other. Overdrilling the hole in the proximal cortex and tapping the hole in the distal cortex is done to prepare for the correct insertion of a lag screw.

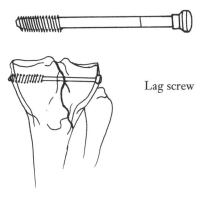

Lag screw

Laguerre's Test (lah-gārz/test) (n.) A means of differentiating hip joint disease from lumbosacral disorders. The patient lies on his or her back with the thigh and knee flexed; the thigh is then abducted and externally rotated. This forces the head of the femur against the anterior capsule of the hip joint. In a positive test, this maneuver produces pain and is indicative of a lesion of the hip joint, iliopsoas muscle spasm, or a sacroiliac lesion, as distinguished from a lumbosacral lesion. See similar **Fabere Test** or **Patrick Test**.

Lambda Chain (lam′dah/chān) (n.) A type of light chain of human immunoglobulins. Lambda chains are distinguished from the other type of light chain (kappa) by the amino acid sequence of the constant region of the light chain in the immunoglobulin molecule.

Lambrinudi Operation (lahm-brē-nū-dē/op-e-ra-shun) (n.) A surgical technique of triple arthrodesis

intended for the treatment of paralytic dropped foot with a fixed equinus deformity. In this procedure, the rest of the foot is dorsiflexed up to the fixed plantar-flexed position of the talus after talar osteotomy. This operation should not be performed on patients younger than 9 years old.

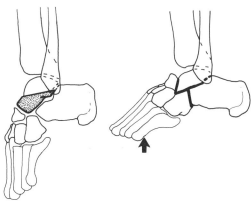

Lambrinudi operation

Lamellar Bone (lah-mel′ar/bōn) (n.) A type of mature bone whose structure is characterized by collagen fibrils running in different directions in each of the multiple layers, known as lamellae. Concentric lamellae constitute the osteons, interstitial lamellae that have been remodeled to form the Haversian system. There are circumferential lamellae in the subperiosteal region.

Lamina (lam′i-nah) (n.) 1. A thin plate or layer of tissue. 2. The flat bone that forms the roof of the posterior vertebral arch. In a typical vertebra, it is a paired structure on either side of the midline that unites posteriorly to form the spinous process. See **Vertebral Lamina**.

Lamina Dura (lam′i-nah/du′rah) (n.) The hard, lining layer of the dental alveoli. It projects radiographically as a radiopaque border of bone surrounding the periodontal ligament. The thickness of the lamina dura varies around different teeth in the same patient, in different areas of the same tooth, and at different times in life. Localized or generalized absence of lamina dura is seen to occur in hyperparathyroidism, osteomalacia, rickets, leukemia, multiple myeloma, Paget's disease, osteoporosis, osteopetrosis, ossifying fibroma, and fibrous dysplasia.

Laminar Airflow System (lam′i-nar/ār′flō/sis′tem) (n.) A system of providing clean air in the operating room by use of high-efficiency particulate air filters. Filtered air flows continuously in a steady, unidirectional straight line, either horizontally or vertically. An increased rate of exchange of air in the room is provided in comparison with ordinary operating room filters. These systems are intended to reduce the number of airborne bacteria-laden particles. In the operating room, units are installed that contain the airflow, filtration, and support systems that isolate the operative field from the periphery of the room. Also called **Clean Air System**.

Laminar Bone (lam'i-nar/bōn) (n.) A type of woven bone that is layered. It is characteristic of the initial subperiosteal diaphyseal and metaphyseal cortices grown during endochondral bone formation. It is interspersed with many vessels and is eventually replaced by mature lamellar bone by progressive remodeling.

Laminar Spreader (lam'i-nar/spred'er) (n.) A self-retaining retractor designed to facilitate exposure of the spinal canal.

Laminectomy (lam"i-nek'to-mē) (n.) The surgical removal of the posterior bony arches of one or more vertebrae in order to expose the neural elements in the spinal cord. Laminectomy allows inspection of the spinal canal as well as identification and removal, of pathologic tissues from the cord and roots.

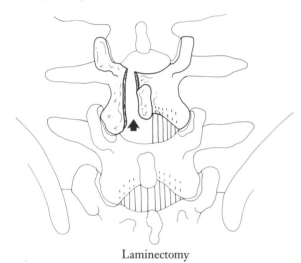

Laminectomy

Laminography (lam"i-nog'rah-fē) (n.) See **Tomography**.

Laminotomy (lam"i-not'ō-mē) (n.) The creation of an opening in one or more laminae.

Landau Reflex (lan-dow'/rē'fleks) (n.) A normal righting reflex found in infants from about 6 to 30 months of age. It is the normal response of an infant held in a horizontal, prone position to maintain a convex arc, with the head raised and the legs slightly flexed. Hold the child prone in your arms, keeping support under the thorax and abdomen, parallel to the floor. First flex and then extend the head, noting the resultant position of the extremities and trunk. The Landau reflex is present when, on passive flexion of the head with the body in extended position, the trunk, arms, and legs go into flexion and, when the head is extended, the trunk and body are brought into the extended position.

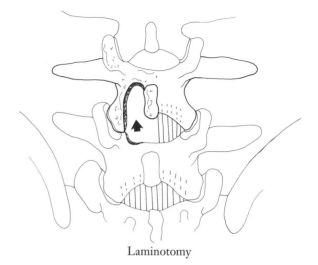

Laminotomy

Landouzy-Déjerine Disease (lan-doo'ze-deh"zher-ēn'/di-zēz') (n.) See **Déjerine-Sota's Disease**.

Landry's Paralysis (lan-drēz'/pah-ral'i-sis) (n.) See **Guillain-Barré Syndrome**.

Landsmeer Ligaments (lahndz-mār/lig'ah-ments) (n.) The retinacular ligaments of the extensor expansion of the finger. The transverse retinacular ligament crosses over the dorsum of the proximal interphalangeal joint and stabilizes it. The oblique retinacular ligaments are paired structures running from the lateral band to the lateral aspect of the distal end of the proximal phalanx. They prevent flexion of the distal interphalangeal joint when the proximal interphalangeal joint is in extension.

Landsteiner's Classification (land'stī-nerz/klas"si-fi-kā'shun) (n.) The classification of human blood groups A, B, AB, and O on the basis of the presence or absence of the two agglutinogens A and B on the erythrocytes.

Langenskiöld Technique (lahn-gen-schōld/tek'nēk) (n.) 1. A surgical resection of bony epiphyseal bridges. 2. A surgical treatment of congenital pseudarthrosis of the fibula. In this procedure, a synostosis between the distal tibial and fibular metaphyses is created to prevent valgus deformity of the ankle.

Langer's Lines (lang'erz/līnz) (n.) Lines of tension within the skin, characteristic for each part of the body, that are caused by the disposition of the cutaneous fibrous tissue. Langer's lines correspond closely to the crease lines on the surface of the skin. They are of particular importance in surgery, as incisions made parallel to them will result in a much narrower scar on healing than will those made perpendicular to them. Synonyms: **Cleavage Line**, **Isotonic Low Tension Lines**.

Langhans-Type Giant Cell (lahng'hahnz/tīp/jī'ant/sel) (n.) A multinucleated giant cell with peripheral, radially arranged nuclei found in certain granulomatous lesions, such as tuberculosis and leprosy.

Laparotomy (lap-ah-rot′ō-mē) (n.) A surgical procedure in which an abdominal incision is made. Referred to commonly as a "Lap."

Lapidus Procedure (lap′i-dus/pro-sē′jur) (n.) 1. Surgical correction of a dorsal bunion. It includes resection of a wedge from the first metatarsocuneiform joint and the first naviculocuneiform joint, if necessary. The tibialis anterior tendon may need to be transferred if it is overactive. The flexor hallucis longus tendon is brought dorsally through a tunnel in the first metatarsal. 2. An operation designed for treatment of severe deformity in the hallux valgus–metatarsus primus varus complex. It is often useful for recurrent varus inclination of the first metatarsal following osteotomy.

Larson Method (lar′sen/meth′ud) (n.) A method of grading the severity of rheumatoid arthritis based on radiographic criteria. The presence or absence of subluxation, dislocation, or ankylosis is not considered in this grading system.

Grade 0: No change. The joints are normal on the roentgenogram.

Grade I: Slight changes. One or more of the following are present: periarticular soft tissue swelling, osteoporosis, slight joint space narrowing. When possible, use for comparison a normal contralateral radiograph or previous radiograph of the involved joint.

Grade II: Definite early changes. Erosions and joint space narrowing. Erosion is obligatory except in the weight-bearing joints.

Grade III: Medium destructive changes. Erosions and joint space narrowing again present but erosion is now obligatory in all joints.

Grade IV: Severe destructive changes. Erosions and joint space narrowing, with bone deformation occurring in the weight-bearing joints.

Grade V: Multilating changes. The original articular surfaces have disappeared and gross bone deformation is present. (Compare with Steinbrocker Scale.)

Larson's Syndrome (lar′senz/sin′drōm) (n.) A congenital disorder in which multiple congenital joint dislocations occur with equinovarus foot deformities, characteristic facial features, and a high incidence of spinal instability.

Larson Procedure (lar′sen/pro-se′jur) (n.) A technique for the surgical repair of a torn anterior cruciate ligament with augmentation using the semitendinosus tendon.

Lasegue Sign (lah-sāg/sīn) (n.) A diagnostic marker in lumbar radiculopathy. With the patient supine and the knee in extension, passively flex the hip. The test is positive if pain is aggravated or reproduced along the course of the sciatic nerve, indicating inflammation of the lower lumbosacral nerve roots. Record the angle of flexion at which pain occurs as well as the site and degree of pain. Also known as **Straight-leg Raising Test**.

Laser (lā′zer) (n.) An acronym derived from Light Amplification by Stimulated Emission of Radiation.

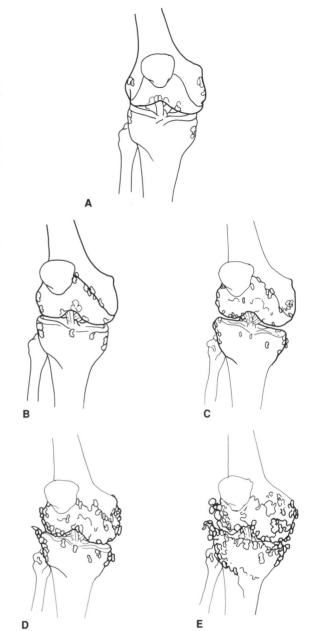

Larson method. **A**, Type 1; **B**, type 2; **C**, type 3; **D**, type 4; **E**, type 5.

Lasers have multiple uses, including the limited application of laser surgery techniques in orthopaedic surgery.

Last (last) (n.) In shoe terminology, a wood, plastic, or metal form or mold over which a shoe is constructed. The last provides the general shape and construction of the shoe with regard to deviations from its longitudinal axis. See also **Straight Last**, **Bunion Last**, and **Reverse Last**.

Lateral (lat′er-al) (adj.)   On the side. Opposite of medial.

Lateral Collateral Ligament of the Knee (lat′er-al/kō-lat′er-al/lig′ah-ment/of/the/nē) (n.)   See **Fibula Collateral of Ligament**.

Lateral Compartment Syndrome (lat′er-al/com-part′ment/sin′drōm) (n.)   A group of disorders involving the lateral compartment of the lower leg. See **Compartment Syndrome**.

Lateral Decubitus Position (lat′er-al/de-kū′bi-tus/po-zish′un) (n.)   A position in which the patient lies on either side. See **Lateral Position**.

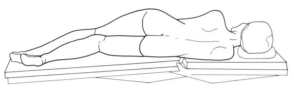

Lateral decubitus position

Lateral Femoral Cutaneous Nerve (lat′er-al/ku-tā′ne-us/nerv) (n.)   A branch of nerve roots L_2 and L_3 and/or the femoral nerve. Supplies sensation to the lateral aspect of the thigh after it pierces the thigh fascia. If traumatized at this point, it produces abnormal sensation to this area. Referred to as **Meralgia Paresthetica**.

Lateral Femoral Subluxation Index (lat′er-al/fem′or-al/sub″luk-sā′shun/in-deks) (n.)   A measurement used for side-to-side comparison of the degree of lateral subluxation of the femoral head from the acetabulum. It is measured by identifying the most medial part of the head of the involved femur and measuring the horizontal distance to the acetabulum. The normal side is then measured at a comparable point, and a ratio is formed by dividing the

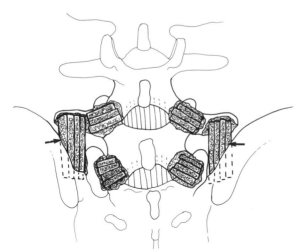

Lateral fusion

involved side by the normal side. The normal ratio is 1.

Lateral Funiculus (lat′er-al/fū-nik′u-lus) (n.)   The lateral mass of fibers on either side of the spinal cord between the anterolateral and posterolateral sulci.

Lateral Fusion (lat′er-al/fū′zhun) (n.)   A technique of spinal fusion in which the arthrodesis of two or more vertebrae is performed by decorticating and bone grafting the lateral surface of the zygapophyseal joint, the pars interarticularis, and the transverse process, either unilaterally or bilaterally.

Lateral Malleolus (lat′er-al/mah-lē′ō-lus) (n.)   The pointed distal extend of the fibula. On its medial surface is an articular surface that makes contact with the lateral side of the talus.

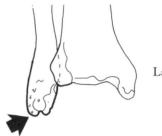

Lateral malleolus

Lateral Meniscus (lat′er-al/me-nis′kus) (n.)   A fibrocartilaginous structure in the lateral compartment of the knee, overlying the lateral articular surface of the tibia. It is more nearly circular than the medial meniscus. Anteriorly, it attaches in the intercondylar area lateral and posterior to the anterior cruciate ligament. Posteriorly, it ends in the intercondylar area anterior to the posterior horn of the medial meniscus. It is loosely attached at the tibial condyle margin, and this attachment is interrupted by the popliteal hiatus through which the popliteus tendon passes. See **Meniscus**.

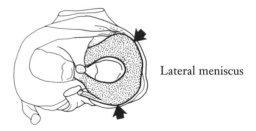

Lateral meniscus

Lateral Oblique (lat′er-al/o-blēk) (n.)   In radiology, a view or projection in which a part is turned a varying number of degrees from a true lateral position in order to more clearly outline a particular structure or organ.

Lateral Patellofemoral Angle (lat-er-al/pah-tel″o-fem′o-ral/ang′g′l) (n.)   A radiographically measured angle used to assess the position of the patella in the

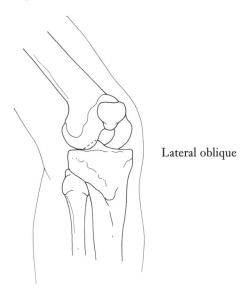

Lateral oblique

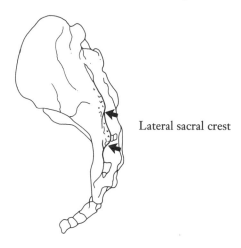

Lateral sacral crest

femoral sulcus. With the patient supine, obtain a tangential view of the knee in 20° of flexion. (The roentgen source is placed below the table top and directed in a cephalad direction with the rays parallel to the anterior border of the tibia and to the patellofemoral interspace. Hold the cassette above the patellofemoral joint, with the plate at 90° to the beam and the patellofemoral joint.) Two lines are then drawn on the radiograph to evaluate the relationship between the femoral sulcus and the patella. The first line joins the peaks of the femoral condyles; the second line joins the two ends of the lateral patellar facet. The angle formed is the lateral patellofemoral angle.

Lateral Pivot Shift Test (lat′er-al/piv′ut/shift/test) (n.) See **MacIntosh Test**.

Lateral Position (lat′er-al/pō-zish′un) (n.) A posture in which the patient is placed on his or her side with both arms forward, knees and hip flexed, with the downside leg more acutely flexed than the other. Weight is borne by the lateral aspects of the patient's ilium as well as the scapula and greater trochanter. This positioning is useful in posterior and lateral approaches to the hip and pelvis. Also called **Lateral Decubitus Position** or **Side-Lying Position**.

Lateral Recumbent Position (lat′er-al/rē-kum′bent/pō-zish′un) (n.) A position in which the patient lies on one side, with the opposite thigh and knee flexed up. Also called **English Position**, **Obstetric Position**.

Lateral Sacral Crest (lat′er-al/sa′kral/krest) A longitudinal excrescence of bone on each side of the posterior surface of the sacrum.

Latex Agglutination Test (lā′teks/ah-gloo″ti-nā′shun/test) (n.) See **Latex Fixation Test**.

Latex Fixation Test (la′teks/fik-sā′shun/test) (n.) A serologic study used in the diagnosis of rheumatoid arthritis. Antigen-coated latex particles agglutinate

with rheumatoid factors in a slide specimen of affected serum or synovial fluid. If positive, the screening slide test is followed by titration. Synonyms: **RA Latex Test**, **RF Test**, **Latex Agglutination Test**.

Latissimus Dorsi Muscle (lah-tis′i-mus/dor′sī/mus′el) (n.) See **Muscle**.

Latitudinal Bone Growth (lat′i-tood′i-nal/bōn/grōth) (n.) Circumferential growth that results in increasing bone diameter.

Lauge-Hansen Classification (lowj-hansen/klas″si-fi-kā′shun) (n.) A detailed binomial classification system for ankle fractures. Four major types of injury are described and several stages within each group. The first word in this system refers to the position of the foot at the time of injury; the second word refers to the direction of the injuring force placed on the foot.

These four groups include supination-external rotation (SE), supination-adduction (SA), pronation-external rotation (PE), and pronation-abduction (PA). The stages are then numbered to denote progressive degrees of damage.

Laugier's Fracture (lō″zhe-āz/frak′chur) (n.) An

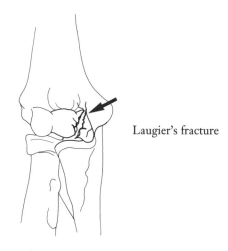

Laugier's fracture

isolated fracture of the trochlea of the distal humerus.

Lavage (lah-vahzh') (v.) The irrigation or washing out of an organ, body cavity, or wound with copious injections of fluid.

Law of Davis (law/of/da'vis) (n.) The law that states that soft tissue remaining uninterruptedly in a loose or lax state will gradually shorten.

Law of Von Schwann (law/of/von-shuahn') (n.) The law that states that the tension of contraction diminishes as muscle fibers shorten.

Lawn Mower Injuries (lawn/mō'er/in'ju-rēz) (n.) A set of injuries involving a rotary lawn mower that creates a "pseudomissile" when a piece of wire or other metal is set into flight by contact with a blade. The wound produced is small, but the "pseudomissile" may become buried in a body cavity or bone as a result of its high kinetic energy. In more direct lawn mower injuries, fragments of dirt, debris, and grass are blown into the wound under pressure. Meticulous attention to debridement of these wounds is mandatory.

LBP Abbreviation for Low Back Pain.

LCPD Abbreviation for Legg-Calvé-Perthes Disease. See **Perthes Disease**.

LD50 The lethal dose of an agent defined as the dose that will kill 50 percent of the population in a test series.

LE Abbreviation for Lower extremity; Lupus Erythematosus.

LE Cell (sel) (n.) A cellular phenomenon characteristically found in patients with systemic lupus erythematosus. Its appearance results from alteration of the nuclei of polymorphonuclear leukocytes by an antinuclear factor present in the gamma globulin fraction. The involved nucleus swells, is extruded from the cell, and is engulfed by another leukocyte. This process continues until one leukocyte may contain several extruded nuclei. The typical LE cell is then an enlarged neutrophilic leukocyte filled with a cytoplasmic inclusion body. This body is an homogeneous globulin mass with a ground-glass appearance; it stains red-purple with Wright's stain. These cells also occur occasionally in other rheumatic diseases, including rheumatoid arthritis, dermatomyositis, and Sjögren's Syndrome.

Le Fort Fracture (lefor'/frak'chur) (n.) 1. A vertical avulsion fracture of the anterior medial aspect of the distal fibula. 2. Bilateral horizontal fractures of the maxilla. They are graded numerically for increasing severity and instability.

Le Fort's Amputation (leforz'/am"pu-tā'shun) (n.) A modification of Pirogoff's amputation through the distal tibia and fibula. The calcaneus is sawed through horizontally instead of vertically, so that the weight-bearing area of calcaneus that is retained is still attached to the same part of the heel that was weight-bearing preamputation.

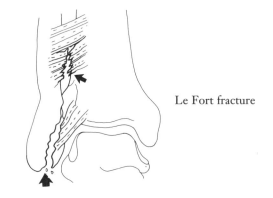

Le Fort fracture

Lead Hand (lēd/hand) (n.) A simple and effective hand-shaped positioning device made of malleable lead, used at the time of surgery to position the hand.

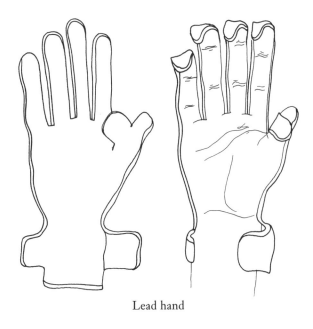

Lead hand

Lead Line (led/līn) (n.) A broad band of radiodensity in the metaphysis of growing bones just adjacent to the epiphyseal plate, caused by lead poisoning. The lead is stored in the metaphyses because the bone is being rapidly laid down in this area.

Lead of a Screw (lēd/of/a/skrū) (n.) The distance through which a screw advances with one turn.

Lead Pipe Fracture (led/pīp/frak'chur) (n.) A fracture in a mature bone in which the cortex is slightly compressed and bulged on one side with a small infraction crack of the opposite cortex. It is so-named for the mechanism of injury—a direct blow with a heavy object, such as a lead pipe.

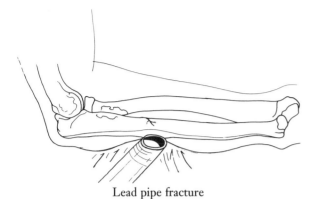

Lead pipe fracture

Leadbetter Maneuver (led'-beter/mah-n͞oo'ver) (n.) A maneuver performed for the reduction of a femoral neck fracture. With the hip flexed to 90°, traction is applied along the axis of the femur (with the hip slightly adducted and the knee flexed to 90°). The hip is then gently internally rotated to engage the fracture fragments. The maneuver is completed by circumducting the hip into abduction and extension. Evaluate the reduction clinically with the heel-palm test by taking the patient's heel, and placing it in the open palm of your hand. If a successful reduction has been obtained, the position of the hip in abduction with slight internal rotation can be maintained. Radiographs should be taken to accurately assess the reduction.

Ledderhose Disease (led-er-hōz/di-zēz') (n.) See **Plantar Fibromatosis**.

Lee-White Clotting Time (lē-wīt/klot'ing/tīm) (n.) A method for estimating the time for blood coagulation. Normal time by this method is 5 to 10 minutes. Synonyms: **Coagulation Time**, **Whole Blood Clotting Time**.

Left Hand Dominance (left/hand/dom'i-nans) (n.) The state in which the left upper extremity is used predominantly for daily activities. Compare to **Right Hand Dominance**.

Leg (leg) (n.) Common name for lower extremity.

Leg Holder (leg/hōl'der) (n.) Any of several com-

mercially available devices used while performing arthroscopy of the knee. It fixes the distal femur to the operating table to allow application of significant varus or valgus stress to the knee joint to maximize exposure. This may obviate the need for a surgical assistant.

Leg Lengthening See **Wagner and Ilizarov Technique** and **Limb Lengthening**.

Leg Ulcer (leg/ul'ser) (n.) Any denudation of the skin between the knee and ankle. Leg ulcers may be acute or chronic, with a varying degree of depth of involvement; they may result from a number of diverse causes, including trauma, insufficient vascularity, and pressure erosion.

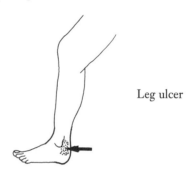

Leg ulcer

Legg-Calvé-Perthes Disease (leg-kal-vā'-per'tez/di-zēz') (n.) An idiopathic osteonecrosis of the femoral capital epiphysis that occurs in children between the ages of 2 and 12 years, but mostly in the 4- to 8-year age group. It occurs more commonly in boys and is bilateral in 10 to 15 percent of cases. Clinically, these patients usually present with a painless limp. On physical examination, decreased range of motion, especially loss of abduction and internal rotation, is found. The radiographic findings, as well as the prognosis and treatment, vary with the extent and stage of involvement. See related **Catterall Classification**. Also called **Perthes Disease**.

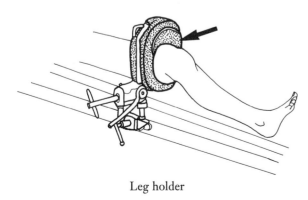

Leg holder

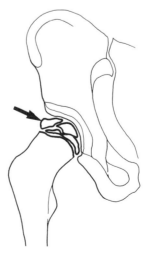

Legg-Calvé-Perthes disease

Lehneis Spiral Orthosis (lā'-nīs/spi'ral/or-thō'sis) (n.) A plastic ankle-foot orthosis used in the bracing of a footdrop. The orthosis slings around the leg in a spiral fashion and cradles the heel. The foot part is applied inside the shoe.

Leinbach Prosthesis (līn'-bahk/pros-the'sis) (n.) A proximal femoral replacement implant that replaces the femoral head, neck, and intertrochanteric areas.

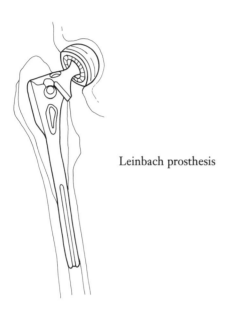

Leinbach prosthesis

Leiomyoma (lī"ō-mī-ō'mah) (n.) A benign tumor of smooth muscle origin.

Leiomyosarcoma (lī"ō-mī"ō-sar-kō'mah) A rare malignant tumor of smooth muscle origin.

Length (length) (n.) 1. The linear distance between two joints. The International System (SI) unit of length is the meter (m). 2. In shoe terminology, the dimension along the last bottom center line, from toe-point to heel-point.

Length of Stay (length/of/stā) (n.) The number of calendar days that elapse between an inpatient's admission and discharge.

Lenox Hill Orthosis (len'ux/hil/or-tho'sis) (n.) A custom-made functional knee brace used for stabilization of ligamentous insufficiency around the knee. The brace was designed at the Lenox Hill Hospital Brace Shop in New York City. Also known as **Lenox Hill Derotation Brace** or **Lenox Hill Brace**.

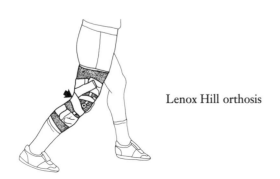

Lenox Hill orthosis

Lentenneur's Fracture (len-tenneur's/frak'chur) (n.) A palmar rim fracture—dislocation of the wrist. Also known as **Volar Fracture**, **Barton's Fracture**, or **Type 2 Smith's Fracture**.

Leprosy (lep'ro-sē) (n.) A chronic, granulomatous infection of skin, peripheral nerves, mucous membranes, and many other organ sites, caused by the acid-fast bacillus *Mycobacterium leprae*. Clinically, pathologically, and immunologically, leprosy has a wide spectrum of manifestations. It may occur as a localized and benign condition that heals spontaneously, or it may become widely disseminated, eventually causing severe deformities. The two principal clinical forms of leprosy are lepromatous and tuberculoid. Extensive skin involvement predominates in lepromatous leprosy, with late and usually partial nerve involvement; tuberculoid leprosy is characterized by neurologic pathology and has much less effect on the skin. Neurologic involvement may result in neuropathic bone and joint destruction. Synonym: **Hansen's Disease**.

Lesion (lē'zhun) (n.) Any wound, trauma, diseased area, or pathologic change in an organ or tissue.

Lesser Trochanter (les'er/tro-kan'ter) (n.) The small, blunt, bony prominence on the medial aspect of the proximal end of the femur at the junction of the femoral neck and shaft. It is joined to the greater trochanter by the intertrochanteric line anteriorly and the intertrochanteric ridge posteriorly. It is the site of insertion of the conjoined iliopsoas tendon. Compare to **Greater Trochanter**.

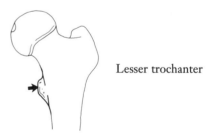

Lesser trochanter

Lesser Tuberosity (les'er/too"be-ros'i-tē) (n.) A small bony prominence on the anterior aspect of the proximal humerus, just proximal to the surgical neck, that is separated from the greater tuberosity by the intertrabecular groove. It is the site of insertion of the subscapularis tendon. It has a distal prolongation, known as the crest of the lesser tubercle, that is the insertion site of the teres major muscle. Also known as the **lesser tubercle**. Compare to **Greater Tuberosity**.

Letterer-Siwe Disease (let'ter-er-si'we/di-zēz') (n.) A disease considered to be one of the histiocytoses.

This is a rare disease seen in infants with a fulminant course. The bony lesions are of minor concern because of the life-threatening visceral lesions. See **Hand-Schüller-Christian Disease**.

Leukemia (loo-kē′mē-ah) (n.) A malignant neoplasm of blood-forming organs, characterized by diffuse replacement of bone marrow with proliferating leukocyte precursors, abnormal numbers and forms of immature white cells in circulation, and infiltration of lymph nodes, the spleen, liver, and other sites. Orthopaedic manifestations include diffuse bone and joint pains, which may be secondary to bone infarct or subperiosteal infiltrates, osteopenia, and osteolytic lesions on radiographs. In affected children, other findings include diffuse periosteal new bone formation, leukemic lines, and rarely, osteosclerosis and arthritis.

Leukemic Lines (loo-kē′mik/līnz) (n.) A radiographic finding in older children with leukemia that may represent a disturbance in endochondral bone formation. These are radiolucent lines in the metaphysis adjacent to the epiphyseal plate.

Leukens' Wrinkle Test (loo-kenz/ring′k′l/test) (n.) A clinical test for finger denervation. The affected hand is totally immersed in a basin of warm water (40°C) for 20 to 30 minutes. The skin of denervated fingers does not wrinkle or shrivel as does normal skin when immersed in warm water, thus, the observation of smooth skin reflects denervation. See **O'Riain's Wrinkle Test**.

Leukocyte (loo′kō-sīt) (n.) A white blood cell. Five morphologic types are identified: neutrophils, monocytes, lymphocytes, eosinophils, and basophils.

Lever Arm (lev′er/arm) (n.) The linear distance over which a load is applied to produce a moment.

Levi-Weill Disease (le′vē-wīl/di-zēz′) (n.) A type of mesomelic dwarfism in which there is usually stunting but not severe dwarfing. It is transmitted as an autosomal dominant trait. Also known as **Dyschondrosteosis**.

Lewin Test (leu′-in/test) (n.) A clinical maneuver used in the evaluation of low back pain and radicular pain. It is a variation of a sciatic stretch test. Have the patient stand with his or her back to you; then cautiously force first the right and then the left knee into complete extension. Both knees are then straightened at the same time. The test is positive if any of these movements are accompanied by pain, with the knee snapping back into flexion to relieve the stretch.

Lewin's Lasegue Rebound Test (le′-vinz/lah-sāg/re′bownd/test) (n.) A clinical manuever used to diagnose sciatica. With the patient supine, locate the exact point where the straight leg raising maneuver produces either recognizable muscle resistance or pain. At this point, allow the leg to drop suddenly onto a pillow. This act will aggravate the back and sciatic pain and increase the degree of muscle spasm. Also called **Rebound Test**.

LFA Abbreviation for Low Friction Arthroplasty.

LHD Abbreviation for Left Hand Dominant.

Lhermitte's Sign (lār′mēts/sīn) (n.) A nonspecific sign elicited in association with cervical cord lesions. A sensation resembling an electrical discharge in the limbs and trunk is experienced when the neck is flexed.

Libman's Test (lib′mans/test) (n.) A test used in evaluation of the pain threshold in the individual patient. It involves pressure on both the tip of the mastoid bone and styloid process and then grading the patient's response to determine sensitivity to painful stimuli.

Lidocaine (lī′do-kān) (n.) A short-acting local anesthetic agent that also has antiarrhythmic and anticonvulsant properties. Marketed as **Xylocaine**.

Ligament (lig′ah-ment) (n.) A cord, band, or sheet of fibrous connective tissue, linking two or more bones, cartilages, or other structures together. A ligament imparts stability, usually to a joint, preventing excessive motion in certain directions.

Ligament Augmentation Device (lig′ah-ment/awg-men′tā-shun/de-vīs′) (n.) Any synthetic material used as a stent to augment the repair or reconstruction of a ligament specifically. Abbreviated **LAD**. See **Kennedy**.

Ligament Calcaneofibular (lig′ah-ment/kal-ka″nē-ō-fib′u-lar) (n.) A cordlike structure that extends from the lateral malleolus downward and backward to the calcaneus. It is part of the lateral ligament of the ankle joint.

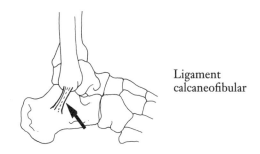

Ligament calcaneofibular

Ligament Fibular Collateral (lig′ah-ment/fib′u-lar/ko-lat′er-al) (n.) A cordlike structure that extends from the lateral epicondyle downward and backward to the head of the fibula. Also called **Lateral Collateral Ligament of the Knee**.

Ligament of Humphry (lig′ah-ment/of/hum′frē) (n.) The inconstant, posterior, lateral meniscofemoral ligament that runs anterior to the posterior cruciate ligament.

Ligament of Struthers (lig′ah-ment/of/stru-therz) (n.) An inconstant fibrous arch that extends from a supracondylar process to the medial epicondyle of the humerus. Because the median nerve and bra-

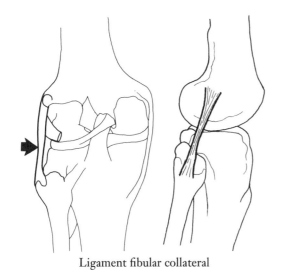

Ligament fibular collateral

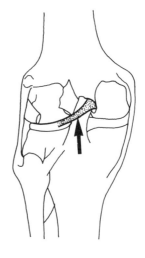

Ligament of Wrisberg

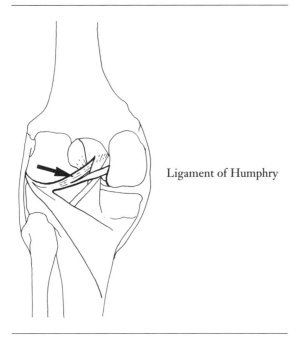

Ligament of Humphry

chial artery will run beneath this ligament, this may be a source of compression for them.

Ligament of Wrisberg (lig′ah-ment/of/rīs′berg) (n.) The inconstant, posterior, lateral meniscofemoral ligament that runs posterior to the posterior cruciate ligament.

Ligament Tibial Collateral (lig′ah-ment/tib′ē-al/ko-lat′er-al) (n.) A thickening in the medial part of the knee joint capsule. It has a deep and a superficial portion. Both take origin from the distal femur. The superficial part bridges the tibial condyle and hollow and inserts into the tibia. The deep part is deltoid-shaped and inserts into the margin of the tibial condyle. Also called the medial collateral ligament of the knee. See **Tibial Collateral Ligament**.

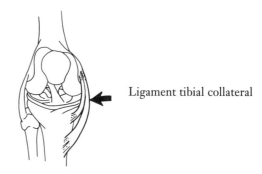

Ligament tibial collateral

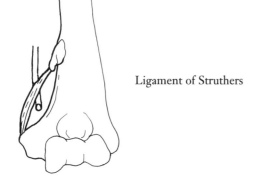

Ligament of Struthers

Ligamentotaxis (lig′ah-men-tō-tak′sis) (n.) A term used to suggest that intra-articular fractures can be successfully reduced by applying traction to the capsular and ligamentous structures around the joint.

Ligamentum Flavum (lig′ah-men′tum/flā′vum) (n.) The yellow-colored ligament connecting the laminae of two adjacent vertebrae. It is a paired structure, located on either side of the spinous process, that extends laterally to blend with the capsule of the joints between the superior and interior articular processes. It runs from the anterior surface of the lamina above, to the leading edge of the lamina below.

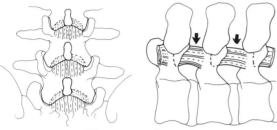

Ligamentum flavum

Ligamentum Nuchae (lig'ah-men'tum/nū-kā) (n.) The large, broad ligament at the back of the neck, which extends from the edges of the external occipital crest bilaterally to the tips of the spinous processes of the cervical vertebrae.

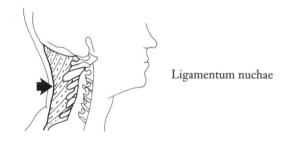

Ligamentum nuchae

Ligamentum Teres (lig'ah-men'tum/ter'-ēz) (n.) An intracapsular ligament of the hip that arises from the margins of the acetabular notch and the lower border of the transverse acetabular ligament and ends in the fossa of the femoral head. Also known as the **Capitis Femoris Ligament** or **Round Ligament of the Hip Joint**.

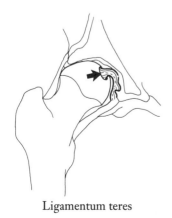

Ligamentum teres

Ligation (lī-gā'shun) (n.) The application of a ligature.

Ligature (lig'ah-chūr) (n.) A thread or strand of material tied around a blood vessel to occlude the lumen and to prevent its bleeding. Commonly called a **Tie**.

Light Chain (līt/chān) (n.) A structural subunit of an immunoglobulin. It is a polypeptide with a molecular weight of 23,000. There are two antigenic types of light chains—*kappa* and *lambda*. Each monomeric immunoglobulin molecule has two light chains. Abbreviated **L Chain**.

Light Microscope (līt/mī'krō-skōp) (n.) A microscope that uses light waves as its illumination source.

Light Source (līt/sōrs) (n.) In orthopaedic surgery, an instrument, remote from the operative field, that provides light for the fiberoptic cable used in arthroscopy.

Lignac-Fanconi Syndrome (lē'-nyahk/fahn-kō-nē/sin'drom) (n.) See **Fanconi Syndrome**.

LLC Abbreviation for Long Leg Cast.

LLE Abbreviation for Left Lower Extremity.

Limb (lim) (n.) An extremity, such as an arm or a leg.

Limb-Girdle Muscular Dystrophy (lim-ger'd'l/mus'ku-lar/dis'tro-fē) (n.) A form of muscular dystrophy, usually transmitted as an autosomal recessive trait, generally less severe than the more common Duchenne type. There is great variability in the age of onset, but it usually begins in the second or third decade of life. The later the age of onset, the more rapid the progression of the disease.

The initial symptoms may present as weakness around the shoulders or the pelvis. The creatinine phosphokinase level is not usually markedly elevated. Electromyographic studies show a myopathic pattern; nerve conduction studies are normal. Intellectual level remains normal in this type of muscular dystrophy. Cardiac involvement is very rare.

There is considerable variation in severity and rate of progression. Severe disability is usually present by 20 years after onset, and death usually occurs before the age of 40 years.

Limb Lengthening (lim/length'en-ing) (n.) Any procedure that results in increased length of an extremity. Apparatuses used for this include **Wagner's Limb Lengthening Apparatus** and the **Iliazarov Frame**.

Limb Salvage (lim/sal'vij) (n.) The process whereby an extremity is maintained through resection and replacement with grafts and implants in a limb that would otherwise be amputated because of extensive trauma or malignant neoplasm. This may require one or a series of complex surgical procedures.

Limb Shortening (lim/short'en-ing) (n.) Any procedure that results in decreased length of an extremity. Examples include resection of a piece of bone or epiphyseal arrest.

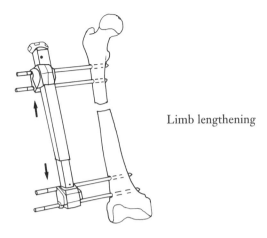

Limb lengthening

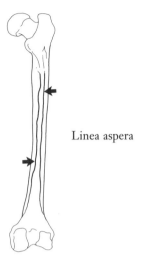

Linea aspera

Limbus (lim′bus) (n.) A fibrous, resilient, sharp-edged, crescent-shaped tissue attached to the bony rim of the acetabulum and the transverse acetabular ligament. Its free edge cups around the head of the femur to increase the stability of the hip joint. Also known as the **Acetabular Labrum**.

Limbus Annulare (lim′bus/an′u-lare) (n.) An inconstant mass of bone situated at the anterosuperior margin of a vertebral body. It results from failure of fusion of the primary and secondary ossification centers.

Limbus Vertebra (lim′bus/ver′te-brah) (n.) The result of an anterior intraosseous herniation of vertebral disc material. In the child, a defect in the anterior margin of the vertebral body adjacent to the end-plate may be seen radiographically. The defect is easily demonstrated by discography with contrast media.

Lindner's Sign (lind′-nerz/sīn) (n.) A diagnostic maneuver in sciatica. With the patient recumbent or seated, place the hip in 90° of flexion with the knee in extension and then effect enforced passive flexion of the neck. In a positive test, pain occurs in the lumbar region and in the sciatic nerve distribution.

Linea Aspera (lin′e-ah/ah′-spā-ra) (n.) A thickened, longitudinal crest on the posterior surface of the shaft of the femur. It is most prominent in the middle third of the femur, where lateral and medial lips are developed. The nutrient foramen of the femur is located along the linea aspera. This crest is an insertion site for the thigh adduction muscles and the origin of much of the vastus musculature.

Linear Fracture (lin′ē-ar/frak′chur) (n.) A narrow fracture line extending nearly parallel to the long axis of a bone that is not displaced.

Liniment (lin′i-ment) (n.) A medicinal preparation that is rubbed into the skin or applied on a surgical dressing.

Lining (līn′ing) (n.) In shoe terminology, a material that covers the inner portions of the shoe in contact with the foot, providing a smooth surface.

Linton's Angle of Inclination (lin-tonz/ang′g′l/of/in″kli-nā′shun) (n.) The angle of inclination of fractures of the neck of the femur as measured on the AP radiograph. The angle is obtained from the intersection of a line drawn through the fractured surface of the distal fragment with a line perpendicular to the longitudinal axis of the femoral shaft. See **Pauwel's Classification**.

Lipid (lip′id) (n.) Any of a group of organic fat or fatlike compounds that are insoluble in water but soluble in alcohol. This includes fats, steroids, phospholipids, carotenes, phosphatides, and other compounds.

Lipid Storage Diseases (lip′id/stōr′ij/dĭ-zēz′ez) (n.) A group of rare, hereditary diseases characterized by the accumulation of lipid complexes due to congenital enzyme deficiencies. These compounds accumulate in the cells of the reticuloendothelial system in various organs, including the liver, the spleen, the lymph nodes, and bone marrow. The major sites of storage differ in different diseases, and the lipids that accumulate are chemically different. Examples include **Gaucher Disease**, **Niemann-Pick Disease**, and the **Amaurotic Familial Idiocies**. Also known as **Lipidoses**.

Lipidoses (lip″i-dō′sēs) (n.) See **Lipid Storage Diseases**.

Lipochondrodystrophy (lip′ō-kon-drō-dis′trō-fē) (n.) See **Hurler Syndrome**.

Lipoma (li-pō′mah) (n.) A benign fatty tumor that is usually soft, generally lobulated, and surrounded by a thin but definite capsule.

Liposarcoma (lip″o-sar-kō′mah) (n.) A malignant tumor of fat cell origin. It is the most common malignant tumor of soft tissue and is found most often in the extremities. Symptoms are usually related to the pressure of a mass.

Lipping (lip′ing) (n.) The formation of a liplike structure, such as the small osteophyte formation on the margins of the articular surfaces of bones. Also called **Bony Spur Formation** or **Spurring**.

Lippmann's Auscultatory Test (lip'-manz/aws-kul″ ah-to″re/test) (n.) A maneuver used to evaluate the presence of a fracture and then to follow the development of bony union. Apply a stethoscope bell to the affected bone and a percussing finger over a bony prominence on the other side of a suspected or known fracture, and compare the sound so elicited with that produced by the same procedure on the uninjured contralateral limb. Sound alteration constitutes the criterion of the test. If you apply auscultatory percussion across two bony prominences separated by a long bone, the sound heard through the stethoscope will have a characteristic "osteal" quality—loud, high-pitched, and moderately resonant. Pitch and quality changes result from free vibration of separate fragments, and accordingly signify complete fracture or incomplete union. Appreciable diminution in sound intensity indicates poor conduction and reflects absence of end-to-end contact. Also called **Osteopathy**.

Lisfranc Amputation (lis-frahnk'/am″pu-tā'shun) (n.) An amputation or disarticulation of the foot through the tarsometatarsal joints. Named for the surgeon general to Napoleon.

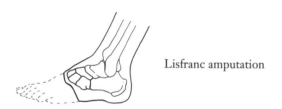

Lisfranc amputation

Lisfranc Fracture (lis-frahnk/frak'chur) (n.) A fracture or fracture dislocation through the tarsometatarsal joints. Named for the Surgeon General to Napoleon. Also called **Lisfranc Fracture Dislocation**.

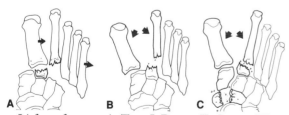

Lisfranc fracture. **A**, Type I; **B**, type II; **C**, type III.

Lisfranc Joint (lis-frahnk/joint) (n.) 1. The tarsometatarsal joints. 2. The articulation between the midfoot and the forefoot. The intrinsic stability of this joint depends on the recessed position of the base of the second metatarsal and the trapezoidal shape of the bases of the middle three metatarsals, which form a "Roman Arch" configuration. Ligamentous stability is provided by transverse metatarsal ligaments and Lisfranc's ligament. Additional stability is provided by the soft tissues in the plantar aspect of the foot.

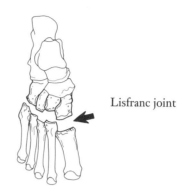

Lisfranc joint

Lisfranc Ligament (lis-frahnk'/lig'ah-ment) (n.) A large ligament that extends between the medial cuneiform and the base of the second metatarsal to help reinforce the bony stability of Lisfranc joint.

List (list) (n.) A tendency to lean to one side, used to refer to the laterally bent trunk. The position may be caused by muscle contraction pulling the spine to one side.

Lister's Tubercle (lis'terz/too'ber-k'l) (n.) A small, bony eminence in the middle of the dorsal aspect of the distal end of the radius. It is the most prominent point on the posterior aspect of the wrist. Its medial side is excavated, providing a shallow shelf and a deep groove for the passage of the tendon of the extensor pollicis longus.

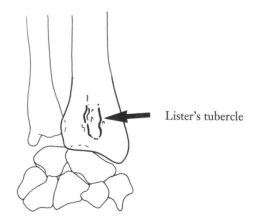

Lister's tubercle

Liter (lē'ter) (n.) The metric measurement of fluid volume. It equals 1000 mL, 1.0567 qt.

Lithotomy Position (li-thot'ō-mē/pō-zish'un) (n.) The patient lies supine with the hips and knees flexed and the thighs abducted and externally rotated. Stirrups may be used to support the feet and legs. Also called the **Dorsosacral Position**.

Little Finger (lit′l/fing′ger) (n.) Common name for the fifth digit of the hand.

Little Leaguer's Elbow (lit′l/lē′gerz/el′bō) (n.) A commonly used term applied to a group of clinical disorders that occur as a result of elbow overuse in growing children. Characterized by pain, tenderness, and swelling on the medial epicondylar area. These injuries appear to be due to repetitive overhand throwing activities that cause a valgus strain to be applied to the elbow, creating compression medially and traction laterally. The spectrum of injury includes osteochondral injuries of the capitellum (with or without associated loose bodies), injury and premature closure of the proximal radial epiphysis (sometimes with associated radial head overgrowth), and inflammation or even avulsion of the medial epicondyle. The management of these injuries depends on the stage at which they are diagnosed.

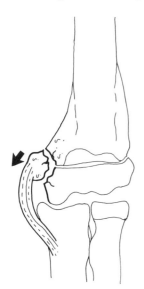

Little Leaguer's elbow

Little Leaguer's Shoulder (lit′l/lē′gerz/shōl′der) (n.) A term applied to a stress fracture of the proximal humeral physis as a result of repetitive throwing.

Little's Disease (lit′lz/di-zēz′) (n.) See **Cerebral Palsy**.

Liverpool Prosthesis (li′-ver-pūl/pros-thē′sis) (n.) A type of two-part unconstrained elbow implant.

Lizar's Line (li′zarz/līn) (n.) A superficial landmark useful in identifying the level at which several arteries exit the pelvis posteriorly. The line is drawn from the posterior superior spine of the ilium to the midpoint between the tuberosity of the ischium and the greater trochanter. The gluteal artery emerges at the point of junction of its superior and middle third; the sciatic and pubic arteries emerge at the point of junction of its middle and lower thirds.

Lloyd's Sensory Fiber Classification (loydz/sen′sor-ē/fī′ber/klas″si-fi-kā′shun) (n.) A Roman numeral classification system sometimes used for sensory neurons.

Number	Origin	Fiber Type
I a	Muscle spindle, annulospiral ending	A
b	Golgi tendon organ	A
II	Muscle spindle, flower-spray ending; touch, pressure	A
III	Pain and temperature receptors; some touch receptors	A
IV	Pain and other receptors	Dorsal root C

Load (lōd) (n.) The application of a force and/or moment (torque) to a structure. The units of measure are newtons (poundforce) for the force, and newton meters (foot-poundforce) for the moment.

Load-Deformation Curve (lōd/de″for-ma′shun/kurv) (n.) A graphic representation used in biomechanics to demonstrate the response of a structure to a given load.

Lobster Claw Hand (lob′ster/klaw/hand) (n.) A developmental anomaly in which a deep central cleft is present in the hand due to the absence of the central ray or rays. The border rays are partially or completely preserved. There is a wide variation of associated soft-tissue involvement. Also called **Cleft Hand**.

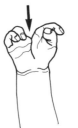

Lobster claw hand

Lobster Claw Foot (lob′ster/klaw/fut) (n.) See **Cleft Foot**.

Local Anesthesia (lo′kal/an″es-the′ze-ah) (n.) The direct administration of an agent to tissues to induce absence of sensation in a small area of the body while the patient remains awake. The agents are applied either topically or injected into the desired area.

Local Anesthetic (lo′kal/an″es-thet′ik) (n.) A substance used to reduce or eliminate neural sensation, specifically pain, in a limited area of the body. Local anesthetics act by blocking transmission of nerve impulses. Many drugs are available for local anesthesia; they are classified as members of the alcohol–ester or the amineamide family.

Local Flap (lo′kal/flap) (n.) A type of flap graft obtained from the immediate vicinity of the soft-tissue defect to be covered. Local flaps include advancement flaps, simple transpositions, Z-plasty, and fillet grafts.

Localizer Cast (lo'kal-īz"er/kast) (n.) See **Risser Localizer Cast**.

Locking (lok'ing) (n.) A mechanical blockage of joint movement.

Lodine (lo-dine) (n.) A proprietary brand of etodolac. A nonsteroidal anti-inflammatory drug.

Lofstrand Crutch (lawf-strand/kruch) (n.) A metal forearm crutch, made from an adjustable aluminum alloy. Attached is a U-shaped metal cuff (arm-band), to accommodate the forearm just below the elbow, and a rubber- or plastic-covered handgrip. The lower end of the crutch is protected by a rubber tip. Also known as the **Canadian Crutch** or the **English Cane**.

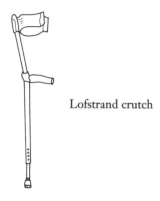

Lofstrand crutch

Long Arm Cast (long/arm/kast) (n.) A circular cast applied for immobilization of the upper extremity. It extends from the lower level of the axillary fold to the proximal palmar crease, with the thumb and fingers remaining free at the level of the metacarpophalangeal joints. The cast is applied with the elbow flexed to 90°. The degree of rotation of the forearm and the position of the wrist vary with the specific fracture under treatment. Compare with **Short Arm Cast**.

Long Arm Splint (long/arm/splint) (n.) A splint used to immobilize a number of injuries involving the elbow and forearm. It is applied to the posterior surface of the upper extremity, extending from the proximal palmar crease to the lower level of the axillary fold. An elastic wrap or gauze bandage may be used to hold the slab of plaster in place. The positioning of the extremity depends on the nature of the underlying injury being treated.

Long Bone (long/bōn) (n.) Any elongated bone of the extremities that consists of a diaphyseal shaft and wider epiphyseal, articulating ends.

Long Extensor Tendons (long/eks-ten'sor/ten'dunz) (n.) The extrinsic finger or toe tendons that function in digital extension.

Long Head of Biceps (long/hed/of/bī'seps) (n.)

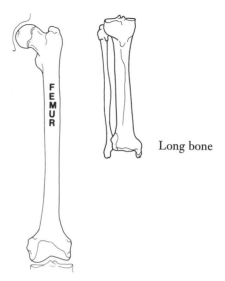

Long bone

That part of the biceps brachii muscle that originates as a rounded tendon from the supraglenoid tubercle of the scapula and runs intracapsularly.

Long Leg Brace (long/leg/brās) (n.) A knee-ankle-foot orthosis—one that extends from the thigh to, and including, the foot. See **Knee-Ankle-Foot Orthosis**.

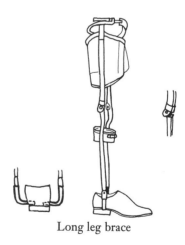

Long leg brace

Long Leg Cast (long/leg/kast) (n.) A circular cast applied for immobilization of the lower extremity. It extends from the junction of the upper and middle third of the thigh to the base of toes. The foot is usually held at a right angle. The version of the foot and the degree of knee flexion placed depend on the nature of the underlying injury and whether the patient is to bear weight on the cast. Compare with **Short Leg Cast**.

Long Leg Splint (long/leg/splint) (n.) A splint used to immobilize the entire lower extremity by applying a posterior plaster slab from the thigh to the base of the toes. The slab is secured in place with an elastic wrap or gauze bandage. The splint may only immobilize the knee, be made of cloth with posterior bones for stiffness, and secured to the extremity with velcro straps.

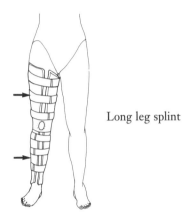

Long leg splint

Long-Term Health Care Facility (long-term/helth/ kar/fah-sil′i-tē) (n.) A facility for inpatient care, with an organized medical staff, medical staff equivalent, or medical director, and continuous nursing service under professional nurse direction. In addition to providing medical needs dictated by diagnoses, such a facility also provides comprehensive preventive, rehabilitative, social, spiritual, and emotional inpatient care to individuals requiring long-term health care as well as to those convalescent patients not in a stable stage of illness or an acute episode of illness who still have a variety of medical conditions with varying needs.

Longitudinal (lon″ji-tū′di-nal) (adj.) Pertaining to the long axis of a structure or part.

Longitudinal Arch of the Foot (lon″ji-tū′di-nal/arch/ of/the/fut) (n.) The anteroposterior arch of the foot formed by the tarsal and metatarsal bones. The arch consists of an inner, or medial, longitudinal arch and an outer, or lateral, longitudinal arch.

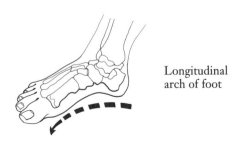

Longitudinal arch of foot

Longitudinal Axis (lon″ji-tū′di-nal/ak′sis) (n.) A line passing through a bone or segment, around which the parts are symmetrically arranged, and which lies in both the frontal and sagittal planes.

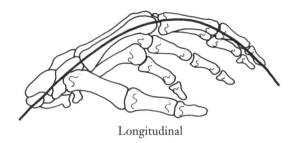

Longitudinal

Longitudinal Bone Growth (lon″ji-tū-di-nal/bōn/ grōth) (n.) The growth of bone that results in increasing length.

Loose Bodies (lo͞os/bod′ēz) (n.) Any separated cartilaginous, osteocartilaginous, or osseous structure found loose within a joint cavity. See related term, **Joint Mice**.

Loosening (lo͞o′sen-ing) (n.) A term used in reference to the loss of fixation of an implant. For example, loosening of a femoral stem is defined roentgenographically by a demonstrated change in the mechanical integrity of the load-carrying cemented femoral component. Definite signs of loosening include a shift in position of the prosthesis or cement, or a fracture of either the prosthesis or cement. Probable loosening is suspected when a continuous radiolucent line is present at the prosthesis-bone or cement-bone interphase.

Looser Lines (lo͞os′er/līnz) (n.) Narrow, transverse lines of rarefaction seen on roentgenograms, which extend incompletely across a bone. They are typically perpendicular to the long axis of the bone and are bilaterally symmetrical. They represent small insufficiency fractures, or regions of pathologic healing, which occur in certain conditions, such as osteomalacia, Paget's disease, and rickets. Also known as **Milkman's Lines**, **Pseudo-fracture Lines**, **Looser's Transformation Zones**, or **Looser's Umbauzonen**.

Lordoscoliosis (lor″dō-skō″lē-ō′sis) (n.) A lateral curvature of the spine associated with either an increased anterior curvature or decreased normal posterior angulation in the sagittal plane for that area of the spine.

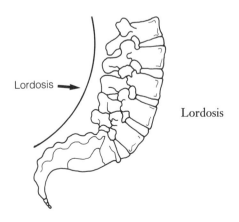

Lordosis

Lordosis

Lordosis (lor-dō'sis) (n.)   1. An anterior angulation of the spine in the sagittal plane. Contast to **Kyphosis**. 2. The angle formed by perpendicular lines drawn from the superior end-plate of L1 and the inferior end-plate of L5 on the lateral radiograph.

Lorenz Bifurcation Osteotomy (lor'ents/bi"fur-ka' shun/os"te-ot'o-me)   An osteotomy of the proximal end of the femur to stabilize a congenitally dislocated hip. The distal portion is placed into the acetabulum. A rarely used procedure.

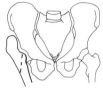
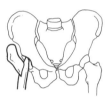

Lorenz bifurcation osteotomy

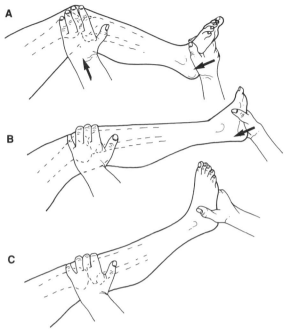

Losee test. **A**, 40° flexion; **B**, 10° flexion and internal rotation; **C**, full extension.

Lorenz Plaster Cast (lor'ents/plas'ter/kast) (n.)   A type of hip spica cast that holds the hips in a position of 90° of abduction-flexion and lateral rotation. The cast extends from the nipple line down to the ankles on both sides, leaving the ankles and feet free.

Lorenz Position (lor'ents/pō-zish'un) (n.)   In this position, the thighs are placed with the hips in 90° to 100° of flexion, 70° of abduction, and full external rotation. Also called the **Frog-Leg Position**.

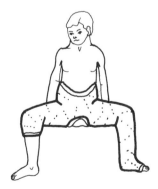

Lorenz position and plaster cast

Lorne-Miller Prosthesis (lorn/mil-er/pros-thē'sis) (n.)   A type of unconstrained surface replacement elbow arthroplasty.

Lorry Driver's Fracture (lorē/drī-verz/frak'chur) (n.)   See **Chauffeur's Fracture**.

Losee Test (lō-zē/test) (n.)   A maneuver used in the evaluation of anterolateral rotatory instability of the knee. This is one variation of the pivot shift phenomenon. With the patient supine, grasp the foot or ankle of the affected extremity with one hand while placing your other hand over the patella, and your thumb beneath the fibular head. First, flex the knee to approximately 40° and then extend the knee, allowing the foot to rotate internally and producing a valgus thrust to the knee. Push the head of the fibula forward with your thumb during extension of the knee, using the fingers over the patella to provide counterpressure. In a positive test, you can palpate and observe the lateral tibial plateau subluxate anteriorly. The patient may recognize this moment as the sensation of the knee "going out." See **Pivot Shift Test**.

Lotion (lō'shun) (n.)   A liquid preparation for external application to the body. Lotions usually have a cooling, soothing, or antiseptic action.

Lottes Nail (lot-ēz/nāl) (n.)   A semirigid, triflanged, nonreamed intramedullary nail; used for closed nailing of the tibia.

Lou Gehrig's Disease (lū/gār-igz/di-zēz') (n.)   See **Amyotrophic Lateral Sclerosis**.

Louis, Angle of (lū-is/ang'g'l/of) (n.)   The angle formed by the body of the sternum and the manubrium. See **Angle of Louis**.

Love's Pin Test (luvz/pin/test) (n.)   A clinical maneuver used to diagnose a glomus tumor. First, press the point of a steel pin against the skin very near the periphery of the lesion, without causing pain. If the pin is then pressed over the lesion, an attack of excruciating pain occurs.

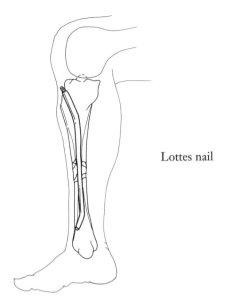

Lottes nail

Lovett Scale (luv′-et/skāl) (n.)   A method of evaluation of muscle strength.
Gone: No contraction felt.
Trace: Muscle can be felt to tighten, but cannot produce movement.
Poor: Produces movement with gravity eliminated but cannot function against gravity.
Fair: Can raise part against gravity.
Good: Can raise part against outside resistance as well as against gravity.
Normal: Can overcome a greater amount of resistance than a "good" muscle.

Low Friction Arthroplasty (low/frik′shun/ar′thro-plas″tē) (n.)   The term coined by Charnley to describe a total hip arthroplasty that combines a small, prosthetic femoral head (22 mm) with a socket of maximum external diameter and thick walls to reduce frictional torque. Abbreviated **LFA**.

Low Median Nerve Palsy (lōw/mē′de-an/nerv/pawl′zē) (n.)   An injury to the median nerve incurred in the forearm, distal to the origin of the anterior interosseous nerve. This results in paralysis of the opponens pollicis, the flexor pollicis brevis, and the first and second lumbrical muscles, with an important functional loss of thumb opposition. There is also a loss of sensation over the sensory distribution of the median nerve in the hand.

Low Molecular Weight Dextran (lō/mo-lek′u-lar/wāt/dek′stran) (n.)   A colloid solution that can effectively expand plasma volume, decrease blood viscosity, and increase microcirculatory flow. It is used in the treatment of hypovolemic shock and for prophylaxis of thromboembolic phenomena. See also **Dextran**.

Low Radial Nerve Palsy (lō/rā′dē-al/nerv/pawl′zē) (n.)   An injury to the radial nerve that occurs distal to the origin of the branches to the radial wrist extensors and the brachioradialis muscles, resulting in paralysis of the digital extensors and the long thumb abductor. The sensory loss is inconsistent because there is usually no autonomous sensory zone. Compare with **High Radial Nerve Palsy**.

Low Ulnar Nerve Palsy (lō/ul′nar/nerv/pawl′zē) (n.)   An injury to the ulnar nerve that occurs in the distal forearm or near the wrist, resulting in paralysis of all ulnar-innervated intrinsic muscles of the hand. Functionally, weakness of pinch and grip are noted. Clawing of the ring and little fingers will result from the unopposed pull of the flexor digitorum profundus to these fingers. There is also a sensory loss over the sensory distribution of the ulnar nerve in the hand.

Low-Velocity Missile (lō/ve-los′i-tē/mis″l) (n.)   Any muzzle velocity under 2,500 ft/sec.

Lowell's S-C Lines (lō-elz/SC/līnz) (n.)   A method for the roentgenographic evaluation of the reduction of femoral neck fractures. In any radiographic projection of an anatomic femoral head-neck junction, the convex outline of the femoral head will meet the concave outline of the femoral neck and form an image of an "S" or reversed "S" curve. In the radiographic projection of a femoral neck fracture that is not anatomically reduced, this image is changed to a "C" curve on one side, with angulation of the opposite cortical outline.

Lowenstein Position (lō′-wen-stīn/pō-zish′un) (n.)   The position to obtain a frog-lateral radiograph of the hips in which the hips are flexed to 90° and then maximally abducted.

Lower Back Pain (lō′er/bak/pān) (n.)   A nonspecific term applied to any of a variety of conditions whose primary symptom is pain in the lumbosacral region.

Lower Extremity (lō′er/eks-trem′i-tē) (n.)   In human anatomy, the lower limb, including the hip, the thigh, the leg, the ankle, and the foot.

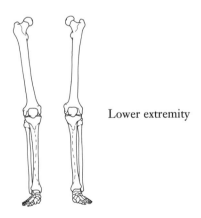

Lower extremity

Lower Leg (lō′er/leg) (n.)   Commonly referred to that part of the lower extremity distal to the knee.

Lower Motor Neuron (lō′er/mō′tor/nū′ron) (n.)   An efferent neuron whose nucleus lies either in the anterior horn of the spinal cord or in the corresponding gray matter of the brain stem (for the cranial nerves). The axons lie in a peripheral nerve and terminate at the end-organ that the nerve innervates.

Lower Motor Neuron Disease (lō′er/mō′tor/nu′ron/di-zēz′) (n.) An injury to the cell bodies or axons of lower motor neurons. It is characterized clinically by weakness accompanied by flaccidity, atrophy, diminution of the deep tendon reflexes, and absence of pathologic reflexes. In addition, there are frequently vasomotor and trophic changes. During the period of degeneration, fasciculations may be noted in involved muscles and fibrillations recorded electromyographically.

Lower Plexus Injury (lo′er/plek′sus/in′ju-re) (n.) See **Klumpke Paralysis**.

LP Abbreviation for Lumbar Puncture.

L-Rod Abbreviation for **Luque Rod**.

Lubricant (loo′bri-kant) (n.) Matter whose function is to allow two bearing surfaces to move on one another with decreased wear and friction.

Ludington's Sign (lud-ing-tonz/sīn) (n.) A clinical test of the integrity of the biceps tendon. If the long head of the biceps tendon is ruptured, it fails to contract when the patient interlocks his or her hands over his or her head.

Ludloff's Sign (lood′lawfs/sīn) (n.) A clinical sign present after fracture of the lesser trochanter. It is characterized by swelling and ecchymosis found at the base of Scarpa's triangle. With Ludloff's sign, it is noted that when the patient is supine, partial flexion of the extended limb may be possible owing to the action of the tensor fasciae and rectus femoris muscles. However, when the patient is in the sitting position, this action cannot be performed owing to insufficiency of the iliopsoas muscle after fracture of the lesser trochanter.

Lues (lū′ĕz) (n.) Any serious infectious disease or plague; commonly used in reference to syphilis.

Luetic (lū′et′ik) (adj.) Syphilitic.

Lumbago (lum-bā′go) (n.) A nonspecific term for a dull, aching pain of the lower back with or without radiation into the buttock and posterior thigh.

Lumbalgia (lum-bal′je-ah) (n.) Low back pain with or without radiation into the buttocks and posterior thigh. See **Lumbago**.

Lumbar Curve (lum′bar/kurv) (n.) A spinal curvature whose apex is between L1 and L4. Also known as **Lumbar Scoliosis**.

Lumbar Disc Syndrome (lum′bar/disk/sin′drōm) (n.) Disorders seen in association with a herniated disc in the lumbar spine; usually characterized by low-back pain and sciatica. The typical history is one of dull, aching low-back pain, developing after a bending or lifting strain. Pain in the lower buttock or radiating to the lower extremity may develop at the

same time but generally develops later in the course of the acute episode. The essential physical findings result from nerve root irritation and muscle spasm caused by disc protrusion. Although these findings vary greatly from patient to patient, flexion and extension of the spine are limited to some degree, the normal lumbar lordosis may be absent, or a list may be evident. Sensory loss, motor weakness, or decreased deep tendon reflexes may occur, and a careful neurologic examination is necessary. The straight-leg raising test or other signs of nerve root irritation are usually present in this syndrome.

Lumbar Index (lum′bar/in′deks) (n.) See **Vallois Lumbar Index**.

Lumbar Plexus (lum′bar/plek′sus) (n.) A nerve plexus formed by the anterior primary rami of the first four lumbar nerves, together with a communication from the twelfth thoracic nerve. It is located deep to the psoas major muscle and lies anterior to the upper lumbar transverse processes. The greater part of the second nerve, third nerve, and upper part of the fourth nerve divide into small anterior and large posterior divisions. The posterior divisions unite to form the femoral nerve whereas the anterior divisions combine to form the obturator nerve. Other branches of the lumbar plexus include the iliohypogastric nerve, the ilioinguinal nerve, the genitofemoral nerve, the lateral femoral cutaneous nerve, the accessory obturator nerve, and the muscular branches to the quadratus lumborum, psoas major, psoas minor, and iliacus muscles.

Lumbar Puncture (lum′bar/pungk′chur) (n.) An invasive procedure in which a hollow needle with a stylet is introduced into the lumbar subarachnoid space of the spinal canal. A sample of cerebrospinal

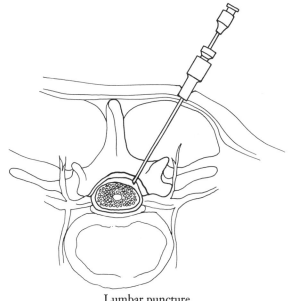

Lumbar puncture

fluid may be obtained for diagnostic purposes; manometric measurements can be made, or injection of medications, anesthetic agents, or contrast media may be given intrathecally. Also known as a **Spinal Tap**.

Lumbar Scoliosis (lum′bar/skō″lē-ō′sis) (n.) See **Lumbar Curve**.

Lumbar Triangle (n.) See **Petit's Triangle**.

Lumbar Vertebrae (lum′bar/ver′te-brē) (n.) The five vertebrae in the lower part of the back, located between the thoracic vertebrae and the sacrum. They are the largest of the unfused vertebrae and are distinguished by the absence of transverse foramina and costal facets. Referred to as L_1, L_2, L_3, L_4, L_5.

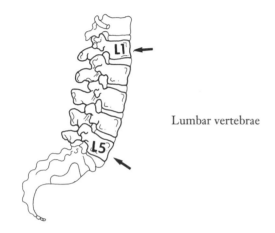

Lumbar vertebrae

Lumbarization (lum″ber-i-zā′shun) (n.) A congenital anomaly of the lumbosacral junction. The first segment of the sacrum is partially or completely separate from the remainder of the sacrum. The sacrum thus consists of only four segments and what appears to be an additional articulating lumbar vertebra. Compare to **Sacralization**.

Lumbering Gait (lum′ber-ing/gāt) (n.) A gait with heavy and clumsy movements, usually seen in individuals with (and as a result of) excessive weight and bulk.

Lumbocostal (lum″bō-kos′tal) (adj.) Pertaining to the lumbar region (loin) and ribs.

Lumbodorsal (lum″bō-dor′sal) (adj.) Pertaining to the thoracic and lumbar regions of the back.

Lumbosacral (lum″bō-sa′kral) (adj.) Pertaining to the lumbar and sacral regions of the back.

Lumbosacral Angle (lum″bō-sa′kral/ang′g′l) (n.) The angle between L5 vertebra and the sacrum. It is measured on a lateral radiograph of the lumbosacral spine by the intersection of two lines drawn through the mid-body of L5 and the sacrum, perpendicular to their end-plates. The normal angle averages about 135°. The lumbosacral angle will vary depending on the load on the spine and the position at the time of

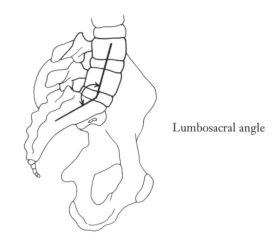

Lumbosacral angle

measurement (recumbency versus sitting versus standing).

Lumbosacral Corset (lum″bō-sa′kral/kor′set) (n.) A flexible, lumbosacral orthosis that consists of a cloth garment that encircles the torso and hips; it is adjusted circumferentially with hooks, laces, or velcro in the front, back, or sides.

Lumbosacral Curve (lum″bō-sa′kral/kurv) (n.) A lateral curvature with its apex at L5 or below. Also known as **Lumbosacral Scoliosis**.

Lumbosacral Disk (lum″bō-sa′kral/disk) (n.) The intervertebral disk between the fifth lumbar vertebra and the sacrum.

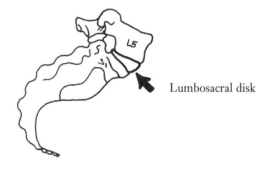

Lumbosacral disk

Lumbosacral Instability (lum″bō-sa′kral/in-sta-bil′ĭ-tē) (n.) A mechanical instability of the lower spine, possibly due to relaxation of ligaments or to faults in the neural arch or articular facets. It may be demonstrated radiographically on flexion-extension or lateral bending views of the lumbosacral junction.

Lumbosacral Joint (lum″bō-sa′kral/joint) (n.) The articulation between the fifth lumbar and the first sacral vertebrae. Also known as the **Lumbosacral Junction**.

Lumbosacral Orthosis (lum″bō-sa′kral/or-tho′sis) (n.) A brace intended for immobilization or stabilization of the lumbosacral spinal region. These or-

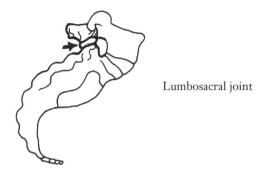

Lumbosacral joint

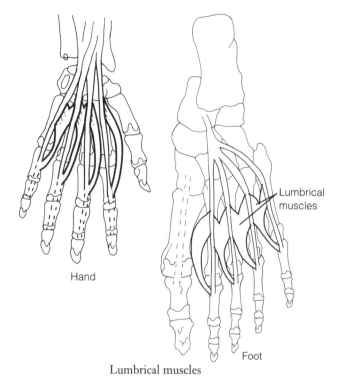

Lumbrical muscles

Hand

Foot

Lumbrical muscles

thoses may be flexible, as in lumbosacral corsets, or they may be rigid.

Lumbosacral Plexus (lum″bō-sa′kral/plek′sus) (n.) The combination of all the ventral primary divisions of the lumbar, sacral, and coccygeal nerves. Usually referred to as separate lumbar and sacrococcygeal plexi. The lumbar and the sacral plexi supply the lower limb. The sacral nerves also supply the perineum through the pudendal plexus and the coccygeal area through the coccygeal plexus. See **Lumbar Plexus** and **Sacral Plexus** for individual details.

Lumbosacral Scoliosis (lum″bō-sa′kral/skō″lē-ō′sis) (n.) See **Lumbosacral Curve**.

Lumbosacral Series (lum″bō-sa′kral/sēr′ēz) (n.) A series of radiographs obtained of the lumbar spine. It includes antero-posterior, lateral, oblique, and coned-down lateral views of the lumbosacral region.

Lumbosacral Sprain (lum″bō-sa′kral/sprān) (n.) A ligamentous injury of the lumbosacral region.

Lumbosacral Strain (lum″bō-sa′kral/strān) (n.) A musculature injury about the lumbosacral region.

Lumbrical Bar (lum′bri-kal/bar) (n.) A flat bar used in making hand orthoses that is placed across the dorsal aspect of the proximal phalanges (II to V) to prevent their extension.

Lumbrical Muscles (lum′bri-kal/mus′els) (n.) The wormlike intrinsic muscles of the hand or foot that arise in association with the flexor digitorum profundus tendons or flexor digitorum longus tendons, respectively, attached to the metacarpals and metatarsals. See **Muscle**.

Lumbrical Plus Finger (lum′bri-kal/plus/fing′ger) (n.) An abnormal posturing of digit that results from relative overpull of a lumbrical muscle in comparison to the deep flexor tendon distal to its origin. This tension produces unwanted secondary extension of the proximal and distal interphalangeal joints. To test for the condition, first demonstrate that full passive flexion of all finger joints is present. Then observe that, on strong flexion or gripping with the distal interphalangeal joints, the involved finger will show incomplete flexion and active partial extension of the interphalangeal joints. See **Intrinsic Plus Deformity** and **Intrinsic Tightness Test**.

Lumen (lū′men) (n.) The cavity, duct, canal, or channel within a vessel or tubular organ.

Lunate Bone (loo′nāt/bōn) (n.) One of the carpal bones of the wrist that is crescent-shaped. The lunate bone lies between the triquetrum and the scaphoid and articulates with the capitate bone distally and the radius proximally.

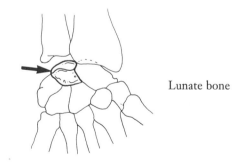

Lunate bone

Lupus Erythematosus (lū′pus/er″-i-thē″-ma-tō-sus) (n.) See **Systemic Lupus Erythematosus**.

Luque Rods (lūk/rodz) (n.) A type of segmental spinal instrumentation system for spinal fixation in the correction of scoliosis and in the treatment of fractures and instability. Sublaminar wires are used at each spinal level and are tied to contoured, L-shaped stainless steel rods. The L-bend of the rod is anchored into a spinous process or the pelvis. This fixation system usually obviates the need for prolonged recumbency or external immobilization postoperatively. Abbreviated **L-Rod**. Invented by Eduardo Luque of Mexico City.

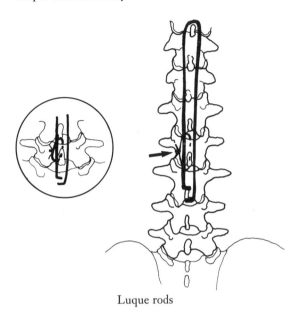

Luque rods

Luschka's Joint (lush′kahz/joint) (n.) Amphiarthrodial joints found in the lower cervical spine from C2 to C7. They are formed just lateral to the intervertebral discs, between the uncus of the inferior vertebra and the lateral inferior surfaces of the superior vertebra. These joints are independent of the disk cartilage and the lateral articulations. They are clinically important if degenerative changes result in overgrowth and osteophyte formation that can impinge on the neural foramina. Also known as **Uncovertebral Joints**.

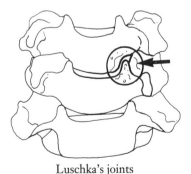

Luschka's joints

Lust's Peroneal Sign (lusts/per″ō-nē′al/sīn) (n.) One of the clinical signs used to diagnose tetany. Tap the peroneal nerve at the lateral aspect of the fibula just below the fibula head. A positive test is evi-

denced by dorsal flexion and abduction of the foot. See **Chvostek's Sign** and **Trousseau's Sign** for other signs of tetany.

Luxatio Erecta (luk-sa′shē-ō/e-rek′ta) (n.) An inferior, subglenoid dislocation of the head of the humerus. The humerus is locked in 110° to 160° of abduction, and the head of the humerus may be palpable on the lateral aspect of the chest wall.

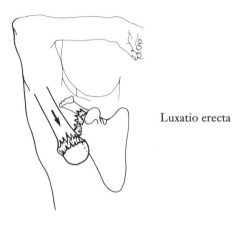

Luxatio erecta

Luxation (luk-sā′shun) (n.) A complete or partial dislocation. Compare with **Subluxation**.

Lyme Arthritis (līm/ar-thrī′tis) (n.) An arthritic condition of infectious origin caused by a spirochete that is transmitted by the minute tick, *Ixodes dammini*. It usually begins in summer with a characteristic rash—erythema chronicum migrans—that may be followed weeks to months later by nervous system, heart, or joint involvement. After periods of intermittent oligoarticular arthritis or migratory polyarthritis, some patients may develop chronic joint involvement accompanied by pannus formation and cartilage erosion. Early administration of penicillin may prevent or minimize the arthritic involvement. The diagnosis is confirmed by serologic tests. The condition was originally described in the community of Lyme, Connecticut.

Lymph (limf) (n.) A transparent, usually slightly yellow fluid, present within the vessels of the lymphatic system. Lymph is about 95 percent water; the remainder consists of plasma proteins and other chemical substances normally contained in blood plasma but at a lower percentage. Its cellular component is chiefly lymphocytes and a few red blood cells.

Lymph Node (limf/nōd) (n.) A discrete, encapsulated aggregate of lymphoid tissue found at intervals along the lymphatic system. It consists of an outer cortical and an inner medullary portion, ranging in size from 1 to 25 mm (some reactive nodes are even larger). Groups of nodes are normally found in many parts of the body, e.g., in the groin and the axilla. These nodes function as filters for the lymph and also in the production of lymphocytes.

Lymphadenography (lim-fad″e-nog′rah-fē) (n.) Roentgenography of lymph nodes after injection of a contrast medium into a lymphatic vessel.

Lymphadenopathy (lim-fad″e-nop′ah-thē) (n.) Any condition or disease that affects one or more lymph nodes.

Lymphangiogram (lim-fan″jē-o-gram) (n.) The radiographic film produced by lymphangiography.

Lymphangiography (lim-fan″jē-og′rah-fē) (n.) The roentgenographic imaging of lymphatic vessels after introduction of a contrast medium or radioisotope tracer.

Lymphangioma (lim-fan″jē-ō′mah) (n.) A benign tumor derived from lymph vessels that usually occurs in skin and subcutaneous tissues. If it contains smooth muscle fibers, it is called a lymphangiomyoma.

Lymphangiosarcoma (lim-fan″je-o-sar-kō′mah) (n.) A rare malignant tumor of lymph vessel origin. It usually occurs in the extremities with chronic lymphedema.

Lymphangitis (lim-fan″ji′tis) (n.) The inflammation of lymphatic vessels, sometimes of infectious origin.

Lymphapheresis (lim″fah-fe-rē′sis) (n.) A technique of lymphocyte removal using venipuncture and passage of blood through automated separators. See **Apheresis**.

Lymphedema (lim″fe-dē′mah) (n.) Swelling of a part due to an accumulation of lymph in the tissues, especially the subcutaneous tissues, secondary to obstruction of lymphatic vessels or lymph nodes. Lymphedema may be divided into primary and secondary forms. *Primary* or *idiopathic* edema may be subdivided into three groups: the congenital type, which is present at birth; *lymphedema praecox*, appearing after birth to age 35 years; and *lymphedema tarda*, seen after the age of 35 years. *Secondary lymphedema* may be secondary to an inflammatory process or it may be noninflammatory, resulting from some extralymphatic process, such as com-

pression by direct invasion of lymphatics or lymph nodes by neoplasms, surgical extirpation of nodes, fibrosis resulting from radiation therapy, and scars. Synonyms: **Elephantiasis, Lymphostasis**.

Lymphocyte (lim′fō-sīt) (n.) A type of white blood cell, characterized by a rounded or kidney-shaped nucleus, formed in lymphoid tissue. These cells produce immunoglobulins and function in the expression of cellular immunity.

Lymphogranuloma Venereum (lim″fo-gran″u-lo′mah/ven-ē-rē-um) (n.) A systemic infectious disease caused by the obligate intracellular bacterium *Chlamydia trachomatis*. Usually transmitted by sexual contact. A small, evanescent, usually genital, primary lesion is followed by regional lymphadenopathy.

Lymphoma (lim-fō′mah) (n.) Any neoplastic disorder of lymphoreticular origin, usually malignant. Neoplastic processes arise in the lymph nodes or the lymphoid tissues of parenchymal organs. Lymphomas are classified by cell type of origin and are described by acuteness or chronicity and then by diffuse or nodular histologic patterns. Commonly, these disorders are grouped as **Hodgkin's Lymphoma** and **Non-Hodgkin's Lymphoma**. Clinically, bone involvement by these tumors is uncommon, and primary lymphomas of bone are extremely rare.

Lyophilization (lī-of″i-li-zā′shun) (n.) The process of quick-freezing a substance and then rapidly dehydrating the frozen material in a high vacuum in order to isolate a solid substance from solution. Also called **Freeze Drying**.

Lysis (lī′sis) (n.) The disintegration or destruction of a cell or tissue.

Lysosome (lī′sō-sōm) (n.) A cytoplasmic organelle consisting of a membrane-bound sac of hydrolyzing enzymes.

Lysozyme (lī′sō-zīm) (n.) A hydrolyzing enzyme that is destructive to cell walls of certain bacteria.

Lytic (lit′ik) A suffix word element used to denote destruction. Pertaining to lysis.

M

M-Band (m-band) (n.) In muscle histology, the darker central line in the H Zone of a sarcomere. Synonym: **M Line**.

Maceration (mas″er-ā′shun) (n.) The softening of a solid by soaking or immersion in a liquid.

Machine Screw (mah-shēn′/skrū) (n.) A usually self-tapping screw that is completely threaded from head to tip. The end of the screw has a flute that cuts the threads as the screw is inserted. Machine screws are used for internal fixation of bone. Compare with an **AO Screw**.

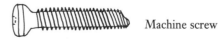
Machine screw

Mackenzie's Amputation (mah-ken′zēz/am″pu-tā′shun) (n.) A modification of Syme's amputation at the ankle joint. The skin flap is taken from the side of the foot instead of the plantar aspect.

MacIntosh Over-the-Top Reconstruction (mak′intosh/over-the-top/re′kon-struk′shun) (n.) A technique for the reconstruction of the anterior cruciate ligament in which the cruciate substitute is passed posteriorly through the intercondylar notch, over the top of the lateral femoral condyle, and then secured in the area of the lateral intermuscular septum and the epicondyle. Synonym: **Over-the-Top Cruciate Ligament Repair**.

MacIntosh Technique (mak′in-tosh/tek′nēk) (n.) A surgical procedure for the extraarticular reconstruction of anterior cruciate ligament insufficiency. A distally based strip of iliotibial band is deeply looped back to the fibular collateral ligament and then secured near the insertion on Gerdy's tubercle.

MacIntosh Test (mak′in-tosh/test) (n.) A clinical test for anterolateral rotatory instability of the knee that represents one of the pivot–shift phenomena. Extend the patient's knee and, with the foot turned inward, apply a valgus stress to the proximal tibia. Slowly flex the knee. In a positive test, the lateral tibial plateau gradually subluxates forward as it comes out of the "locked home" position, owing to anterior cruciate ligament insufficiency. As the knee is pushed into further flexion, the tibia reduces suddenly, owing to the pull of the iliotibial tract as it moves posteriorly. Like weight-bearing, the valgus thrust to the knee enhances the speed of the reduction and accentuates the reduction. This is also known as the **MacIntosh Lateral Pivot Shift Test**. See **Pivot Shift Test**.

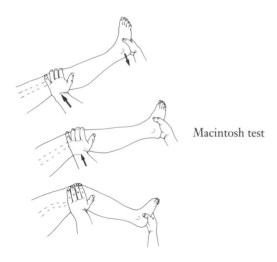

Macintosh test

Macrodactyly (mak″ro-dak′ti-lē) (n.) A rare congenital anomaly of gigantism in fingers or, less commonly, toes. There is enlargement of all structures of the involved digit.

Macroglobulin (mak″ro-glob′ū-lin) (n.) A large protein molecule of the globulin series found in the blood that functions as an antibody. Synonym: **Immunoglobulin**.

Macroglobulinemia (mak″ro-glob″u-li-nē′mē-ah) (n.) A hematologic disorder characterized by an abnor-

mal form of immunoglobulin in the blood. See **Waldenström's Macroglobulinemia**.

Macromolecule (mak″rō-mol′e-kūl) (n.) A molecule of very high molecular weight; specifically, proteins, nucleic acids, polysaccharides, and their complexes.

Macule (mak′ūl) (n.) A circumscribed, nonelevated discoloration on the skin up to 1 cm in diameter. It may be described by its appearance, for example, "depigmented" or "erythematous." Compare with **Papule**.

Madelung Deformity (mahd-luhng/de-for′mi-tē) (n.) A volar and ulnar subluxation of the carpus on the radius. The wrist deformity may arise from several etiologies. The distal end of the ulna appears prominent on the dorsal aspect of the wrist, and the ulna attains greater length overall. This results in limited wrist dorsiflexion and a loss of supination of the forearm.

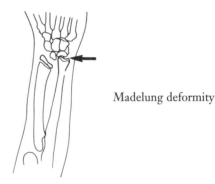

Madelung deformity

Madura Foot (mad′ū-rah/fut) (n.) A progressive, destructive, tropical infection of the foot that produces chronic inflammation. It is caused by various filamentous fungi (e.g., Madurella) and certain bacteria of the genera Nocardia and Streptomyces. Madura foot is characterized by nodules, abscesses, draining sinuses, and marked edema. Synonyms: **Maduramycosis of the Foot, Mycetoma**.

Madurella (mad″u-rel′ah) (n.) One of several fungi that can cause maduramycosis See **Mycetoma, Madura Foot**.

Maffuci's Syndrome (mah-fu′chēz/sin′drōm) (n.) A rare, congenital disorder characterized by enchondromatosis in association with hemangiomatosis.

Magilligan Technique (mah-gil-i-gan/tek′nēk) (n.) A radiographic evaluation of femoral anteversion. Place the patient supine on either a fracture or a roentgenographic table. Hold the femur in neutral rotation and comfortable abduction, parallel to the table surface; maintain the hip in this position throughout the examination. First, take an AP roentgenogram and determine the cervicofemoral angle, which is designated O. Next, take a lateral roentgenogram by placing the x-ray tube between the thighs, pointed at the hip joint, and place the cassette against the lateral side of the trunk, parallel to the long axis of the femoral neck. Determine the apparent angle of anteversion, designated as B, from this roentgenogram. Then, to determine the true angle of anteversion, use the radiograph of Magilligan with the trigonometric function of the O and B angles. The true anteversion always equals or exceeds the apparent angle of anteversion.

Magnetic Resonance Imaging (mag-net′ik/rez′o-nans/im′ah-jing) (n.) An imaging technique that employs radio frequency waves and a strong magnetic field to produce clinically useful images. It is derived from the density and magnetic properties of nuclei rather than nuclear mass, which is the case with conventional x-rays. No ionizing radiation is used. It is based on the principle that nuclei with an odd number of protons or neutrons exhibit spin. To induce spin, a strong static magnetic field and then a radiofrequency pulse are applied; a relaxation or return to equilibrium then occurs. The proton density and the relaxation times provide the basis for image formation. Different pulse sequences are designed to measure different factors in the tissue to be imaged. The resulting image gives excellent soft tissue contrast without bony artifact, and there is no known biologic hazard (as is found with radiation imaging). The major disadvantage for musculoskeletal imaging is the lack of cortical bone detail, but there is excellent imaging of intramedullary bone. Abbreviated **MRI**.

Magnification Radiography (mag″ni-fi-kā′shun/rā″-de-og′rah-fē) (n.) A roentgenographic technique that can provide accurate and detailed assessment of a limited area by providing an enlarged, sharper x-ray image. This requires three techniques: using a smaller focal spot, decreasing the distance between the focal spot and the object, and increasing the distance between the object and the image.

Magnuson Procedure (mag′nu-son/pro-sē′jur) (n.) A surgical technique for systematic debridement or "housecleaning" of the knee through an anteromedial incision.

Magnuson-Stack Procedure (mag′nu-son/stak/pro-sē′jur) (n.) A surgical treatment of recurrent anterior dislocation of the shoulder. It involves laterally advancing the anterior capsule and the subscapularis tendon.

Magnuson's Test (mag′nu-sonz/test) (n.) An evaluation procedure for low back pain intended to differentiate patients with true pain from malingerers. Mark the pain site as indicated by the patient. Then, distract the patient by performing a relevant examination elsewhere. Resume the back examination. The site of real pain will remain unchanged.

Maisonneuve Fracture (ma″zo-nev′/frak′chur) (n.) An external rotation injury of the ankle that produces a fracture of the proximal third of the fibula. This is associated with tearing of the distal tibiofibular ligament and interosseous membrane. On the medial side of the ankle, a disruption of the deltoid ligament or fracture through the medial malleolus occurs.

Major (mā′jer) (adj.) Greater in size or importance.

Major Amputation (mā′jer/am″pu-tā′shun) (n.) Any traumatic or surgical amputation through a long bone of the upper or lower extremity; a disarticulation at the hip or shoulder joint.

Major Curve (mā′jer/kerv) (n.) In describing scoliosis, the larger curve. It is usually structural.

Major Thread Diameter (mā′jer/thred/dī-am′e-ter) (n.) The largest diameter of a screw thread in any given plane normal to the screw axis.

Mal (mahl) Prefix meaning bad or ill.

Malacia (mah-lā′she-ah) (n.) Abnormal softening of a part, organ, or tissue (e.g., bone or cartilage). Also used as a suffix.

Malaise (mal-āz′) (n.) A general, conditional symptom described as a feeling of uneasiness, discomfort, and weakness. It often marks the onset of a disease process.

Malgaigne Fracture (mal-gān′/frak′chur) (n.) An eponym commonly used for complex fractures and dislocations of the pelvis in which there are breaks

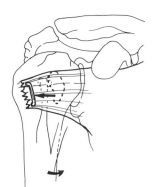

Magnuson Stack procedure

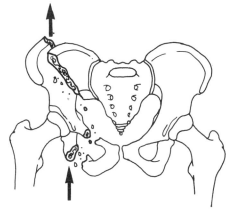

Malgaigne fracture. *Arrows,* Two vertical fractures of the pelvic ring.

in the anterior and posterior portions of the pelvic ring. This is an unstable injury with vertical fractures produced by a vertical shear force. Anteriorly, there may be fractures through the inferior and superior pubic rami or a disruption of the pubic symphysis, or both. Posteriorly, there is an ipsilateral fracture through the ilium and the sacrum or disruption of the sacroiliac joint. As a result of these fractures, the intervening fragment, which contains the hip joint, is potentially displaceable. Also known as a **Double Vertical Fracture of the Pelvis.**

Malignancy (mah-lig′nan-sē) (n.) 1. Of or pertaining to a malignant condition. 2. The common reference to a cancerous neoplasm.

Malignant (mah-lig′nant) (adj.) Severe, usually fatal. Used to describe any medical condition that is resistant to treatment and/or is rapidly progressive; a neoplasm that will grow uncontrollably and metastasize.

Malignant Hyperthermia (mah-lig′nant/hī″per-ther′mē-ah) (n.) A heritable disorder characterized by a rapid rise in body temperature (up to 39° to 42°C) after the use of inhalation anesthetic agents. This is an emergency condition; its mortality has been decreased markedly by the use of dantrolene sodium.

Malingering (mah-ling′ger-ing) (n.) A willful, conscious, and deliberate attempt by a patient to distort, feign, and exaggerate the degree of physical and psychologic difficulties present. Possibility of secondary gain may be a motivating factor.

Malleolar (mal-e′ō-lar) (adj.) Of or pertaining to a malleolus.

Malleolus (mah-le′ō-lus) (n.) One of the three rounded bony protuberances of the ankle. The lateral malleolus, which is at the distal end of the fibula, and the medial malleolus, which is at the distal end of the tibia, are both palpable subcutaneously on either side of the ankle. The posterior malleolus is at the posterior, distal aspect of the tibia and is not palpable. See **Medial** and **Lateral Malleolus.**

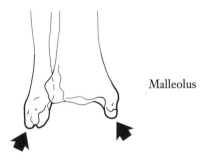

Malleolus

Mallet Finger (mal′et/fing′ger) (n.) A deformity of the finger in which the distal interphalangeal joint has an extension lag; this results from a disruption of the extensor tendon mechanism at or near its site of insertion into the distal phalanx. The patient can passively (but not actively) extend the distal phalanx at the distal interphalangeal joint. The injury is caused by a sharp blow on the end of the finger, as when struck by a baseball (hence its popular name *baseball finger*), or it may result from an open laceration. A radiographic examination is needed to rule out the association of an avulsion fracture.

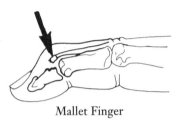

Mallet Finger

Mallet Toe (mal′et/tō) (n.) A flexion deformity at the distal interphalangeal joint of any of the lesser toes.

Malmo Splint (mal′mō/splint) (n.) See **Von Rosen Splint.**

Malposition (mal″pō-zish′un) (n.) An abnormal position or placement. Used in reference to limb alignment or fracture fragments.

Malpractice (mal-prak′tis) (n.) Inappropriate medical treatment due to negligence, ignorance, or criminal intent.

Malpractice Insurance (mal-prak′tis/in′shur-ans) (n.) The insurance carried by a physician or other health care professional to provide payment if that professional is found guilty of malpractice.

Malreduction (mal″re-duk′shun) (n.) The reduction of fracture fragments into an abnormal position or alignment.

Malum Coxae Senilis (mal′um/kok′sā/se′nil-is) (n.) An outdated term for osteoarthritis of the hip.

Malunion (mal-ūn′yon) (n.) A common reference to a malunited fracture.

Malunited Fracture (mal′ū′nī-ted/frak′chur) (n.) A fracture whose fragments have healed in an abnormal position or placement. Also known as a **Malunion.**

Mandible (man′dĭ-b′l) (n.) The lower jawbone. The bone comprises the tooth-bearing, horseshoe shaped body and two upright plates of bone, the rami, each of which is surmounted by two processes, an anterior process called coronoid and a posterior, or condyloid process and articulates with the temporal bone.

Manipulation (mah-nip″u-la′shun) (n.) The application of passive movement to a peripheral joint for therapeutic purposes. Manipulation increases the range of motion by stretching tight ligaments and, in some cases, by helping to break adhesions. Movements often include a gliding motion (either anteri-

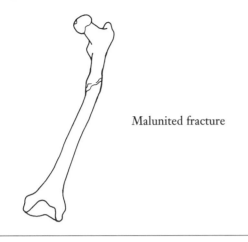

Malunited fracture

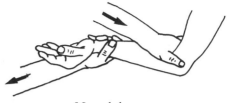

Manual therapy

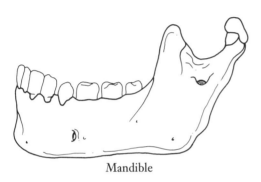

Mandible

orly, posteriorly, or laterally), rotation, flexion, and extension.

Manipulation Under Anesthesia (mah-nip″u-la′ shun/un′der/an″ēs-the′zē-ah) (n.) An extreme, effective, passive stretching used to treat restricted motion from intraarticular adhesions or other soft-tissue limitations. In this technique, gentle, forceful manipulation is performed after anesthesia is given to induce profound muscle relaxation or paralysis. Abbreviated **MUA**.

Mankin Score (man′kin/skor) (n.) A severity classification scale for the disease course of osteoarthritis. Described by Henry Mankin of Boston, Massachusetts.

Manual Muscle Testing (man′ū-al/mus′el/test′ing) (n.) A method of testing muscle strength by resistance. The strength is graded from 0 to 5 as follows:
Grade 0 or Zero: no contraction
1 or Trace: palpable contraction only
2 or Poor: moves joint with gravity eliminated
3 or Fair: moves against gravity
4 or Good: moves joint against gravity and some resistance
5 or Normal: normal strength

Manual Therapy (man′u-al/ther′ah-pē) (n.) A collective term for treatment by hands; this includes massage manipulation, mobilization, and manual traction.

Maquet Procedure (mah-kē/pro-se′jur) (n.) Surgical treatment of chondromalacia patella in which anterior displacement of the tibial tubercle is performed in order to decompress the patellofemoral joint.

Marateux-Lamy Syndrome (mar-a′-tō/lam-ē′/ sin′drōm) (n.) See **Polydystrophic Dwarfism**.

Marble Bones Disease (mar′bl/bōnz/di-zēz) (n.) See **Albers-Schonberg Syndrome**.

Marcaine (mar-kan′) (n.) A proprietary name for bupivacaine, a long-acting local anesthetic agent.

March Fracture (march/frak′chur) (n.) A stress fracture caused by repetitive overuse of the lower extremity. It can occur in any bone but is most commonly seen in the metatarsal bones of the foot. Clinical characteristics include swelling of the soft tissue in the dorsum of the foot, with pain and tenderness over the involved bone. The condition is named for its prevalence among army recruits after prolonged marching.

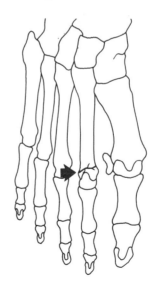

March fracture

March Gangrene (march/gang′grēn) (n.) An anterior tibial compartment syndrome that results in muscle ischemia. It is named for reports of this condition occurring in young soldiers after strenuous marching.

March à Petits Pas (march/a/pe′tē/pah) (n.) An abnormal gait with very short steps, as is seen in parkinsonism. Its name is derived from the French for "walking with small steps."

Marfan Syndrome (mar-fahn′/sin′drōm) (n.) A heterogeneous group of congenital disorders of connective tissues. These all have similar clinical characteristics and presumably autosomal dominant inheritance. Commonly, there are affections of the musculoskeletal, cardiovascular, and ocular systems. These include excessive height; long, thin, spidery digits (arachnodactyly), hypermobility; dolichosteonomalia; and scoliosis; aortic and valvular disorders; and myopia and superior dislocations of the lens.

Marginal Spurs (mar′ji-nal/sperz) (n.) Bony excrescences on the edges of articulating surfaces. These are found in association with arthritis, especially osteoarthritis. See **Osteophytes** and **Syndesmophytes**.

Maria-Stanton Disease (mah-rē′/stan′ton/di-zēz′) (n.) See **Cleidocranial Dysplasia**.

Marie-Strumpell Disease (mah-rē′/strim′pel/di-zēz′) (n.) See **Ankylosing Spondylitis**.

Marique and Taillard Method (mah-rēk′/and/tā-lard′/meth′ud) (n.) A radiographic measurement of the degree of slipping in spondylolisthesis. The olisthy is described as a percentage of the subjacent vertebral body.

Marmor Knee Replacement (mar′mor/nē/rē-plās′ment) (n.) A unicompartmental knee replacement system.

Marrow Cavity (mar′o/kav′i-tē) (n.) The central space in most bones that contains the mixture of fat and blood-forming cells called marrow. Also known as the **Medullary Canal**. See also **Bone Marrow**.

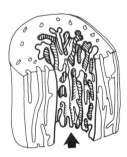

Marrow cavity

Marshall Technique (mar′shal/tek-nēk′) (n.) 1. A surgical technique for the primary repair of anterior cruciate ligament tears. Multiple sutures are placed in the ACL stump and brought out through holes in the lateral femoral condyle as two groups, which are then tied down as one unit. 2. A surgical technique for the reconstruction of anterior cruciate ligament insufficiency that uses the patelloquadriceps tendon as a substitute. The graft is passed first through a tibial tunnel, then through the intercondylar notch, and then either through a femoral tunnel or over the top of the lateral femoral canal.

Martin Clamp (mar′tin/klamp) (n.) A strong surgical forceps used to help in the open excision of a meniscus. This well-built clamp has a T-square cut at the points with which it is intended to grasp the meniscus.

Martin-Gruber Anastomosis (mar′tin/grū′ber/ah-nas″tō-mō′sis) (n.) An anomalous neural communication involving fiber cross-over from the median to the ulnar nerve in the forearm. It occurs in about 15 percent of the general population. Martin-Gruber anastomosis may possibly cause investigative error in nerve conduction studies.

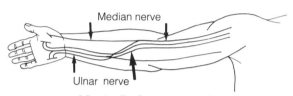

Martin-Gruber anastomosis

Marval Test (mar′val/test) (n.) A maneuver used to assess the integrity of the transverse humeral ligament. Apply pressure to the bicipital groove while rotating the patient's arm internally and externally. During external rotation abduct the arm. Pain with an audible snap or pop indicates rupture of the transverse ligament with bicipital tendon subluxation.

Mass (mas) (n.) 1. The quantitative measure of inertia for linear motion. The unit of measure is kilograms (pounds). 2. A general term applied to describe a tumor or growth.

Massage (mah-sahzh′) (n.) The systematic manual manipulation of the soft tissues of the body for the purpose of affecting the nervous and muscular system and the general circulation. The five classical maneuvers are effleurage, friction, petrissage, tapotement, and vibration.

Massie Nail (mas′ē/nāl) (n.) A three-part, telescoping nail-plate assembly used for the internal stabili-

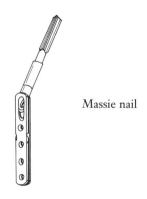

Massie nail

zation of intertrochanteric fractures. It consists of a standard-length tube, nails with varying triflanged portions, and plates with a slot on the proximal cortical aspect, which grip the tube laterally and distally for increased support. When assembled, the plate and the nail tube form an angle of 150 degrees.

MAST Suit (mast/sūt) (n.) Abbreviation for Military Antishock Trousers. A device used for raising blood pressure or controlling hemorrhage in patients with severe hypotension or bleeding.

Master Knot of Henry (mas′ter/not/of/hen′rē) (n.) A fascial thickening in the foot in which the flexor hallucis longus and flexor digitorum longus cross in the medioplantar aspect of the foot.

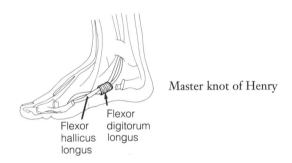

Master knot of Henry

Flexor hallicus longus

Flexor digitorum longus

Mat Crutch (mat/kruch) (n.) A shortened axillary device used for preparing paraplegics or bilateral lower limb amputees for regular crutches. The lower part reaches floor level, which is where the user sits.

Matchett-Brown Hip Endoprosthesis System (mach-et / brown / hip / en″do-pros-thē′sis / sis′tem) (n.) A type of long-stem intramedullary replacement of the femoral head.

Mathematical Model (ma-the-mat-i-kl/mod′el) (n.) A set of equations that quantitatively describes how a given physical system behaves.

Matthews-Green Pin (ma-thūz/grēn/pin) (n.) A skeletal pin that has a half drill-point.

Matrix (ma′triks) (n.) 1. The groundwork or basic material on which or from which something new develops. 2. An intercellular substance.

Matrix Vesicles (ma′triks/ves′i-k′lz) (n.) In the normal mineralization process of bone, globules, bounded by unit membranes and believed to be cellular extrusions, contained electron-dense particles that appear to be calcium. These vesicles are throught to be the site of initial calcification.

Maximum (mak′si-mum) (n.) The greatest value that can be obtained.

Maximum Permissible Dose (mak′si-mum/per′mis-i-b′l/dōs) (n.) The most ionizing radiation an individual can receive within a specified period without harm. This dose is established by authorities and is below the lowest level of any definite hazard. Abbreviated as **MPD**.

Mayer Orthosis (mā′er/or-thō′sis) (n.) A device for metatarsal elevation and compensation that consists of a shell that conforms to the plantar surface of the foot from the heel to a point just posterior to the metatarsophalangeal joints. There is no medial or lateral flange.

Mayo Orthosis (mā′ō/or-thō′-sis) (n.) In shoe terminology, a metatarsal bar with the anterior edge curved to approximate the position of the metatarsal heads.

Mazet Technique (mah-zā′/tek′nēk) (n.) A knee disarticulation in which the protruding medial, lateral, and posterior aspects of the femoral condyles are resected to create a stump onto which a better appearing and fitting prosthesis can be constructed.

McArdle Disease (mik-ar′-dl/di-zēz′) (n.) A congenital glycogen storage disease resulting from a deficiency of muscle phosphorylase. It is characterized by muscular weakness, pain, and stiffness after exercise. The exercised muscles remain partly flexed and firm and cannot be voluntarily extended. Symptoms begin in adolescence and are slowly progressive. Also known as **Glycogen Storage Disease Type V** or **Myophosphorylase Deficiency**.

McBride Procedure (mik-brīd′/pro-sē′jur) (n.) A surgical correction of hallux valgus. After the medial eminence is excised, what remains is mostly a soft tissue procedure, with release of the adductor tendon and lateral capsule and excision of the lateral sesamoid.

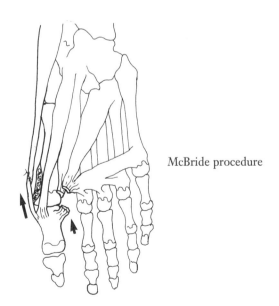

McBride procedure

McBride Test (mik-brīd′/test) (n.) An evaluation technique in patients with hallux valgus for contracture of the capsule or adductor hallucis. Seat the patient with the foot relaxed. Attempt to passively correct the deformity of the great toe. If the toe cannot be placed in a neutral or slight varus position, the capsule is contracted. If capsular contracture is not demonstrated, have the patient stand and actively move the adductor hallucis. Again, try to passively correct the deformity. If the toe cannot be placed in a neutral or slight varus position, the adductor hallucis muscle is contracted. The test also may show contraction of both the capsule and adductor hallucis.

McBride Toe-To-Mouth Test (mik-brīd/tō/to/mouth/test) (n.) A test used in the evaluation of sacroiliac joint disease. Have the patient stand on the affected leg and draw the toes of the opposite foot forward toward his or her mouth, bending his or her head forcibly forward. The test is positive if pain occurs in the sacroiliac joint opposite the lifted leg.

Mcg (n.) An abbreviation for microgram; also μg.

McGill-Melzack Pain Questionnaire (muh-gil'-mel-zak/pān/kwes'chun-ār) (n.) An assessment device used to measure a patient's perception of the sensory, affective, evaluative, or intensity dimensions of pain.

McGregor's Line (muh-greg'-orz/līn) (n.) A landmark used in the radiologic evaluation of basilar invagination. On a true lateral radiograph centered over C2, draw a line from the posterosuperior margin of the hard palate to the lowermost point on the midline occipital curve. The apex of the dens should not rise more than 4.5 mm above this line. Basilar invagination is present if this measurement is greater than 4.5 mm.

McKee-Farrar Hip Arthroplasty (muh-ke'-far-ar'/hip/ar'thro-plas"tē) (n.) A type of metal-on-metal total hip prosthesis. Designed for cement fixation.

McKibben Muscle (muh-kib'-ben/mus'el) (n.) An inflatable rubber tube encased in a woven nylon cover used to supply external power for an orthosis. Also called a **Pneumatic** or **Artificial Muscle**.

McLaughlin Nail-Plate (mik-lawk'-lin/nāl-plāt) (n.) A four-flanged, cannulated device for the fixation of hip fractures.

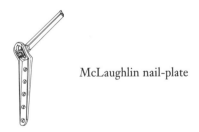

McLaughlin nail-plate

McMurray Osteotomy (mik-mur'-ā/os"te-ot'ō-me) (n.) A proximal femoral osteotomy described for the treatment of osteoarthritis of the hip. In this procedure, the distal fragment is displaced medially, and the proximal fragment is adducted.

McMurray Sign (mik-mur'-ā/sīn) (n.) A test used in the evaluation of meniscal tears. With the patient supine, palpate the posteromedial margin of the knee joint with one hand. With the other hand, grasp the foot and passively flex the patient's knee and hip to an acute angle. Keep the knee flexed and the leg externally rotated as far as possible. While gently rotating the leg, slowly extend the knee. Repeat the examination by palpating the lateral joint line and internally rotating the leg. if a mensical tear is present as the femoral condyle passes over the tear, a click may be audible or palpable.

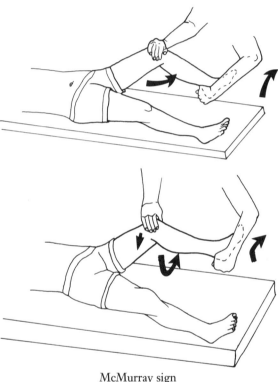

McMurray sign

McRae's Line (mik-rāz'/līn) (n.) A radiologic line used in the clinical assessment of patients with basilar impression. On a true lateral radiograph, with the central ray perpendicular to the skull, draw a line from the anterior margin of the foramen magnum to its posterior border. If the tip of the odontoid process remains above this line, basilar impression is present.

Mean (mēn) (n.) An average as determined by a sum of numbers divided by their number.

Mean Corpuscular Hemoglobin (mēn/kor-pus'ku-lar/hē'mō-glō"bin) (n.) The amount of hemoglobin per cell, as expressed in picograms. The average normal is 29.5, with a range of 27 to 32. Abbreviated **MCH**.

Mean Corpuscular Hemoglobin Concentration

(mēn / kor-pus′ku-lar / he′mo-glo″bin / kon″sen-tra′ shun) (n.) The percentage expression of the concentration of hemoglobin in grams per 100 mL (dL) of erythrocytes. The normal average is 35 percent, with a range of 33 to 38 percent. Abbreviated **MCHC**.

Mean Corpuscular Volume (mēn/kor-pus′ku-lar/ vol′ūm) (n.) The average erythrocyte volume as measured in cubic micrometers. The normal average is 87, with a range of 80 to 94. Abbreviated **MCV**.

Mean Inhibitory Concentration (mēn/in-hib′ĭ-tor″ē/kon″sen-tra′shun) (n.) A measure of the antibiotic susceptibility of a microorganism. An effective antibiotic should have serum levels of four to eight times that of the MIC as determined in a laboratory setting.

Meary's Angle (mēr-ēz/ang′g′l) (n.) A measurement of degree of pes cavus. On a lateral radiograph of the foot, draw two lines, one through the center of the longitudinal axis of the talus and the other through the long axis of the first metatarsal. The angle is formed by the intersection of these lines.

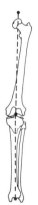

Mechanical axis

Mechanical Axis (me-kan′i-kal/ak′sis) (n.) The line that is perpendicular to the transverse axis of a joint. It runs from the center of the head of the proximal end of the proximal bone involved in the articulation to the center of the distal aspect of the distal bone of the articulation.

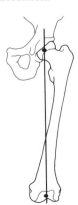

Mechanical axis of femur

Mechanical Axis of Femur (me-kan′i-kal/ak′sis/of/ fē′mur) (n.) The axis represented by a line drawn between the centers of the femoral head and the intercondylar notch. Normally, the mechanical axis or the femur and tibia intersect at 180 degrees to form a straight line. In the varus knee, the line falls medial to the center of the knee joint. In the valgus knee, the line falls lateral to the center of the joint. Compare this with the **Anatomic Axis of Femur**.

Mechanical Axis of Lower Extremity (me-kan′i-kal/ ak′sis/of/lō′er/eks-trem′i-tē) (n.) The axis represented by a straight line drawn from the center of the femoral head to the center of the tibial plafond, passing near or at the center of the lower extremity. It is usually in 3 degrees of valgus from the true vertical axis of the lower extremity. See **Anatomic Axis**.

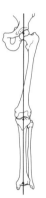

Mechanical axis of lower extremity

Mechanical Axis of Tibia (me-kan′i-kal/ak′sis/of/ tib′ē-ah) (n.) The axis represented by a line drawn between the centers of the tibial spines and the ankle plafond. Compare this with the **Anatomic Axis Tibia**.

Meclofenamate Sodium (me-klō″fen-am′āt/sō′de-um) (n.) A nonsteroidal, antiinflammatory drug marketed under the brand name Meclomen.

Meclomen (mĕ-klo′men) (n.) The proprietary name for meclofenamate sodium, a nonsteroidal, antiinflammatory drug.

MED (n.) Abbreviation for Multiple Epiphyseal Dysplasia.

Medial (me′de-al) (adj.) Of or pertaining to the side toward the midline.

Medial Hamstrings (mē′dē-al/ham′stringz) (n.) The more medial of the hamstring muscle groups that pass along the medial aspect of the back of the knee. This group includes the semitendinosus and semimembranosus muscles and part of the adductor magnus muscles. See **Muscle**.

Medial Malleolus (mē′dē-al/mah-le′ō-lus) (n.) A bony process on the inner surface of the distal aspect of the tibia. See **Malleolus**.

Medial Meniscus (mē′dē-al/me-nis′kus) (n.) See **Meniscus**.

Medial Patellar Plica (mē′dē-al/pah-tel′ar/plī′kah)

(n.) A synovial fold that runs from the medial side of the suprapatellar pouch down over the medial femoral condyle. It lies in a plane roughly at right angles to the suprapatellar plica. See **Plica**.

Medial Plica Syndrome (mē′dē-al/plī′kah/sin′drōm) (n.) A disorder caused by a persistent synovial fold running along the medial and superior borders of the patella that may have become thickened, especially posttraumatically. The syndrome is characterized by pain localized at the medial border of the patella over the medial femoral condyle. The synovial fold may be palpably thickened. A symptomatic plica may lead to erosive cartilage changes on the adjacent surface of the patella or medial femoral condyle. Also known as **Pathological Plica Syndrome**.

Medial Shelf (mē′dē-al/shelf) (n.) A medial patellar plica.

Medial Subluxation Test (mē′dē-al/sub″luk-sā′shun/ test) (n.) A means to determine the tightness of the lateral retinacular structures of the patella. With the patient supine, flex the knee to 30 degrees. Push the patella medially with your thumbs, and estimate the amount of medial translation. The width of the exposed lateral femoral condyle can be easily palpated. Repeat the test with the knee in full extension. This test is more significant if tightness occurs with a flexed knee because this is when the patella is in the femoral sulcus. Normally, no more than 15 mm of medial patellar translation occurs.

Median Lethal Dose (mē′dē-an/lē′thal/dōs) (n.) The amount of radiation received by an individual that would be fatal to about 50 percent of all living organisms. Abbreviated **MLD**.

Medicaid (med′i-kād) (n.) A federally funded, state-administered program of health care benefits for the indigent. It was created by Title XIX, a 1965 amendment to the Social Security Act.

Medical (med′i-kal) (adj.) Of or related to medicine.

Medical Consultation (med′i-kal/kon′sul-tā′shun) (n.) The response by one member of the medical staff to a request for medical advice by another member of the medical staff to further evaluate and treat a patient. It is characterized by a review of the patient's history, an examination of the patient, and a completion of a consultation report giving recommendations and/or opinions.

Medical Determination Related to Employability (med′i-kal/dĕ-ter″mi-na′shun/re-lā′ted/to/ em-ploy-a-bil-i-tē) (n.) A physician's statement about the relationship of an individual's health to the demands of a specific job. It includes performance, reliability, integrity, durability, and overall useful service as defined by the employer. The physician must ensure that the medical evaluation is complete and detailed enough to provide the clinical information needed to draw valid conclusions. The physician must: (1) identify impairments that could affect performance; (2) determine whether the impairments are permanent; (3) identify impairments that could lead to sudden or gradual incapacitation, further impairment, transmission of a communicable disease, or other adverse conditions. The physician should indicate whether the individual represents a greater risk to the employer than a nonimpaired person. The physician should also indicate his or her inability to predict a possibly unexpected occurrence.

Medical Impairment (med′i-kal/im-pār′ment) (n.) An alteration of health status assessed by medical means.

Medical Record Department (med′i-kal/rek′ord/dē-part′ment) (n.) A department of a hospital or medical office that provides systems and services for filing, maintenance, security, and retrieval of primary and secondary medical records. Its personnel collect, code, and index health care data and prepare administrative and clinical statistical reports. They also process authorized disclosure of medical record information and quantitative analysis of medical records.

Medical Services (med′i-kal/ser′vi-ses) (n.) Medical care performed by physicians, nurses, and other professional and technical personnel under the direction of a physician.

Medical Staff (med′i-kal/staf) (n.) An aggregate body of licensed medical and osteopathic physicians and dentists who take care of the patients of a hospital.

Medical Technologist (med′i-kal/tek-nol′o-jist) (n.) A technologist who performs specialized chemical, microscopic, and bacteriologic tests on human blood, tissue, and fluids under the direction of a pathologist, physician, or scientist.

Medicare (med′i-kār) (n.) A federally funded program that provides health insurance benefits to those patients over 65 years of age or those eligible for Social Security benefits. Part A provides for hospital care; Part B is a voluntary medical insurance program. Medicare was created by the Title XVIII Health Insurance for the Aged, a 1965 amendment to the Social Security Act.

Medicolegal (med″i-ko-lē′gal) (adj.) Of or pertaining to a situation involving both medical and legal considerations.

Mediloy (med′-i-loy) (n.) A trade name for a cast cobalt-chromium-molybdenum alloy used to make orthopaedic implants. It is manufactured by 3M/Medtec.

Medium (mē-dē-um) (n.) A substance that provides nutrients for the growth and multiplication of microorganisms.

MEDLARS (n.) A registered acronym for the Medical Literature Analysis and Retrieval System, a computerized system that aids in the search and retrieval of articles published in medical journals or journals related to medical topics. MEDLARS is based on the citations in *Index Medicus* and is made available through the United States National Library of Medicine in Bethesda, Maryland.

Medulla (me-dul′ah) (n.) An inner part of an organ.

Medullary Cavity (med′u-lār″ē/kav′i-tē) (n.) A marrow-filled space within the diaphysis of a long bone. It is also known as the marrow cavity or intramedullary cavity.

Medullary Fixation (med′u-lār″ē/fik-sā′shun) (n.) Any type of internal fixation that uses a rod placed in the intramedullary canal of a long bone for stability. See related term, **Intramedullary rod**.

Mehta Angle (mā′-tah/ang′g′l) (n.) A radiographic measurement of the rib vertebral angle difference used to predict the possibility of progression in infantile scoliosis. The rib-vertebral angle is measured by drawing a line to the middle of either upper or lower border of a selected thoracic vertebra (in a scoliotic curve, the apical vertebra). Another line is drawn from the midpoint of the head of the rib to the midpoint of the neck of the rib, just medial to the region where the neck widens into the shaft of the rib. This rib line is extended medially to intersect the vertebral line to make the rib-vertebral (R-V) angle. If this angle difference is greater than 20 degrees at the apex of the curve, the scoliosis is likely to be progressive. Also called **Rib-Vertebral Angle Difference**.

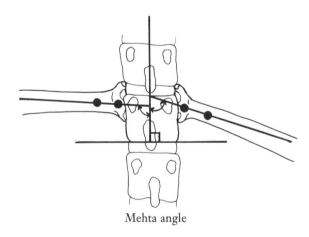

Mehta angle

Meiosis (mī-ō′sis) (n.) Cell division that involves two successive cell divisions with only one duplication of the chromosomes. The division produces four cells, each containing half the number of chromosomes in the original cell. Compare with **Mitosis**.

Melanin (mel′ah-nin) (n.) A dark pigment occurring naturally in the skin and hair. Melanin is an insoluble polymer of high molecular weight. It is produced in the basal layers of the epidermis by melanocytes through a series of oxidations of its precursor by the enzyme tyrosine. Sunlight exposure increases the amount of melanin in the skin.

Melnick-Needles Syndrome (mel-nik′-nē′-dlz/sin′drōm) (n.) See **Osteodysplasty**.

Melorheostosis (mel″o-rē″os-tō′sis) (n.) A rare bone

dysplasia of unknown etiology that usually affects only one side of the body. It may be monostotic, polyostotic, or monomelic. It usually affects the extremities, but on rare occasions it can affect the spine, ribs, skull, and facial bones.

The lesions associated with this illness are characterized radiographically by a wavy hyperostosis resembling melted wax that has dripped down one side of a candle. The presenting symptom is pain exaggerated by activity. Limited joint motion and stiffness caused by contractures, soft-tissue fibrosis, and ectopic periarticular bone formation are common. Indurated, shiny, erythematous and/or edematous skin may be present over the affected bone. Also known as the **Leri Osteopetrosis**.

Menard's Lines (men′arz/līnz) (n.) See **Shenton's Line**.

Meninges (me-nin′jēz) (n.) Any one of the three membranes (the dura mater, the arachnoid, and the pia mater) that encloses the central nervous system.

Meningioma (me-nin″jē-ō′mah) (n.) A benign tumor composed of the cells that line the arachnoid mater. These cells may penetrate through the dura mater and appear to originate there. They can occur throughout the central nervous system.

Meningitis (men″in-jī′tis) (n.) An inflammation of the pia-arachnoid membranes covering the brain and the spinal cord.

Meningocele (me-ning′gō-sēl) (n.) A saclike meningeal protrusion through a neural tube defect. Neural elements are not an integral part of the sac. Compare this with **Myelomeningocele**.

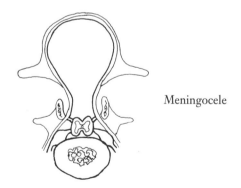

Meningocele

Meningomyelocele (mĕ-ning″go-mi′ĕ-lo-sēl″) (n.) See **Myelomeningocele**.

Meniscal Flap Tear (me-nis′kal/flap/tār) (n.) A split that extends obliquely into the substance of the meniscus from its inner margin, creating an unstable segment.

Meniscal Interstitial Tear (me-nis′kal/in-ter-stish′-al/tār) (n.) A disruption within the substance of the meniscus that does not propagate to the surfaces of the meniscus.

231

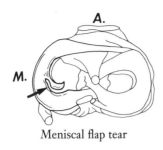

Meniscal flap tear

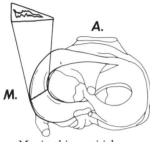

Meniscal interstitial tear

Meniscal Longitudinal Tear (me-nis′kal/lon″ju-tū′di-nal/tār) (n.) A vertical split in the meniscus that is in line with its concentric collagen fiber network. Most common in the medial meniscus of the knee.

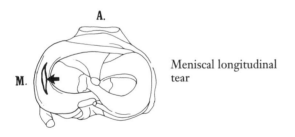

Meniscal longitudinal tear

Meniscal Radial Tear (mĕ-nis′-kal/ra′-dē-al/tār) (n.) A linear disruption of the meniscus that runs perpendicular to its margins emanating from the inner or mesial margin.

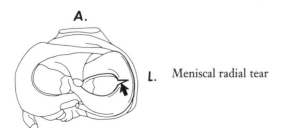

Meniscal radial tear

Meniscectomy (men″i-sek′tō-mē) (n.) The surgical removal of a meniscal cartilage. This term is usually modified by the side of resection (medial or lateral) and by the extent of resection (partial, subtotal, or complete).

Meniscorrhesis (me-nis″kō-rē′sis) (n.) The repair of a meniscus. Also called **Meniscorraphy**.

Meniscus (me-nis′kus) (n.) A crescent-shaped fibrocartilaginous wedge that sits on top of the periphery of the tibial articular surface. It is thicker peripherally and tapers to a thin, unattached edge centrally. The menisci serve to deepen the articular fossae of the tibial condyles, allowing them to receive the femoral condyles and function in joint stabilization, shock absorption, and weight-bearing in the knee. Peripherally, the edges of the menisci are attached by short coronary ligaments to the margin of the tibial condyles and to the inner surface of the joint capsule, except where the popliteus tendon crosses laterally. At either end, the menisci attach anterior and posterior to the tibial eminence.

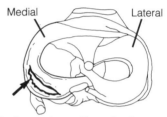

Meniscus. *Arrow*, Posterior horn tear.

Meniscus, Lateral (me-nis′kus/lat′er-al) (n.) The knee meniscus in the lateral compartment. It is more circular in form than the medial meniscus.

Meniscus, Medial (me-nis′kus/me′dē-al) (n.) The knee meniscus in the medial compartment. It is a crescent-shaped, fibrocartilaginous structure, triangular in the vertical section, and having a complete peripheral capsular attachment. It is wider posteriorly than anteriorly.

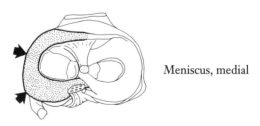

Meniscus, medial

Meniscus Shaver (me-nis′kus/shā′ver) (n.) A motorized, intraarticular soft-tissue shaver intended to cut meniscal tissue during arthroscopic surgery.

Menopause (men′ō-pawz) (n.) The cessation of menstrual activity.

Meralgia Paresthetica (me-ral′je-ah/par″es-thet′ik-ah) (n.) A painful paresthesia-dysesthesia in the lateral femoral cutaneous nerve of the thigh. It is manifested by a burning, tingling, and numbness in the distribution of this nerve on the outer side of the thigh, with a variable decrease in sensation. The nerve may be irritated by various factors, such as a tight belt or corset, prolonged walking, or pregnancy. Occasionally, the nerve is affected by a local surgical incision. The clinical course varies, but the symptoms usually resolve spontaneously, especially if the cause is identified and removed.

Mercedes Sign/View (mer-sa′dez/sīn/vū) (n.) A lateral x-ray of the scapula to determine if the humeral head is dislocated either anterior or posterior to the glenoid.

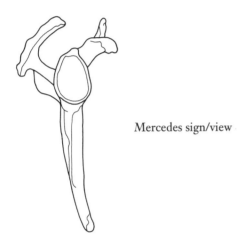

Mercedes sign/view

Merchant View (mer′chant/vū) (n.) An axial radiographic view of the patellofemoral joint. To obtain the view, have patient lie supine with the knees flexed at 45 degrees. Place the cassette distal to the patella, with the central ray inclined inferiorly 30 degrees from the horizontal. In order to minimize the lateral divergence of the x-ray beam, examine each knee separately. The following measurements may be determined on this view: (1) sulcus angle, (2) patellofemoral angle, (3) congruence angle, and (4) patellofemoral index.

    Also called the **Patellofemoral View** or **Mountain View**. See individual angles for related terms.

Merke's Sign (mer-kēz/sīn) (n.) A diagnostic marker in meniscal tears. Have the standing patient rotate his or her body on the fixed leg internally and externally. With internal rotation, pain in the medial joint space suggests a lesion of the medial meniscus; pain on external rotation suggests a lesion of the lateral meniscus.

Meromelia (mer″o-mē′lē-ah) (n.) Congenital absence of any body part; this does not include the entire limb.

Meromyosin (mer″o-mī′ō-sin) (n.) The two smaller molecules that result when myosin is broken down by the enzymatic action of papain. "Heavy meromyosin" is that portion containing the head group and a small portion of the rod. "Light meromyosin" is the portion containing most of the rod.

Meryon's Sign (mer′-yōnz/sīn) (n.) A diagnostic marker in patients with Duchenne-type muscular dystrophy. Owing to shoulder girdle weakness, if the child is lifted from under the arms, he or she will slide through the examiner's hands.

Meschan Angle (mē-shun/ang′g′l) (n.) A method for measuring the degree of spondylolisthesis at L5–S1. On the lateral radiograph, draw the two Meschan lines: the first connecting the posterior proximal and distal margins of L5; the second connecting the posterior distal margin of L4 and the posterior proximal margin of S1. Extend both lines to create a measurable angle where they meet. If the lines are parallel, a distance of more than 3 mm is considered abnormal. If the lines intersect, an angle of 3 degrees or less is normal. If the angle is less than 10 degrees, the spondylolisthesis is slight; if the angle is between 11 degrees and 20 degrees, moderate; if the angle is greater than 20 degrees, severe.

Mesenchymal Chondrosarcoma (me-seng′ki-mal/kon″drō-sar-kō′mah) (n.) A subset of malignant cartilage tumors with a biphasic histology—they contain a cartilaginous component and a mesenchymal component. This is a high-grade, highly lethal lesion.

Mesenchyme (mes′eng-kīm) (n.) The primordial embryonic tissue that has no epithelial configuration; it is derived from the mesoderm. The cells of this tissue, the mesenchymal cells, give rise to the connective tissue, the musculature, the blood cells and vessels, the lymphatic system, and major portions of the genitourinary system.

Meso (mēs′o) Prefix meaning middle.

Mesoderm (mēs′o-derm) (n.) The middle of the three embryonic tissue layers; it is found between the ectoderm and the endoderm. The mesoderm gives rise to many embryonic tissues, one of which is the mesenchyme, which in turn gives rise to the connective tissues, muscle, blood cells and vessels, lymphatics, and part of the genitourinary system. Also called the **Mesoblast.**

Mesoneurium (mēs″o-nū-rē′um) (n.) The thin, connective tissue that anchors a peripheral nerve to its surrounding tissues and through which its vascular supply passes.

Mesotendon (mēs″o-ten′don) (n.) A delicate fold of connective tissue that extends to a tendon from its synovial-tendon sheath.

Metabolic Disease (met″ah-bol′ik/di-zēz′) (n.) Any dysfunction caused by a defect in the hormonal or chemical reactions of body cells.

Metabolism (mĕ-tab′o-lizm) (n.) The combination

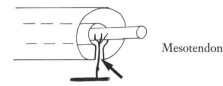

Mesotendon

of all physical and chemical processes in the organism. The success of their integration affects the growth, maintenance, and transformation of organized substances in living systems.

Metabolite (me-tab'o-līt) (n.) A substance used in or produced by the metabolism of an organism.

Metacarpal (met″ah-kar'pal) 1.(adj.) Of or pertaining to the bones of the hand that form the metacarpus. 2.(n.) Any of the bones forming the metacarpus.

Metacarpal Block (met″ah-kar'pal/blok) (n.) A technique for digital anesthesia in which the agent is injected at the level of the distal palmar crease of the hand.

Metacarpal Index (met″ah-kar'pal/in'deks) (n.) The average of the ratios of length to width at the midpoint of the second to the fifth metacarpals. Normal values vary from 5.4 to 7.9.

Metacarpal Sign (met″ah-kar'pal/sīn) (n.) An accessory sign of gonadal dysgenesis. The sign is positive if a line tangent to the distal ends of the heads of the fourth and fifth metacarpals extends through the head of the third metacarpal.

Metacarpophalangeal (met″ah-kar″po-fah-lang'jē-al) (adj.) Of or relating to the metacarpophalangeal joint.

Metacarpus (met″ah-kar'pus) (n.) The five bones of the hand that connect the carpus to the phalanges.

Metal (met″l) (n.) One of the electropositive elements from which many orthopaedic implants are created. Depending on the specific chemical composition, different metals have varying biocompatibility, strength and wear characteristics, and corrosiveness. Most commonly used implants are made of iron-based, titanium-based, or cobalt-based metals.

Metaphase (met'ah-fāz) (n.) A stage during mitotic division when the chromosomes line up in a plane at right angles to the spindle axis.

Metaphyseal (met″ah-fiz'ē-al) (adj.) Of or relating to the metaphysis.

Metaphyseal Chondrodysplasia (met″ah-fiz'ē-al/kon″dro-dis-plā'ze-ah) (n.) A bone dysplasia whose primary defect is thought to be in the distal or metaphyseal aspect of the growth plate. There are five types of metaphyseal chondrodysplasia, all of which are manifested after birth and result in short-limbed dwarfism. They are differentiated by the actual age of evidence, the pattern of inheritance, and the presence of other associated disorders. These types are: Jansen Type, Schmid Type, McKusick Type, metaphyseal chondrodysplasia with thymo-

lymphopenia, metaphyseal chondrodysplasia with malabsorption and neutropenia. This is also known as the syndrome of pancreatic exocrine insufficiency.

Metaphyseal Fibrous Defects (met″ah-fiz'e-al/fī'brus/dē'fekts) (n.) See **Nonossifying Fibroma.**

Metaphyseal Flaring (met″ah-fiz'e-al/flār'ing) (n.) An abnormal enlargement of the metaphyseal ends of the long bones proximal to the epiphysis. This may be seen in rickets.

Metaphysis (me-taf'i-sis) (n.) The widened end of the tubular bone shaft; this is where active bone formation occurs. It is found between the diaphysis and the epiphysis. In growing bones, it is composed of the primary and secondary spongiosa. Contrast **Diaphysis.**

Metaplasia (met″ah-plā'ze-ah) (n.) An abnormal change of one fully differentiated tissue into another type of fully differentiated tissue.

Metastability (met'ah-sta″bil-i-tē) (n.) In discussing calcium and phosphate homeostasis, the state in which the calcium and phosphate concentrations exceed the critical solubility product but are presumably held in solution by an unknown inhibitor system. This allows for rapid "metastasis" into hydroxyapatite crystals during bone formation.

Metastasis (me-tas'tah-sis) (n.) The transfer of pathogenic microorganisms or abnormal cells distant from the site primarily involved by the morbid process; this is secondary to metastasizing.

Metastasize (me-tas'tah-sīz) (v.) Transfer of disease from a primary site or part to another part not directly connected to it. Either pathogenic microorganisms (e.g., tubercle bacilli) or malignant cells may metastasize.

Metastatic Calcification (met″ah-stat'ik/kal″si-fi-kā'shun) (n.) The formation of calcified material in soft tissues as a result of hypercalcemia and hyperphosphatemia that cause an increased calcium-phosphate product in the blood.

Metastatic Tumor (met″ah-stat'ik/too'mor) (n.) A growth of malignant tumor cells distant to the primary site of malignancy.

Metatarsal (me″ah-tar'sal) 1. (adj.) Of or relating to the bones of the foot that form the metatarsus. 2. (n.) Any of the bones forming the metatarsus.

Metatarsal Bar (met″ah-tar'sal/bar) (n.) In shoe terminology, a strip of material applied to the outersole across the distal aspect of the shaft of the metatarsal bones to relieve pressure on the metatarsal heads.

Metatarsal Break (met″ah-tar'sal/brāk) (n.) The obliquity created by a line drawn through the metatarsal heads. The line slopes laterally, and its average deviation is approximately 62 degrees through the long axis of the foot. Clinically, one notes the metatarsal break by observing the crease pattern present on the top of a leather shoe. As a person rises onto the ball of the foot at the end of stance phase, the metatarsal break allows for external rotation of the tibia and thus the entire lower extremity at toe-off.

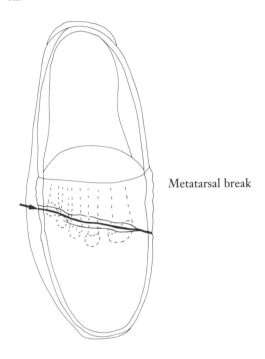

Metatarsal break

Metatarsal Formula (met″ah-tar′sal/for′mu-lah) (n.) A description of three metatarsal types according to their length: (1) The "index plus minus" type, in which the first metatarsal is equal in length to the second; (2) the "index minus" type, in which the first metatarsal is shorter than the second; (3) The "index plus" type, in which the first metatarsal is longer than the second.

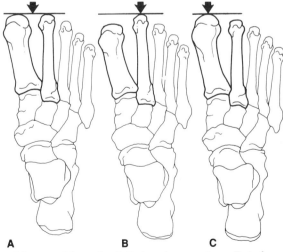

Metatarsal formula. **A**, Index plus = minus; **B**, index minus; **C**, index plus.

Metatarsal Pad (met″ah-tar′sal/pad) (n.) A cushion applied to the sole of the foot or inside of the shoe just proximal to some or all of the metatarsal heads that relieves metatarsalgia by redistributing weight bearing. This triangular-shaped, soft insert has rounded corners and thinned, tapered edges.

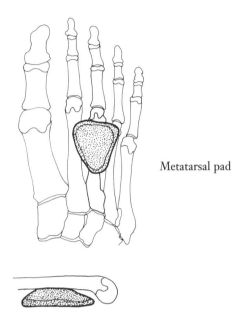

Metatarsal pad

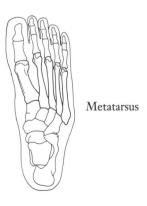

Metatarsalgia (met″ah-tar-sal′je-ah) (n.) Discomfort or pain in the region of the metatarsal heads and metatarsophalangeal joints. Pain only on weight-bearing is called **Pressure Metatarsalgia.**

Metatarsophalangeal (met″ah-tar″so-fah-lan′je-al) (adj.) Of or relating to the metatarsophalangeal joint.

Metatarsus (met″ah-tar-sus) (n.) The five bones of the foot that connect the tarsus to the phalanges; the cuboid, navicular, and the three cuneiform bones.

Metatarsus

Metatarsus Abductus (met″ah-tar′sus/ab-duk′tus) (n.) A congenital deviation of the forefoot away from the body midline. The heel remains in a neutral

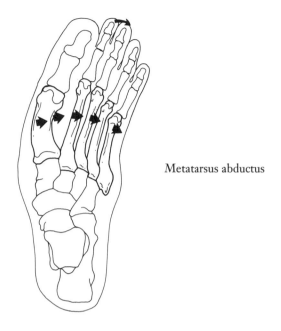

Metatarsus abductus

usually responds to conservative treatment with passive stretching and/or serial casting. Also known as **Metatarsus Varus, Pes Varus, Skewfoot,** and **Metatarsus Adductovarus.**

Metatarsus Primus Atavicus (met″ah-tar′sus/prī′mus/atah-vī′kus) (n.)   A congenital foot deformity in which there is abnormal shortening of the first metatarsal bone. Also known as **Congenital Short First Metatarsal.**

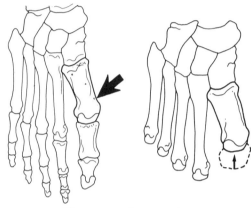

Metatarsus primus atavicus

or slightly valgus position. The deviation is caused by soft tissue contracture; therefore, no bone deformity exists at birth. Bone deformity may develop, with growth due to secondary adaptation.

Metatarsus Adductus (met″ah-tar′sus/ad-duk′tus) (n.)   A relatively common congenital condition in which the forefoot is deviated toward the midline of the body. The forefoot is usually supinated as well as being in varus. The lateral border of the foot is convex. The hindfoot is usually in neutral position, but a valgus heel is not uncommon. Internal tibial torsion is also commonly associated. This condition

Metatarsus Primus Varus (met″ah-tar′sus/prī′mus/vā′rus) (n.)   A structural deformity of the foot in which the first metatarsal diverges from its normal position in relation to the second metatarsal. The first metatarsal deviates toward the midline. The AP roentgenogram of the standing foot shows the angle between the first and second metatarsals measuring about 7 degrees in the normal foot. An angle greater than 10 degrees is abnormal and is diagnostic for this condition.

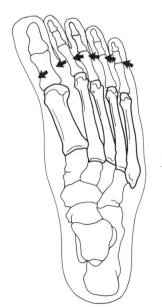

Metatarsus adductus

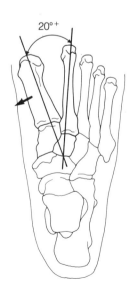

Metatarsus primus varus

Metatarsus Varus (met″ah-tar′sus/vār′us) (n.) See **Metatarsus Adductus**.

Metatropic Dwarfism (met-ah-trof′ik/dwarf′izm) (n.) A short-limbed, disproportionate dwarfism evident at birth. Common findings are metaphyseal flattening and flaring, severe kyphoscoliosis, ligamentous laxity, and odontoid hypoplasia. Longevity is significantly decreased because of serious neurologic sequelae of cervical compression, which is due to a hypoplastic odontoid and atlantoaxial instability or cardiopulmonary complications of kyphoscoliosis.

Methyl Methacrylate (meth′il/meth-ak′ri-lāt) (n.) An abbreviated term for polymethylmethacrylate or bone cement.

Methylprednisolone (meth″il-pred-nis′o-lōn) (n.) A long-acting steroid preparation used for injection. It is marketed under the proprietary name Depo-Medrol.

Metrizamide (me-triz′ah-mīd) (n.) A nonionic, water-soluble, iodinated contrast medium with relatively low toxicity used for myelographic examinations. Its brand name is Amipaque.

Meurig-Williams Plate (mur-ig-wil-yumz/plāt) (n.) A type of plate designed for internal fixation of the spine; no longer widely used.

Meyerding Method (mī′er-ding/meth′ud) (n.) A radiographic method for classification of spondylolisthesis, based on the position of the inferior surface of the fifth vertebral body, relative to the superior surface of the first segment of the sacrum.

Meyers Graft (mī′erz/graft) (n.) A technique of open reduction and internal fixation of femoral neck fractures. Cancellous bone is grafted to the defect on the posterior aspect of the neck, and a primary muscle pedicle graft is placed over the posterior head and fixed to the posterior neck. The graft is intended to improve the rate of bony union and decrease the incidence of avascular necrosis of the femoral head.

Michele Buckling Sign (me-shel′/buk′l′ing/sīn) (n.) A diagnostic marker used in determining sciatic nerve tension on the extrathecal nerve root. It also can be helpful in differentiating between the genuine tension case and the simulator. With the patient supine, place the palm of your hand under the heel of the affected extremity. Gradually elevate the limb with the knee in full extension. With true sciatic nerve tension, there is a point in the arc of elevation at which the patient's knee will buckle instinctively in order to avoid pain; this point depends on the degree of sciatic tension. Continuing the excursion with the knee extended inevitably increases the pain. In a simulator without true sciatic nerve tension, no buckling point exists, and any elicited response is purely voluntary.

Michele Flip Sign (me-shel′/flip/sīn) (n.) A clinical sign used in the evaluation of sciatic nerve root tension. Have the patient sit as squarely and erect as possible on the examining table, with his or her legs dangling off the edge and his or her arms hanging at the side of his or her body. Alternatively, have the patient place his or her arms against the table for supplemental support of the thigh to be tested. Place the open palm of one hand on the suprapatellar area of the affected extremity and depress the thigh against the table, keeping the other hand under the heel cord so that the heel rests in the palm. Gradually extend the affected limb at the knee. With genuine sciatic tension, the patient offers no resistance until approximately 45 degrees of extension is reached. Continued elevation past that point causes no acute reversal of the lumbar lordosis. Also, the patient tends to fall backward frequently, using the hands braced against the table to prevent a complete backward fall.

As a corollary, if there is a positive flip sign, the patient is unable to sit erect with both knees fully extended. In order to avoid the pain of nerve root tension, either the affected knee flexes or the trunk sags due to reversal of the lumbar lordosis.

Microcrystalline Collagen (mī″kro-kris′tal-īn/kol′ah-jen) (n.) A topical hemostatic agent that is off-white, fluffy, and flourlike in consistency. It functions only when applied directly to raw, oozing surfaces, including bone and friable tissues, or around vascular anastomoses. Hemostasis occurs on direct contact with the agent by adhesion of platelets and prompt fibrin deposition within the interstices of the collagen.

Microdamage (mī″kro-dam′ij) (n.) The microscopic damage to the physical properties of a biologic material, usually due to a fatiguelike phenomena.

Microfatigue (mī″kro-fah′tēg) (n.) The microscopic changes seen in the development of fatigue failure, e.g., those seen in bone prior to actual fatigue fracture.

Microfracture (mī″kro-frak′chur) (n.) Microscopic cracks in bone or other materials due to fatigue or abnormal loading. These form stress risers from which complete fatigue fractures may result.

Micron (mī′kron) (n.) A metric unit of length equalling one one-thousandth of a millimeter. Usually designated by the Greek letter μ, or mu.

Microorganism (mī″kro-or′gan-izm) (n.) Any organism of microscopic size. This includes bacteria, viruses, protozoans, and many large algae. Also known as a **Microbe**.

Microsurgery (mi′kro-ser″jer-ē) (n.) 1. The branch of surgery in which ocular adjuncts are used to improve visual acuity, thus allowing the application of Halstedian principles to small structures. 2. Surgical procedures performed with highly refined operating microscopes and miniature precision instruments.

Microtome (mī′kro-tōm) (n.) An instrument used to make thin tissue sections for histologic study.

Mid Prefix: in the center of.

Midclavicular Line (mid′klah-vik′u-lar/līn) (n.) A vertical line parallel to and midway between the midsternal line and a vertical line drawn downward through the outer end of the clavicle.

Midget (mij′et) (n.) An undersized person who is normally formed. This person is also known as a proportionate dwarf.

Midline (mid′līn) (n.) Any line that bisects a figure symmetrically.

Midline Disk Herniation (mid′līn/disk/her″nē-ā′ shun) (n.) A herniated nucleus pulposus found in the midline of the spinal canal. This can result from compression of the spinal cord without the involvement of the nerve root.

Midpalmar (mid′pal-mar) (n.) A potential space in the palm of the hand that lies between the radial and ulnar septa of the palmar aponeurosis and separates the thenar and hypothenar spaces.

Midsole (mid′sōl) (n.) In shoe terminology, a piece of material interposed between the innersole and outersole.

Midsagittal Plane (mid-saj′i-tal/plān) (n.) A vertical plane at the midline that divides the body into left and right portions. Also called the **median plane** and **median sagittal plane**.

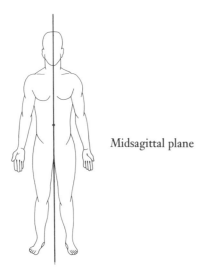

Midsagittal plane

Midsternal Line (mid′ster′nal/līn) (n.) A line that passes down the middle of the sternum from the suprasternal notch to the xiphoid.

Midtarsal Joint (mid-tar′sal/joint) (n.) The transverse tarsal joint. Also known as **Chopart's Joint**.

Migration (mi-grā′shun) (n.) Movement out of place. This applies specifically to the movement of prosthetic components from their initial points of fixation, as seen radiographically. This is indicative of component loosening.

Mikulicz's Angle (mik′u-lich″ez/ang′g′l) (n.) The

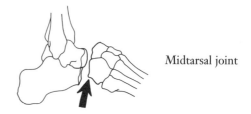

Midtarsal joint

angle of decline of the proximal femur determined by a line passing through the long axis of the proximal epiphysis of the femur intersecting a line passing through the long axis of the diaphysis. The normal angle is 137 degrees. More commonly known as the **neck–shaft angle**.

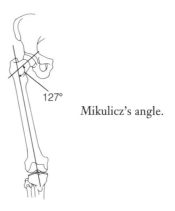

127°

Mikulicz's angle.

Milch Disease (milch/di-zēz′) (n.) An eponym for osteochondrosis of the ischial apophysis.

Milch Method (milch/meth′ud) (n.) A method of determining the degree of hip flexion deformity in stance. Draw a line from the ischial tuberosity to the anterior superior iliac spine. Draw a second line along the axis of the femoral shaft. The angle formed by the intersection of these two lines is the pelvifemoral angle, which normally measures 55 degrees. Then determine the pelvifemoral angle on the unaffected side. The difference between the two sides is the degree of flexion deformity.

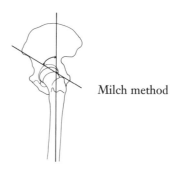

Milch method

Milch Technique (milch/tek′nēk) (n.) A maneuver used in the reduction of anterior shoulder dislocation. With the patient supine, place your hand over the top of the acromion. Put your thumb in the axilla in order to support the dislocated humeral head. Flex the humeral head with your thumb while the other hand gently abducts and externally rotates the arm overhead. When the arm reaches complete abduction, gently push the head over the glenoid rim and into place.

Milgram Test (mil′grim/test) (n.) A maneuver used in the evaluation of radiculopathy. Instruct the supine patient to keep both legs straight and to raise them to a position about 2 inches from the table. If the patient can hold this position for at least 30 seconds without pain, intrathecal pathology usually is not present.

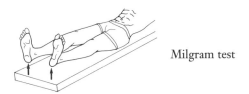

Milgram test

Milk-Alkali Syndrome (milk-al/kah-lī/sin′drōm) (n.) A cause of metabolic alkalosis in which a small exogenous load of alkali (milk products and antacids with calcium) will cause sustained alkalosis because of impaired renal function. Excessive intake of absorbable alkali will therefore result in hypercalcemic nephropathy and alkalosis.

Milkmaid's Elbow (milk′mādz/el′bo) (n.) A subluxation of the radial head in children. More commonly known as **Nursemaid's Elbow**. See **Nursemaid's Elbow**.

Milkman Pseudofractures (milk′man/soo″do-frak′ churs) (n.) See **Looser Lines**.

Milkman's Syndrome (milk′manz/sin′drōm) (n.) An eponym for rachitic and osteomalacic syndromes characterized by multiple symmetric areas of absorption in various bones. Named for the radiographic presence of multiple milkman's pseudofractures. See **Rickets** and **Osteomalacia**.

Mill's Maneuver (milz/mah-noo′ver) (n.) A diagnostic test in tennis elbow. Place the patient's elbow in full extension with the wrist flexed. Pronating the forearm in this position elicits the characteristic pain of tennis elbow.

Millbank Cup (mil′bank/kup) (n.) A metallic device that grasps the heel of the shoe used with a Thomas splint to provide distal traction during emergency transport.

Millender Technique (mil-en-der/tek′nēk) (n.) Surgical interpositional arthroplasty of the first carpometacarpal joint in rheumatoid arthritis.

Millender and Nailbuff Technique (mil-en-der/ nāl′-buf/tek-nēk) (n.) A wrist arthrodesis performed through a dorsal, longitudinal incision and stabilized with an intramedullary smooth Steinmann pin across the wrist into the shaft of the third metacarpal.

Miller Twister (mil′er/twist′er) (n.) A torsion cable that rotates the lower limb in order to correct internal or external rotation. The Miller twister is attached to a belt at one end and a shoe at the other. It may be used alone or in combination with a hip-knee-ankle-foot orthosis. Also known as a **Twister Cable**.

Milligram (mil′i-gram) (n.) Metric unit of weight equal to one one-thousandth of a gram. Abbreviated mg.

Millimeter (mil′i-me-ter) (n.) Metric unit of length equal to one one-thousandth of a meter (one meter equalling 39.36 inches). Abbreviated **mm**.

Milwaukee Brace (mil-waw′-kē/brās) (n.) A corrective spinal orthosis for skeletally immature scoliosis, lordosis, and kyphosis. It presumably redirects spinal growth by stimulating trunk muscle patterns, with the three-point pressure systems playing a lesser role. The device extends from the occiput and chin to the pelvis; it consists of a contoured pelvic girdle attached by three uprights to an occipital pad and a throat mold or chin piece. Lumbar and thoracic and other accessories, such as shoulder flanges, axillary slings, or subclavicular pads, hang from the uprights. Developed by doctors Blount and Schmidt of Milwaukee.

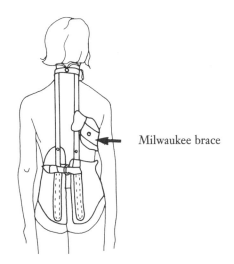

Milwaukee brace

Mineral Phase (min′er-al/fāz) (n.) The inorganic component in bone.

Mineralization (min″er-al-ī′zā′shun) (n.) The addition of any mineral matter to the body; commonly used to refer to the deposition of hydroxyapatite crystals to osteoid to form normal, mineralized bone.

Minerva Jacket (min′er-vah/jak′et) (n.) A body cast

to support fractures of the cervical or upper thoracic vertebrae. The Minerva jacket envelopes and immobilizes the trunk and is molded to fit around the face and lower jaw. The name is taken from the armor-clad Roman goddess.

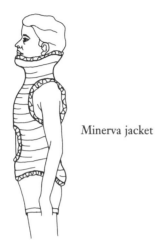

Minerva jacket

Minnesota Multiphasic Personality Inventory (min′e-sōt′e / mul′ti-fā-zik / per′su-nal′i-te / / in′ventor′e) (n.)   An objective, empirical psychometric test consisting of 550 written statements. The person taking the test assesses each statement as true or false as it pertains to him or her. Test scores show four validity scales and basic clinical or personality scales.

The validity scales include: measures of items omitted or marked both true or false, a lie scale, a measure of deviant approach to test taking, and a correction factor for clinical defensiveness.

The clinical response scales—previously identified characteristics found through research and clinical experience—are identified with similar scores on that scale and then attributed to the patient. This test is used in orthopaedics as a predictor of surgical and conservative treatment results in patients with spine pathology. Abbreviated MMPI.

Minor (mī′nor) (adj.)   The lesser in size or importance.

Minor Curve (mī′nor/kerv) (n.)   In scoliosis, the smaller curve.

Minor's Sign (mi′norz/sīn) (n.)   A diagnostic marker in sciatica. The patient arises from a supine position by supporting himself or herself on the unaffected side, and then places one hand on his or her back while bending the affected leg.

Minor's Sweating Test (mi′norz/swet′ing/test) (n.)   An evaluation of the intactness of the sympathetic nervous system. Prepare a solution of 2.0 g metallic iodine, 10 mL castor oil and 90 mL abosolute alcohol. Completely clean and dry the patient's skin. Paint the test areas with the solution, avoiding trans-

fer of any insensible sweating from one area to another. Then dust on some fine rice starch with a cotton powder puff or a blower. Fan or blow off all excess starch; then cover the patient with blankets or place him or her under a heat lamp. After 10 to 15 minutes, small, fine, bluish black spots resembling poppy seeds will appear in the normally perspiring areas. As perspiration increases, the fine dots gradually enlarge until they form violet-color.

Mitochondrion (mi″to-kon′drē-on) (n.)   A small, threadlike, rod-shaped, intracellular organelle in the cytoplasm that contains the electron transport system and certain other enzymes. It is the site of oxidative phosphorylation.

Mitogen (mī′tō-gen) (n.)   A substance that stimulates mitosis and lymphocyte transformation.

Mitosis (mī′tō-sis) (n.)   A form of nuclear division in which exact chromosome duplication results in the creation of two daughter cells identical to the original cell. It is a continuous process, consisting of five stages: (1) interphase, (2) prophase, (3) metaphase, (4) anaphase, and (5) telophase.

Mixed Connective Tissue Disorder (mixt/konek′tiv/tish′u/dis-or′der) (n.)   A syndrome having the clinical features of systemic sclerosis, systemic lupus erythematosis, and polymyositis.

mm   Abbreviation for millimeter.

MMPI (n.)   Abbreviation for Minnesota Multiphasic Personality Inventory.

Moberg's Pick-up Test (mō′-bergz/pik-up/test) (n.)   An evaluation of coordination and tactile gnosis. Ask the patient to gather a number of small objects (paper clip, coin, key, screw, nut and bolt, marble, etc.) from a table and to put them into a small container, using first the normal hand and then the affected hand. Time the patient with a stopwatch each time he or she performs the test and note the functional aptitude for picking up objects. Record the results. Periodically reassess the patient to determine change in functional status.

Mobility (mō-bil′i-tē) (n.)   The degree of motion; used in reference to the entire body or a specific body part. Abnormal mobility refers to any motion of a joint short of or beyond the anticipated range, or in any plane other than normal.

Mobilization (mō″bi-li-zā′shun) (n.)   The act of increasing the motion of part or all of a body.

Moccasin (mok′ah-sin) (n.)   1. A shoe made of one-piece vamp quarter and sole, a stitched back seam, and tongue. 2. A stitched and/or perforated circular decorative design on the vamp of a shoe.

Modulus (mod′ū-lus) (n.)   A specific property of a substance.

Modulus of Elasticity (mod-ū-lus/of/ē″las-tis′i-tē) (n.)   The slope of a stress-strain curve in the elastic region. It is indicative of the stiffness of a material. The steeper the curve, the higher modulus of elasticity; therefore, the stiffer the material. A low modulus indicates a more elastic material. The rigidity of a structure depends on the modulus of elasticity and the structure's geometry. The unit of measure for the modulus of elasticity (e) is newtons per square meter (poundforce per square foot). Also known as **Young's Modulus**.

Moe Technique (mō/tek′nēk) (n.)   A procedure for posterior spinal fusion that uses the intra-articular fusion of the lateral articulation.

Moiré Topography (mwa-rā′/to-pog′rah-fē) (n.)   A biostereometric method that produces a three-dimensional image of the shape of the trunk. It can be used to show the asymmetry of the two halves of the back in structural scoliosis. "Moiré" refers to the pattern of shadows produced by interference when periodic or quasiperiodic grids are placed on top of one another—the width of the lines should equal the space between them. The moire effect can also arise through interference between a screen and its shadow falling on an object behind. An asymmetry of at least one fringe interval is considered proof of trunk asymmetry.

Mold Arthroplasty (mōld/ar′thrō-plas″tē) (n.)   A resurfacing procedure in ball and socket joints, such as the hip. The ball is resurfaced with a smooth, usually metallic component that articulates with the native socket. The intent is to remold or mold the surface of the socket to conform to the prosthesis. An example is the **Smith-Petersen Cup**.

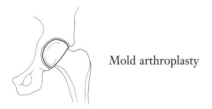

Mold arthroplasty

Molecular Weight (mō-lek′ū-lar/wāt) (n.)   The sum of the atomic weights of the atoms in a molecule.

Molecule (mol′e-kūl) (n.)   The smallest particle of a covalently bonded element or compound that retains the properties of that substance. A molecule is composed of two or more atoms chemically combined; examples are O_2 and H_2O.

Moloney's Line (mō-lō-nēz/līn) (n.)   An eponym for the scapulohumeral arch in the shoulder girdle. It is formed by the axillary border of the scapula, the inferior portion of the humeral neck, and the shaft of the humerus. Moloney's line is outlined in the lateral thoracic view of the glenohumeral joint. A break in the normal, smooth scapulohumeral arch indicates shoulder dislocation.

Moment (mō′ment) (n.)   1. A force acting through a lever arm to produce perpendicular rotation. Also called a **Torque**. 2. The force needed to impart an-

gular acceleration to a mass. The unit of measurement is newton meters.

Momentum (mō′men′tum) (n.)   The product of mass and velocity of a particle or rigid body. The unit of measure is kilogram meters per second (pound feet per second).

Mongolism (mon′go-lizm) (n.)   Another name for **Down syndrome**; the result of trisomy of a G group chromosome.

Monomer (mon-o-mer) (n.)   A simple molecular unit linked with others to form a polymer.

Monoplegia (mon″o-plē′je-ah) (n.)   Paralysis or weakness that involves only one extremity.

Monosodium Urate (mon″o-sō′dē-um/u-rāt) (n.)   The crystalline form of uric acid that is deposited in and around joints and tendon sheaths in gout.

Monostotic (mon″os-tot-ik) (adj.)   Of or related to only one bone. Compare with **Polyostotic**.

Monteggia Equivalent (mon-tej′ah/e-kwiv′ah-lent) (n.)   Clinical variants of Type I Monteggia Fractures. There are four types: (1) isolated anterior dislocation of the radial head without a fracture of the ulna, (2) single or segmental ulnar fracture with a fracture of the radial neck, (3) fractures of both bones—fracture of the forearm at the middle third with fracture of the radial shaft proximal to that of the ulnar shaft, and (4) fracture of the ulnar shaft and radial neck with dislocation of the radial shaft but maintenance of the anatomic position of the radial head.

Monteggia Fracture (mon-tej′ah/frak′chur) (n.)   A fracture of the ulna near the junction of its proximal and middle thirds associated with a dislocation of the radial head. These fractures are often classified by the direction of radial head dislocation:

Type I: The radial head is dislocated anteriorly, with volar angulation of the fractured shaft of the ulna.

Type II: The radial head is dislocated posteriorly, with dorsal angulation of the fractured shaft of the ulna.

Type III: The radial head is dislocated laterally, with lateral angulation of the fractured shaft of the ulna.

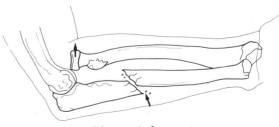

Monteggia fracture,
Type I 60%.

Montercaus Fracture (mon′-ter-kaus/frak′chur) (n.)   Fracture of the fibula neck with diastasis of the ankle mortise.

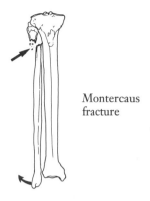

Montercaus fracture

Moore Fracture (moor/frak′chur) (n.) A fracture of the distal radius, with dorsal subluxation of the ulna and incarceration of the ulnar styloid process under the annular ligaments of the wrist.

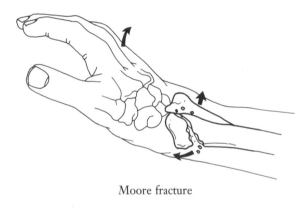

Moore fracture

Moore Pin (moor/pin) (n.) A type of metallic pin designed for internal fixation of femoral neck fractures.

Moore Procedure (moor/pro-sē′jur) (n.) An operation intended to prevent recurrent posterior subluxation of the humeral head by placing a graft in the posterior aspect of the glenoid.

Moore Prosthesis (moor/pros-thē′sis) (n.) See **Austin Moore Prosthesis**.

Morbidity (mor-bid′i-tē) (n.) A diseased or pathologic state.

Morning Stiffness (mor′ning/stif′nes) (n.) The subjective complaint of local or general joint immobility on arising from bed in the morning. The stiffness is a nonspecific indication of inflammation and is manifest in most types of inflammatory arthritis (e.g., rheumatoid arthritis) as well as in polymyalgia rheumatica. Duration is variable and directly proportional to the severity of the inflammatory process.

Moro Reflex (mo′ro/rē′fleks) (n.) An immature reflex that is pathologic if it persists after 3 months of age. On hearing a loud noise or otherwise being star-

tled, an infant abducts and extends all four extremities, extends the spine, and extends and fans the digits. Also known as the **Startle Reflex**.

Morphogenesis (mor′fō-jen′e-sis) (n.) The development of size, form, and other structural features of organisms.

Morphology (mor-fol′o-jē) (n.) The study of the structure of organisms.

Morquio Syndrome (mor-kē′ō/sin′drōm) (n.) One of the mucopolysaccharidoses; transmitted as an autosomal recessive trait. Patients are usually diagnosed between 18 months and 2 years of age. Keratan sulfate is the characteristic protein-sugar molecule that accumulates; it is found in the urine. These patients usually have normal mentation, but there is mild corneal clouding and significant skeletal dysplasia. Common findings include marked platyspondyly, hypoplasia of the anterior portion of one or several vertebrae (which results in kyphosis), genu valgum and coxa valga, acetabulum dysplasia, and obliquity of the distal radius and ulna, with narrowing of the proximal metacarpal shafts. Also known as **Mucopolysaccharidosis IV**, **Brailsford Syndrome**, and **Ullrich Disease**.

Morrey System (mor′-ē/sis′tem) (n.) A rating scheme for evaluating the results of total elbow arthroplasties. It uses three criteria to determine results: radiographic appearance, subjective pain, and objective evaluation of motion. The results are classified as good, fair, or poor.

Morse-Type Taper (mors-tīp/tā′per) (n.) A slightly tapered post on the proximal aspect of a femoral stem on which modular components with varying neck lengths and head diameter can be interchangeably attached.

Mortality (mor-tal′i-tē) (n.) Fatality.

Mortise Joint (mor′tēs/joint) (n.) A type of joint, e.g., the ankle joint

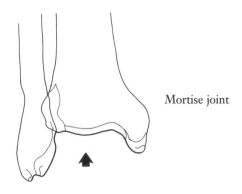

Mortise joint

Mortise View (mor′-tis/vū) (n.) A radiographic view of the ankle in which the AP projection is taken with the medial and lateral malleoli on a plane horizontal to the table. To achieve this, the foot is internally rotated 10 degrees to 15 degrees. This view permits visualization of the distal tibiofibular joint and an accurate assessment of the medial clear space.

Morton's Foot (mor′tonz/fut) (n.) A foot with a short big toe and a long second toe. The congenitally short first metatarsal bone changes the weight-bearing pattern of the foot, resulting in callosities beneath the second and third metatarsals and hypertrophy of the second metatarsal. The additional pressure on the second metatarsal causes pain, especially during rollover of the stance phase of walking or toe spring at push-off. Also called **Morton's Syndrome**.

Morton's Metatarsalgia (mor′tonz/met″ah-tar-sal′je-ah) (n.) See **Morton's Neuroma**.

Morton's Neuroma (mor′tonz/nū′rō-mah) (n.) An interdigital neuroma of the foot, most commonly seen in the third webspace. It is caused by an apparently degenerative pseudoneuroma of the most lateral branch of the medial plantar nerve. Patients usually present with a burning or aching pain in the region of the metatarsal heads; this pain is usually increased with walking. On examination, tenderness to palpation is elicited and a click on compression of the metatarsal heads may be heard. Although subjective complaints of numbness are common, objective signs of decreased sensation usually are not found. Also known as **Morton's Toe**, **Morton's Metatarsalgia**, and **Interdigital Neuroma**.

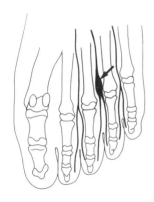

Morton's neuroma

Morton's Test (mor′tonz/test) (n.) A method used in evaluation of a foot for Morton's neuroma. Transverse compression across the heads of the metatarsals causes a sharp pain and possibly a clicking noise between the involved metatarsals.

Morton's Toe (mor′tonz/tō) (n.) See **Morton's Neuroma**.

Mosaic Bone (mo-zā′ik/bōn) (n.) A descriptive term for bone that has a disorganized structural pattern. This pattern is the histologic hallmark of the altered bone in Paget's disease. Microscopically, the osseous fragments are faceted together and bounded by numerous irregular cement lines.

Mose Template (mōz/tem′plat) (n.) A radiographic measurement to evaluate the roundness of the femoral head. A grid ruled with a series of 28 concentric circles 2 mm apart that is superimposed onto the femoral head on an AP and a lateral radiograph of the hip. If the head constitutes a circle in both views and both circles have the same radius, the head is spherical. The deviation from circularity can be measured by using the overlay. If the outline of these two circles varies by 2 mm or less, the head is termed elliptical. If the variation is greater than 2 mm on frontal and lateral x-rays, the head is considered irregular. This template is used to evaluate the final shape of the femoral head after such affections as Legg-Calvé-Perthes disease or slipped capital femoral epiphysis. Also called **Moses' Concentric Circles**.

Moskowicz Test (mos′ko-witz/test) (n.) A means of determining the adequacy of collateral circulation in the presence of an arteriovenous fistula. For this test, first elevate the extremity. Then apply a tight bandage for 5 minutes. Next, place the extremity in a horizontal position and quickly remove the bandage. With adequate circulation, a hyperemic blush occurs promptly. With inadequate circulation, the blush is absent or slight and progresses slowly to the periphery.

Mosquito (mos-kē′tō) (n.) An abbreviated reference to a mosquito hemostat, which is a small, cured surgical clamp used on blood vessels. Also called a **Mosquito Clamp**.

Most Significant Diagnosis (most/sig-nif′i-kant/dī″ag-nō′sis) (n.) The one diagnosis that describes the most important or significant condition of a patient. It is used in the provision of medical care, in hospitals, and for monitoring the patient's health.

Motion (mō′shun) (n.) The relative displacement over time of a body in space with respect to other bodies or reference systems.

Motor Ataxia (mo′tor/ah-tak′sē-ah) (n.) The inability to perform coordinated muscular activity.

Motor End-Plate (mo′tor/end-plate) (n.) The junction between the terminal branch of the nerve fiber and a skeletal muscle fiber. Also called a **Myoneural Junction**.

Motor Neuron (mo′tor/nū′ron) (n.) An efferent neuron that conducts motor impulses away from the central nervous system. There are two types of motor neurons: upper and lower. The cell body of an upper motor neuron is in the brain; the axon, which ends in synapses, extends only into the spinal cord. It is thus entirely within the central nervous system. The cell body of the lower motor neuron is in the spinal cord; its axon, extending outward, becomes a cranial or spinal motor nerve in order to reach an effector. This is also known as a motor neuron.

Motor Neuron Disease (mo′tor/nu′ron/di-zēz′) (n.) A neurologic disorder of widespread degeneration of motor neurons at all levels that results in wasting, weakness, and fasciculation of skeletal muscles. In the restricted sense, motor neuron disease is divided into separate syndromes, which depend solely on the sites of maximal stress of the pathologic process. Examples include amyotrophic lateral sclerosis, lateral sclerosis, peroneal and spinal muscular atrophy, and progressive bulbar paralysis.

Motor Nerve (mo′tor/nerv) (n.) A nerve consisting of different fibers that carry impulses outward from the central nervous system to activate a muscle, gland, or organ. Compare with **Sensory Nerve**.

Motor Paralysis (mo′tor/pah′ral-i-sis) (n.) Paralysis of the voluntary muscles.

Motor Point (mo′tor/point) (n.) 1. The local region within a muscle where the motor nerve provides innervation. 2. A point on the skin where low voltage electric stimulation in short doses elicits contraction of a specific muscle. This is used in electromyography.

Motor Unit (mo′tor/ū′nit) (n.) The functional unit of the neuromuscular system. It consists of the anterior horn cell, its axon, and all the muscle fibers innervated by that axon.

Motorized Shaver (mo′tor-ized/sha′ver) (n.) An externally powered, high- or low-speed instrument used in arthroscopic surgery to debride soft tissues and suction loose debris from a joint. These shavers have a variety of cutting tips that spin about a hollow, fenestrated cylinder, also of variable size and shape.

Motrin (mo′trin) (n.) A proprietary name for ibuprofen, a nonsteroidal, antiinflammatory drug.

Mountain View (mown′ten/vū) (n.) A simple, axial radiographic view of the patellofemoral joint. To obtain this view, lean a chair against the end of a standard x-ray table at a 45 degree angle. Have the patient lie supine, with the knee flexed to 45 degrees over the table edge and supported by the chair back, which in turn is supported by the handle of a stepstool. Strap the patient's calves together to prevent rotation. Lean the film cassette against the patient's ankles and the handle of the stepstool. Aim the beam caudally and 30 degrees down from the horizontal.

This view was first described by MacNab and then modified by Merchant and his colleagues, all of whom work in Mountain View, California. Compare with **Skyline** or **Sunrise View**.

Movie Sign (n.) See **Theatre Sign**.

MPS (n.) Abbreviation for Mucopolysaccharide.

MRI (n.) Abbreviation for Magnetic resonance imaging.

Mouchet Fracture (mu-shay′/frak′chur) (n.) A fracture of the capitellum of the humerus.

Mucin Clot Test (mu′sin/klot/test) (n.) A way to estimate the quality and quantity of hyaluronate in a sample of synovial fluid. Add a few drops of synovial fluid to 20 mL of 5% acetic acid. A clot should form within minutes. Normal or "good" mucin is present if a tight mass forms in the clear solution. A softer threading mass indicates a "fair" mucin. A turbid so-

lution with threads is a "poor" mucin. A cloudy solution with a few flecks is a "very poor" mucin. Firm clot formation indicates integrity of the high molecular weight hyaluronate-protein complexes; a friable clot indicates smaller polymer chains. Also called the **Ropes Test**.

Mucopolysaccharide (mu″ko-pol″ē-sak′ah-rīd) (n.) A group of polysaccharides that contain hexosamine. Mucopolysaccharides may or may not be found in combination with a protein.

Mucopolysaccharidosis (mu″ko-pol″ē-sak″ah-ri-dō′sis) (n.) One of several inborn errors in the metabolism of mucopolysaccharides. These protein-sugar molecules accumulate within cells, which results in disease and deformity.

The errors are differentiated by clinical, genetic, and biomechanical findings into different types. These include: MPS I (Hurler syndrome; also known as MPS-IH), MPS II (Hunter syndrome), MPS III (Sanfilippo syndrome), MPS IV (Morquio syndrome), MPS V: (Scheie syndrome), MPS VI (Maroteaux-Lamy syndrome), pseudopolydystrophy, generalized gangliodosis. See individual diseases.

Mucoprotein (mu″ko-pro′tē-in) (n.) One of a group of proteins found in the globulin fraction of blood plasma. Mucoproteins are globulins combined with a carbohydrate group.

Mucous Cyst (mu′kus/sist) (n.) A benign cyst that typically appears in the skin on the dorsum and to one side of the distal finger joint in adults. The cyst is filled with a clear mucoid fluid that may be seen through the thin, transparent overlying skin. These cysts are believed to result from the myxomatous degeneration of the corneum layer and are frequently associated with Heberden's nodes in osteoarthritis. A bony osteophyte near the cyst is almost always identified radiographically.

Muenster Socket (muhn-ster/sok′et) (n.) A preflexed arm prosthesis designed to fit amputees with short below-elbow stumps. It consists of an intimately fitted suction socket extending above the condyles of the humerus. It was developed in 1956 in Muenster, Germany.

Muller Approach (mul′er/ah-prōch′) (n.) A modification of the anterolateral surgical approach to the hip in which, with the patient supine, the hip is dislocated anteriorly, but a trochanteric osteotomy is not done. The deep dissection plane is between the fascia lata and the gluteus medius muscles.

Muller Total Hip Prosthesis (mul′er/tō′tal/hip/pros-thē′sis) (n.) One of the early femoral stem designs that modified the original Charnley prosthesis by increasing the head diameter, adding a collar, and changing the contour to a curved saber shape.

Multifocal Osteomyelitis (mul″ti-fō′kal/os″te-ō-mī″e-lī-tis) (n.) The simultaneous occurence of acute or chronic bone infections at multiple bone sites.

Multiple Enchondromatosis (mul′ti-p′l/en-kon″drō-mah-tō′sis) (n.) See **Enchondromatosis**.

Multiple Epiphyseal Dysplasia (mul′ti-p′l/ep″i-fiz′ē-al/dis-plā′se-ah) (n.)   An osteochondrodysplasia that results in short-limbed disproportionate dwarfism. Inherited as an autosomal dominant condition, it is not apparent at birth. Radiographically, the epiphyses are noted to have delayed, irregular, or fragmented ossification centers. This results in leg length discrepancy, angular deformities, scoliosis, and early degenerative joint disease. Commonly known as **Fairbank's Disease**.

Multiple Exostoses (mul′ti-p′l/ek″sos-tō′sēs) (n.) See **Osteochondromatosis**.

Multiple Fractures (mul′ti-p′l/frak′churz) (n.)   A descriptive term for the occurrence in one patient of two or more complete bone fractures involving more than one bone (with fractures of the forearm or lower leg counted as one fracture).

Multiple Myeloma (mul-ti-p′l/mi″e-lō′mah) (n.)   A primary malignant tumor of bone. A neoplastic proliferation of plasma cells within the bone marrow produces a monoclonal immunoglobulin, which is identifiable in the serum or urine. Clinically, symptoms result from pathologic fracture and bone marrow dysfunction. Radiographically, one sees either multiple rounded, osteolytic, or punched-out lesions without sclerotic borders or generalized osteopenia. The diagnosis is confirmed by the presence of a monoclonal spike on serum or urine immunoelectrophoresis. Also known as **Plasma Cell Myeloma**.

Multiple Pin Fixation (mul′ti-p′l/pin/fik-sā′shun) (n.)   A descriptive term for a technique of internal fixation across the femoral neck and into the femoral head, into which more than one threaded pin is placed. This procedure is used in the treatment of femoral neck fractures and slipped capital femoral epiphyses.

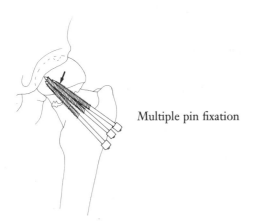

Multiple pin fixation

Mumford Procedure (mum-ford/pro-se′jur) (n.)   A surgical technique for the treatment of chronic, symptomatic acromioclavicular joint dislocation and disorders. In this procedure, the lateral end of the

clavicle is resected. Also known as the **Gurd** or **Mumford-Gurd Procedure**.

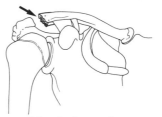

Mumford procedure

Munchhausen's Syndrome (men-chow′zenz/sin′drōm) (n.)   A psychiatric disorder in which a patient persistently seeks hospital care for a nonexistent illness. The patient can describe the disease vividly and may deliberately inflict injury on himself or herself to substantiate the claims.

Murphy's Sign (mur′fēz/sīn) (n.)   A technique used in evaluation of a fracture of the carpal navicular bone. With the patient's wrist in neutral position, pound on the head of the index metacarpal bone. If a navicular fracture is present, pain will be pronounced over the ray. If a lunate dislocation is present, pain will be more pronounced on the middle ray.

Muscle (mus′el) (n.)   One of the contractile organs of the body that effects movement of various body parts. Muscle is classified as skeletal, cardiac, or smooth. On histologic examination, the two former types are transversely striated. Skeletal muculature is voluntary; typically it is composed of a muscle belly attached at either end to bone by a tendon, aponeurosis, or other fascial tissue. A list of muscles follows:

Muscles, Abdominal (mus′elz/ab-dom′i-nal) (n.) Muscles of the abdominal wall: Rectus abdominous, External oblique, Internal oblique, and Transverse abdominous muscle.

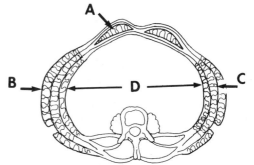

Muscle, Abdominal: **A**, rectus abdominus; **B**, external obliques; **C**, internal obliques; **D**, transversus abdominis.

Abductor Digiti Minimi (Manus)

Origin: Pisiform bone tendon of ulnar flexor muscle of wrist.

Insertion: Proximal phalanx of fifth digit.

Action: Abducts little finger.

Innervation: Ulnar nerve.

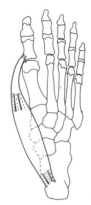

Muscle, Abductor hallucis

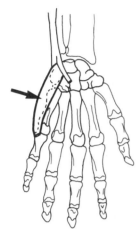

Muscle, Abductor digiti minimi (manus)

Abductor Digiti Minimi (Pedis)

Origin: Lateral tubercle of calcaneus.

Insertion: Proximal phalanx of little toe.

Action: Abducts little toe.

Innervation: Superficial branch of lateral plantar nerve.

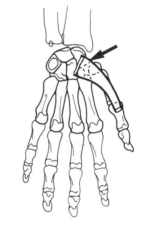

Muscle, Abductor pollicis brevis

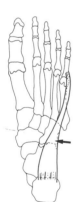

Muscle, Abductor digiti minimi (pedis).

Abductor Pollicis Longus

Origin: Posterior surface of ulna, middle third of radius.

Insertion: First metacarpal bone.

Action: Abducts thumb and hand.

Innervation: Posterior interosseous nerve.

Adductor Brevis

Origin: Pubis, below origin of the long adductor muscle.

Abductor Hallucis

Origin: Calcaneus, plantar aponeurosis.

Insertion: Proximal phalanx of great toe (joined by flexor muscle of great toe).

Action: Abducts and aids in flexion of great toe.

Innervation: Medial plantar nerve.

Abductor Pollicis Brevis

Origin: Flexor retinaculum of hand, scaphoid, and trapezium.

Insertion: Proximal phalanx of thumb.

Action: Abducts and aids in flexion of thumb.

Innervation: Median nerve.

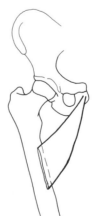

Muscle, Adductor brevis

246

Insertion: Upper part of linea aspera of femur.
Action: Adducts, flexes, and rotates thigh laterally.
Innervation: Obturator nerve.

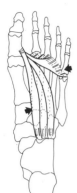

Muscle, Adductor hallucis

Adductor Hallucis
Origin: Oblique head: long plantar ligament, transverse head, capsules of metacarpophalangeal joints.
Insertion: Proximal phalanx of great toe (joined by flexor muscle of great toe).
Action: Oblique head adducts and flexes great toe; transverse head supports transverse arch, adducts great toe.
Innervation: Lateral plantar nerve.

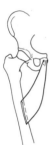

Muscle, Adductor longus

Adductor Longus
Origin: Pubis, below pubic crest.
Insertion: Linea aspera of femur.
Action: Adducts, flexes, and rotates thigh laterally.
Innervation: Anterior division of obturator nerve.

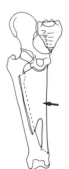

Muscle, Adductor magnus

Adductor Magnus
Origin: Adductor part: inferior ramus of pubis, ramus of ischium. Extensor part: ischial tuberosity.
Insertion: Adductor part: linea aspera of femur. Extensor part: adductor tubercle of femur.
Action: Adducts, flexes, and laterally rotates thigh.
Innervation: Posterior division of obturator nerve.

Adductor Pollicis
Origin: Capitate, second, and third metacarpal bones.
Insertion: Proximal phalanx of thumb.
Action: Adducts and aids in apposition of thumb.
Innervation: Deep palmar branch of ulnar nerve.

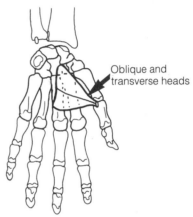

Oblique and transverse heads

Muscle, Adductor pollicis

Anconeus
Origin: Back of lateral epicondyle of humerus.
Insertion: Olecranon process, posterior surface of ulna.
Action: Extends forearm, abducts ulna in pronation of wrist.
Innervation: Radial nerve.

Articularis Cubiti
Origin: Posterior distal surface of humerus.
Insertion: Posterior aspect of elbow joint.
Action: Elevates capsule in extension of elbow joint.
Innervation: Radial nerve.

Articularis Genus
Origin: Lower part of anterior surface of femur.
Insertion: Synovial membrane of knee joint.
Action: Elevates capsule of knee joint.
Innervation: A branch of the femoral nerve.

Biceps Brachii
Origin: Long head: supraglenoid tubercle of scapula. Short head: apex of coracoid process.
Insertion: Tuberosity of radius.
Action: Flexes forearm and arm, supinates hand.
Innervation: Musculocutaneous nerve.

Biceps Femoris
Origin: Long head: ischial tuberosity (in common with semitendinosus muscle). Short head: supracondylar ridge of femur.
Insertion: Head of fibula, lateral condyle of tibia.

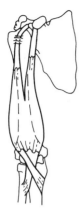

Muscle, Biceps brachii

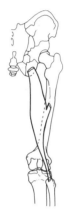

Muscle, Biceps femoris

Action: Flexes knee, rotates leg laterally; long head extends thigh.

Innervation: Long head by tibial nerve; short head by peroneal nerve.

Brachialis

Origin: Distal two thirds of humerus.
Insertion: Coronoid process of ulna.
Action: Flexes forearm.
Innervation: Musculocutaneous nerve.

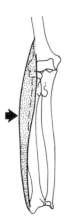

Muscle, Brachioradialis

Brachioradialis

Origin: Lateral supracondylar ridge and intermuscular septum of humerus.
Insertion: Styloid process of radius.
Action: Flexes forearm.
Innervation: Radial nerve.

Coccygeus

Origin: Ischial spine and sacrospinous ligament.
Insertion: Coccyx, lower part of lateral border of sacrum.
Action: Aids in raising and supporting pelvic floor.
Innervation: Pudendal nerve.

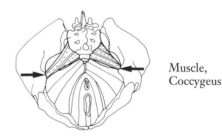

Muscle, Coccygeus

Coracobrachialis

Origin: Scapula (coracoid process).
Insertion: Humerus (middle third, medial surface).
Action: Adduction: assists in flexion and medial rotation of arm.
Innervation: Musculocutaneous nerve.

Deltoid

Origin: Lateral third of clavicle, acromion process, and spine of scapula.
Insertion: Deltoid tuberosity of humerus.
Action: Abductor of arm; aids in flexion and extension.
Innervation: Axillary nerve.

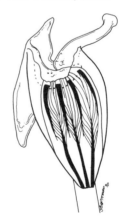

Muscle, Deltoid

Diaphragm

Origin: Xiphoid process, six lower costal cartilages, four lower ribs, lumbar vertebrae arcuate ligaments.
Insertion: Central tendon of diaphragm.
Action: Increases capacity of thorax in inspiration; the main muscle of inhalation.
Innervation: Phrenic nerve.

Erector Spinae

Origin: Deep muscle arising from the broad and thick ten-

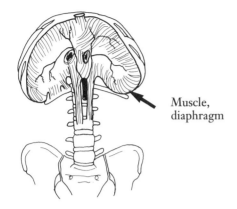

Muscle, diaphragm

Origin: Lateral condyle of tibia, upper three fourths of fibula, interosseous membrane.
Insertion: Extensor expansion of four lateral toes (by four slips).
Action: Extends toes.
Innervation: Deep peroneal nerve.

Extensor Hallucis Brevis

Origin: Dorsal surface of calcaneus.
Insertion: Base of proximal phalanx of great toe.
Action: Dorsiflexes great toe.
Innervation: Deep peroneal nerve.

Extensor Hallucis Longus

Origin: Middle of fibula, interosseous membrane.
Insertion: Distal phalanx of great toe.
Action: Extends great toe, dorsiflexes foot.
Innervation: Deep peroneal nerve.

Extensor Indicis

Origin: Posterior surface of ulna.
Insertion: Extensor expansion of index finger.
Action: Extends index finger and hand.
Innervation: Deep radial nerve.

Extensor Pollicis Brevis

Origin: Middle third of radius.
Insertion: Proximal phalanx of thumb.
Action: Extends and abducts hand.
Innervation: Deep radial nerve.

Extensor Pollicis Longus

Origin: Middle third of ulna, adjacent interosseous membrane.
Insertion: Distal phalanx of thumb.
Action: Extends distal phalanx of thumb, abducts hand.
Innervation: Deep radial nerve.

External Intercostal

Origin: Rib (lower border; forward fibers).
Insertion: Rib (upper border of rib below origin).
Action: Elevate ribs.
Innervation: Intercostal nerves.

Flexor Carpi Radialis

Origin: Medial epicondyle of humerus.

don attached to the middle crest of sacrum, spinous processes of lumbar and 11th and 12th thoracic vertebrae and back part of the iliac crest. It splits in the upper lumbar region into three columns of muscles: iliocostal (lateral division), longissimus (intermediate division), and spinal (medial division).
Action: Extends vertebral column and bends trunk to one side.
Innervation: Branches of dorsal primary divisions of spinal nerves.

Extensor Carpi Radialis Brevis

Origin: Lateral epicondyle of humerus, radial collateral ligament.
Insertion: Third metacarpal.
Action: Extends and abducts wrist.
Innervation: Radial nerve.

Extensor Carpi Radialis Longus

Origin: Lateral surpacondylar ridge of humerus.
Insertion: Second metacarpal bone.
Action: Extends and abducts wrist.
Innervation: Radial nerve.

Extensor Carpi Ulnaris

Origin: Humeral head: lateral epicondyle of humerus. Ulnar head: posterior border of ulna.
Insertion: Fifth metacarpal bone.
Action: Extends and abducts wrist.
Innervation: Radial nerve.

Extensor Digiti Minimi (Manus)

Origin: Lateral epicondyle of humerus.
Insertion: Extensor expansion of little finger.
Action: Extends little finger.
Innervation: Deep radial nerve.

Extensor Digitorum Brevis (Pedis)

Origin: Dorsal surface of calcaneus.
Insertion: Extensor tendons of first, second, third, and fourth toes.
Action: Extends toes.
Innervation: Deep peroneal nerve.

Extensor Digitorum Communis

Origin: Lateral epicondyle of humerus.
Insertion: Forms extensor expansion over fingers.
Action: Extends fingers, hand, and forearm.
Innervation: Deep radial nerve.

Extensor Digitorum Longus (Pedis)

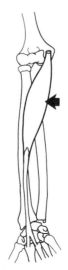

Muscle, flexor carpi radialis

Insertion: Bases of second and third metacarpal bones.
Action: Flexes hand and forearm, aids in pronation and abduction of hand.
Innervation: Median nerve.

Flexor Carpi Ulnaris

Origin: Humeral head: medial epicondyle of humerus. Ulnar head: olecranon and posterior border or ulnar.
Insertion: Pisiform, hamate, and fifth metacarpal bones.
Action: Flexes and adducts hand.
Innervation: Ulnar nerve.

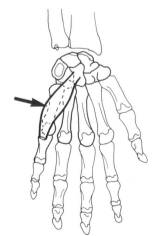

Muscle, flexor carpi ulnaris

Flexor Digiti Minimi Brevis (Manus)

Origin: Hook of hamate, flexor retinaculum.
Insertion: Proximal phalanx of little finger.
Action: Flexes proximal phalanx of little finger.
Innervation: Ulnar nerve.

Muscle, flexor digiti minimi brevis (manus)

Flexor Digiti Minimi Brevis (Pedis)

Origin: Base of fifth metatarsal and plantar fascia.
Insertion: Lateral surface of proximal phalanx of little toe.

Action: Flexes little toe.
Innervation: Lateral plantar nerve.

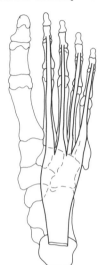

Muscle, flexor digitorum brevis (pedis)

Flexor Digitorum Brevis (Pedis)

Origin: Calcaneus and plantar fascia.
Insertion: Middle phalanges of four lateral toes.
Action: Flexes four lateral toes.
Innervation: Medial plantar nerve.

Flexor Digitorum Longus (Pedis)

Origin: Middle half of tibia.
Insertion: Distal phalanges of lateral four toes (by four tendons).
Action: Flexes second to fifth toes.
Innervation: Tibial nerve.

Flexor Digitorum Profundus (Manus)

Origin: Proximal three fourths of ulna and adjacent interosseous membrane.
Insertion: Distal phalanges of fingers.
Action: Flexes terminal phalanges and hand.
Innervation: Palmar interosseous nerve.

Flexor Digitorum Superficialis (Manus)

Origin: Humeroulnar head: medial epicondyle of humerus, coronoid process of ulna. Radial head: anterior border of radius.
Insertion: Middle phalanges of fingers.
Action: Flexes phalanges, hand, and forearm.
Innervation: Median nerve.

Flexor Hallucis Brevis

Origin: Cuboid and third cuneiform bones.
Insertion: Both sides of proximal phalanx of great toe.
Action: Flexes great toe.
Innervation: Medial plantar nerve.

Flexor Hallucis Longus

Origin: Lower two thirds of posterior surface of fibula, intermuscular septum.
Insertion: Distal phalanx of great toe.
Action: Flexes great toe.
Innervation: Tibial nerve.

Flexor Pollicis Brevis

Origin: Tubercle of trapezium, flexor retinaculum.

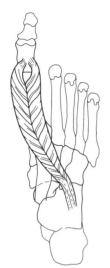

Muscle, flexor hallicis brevis

Action: Rotates thigh laterally.
Innervation: Sacral plexus.

Gemellus Superior
   Origin: Upper margin of lesser sciatic notch.
   Insertion: Internal obturator tendon.
   Action: Rotates thigh laterally.
   Innervation: Sacral plexus.

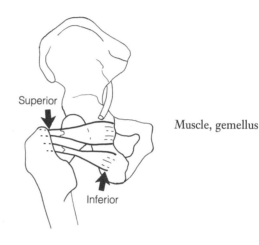

Muscle, gemellus

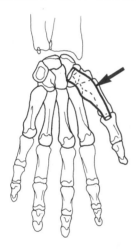

Muscle, flexor pollicis brevis

Gluteus Maximus
   Origin: Upper portion of ilium, sacrum, and coccyx, sacrotuberous ligament.
   Insertion: Gluteal tuberosity of femur, iliotibial tract (band of fascia lata).
   Action: Chief extensor; powerful lateral rotator of thigh.
   Innervation: Inferior gluteal nerve.

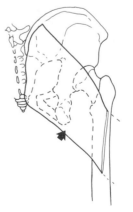

Muscle, gluteus maximus

Insertion: Proximal phalanx of thumb.
Action: Flexes and adducts thumb.
Innervation: Lateral portion, branch of median nerve; medial portion, deep branch of ulnar nerve.

Flexor Pollicis Longus
   Origin: Radius, adjacent interosseous membrane, coronoid process of ulna.
   Insertion: Distal phalanx of thumb.
   Action: Flexes thumb.
   Innervation: Palmar interosseous nerve.

Gastrocnemius
   Origin: Medial head: popliteal surface of femur, upper part of medial condyle of femur. Lateral head: lateral condyle of femur.
   Insertion: Calcaneus via calcaneal tendon (tendo calcaneus)—in common with soleus muscle.
   Action: Flexes foot and leg.
   Innervation: Tibial nerve.

Gemellus Inferior
   Origin: Lower margin of lesser sciatic notch.
   Insertion: Internal obturator tendon.

Gluteus Medius
   Origin: Midportion of ilium.
   Insertion: Greater trochanter and oblique ridge of femur.
   Action: Abducts, rotates thigh medially.
   Innervation: Superior gluteal nerve.

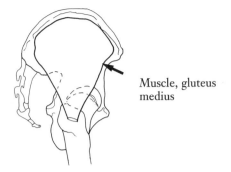

Muscle, gluteus medius

Gluteus Minimus

Origin: Lower portion of ilium.
Insertion: Greater trochanter of femur, capsule of hip joint.
Action: Abducts, rotates thigh medially.
Innervation: Superior gluteal nerve.

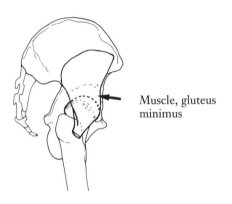

Muscle, gluteus minimus

Gracilis

Origin: Pubic bone (just below symphysis).
Insertion: Tibia (medial surface behind sartorius).
Action: Adducts thigh and flexes and adducts leg.
Innervation: Obturator nerve.

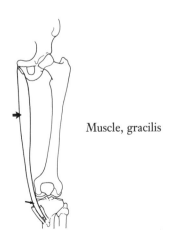

Muscle, gracilis

Iliacus

Origin: Iliac fossa, lateral aspect of sacrum.
Insertion: Greater psoas tendon, lesser trochanter of femur.
Action: Flexes and rotates thigh medially.
Innervation: Femoral nerve.

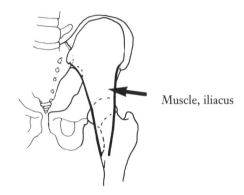

Muscle, iliacus

Iliocostalis Cervicis

Origin: Upper six ribs.
Insertion: Transverse processes of fourth, fifth, and sixth cervical vertebrae.
Action: Extends cervical vertebral column.
Innervation: Branches of dorsal primary divisions of spinal nerves.

Iliocostalis Lumborum

Origin: Iliac crest and sacrospinal aponeurosis.
Insertion: Lumbodorsal fascia, transverse processes of lumbar vertebrae, angles of lower six ribs.
Action: Extends lumbar spine.
Innervation: Branches of dorsal primary divisions of spinal nerves.

Iliocostalis Thoracis

Origin: Lower seven ribs, medial to the angles of the ribs.
Insertion: Angles of upper seven ribs, transverse process of seventh cervical vertebra.
Action: Keeps thoracic spine erect.
Innervation: Branches of dorsal primary divisions of spinal nerves.

Iliopsoas

Origin: Ilium (iliac fossa); Vertebrae (bodies of twelfth thoracic to fifth lumbar).
Insertion: Femur (lesser trochanter); a compound muscle consisting of the iliac and greater psoas muscles, which join to form the iliopsoas tendon.
Action: Flexes thigh; flexes trunk (when femur acts as origin).
Innervation: Femoral and second to fourth lumbar nerves.

Infraspinatus

Origin: Infraspinous fossa of scapula.
Insertion: Midportion of greater tubercle of humerus.
Action: Rotates arm laterally.
Innervation: Suprascapular nerve.

Intercostales Externi

Origin: Inferior border of rib.
Insertion: Superior border of rib below origin.

Action: Draw ribs together.

Innervation: Intercostal nerves.

Intercostales Interni

Origin: Superior border of rib.

Insertion: Interior border of rib above origin.

Action: Draw ribs together.

Innervation: Intercostal nerves.

Internal Oblique

Origin: Ossa coxae (iliac crest and inguinal ligament); lumbodorsal fossa.

Insertion: Ribs (lower three), pubic bone, linea alba.

Action: Same as external oblique.

Innervation: Last three intercostal nerves, iliohypogastric and ilioinguinal nerves.

Interossei Dorsales (Manus)

Origin: Adjacent sides of metacarpal bones.

Insertion: Extensor tendons of second, third, and fourth fingers.

Action: Abduct, flex proximal phalanges.

Innervation: Deep palmar branch of ulnar nerve.

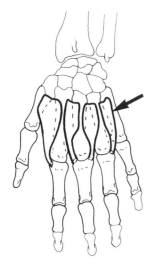

Muscle, interossei dorsales (manus)

Interossei Dorsales (Pedis)

Origin: Adjacent sides of metatarsal bones.

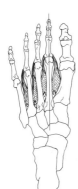

Muscle, interossei dorsales (pedis)

Insertion: Proximal phalanges of both sides of second toe, lateral side of third and fourth toes.

Action: Abduct lateral toes, move second toe from side to side.

Innervation: Deep branch of lateral plantar nerve.

Interossei Palmares

Origin: Medial side of second lateral side of fourth and fifth metacarpals.

Insertion: Base of proximal phalanx in line with its origin.

Action: Adduct index, ring, and litle fingers; aid in extension of fingers.

Innervation: Deep palmar branch of ulnar nerve.

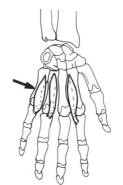

Muscle, interossei palmares

Interossei Plantares

Origin: Medial side of third, fourth, and fifth metatarsal bones.

Insertion: Medial side of proximal phalanges of third, fourth, and fifth toes.

Action: Adduct three lateral toes toward second toe.

Innervation: Lateral plantar nerve.

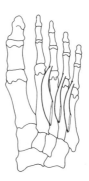

Muscle, interossei plantares

Interspinales

Origin: Superior surface of spinous process of each vertebra.

Insertion: Inferior surface of spinous process of vertebra above vertebra of origin.

Action: Extend vertebral column.

Innervation: Dorsal primary divisions of spinal curves.

Intertransversarii

Origin: Extends between transverse process of adjacent vertebrae.

Action: Bend vertebral column laterally.

Innervation: Anteriores, posteriores, and laterales by branches of ventral primary divisions of spinal nerves; the mediales by branches of the dorsal primary divisions.

Ischiocavernosus

Origin: Ramus of ischium adjacent to crus of penis or clitoris.

Insertion: Crus near pubic symphysis.

Action: Maintains erection of penis or clitoris.

Innervation: Perineal branch of pudendal nerve.

Latissimus Dorsi

Origin: Spinous processes of lower six thoracic vertebrae, lumbodorsal fascia, crest of ilium.

Insertion: Floor of intertubercular groove of humerus.

Action: Adducts, extends, medially rotates arm.

Innervation: Thoracodorsal nerve.

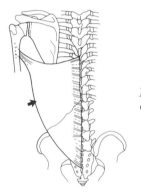

Muscle, latissimus dorsi

Levator Ani

Origin: Pubococcygeus m. part: pubis and pelvic fascia; puborectal m. part: pubis; iliococcygeus m. part: pelvic surface of ischial spine and pelvic fascia.

Insertion: Third and fourth sacral and perineal.

Action: Supports pelvic viscera.

Innervation: Pudendal nerve.

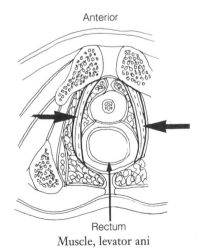

Anterior

Rectum

Muscle, levator ani

Levator Scapulae

Origin: Transverse processes of first four cervical vertebrae.

Insertion: Vertebral border of scapula.

Action: Raises scapula.

Innervation: Branches of third and fourth cervical nerves from the cervical plexus and frequently the lower portion by a branch of the dorsal scapular nerve.

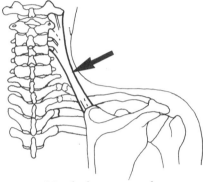

Muscle, levator scapulae

Longissimus Capitis

Origin: Transverse processes of cervical vertebrae.

Insertion: Mastoid process of temporal bone.

Action: Draws head backward, rotates head.

Innervation: Branches of dorsal primary divisions of the middle and lower cervical nerves.

Longissimus Cervicis

Origin: Transverse process of upper six thoracic vertebrae.

Insertion: Transverse processes of second through sixth vertebrae.

Action: Extends cervical vertebrae.

Innervation: Branches of dorsal primary divisions of spinal nerves.

Longus Capitis

Origin: Transverse processes of third and sixth cervical vertebrae.

Insertion: Basal part of occipital bone.

Action: Flexes head.

Innervation: First, second, and third cervical nerves.

Longus Colli

Origin: Superior oblique part: anterior tubercle of transverse processes of third, fourth, and fifth cervical vertebrae.

Insertion: Superior oblique part: anterolateral surface of tubercle on anterior arch of first vertebra (atlas).

Action: Bends neck forward and slightly rotates the cervical portion of the vertebral column.

Innervation: Branches from second to seventh cervical nerves.

Lumbricales (Manus)

Origin: Tendons of deep flexor muscle of fingers.

Insertion: Extensor tendons of four lateral fingers.

Action: Flexes proximal, extends middle and distal phalanges.

Innervation: First and second lumbricales by branches of

the third and fourth digital branches of the median nerve; the third and fourth lumbricales by branches of the deep palmar branch of the ulnar. The third lumbricalis may receive twigs from both nerves or all its fibers from the median nerve.

Lumbricales (Pedis)

Origin: Tendons of long flexor muscle of toes.

Insertion: Medial side of proximal phalanges of four lateral toes.

Action: Aids in flexion of toes.

Innervation: First lumbricalis by a branch of the medial plantar nerve; other three lumbricales by branches of the lateral plantar nerve.

Masseter

Origin: Superficial part: zygomatic process and arch; deep part: zygomatic arch.

Insertion: Superficial part: ramus and angle of lower jaw; deep part: upper half of ramus, coronoid process of lower jaw.

Action: Closes mouth, clenches teeth (muscle of mastication).

Innervation: Masseteric nerve from mandibular division of the trigeminal nerve.

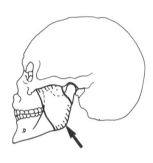

Muscle, masseter

Multifidus

Origin: Sacrum and transverse processes of lumbar, thoracic, and lower cervical vertebrae.

Insertion: Spinous processes of lumbar, thoracic, and lower cervical vertebrae.

Action: Extends, rotates vertebral column.

Innervation: Dorsal primary divisions of spinal nerves.

Oblique Capitis Superior

Origin: Transverse process of atlas vertebra.

Insertion: Outer third of inferior curved line of occipital bone.

Action: Rotates head.

Innervation: Branch of dorsal primary division of suboccipital nerve.

Obliquus Internus Abdominis

Origin: Iliac crest, lumbodorsal fascia, inguinal ligament.

Insertion: Lower three or four costal cartilages, linea alba by conjoint tendon to pubis.

Action: Flexes and rotates vertebral column, tenses abdominal wall.

Innervation: Branches of the eighth to twelfth intercostal and the iliohypogastric and ilioinguinal nerves.

Obliquus Capitis Inferior

Origin: Spine of axis vertebra.

Insertion: Transverse process of atlas vertebra.

Action: Rotates head.

Innervation: Branch of dorsal primary division of suboccipital nerve.

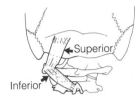

Muscle, obliquus capitis inferior

Obliquus Externus Abdominis

Origin: External surface of lower eight ribs at costal cartilages.

Insertion: Anterior half of crest of ilium, linea alba through rectus sheath.

Action: Flexes and rotates vertebral column, tenses abdominal wall.

Innervation: Branches of the eighth to twelfth intercostal and the iliohypogastric and ilioinguinal nerves.

Obturatorius Externus

Origin: Margin of obturator foramen of pelvis, obturator membrane.

Insertion: Intertrochanteric fossa of femur.

Action: Flexes and rotates thigh laterally.

Innervation: Obturator nerve.

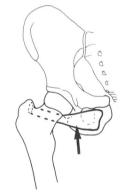

Muscle, obturatorius externus

Obturatorius Internus

Origin: Pelvis surface of hipbone and obturator membrane, margin of obturator foramen.

Insertion: Greater trochanter of femur.

Action: Abducts and laterally rotates thigh.

Innervation: A special nerve from the sacral plexus containing fibers from the lumbosacral trunk (fifth lumbar) and first and second sacral nerves.

Opponens Digiti Minimi (Manus)

Origin: Hook of hamate bone, flexor retinaculum.

Insertion: Fifth metacarpal.

Action: Draws fifth metacarpal bone toward palm.

Innervation: Ulnar nerve.

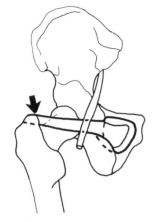

Muscle, obturator internus

Insertion: Lateral border of first metacarpal bone.
Action: Draws first metacarpal bone toward palm, opposes thumb.
Innervation: Median nerve.

Palmaris Brevis

Origin: Flexor retinaculum.
Insertion: Skin of palm.
Action: Aids in deepening hollow of palm; wrinkles skin of palm.
Innervation: Ulnar nerve.

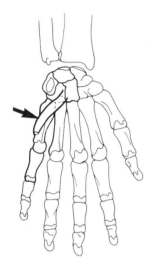

Muscle, opponens digiti minimi (manus)

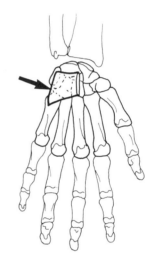

Muscle, palmaris brevis

Palmaris Longus

Origin: Medial epicondyle of humerus.
Insertion: Flexor retinaculum, palmar aponeurosis.
Action: Flexes hand.
Innervation: Median nerve.

Pectineus

Origin: Pectineal line of pubis.
Insertion: Pectineal line of femur between lesser trochanter and linea aspera.
Action: Adducts and aids in flexion of thigh.
Innervation: Usually a branch of femoral nerve containing fibers from second, third, and fourth lumbar nerves.

Opponens Pollicis

Origin: Tubercle of trapezium, flexor retinaculum.

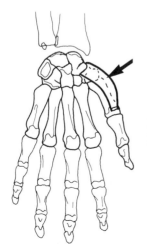

Muscle, opponens pollicis

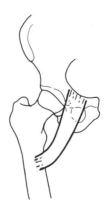

Muscle, pectineus

When accessory obturator is present, one of its branches is distributed to the pectineus. It may receive a branch from the obturator nerve.

Pectoralis Major

Origin: Medial half of clavicle, sternum, and costal cartilages; aponeurosis of external oblique muscle of abdomen.

Insertion: Lateral lip intertubercular groove of humerus.

Action: Flexes, adducts, and rotates arm medially.

Innervation: Medial and lateral anterior thoracic nerves.

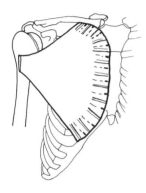

Muscle, pectoralis major

Pectoralis Minor

Origin: Anterior aspect of second through fifth ribs.

Insertion: Coracoid process of scapula.

Action: Draws scapula downward, elevates ribs.

Innervation: Medial and lateral anterior thoracic nerves.

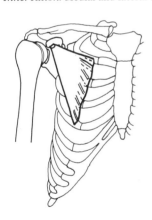

Muscle, pectoralis minor

Peroneus Brevis

Origin: Lower two thirds of fibula.

Insertion: Tuberosity of fifth metatarsal bone.

Action: Flexes and everts foot.

Innervation: Superficial peroneal nerve.

Peroneus Longus

Origin: Upper aspect of tibia and fibula.

Insertion: First metatarsal bone, first cuneiform bone.

Action: Flexes and everts foot.

Innervation: Common peroneal nerve.

Peroneus Tertius

Origin: Distal fourth of fibula, interosseous membrane.

Insertion: Fascia of fifth metatarsal bone on dorsum of foot.

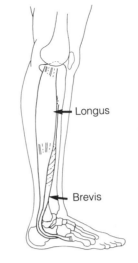

Muscle, peroneus brevis

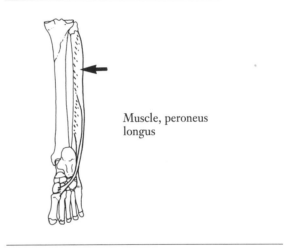

Muscle, peroneus longus

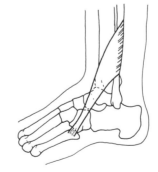

Muscle, peroneus tertius

Action: Extends and everts foot.

Innervation: Deep peroneal nerve.

Piriformis

Origin: Internal aspect of sacrum, sacrotuberous ligament.

Insertion: Upper portion of greater trochanter of femur.

Action: Rotates thigh laterally.

Innervation: First or second sacral nerves.

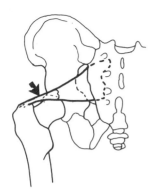

Muscle, piriformis

Plantaris

Origin: Popliteal groove of lateral condyle of femur.
Insertion: Medial side of calcaneal tendon.
Action: Extends foot (plantar flexion).
Innervation: Tibial nerve.

Popliteus

Origin: Popliteal groove of lateral condyle of femur.
Insertion: Medial two thirds of popliteal line on posterior surface of tibia.
Action: Flexes leg and rotates it medially.
Innervation: Tibial nerve.

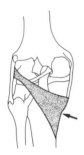

Muscle, popliteus

Pronator Quadratus

Origin: Distal fourth of shaft of ulna.
Insertion: Distal fourth of shaft of radius.
Action: Pronates forearm.
Innervation: Median nerve.

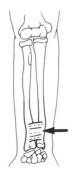

Muscle, pronator quadratus

Pronator Teres

Origin: Humeral part: medial epicondyle of humerus; ulnar part: coronoid ulna.
Insertion: Lateral aspect of radius bone.
Action: Pronates and flexes forearm.
Innervation: Median nerve.

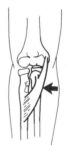

Muscle, pronator teres

Psoas Major

Origin: Transverse processes of bodies of lumbar vertebrae.
Insertion: Lesser trochanter of femur.
Action: Flexes and medially rotates thigh.
Innervation: Lumbar plexus.

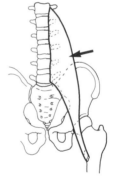

Muscle, psoas major

Psoas Minor

Origin: Bodies of last thoracic and first lumbar vertebrae.
Insertion: Pectineal line of hipbone.

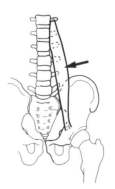

Muscle, psoas minor

Action: Flexes vertebral column.

Innervation: First lumbar nerve.

Quadratus Femoris

Origin: Proximal part of the external border of the tuberosity of the ischium.

Insertion: Proximal part of the linea quadrata (line extending vertically and distally from the intertrochanteric crest of femur).

Action: Rotates thigh laterally.

Innervation: Special branch from sacral plexus, which contains fibers from the lumbosacral trunk (fourth and fifth lumbar) and the first sacral nerves.

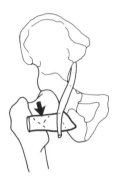

Muscle, quadratus femoris

Quadratus Lumborum

Origin: Iliac crest, lumbodorsal fascia, lumbar vertebrae.

Insertion: Twelfth rib, transverse processes of upper lumbar vertebrae.

Action: Draws rib cage inferiorly, bends vertebral column laterally.

Innervation: First three or four lumbar nerves.

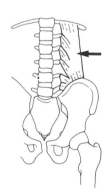

Muscle, quadratus lumborum

Quadratus Plantae

Origin: Calcaneus and plantar fascia.

Insertion: Tendons of long flexor muscle of toes (m. flexor digitorum longus).

Action: Straightens tendon pull of the long flexor muscle of toes.

Innervation: Lateral plantar nerve.

Quadriceps Femoris

Origin: Ilium (anterior, inferior spine).

Insertion: Tibia (by way of patellar tendon).

Action: Flexes thigh; extends leg.

Innervation: Femoral nerve.

Rectus Capitis Anterior

Origin: Lateral portion of first vertebra (atlas).

Insertion: Basilar portion of occipital bone.

Action: Flexes and supports head.

Innervation: Branch of loop between first and second cervical nerves.

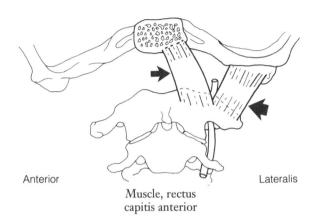

Anterior   Lateralis

Muscle, rectus capitis anterior

Rectus Capitis Lateralis

Origin: Transverse process of first vertebra (atlas).

Insertion: Jugular process of occipital bone.

Action: Aids in lateral movements of head, supports head.

Innervation: Branch of the loop between the first and second cervical nerves.

Rectus Capitis Posterior Major

Origin: Spinous process of second vertebra (atlas).

Insertion: Occipital bone.

Action: Extends head.

Innervation: Branch of dorsal ramus of suboccipital nerve.

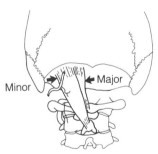

Minor   Major

Muscle, rectus capitis posterior major and minor

Rectus Capitis Posterior Minor

Origin: Posterior tubercle of first vertebra (atlas).

Insertion: Occipital bone.

Action: Extends head.

Innervation: Branch of dorsal primary division of suboccipital nerve.

Rectus Femoris

Origin: Anterior interior iliac spine, rim of acetabulum.

Insertion: Tibial tuberosity, base of patella (kneecap).
Action: Extends leg and flexes thigh.
Innervation: Femoral nerve.

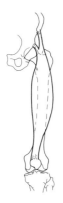

Muscle, rectus femoris

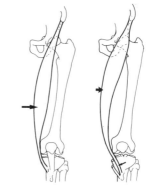

Muscle, sartorius

Rhomboideus Major

Origin: Spinous processes of second through fifth thoracic vertebrae.
Insertion: Vertebral margin of scapular.
Action: Adducts and laterally rotates scapula.
Innervation: Dorsal scapular nerve from brachial plexus.

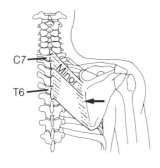

Muscle, rhomboideus major and minor

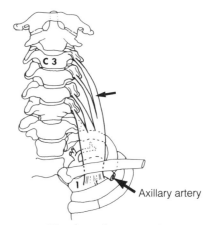

Muscle, scalenus anterior

Scalenus Medius

Origin: Transverse processes of first six cervical vertebrae.
Insertion: Upper surface of first and second ribs.
Action: Raises first rib, stabilizes or inclines neck to the side.
Innervation: Lower cervical nerves.

Rhomboideus Minor

Origin: Spinous processes of seventh cervical and first thoracic vertebrae and lower part of nuchal ligament.
Insertion: Vertebral margin of root of scapular spine.
Action: Adducts and laterally rotates scapula.
Innervation: Dorsal scapular nerve from brachial plexus.

Sartorius

Origin: Anterior superior iliac spine.
Insertion: Upper medial surface of tibia.
Action: Flexes thigh and leg.
Innervation: Femoral nerve.

Scalenus Anterior Muscle

Origin: Transverse processes of third to sixth cervical vertebrae.
Insertion: Scalene tubercle of first rib.
Action: Raises first rib, stabilizes or inclines neck to the side.
Innervation: Lower cervical nerves.

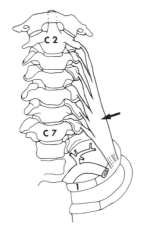

Muscle, scalenus medius

Scalenus Posterior

Origin: Transverse processes of fifth to seventh cervical vertebrae.

Insertion: Outer surface of upper border of second rib.

Action: Raises second rib, stabilizes or inclines neck to the side.

Innervation: Ventral primary divisions of last three cervical nerves.

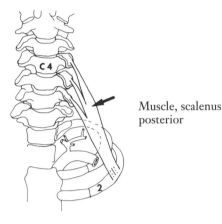

Muscle, scalenus posterior

Semimembranous

Origin: Tuberosity of ischium.

Insertion: Upper and posterior portion of tibia.

Action: Extends thigh, flexes and rotates leg medially.

Innervation: Tibial nerve.

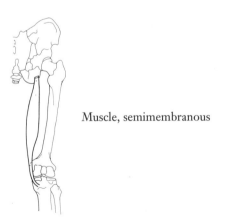

Muscle, semimembranous

Semispinalis Capitis

Origin: Transverse processes of six upper thoracic and four lower cervical vertebrae.

Insertion: Occipital bone between superior and inferior nuchal lines.

Action: Rotates head and draws it backward.

Innervation: First five cervical nerves.

Semispinalis Cervicis

Origin: Transverse processes of upper six thoracic vertebrae.

Insertion: Spinous processes of second through sixth cervical vertebrae.

Action: Extends and rotates vertebral column.

Innervation: Dorsal primary divisions of spinal nerves.

Semispinalis Thoracis

Origin: Transverse processes of lower six thoracic vertebrae.

Insertion: Spinous processes of upper six thoracic and lower two cervical vertebrae.

Action: Extends and rotates vertebral column.

Innervation: Dorsal primary divisions of spinal nerves.

Semitendinosus

Origin: Tuberosity of ischium (in common with biceps muscle of thigh).

Insertion: Upper part of tibia.

Action: Flexes and rotates leg medially, extends thigh.

Innervation: Tibial nerve.

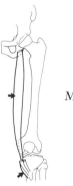

Muscle, semitendinosus

Serratus Anterior

Origin: Lateral surface of eight or nine uppermost ribs.

Insertion: Vertebral border of scapula.

Action: Draws scapula forward and laterally rotates scapula in raising arm.

Innervation: Long thoracic nerve.

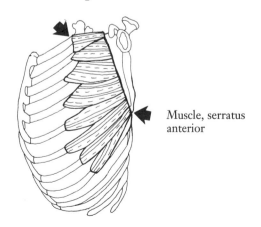

Muscle, serratus anterior

Serratus Posterior Inferior

Origin: Spinous processes of last two thoracic and first two or three lumbar vertebrae, supraspinal ligament.

Insertion: Inferior borders of the last four ribs, slightly beyond their angles.

Action: Draws the ribs outward and downward (counteracting the inward pull of the diaphragm).

Innervation: Branches of ventral primary divisions of ninth to twelfth thoracic nerves.

Serratus Posterior Superior

Origin: Caudal part of nuchal ligament, spinous processes of the seventh cervical and first two or three thoracic vertebrae, supraspinal ligament.

Insertion: Upper borders of the second, third, fourth, and fifth ribs, slightly beyond their angles.

Action: Raises the ribs.

Innervation: Branches of ventral primary divisions of first four thoracic nerves.

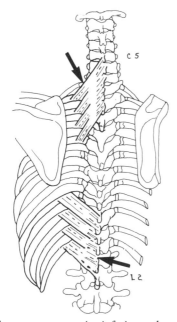

Muscle, serratus posterior inferior and superior

Soleus

Origin: Upper third of fibula, soleal line of tibia, tendinous arch.

Insertion: Calcaneus by calcaneal tendon (tendon calcaneus).

Action: Flexes foot.

Innervation: Tibial nerve.

Spinalis Thoracis

Origin: Spinous processes of upper two lumbar and lower two thoracic vertebrae.

Insertion: Spinous processes of second through ninth thoracic vertebrae.

Action: Extends vertebral column.

Innervation: Branches of the dorsal primary divisions of the spinal nerves.

Splenius Capitis

Origin: Spinous processes of upper thoracic vertebrae.

Insertion: Mastoid process and superior nuchal line.

Action: Inclines and rotates head.

Innervation: Lateral branches of dorsal primary divisions of middle and lower cervical nerves.

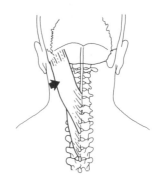

Muscle, splenius capitis

Splenius Cervicis

Origin: Transverse processes of upper six thoracic and seventh cervical vertebrae.

Insertion: Spinous processes of second, third, and fourth cervical vertebrae.

Action: Extends vertebral column.

Innervation: Lateral branches of dorsal primary divisions of middle and lower cervical nerves.

Sternocleidomastoideus

Origin: Sternal head: anterior surface of manubrium; clavicular head: medial third of clavicle.

Insertion: Mastoid process, superior nuchal line of occipital bone.

Action: Rotates and extends head, flexes vertebral column.

Innervation: The spinal part of the accessory nerve and branches from the anterior rami of the second and third cervical nerves.

Subclavius

Origin: Junction of first rib and costal cartilages.

Insertion: Lower surface of clavicle.

Action: Depresses lateral end of clavicle.

Innervation: Fifth and sixth cervical nerves.

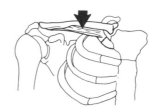

Muscle, subclavius

Subcostales

Origin: Inner surface of ribs near angle.

Insertion: Lower inner surface of second or third rib below rib of origin.

Action: Draws adjacent ribs together.

Innervation: Intercostal nerves.

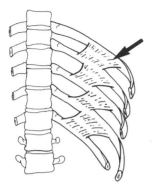

Muscle, subcostales

Subscapularis

Origin: Subscapular fossa.
Insertion: Lesser tubercle of humerus.
Action: Rotates arm medially.
Innervation: Upper and lower subscapular nerves from brachial plexus.

Supinator

Origin: Lateral epicondyle of humerus, supinator crest of ulna.
Insertion: Upper third of radius.
Action: Supinates the forearm.
Innervation: Radial nerve.

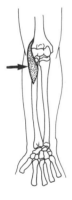

Muscle, supinator

Supraspinatus

Origin: Supraspinous fossa.
Insertion: Superior aspect of greater tubercle of humerus.
Action: Abducts arm.
Innervation: Suprascapular nerve.

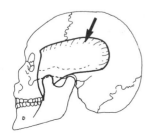

Muscle, temporalis

Temporalis

Origin: From temporal fascia and entire temporal fossa from temporal lines to infratemporal crest.
Insertion: Coronoid process and anterior border of ramus of mandible.
Action: Closes jaw, posterior part retracts jaw.
Innervation: Trigeminal nerve.

Tensor Fasciae Latae

Origin: Iliac crest.
Insertion: Iliotibial tract of fascia lata.
Action: Tenses fascia lata.
Innervation: Superior gluteal nerve.

Teres Major

Origin: Inferior axillary border of scapula.
Insertion: Crest of lesser tubercle of humerus.
Action: Adducts and rotates arm medially.
Innervation: Lower subscapular nerve.

Teres Minor

Origin: Axillary border of scapula.
Insertion: Inferior aspect of greater tubercle of humerus.
Action: Rotates arm laterally.
Innervation: Axillary nerve.

Tibialis Anterior

Origin: Upper two thirds of tibia, interosseous membrane.
Insertion: First metatarsal bone, first cuneiform bone.
Action: Extends and inverts foot.
Innervation: Common and deep peroneal nerves.

Tibialis Posterior

Origin: Interosseous membrane adjoining tibia and fibula.
Insertion: Navicular, with slips to three cuneiform bones; cuboid, second, third, and fourth metatarsals.
Action: Principal inverter of foot; aids in flexion of foot.
Innervation: Tibial nerve.

Transversus Abdominis

Origin: Seventh through twelfth costal cartilages, lumbar fascia, iliac crest, inguinal ligament.
Insertion: Xiphoid process, linea alba, conjoint tendon to pubis.
Action: Supports abdominal viscera.
Innervation: Branches of the seventh to twelfth intercostal, and the iliohypogastric and ilioinguinal nerves.

Transversus Perinei Profundus

Origin: Inferior ramus of ischium.
Insertion: Central tendon of perineum, external anal sphincter.
Action: Fixes central tendon of perineum.
Innervation: Perineal branch of pudendal nerve.

Transversus Thoracis

Origin: Xiphoid process, posterior surface of lower part of sternum.
Insertion: Second to sixth costal cartilages.
Action: Narrows chest, draws costal cartilages downward.
Innervation: Branches of the intercostal nerves.

Trapezius

Origin: Superior nuchal line of occipital bone, nuchal ligament, spinous processes of seventh cervical and all thoracic vertebrae.
Insertion: Superior part: posterior border of lateral third of clavicle; middle part: median margin of acromion, supe-

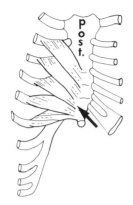

Muscle, transversus
thoracis

Action: Flexes foot and leg.
Innervation: Branches of tibial nerve (tibialis).

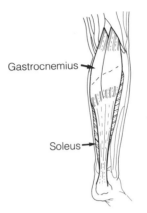

Muscle, triceps surae

rior lip of posterior border of scapular spine; inferior part: tubercle at apex of median end of scapular spine.
Action: Elevates shoulder, rotates scapula to raise shoulder in full abduction and flexion of arms, draws scapula backward.
Innervation: Spinal accessory, second, third, and fourth cervical nerves.

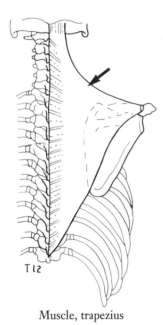

Muscle, trapezius

Triceps Brachii
Origin: Long head: infraglenoid tubercle of scapula; lateral head: proximal portion of humerus; medial head: distal half of humerus.
Insertion: Olecranon process of ulna.
Action: Extends arm and forearm.
Innervation: Radial nerve.

Triceps Surae
Origin: Combined gastrocnemius and soleus muscles.
Insertion: Calcaneal tendon.

Vastus Intermedius
Origin: Anterior and lateral surface of femur.
Insertion: Common tendon of quadriceps muscle of thigh, patella.
Action: Extends leg.
Innervation: Femoral nerve.

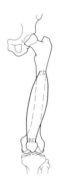

Muscle, vastus
intermedius

Vastus Lateralis
Origin: Lateral aspect of femur.
Insertion: Common tendon of quadriceps muscle of thigh, patella.

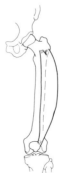

Muscle, vastus
lateralis

Action: Extends leg.
Innervation: Femoral nerve.

Vastus Medialis

Origin: Medial aspect of femur.
Insertion: Common tendon of quadriceps muscle of thigh, patella.
Action: Extends leg.
Innervation: Femoral nerve.

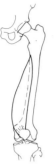

Muscle, vastus medialis

Muscle Atrophy (mus'el/at-rō-fē) (n.) See **Muscular Atrophy**.

Muscle Cylinder Ratio (mus'el/sil'in-der/rā'shē-o) (n.) The ratio of muscle diameter to the total cylindrical diameter of the extremity containing that muscle.

Muscle Fibers (mus'el/fī'berz) (n.) Long, multinucleated cells that are the basic cellular unit of muscle. In skeletal muscle, these fibers are grouped into fascicles by the perimysium. Microscopically, the fiber's contractile apparatus is subdivided into myofibrils.

Muscle Load (mus'el/lōd) (n.) The actual resistance an exercised muscle overcomes. The unit of measurement is a newton.

Muscle Pedicle Bone Graft (mus'el/ped'i-k'l/bōn/graft) (n.) Any local bone graft transplanted with a piece of muscle that retains its vascularity, thereby maintaining vascularity in the bone that is being grafted. A **Meyers Graft** is an example.

Muscle Relaxant (mus'el/re-lak'sant) (n.) A pharmacologic agent used specifically to reduce muscle tension.

Muscle Spasm (mus'el/spazm) (n.) An involuntary, sustained muscle contraction of a specific muscle or group of muscles. This is usually transient but may be painful.

Muscle Spindle (mus'el/spin'd'l) (n.) A specialized sensory receptor found between skeletal muscle fibers. It is important for coordinated muscular movement and is responsible for the muscle stretch reflex.

The muscle spindle is composed of two specialized types of muscle fibers enclosed in a fibrous capsule and is innervated by two types of sensory fibers and two types of gamma motor neurons. Muscle spindles are usually located at or near the ends of fascicles in the muscle and are arranged parallel to muscle fibers. They are attached to a tendon, an aponeurosis, or a perimysium at one end. The muscle spindle responds to the passive stretching of the muscle.

Muscle Stretch Reflex (mus'el/strech/re'fleks) (n.) A reflex contraction of a muscle resulting from a sudden muscle stretch. Also known as **Deep Tendon Reflex** or **Myotatic Reflex**.

Muscle-Tendon Imbalance (mus'el-ten'don/im-bal'ans) (n.) A risk factor associated with the occurrence of overuse injuries in children and adults. This may be an imbalance of strength, flexibility, or mass. Proper athletic training to emphasize strengthening, stretching, and range of motion should prevent its occurrence.

Muscle Tone (mus'el/tōn) (n.) The apparent resting tension of a muscle or muscle groups. This may be normal, decreased (hypotonic), or increased (hypertonic).

Muscular Atrophy (mus'ku-lar/at'ro-fē) (n.) A loss of muscle mass or bulk. Muscular atrophy may be caused by a number of factors: by a neurologic lesion involving either the cell body or axon of the lower motor neuron; by aging, disuse, or deficiency states; or by a variety of degenerative, toxic, inflammatory, vascular, or metabolic disorders of the muscle fibers themselves. It may be localized or generalized, symmetrical or asymmetrical. it is usually accompanied by weakness.

Muscular Dystrophy (mus'ku-lar/dis'tro-fē) (n.) Hereditary disorders characterized by progressive weakness and wasting of muscle; they are defined as primary myopathies because the muscle fiber itself is primarily diseased. The etiology of muscular dystrophy is unknown. Its classification is divided into cases of pure muscular dystrophies and those associated with myotonia. Further subdivision is based on mode of inheritance, age of onset of symptoms, and distribution of the weakness. Diagnosis and disease management is aided by clinical and laboratory tests that include manual muscle testing, the determination of the serum enzymes aldolase or creatine phosphokinase (or both), electromyography, and muscle biopsy.

Muscular Endurance (mus'ku-lar/en-dūr'ans) (n.) The capacity of a muscle either to perform at a submaximal level to fatigue or to hold a maximum contraction.

Muscular Irritability (mus'ku-lar/ir"i-tah-bil'i-tē) (n.) The inherent capacity of a muscle to merely respond, or to respond to threshold or suprathreshold stimuli by means of contraction.

Muscular Strength (mus'ku-lar/strenth) (n.) The contractile force generated by a muscle or muscle group in one, brief, maximal effort.

Muscular Tripod (mus'ku-lar/tri'pod) (n.) A group of three muscles, the sartorius, the gracilis, and the semitendinosus, that form a tripod to support the medial side of the knee. Each muscle has a different nerve supply.

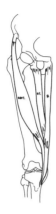

Muscular tripod

Musculature (mus'ku-lah'chur) (n.) The muscles arranged in a part of the body or the body as a whole.

Musculo (mus'ku-lō) A prefix meaning muscle.

Musculoaponeurotic (mus"ku-lō-ap"ō-nu-rot'ik) (adj.) Of or related to muscle and its fibrous connective tissue of origin or insertion.

Musculocutaneous (mus"ku-lō-ku-tā'ne-us) (adj.) Of or related to the muscles and skin.

Musculocutaneous Nerve (mus"ku-lō-ku-ta'ne-us/nerv) (n.) See **Nerve**.

Musculofascial (mus"ku-lō-fash'ē-al) (adj.) Consisting of both muscular and fascial elements; an amputation flap is an example.

Musculofibrous (mus"ku-lō-fī'brus) (adj.) Of or pertaining to tissue that is partly muscular and partly fibrous.

Musculoskeletal (mus"ku-lō-skel'e-tal) (adj.) Of, pertaining to, or composed of the muscles and bony skeleton.

Musculospiral Paralysis (mus"ku-lō-spī'ral/pah-ral'i-sis) (n.) A term for radial nerve palsy no longer commonly used. See **Saturday Night Palsy**.

Mustard Procedure (mus'tard/pro-sē'jur) (n.) A surgical operation to restore stability and abduction of the hip due to paralysis of the gluteus medius and maximus muscles. In this technique, the tendon of the iliopsoas muscle is transferred laterally to the greater trochanter.

Myalgia (mī"al-jē'ah) (n.) Muscle pain.

Myasthenia Gravis (mī"as-thē'nē-ah/grav'vis) (n.) A chronic disorder of neuromuscular transmission in voluntary muscle groups. The most outstanding characteristic of this disorder is the fluctuant or episodic weakness. Other associated characteristics include excessive fatigue of muscle, which is marked by the onset of abnormal weakness after repetitive or sustained contractions; partial recovery of power after a short interval of rest; and partial recovery following administration of anticholinesterases, such as Tensilon.

Myatonia Congenita (mī"ah-tō'nē-ah/kon"jen-i"tah) (n.) See **Myotonia**.

Mycetoma (mī'se-to'mah) (n.) A chronic, localized, granulomatous infection or abscess that is caused by true fungi or certain aerobic actinomycetes. Characteristics include the formation of fistulae and intercommunicating sinus tracts, from which purulent drainage with small granules of variable size and color may be expressed.

Mycetoma generally occur on the feet and hands but may occur elsewhere. The skin and subcutaneous tissues are primarily involved during the early stages of infection; in the next stage, the fascia, muscle, and bone are invaded as the lesion progresses. Synonym: **Madura Foot**.

Mycobacterium (mī"ko-bak-te're-um) (n.) A genus of relatively slow-growing, gram-positive rods of the family Mycobacteriaceae, with acid-fast staining. The genus contains both saprophytic and pathogenic species. Mycobacterium includes the highly pathogenic organisms that cause tuberculosis and leprosy.

Mycosis (mī-kō'sis) (n.) Any disease caused by fungi.

Myelin (mī'e-lin) (n.) The phospholipid substance that forms a spiral-wrap sheath around the axons of certain neurons. This sheath is formed by Schwann cells. These wrapped neurons are called myelinated or medullated fibers. Also known as the **White Substance of Schwann**.

Myelin Sheath (mī'e-lin/shēth) (n.) Short segments of myelin surrounding an axon interrupted by the nodes of Ranvier and enveloped by a Schwann cell plasma membrane.

Myelination (mī"e-li-na'shun) (n.) The process by which myelin is deposited around the axons of certain neurons.

Myelitis (mī"e-li'tis) (n.) Any inflammatory process involving the spinal cord. These diseases produce symptoms and signs of cord dysfunction.

Myelo (mī'e-lo) Prefix pertaining to the spinal cord or bone marrow.

Myelodysplasia (mī"e-lo-dis-plā'se-ah) (n.) A generic term for congenital neural tube defects, including meningocele, myelomeningocoele, and rachischisis. Also known as **Spinal Dysraphism**.

Myelofibrosis (mī"e-lō-fī-brō'sis) (n.) 1. Fibrosis of the bone marrow. 2. Specifically, chronic, progressive myeloproliferative disease characterized clinically by marked anemia and histologically by fibrosis of the bone marrow. Radiographically, the bone appears dense and sclerotic. The common sites of adult hematopoiesis are usually the bony sites involved.

Myelogram (mī'e-lō-gram) (n.) The roentgenograms produced by myelography.

Myelography (mī"e-log'rah-fē) (n.) The introduction of a radiopaque substance, such as Metrizamide or Pantopaque, or a negative contrast medium, such as air, into the subarachnoid space for a special radiographic study of the spinal canal.

Myeloid (mī'e-loid) (adj.)   1. Of, pertaining to, or derived from elements formed in bone marrow. 2. Resembling marrow.

Myeloma (mī"e-lō'mah) (n.)   A tumor composed of cells derived from bone marrow hematopoietic tissues. See also **Multiple Myeloma**.

Myelomeningocele (mī'e-lō-me-ning'gō-sēl) (n.)   A type of myelodysplasia in which the neural tube defects contain abnormal neural elements within the protruding sac. It is usually not epithelialized, and the cord elements are visible beneath the thin membrane covering the sac at birth.

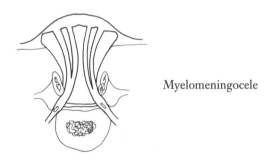

Myelomeningocele

Myelopathy (mī"e-lop'ah-thē) (n.)   Any disorder of the spinal cord or myeloid tissues, usually producing signs and symptoms of cord dysfunction.

Myelophthisis (mī"e-lof'thi-sis) (n.)   1. Replacement of bone marrow tissue by bone, fibrous tissue, or neoplastic growth. 2. Spinal cord atrophy or wasting, as seen in tabes dorsalis.

Myeloproliferative (mī"e-lō-prō-lif'er-ah-tiv) (adj.)   Pertaining to or characterized by abnormal proliferation of bone marrow constituents.

Myeloproliferative Disorders (mī"e-lō-prō-lif'er-ah-tiv/dis-or'-derz) (n.)   A proliferation of one or more bone marrow elements without definite evidence of neoplasia. It is accompanied by extramedullary hematopoiesis release of immature blood cells into the peripheral circulation.

Myeloradiculitis (mī"e-lō-rah-dik"u-lī'tis) (n.)   An inflammation of the spinal cord and roots of the spinal nerves.

Myeloradiculopathy (mī"e-lō-rah-dik"u-lop'ah-the) (n.)   A disease of the spinal cord and roots of the spinal nerves.

Myo (mī'ō)   Prefix indicating muscle.

Myoclonus (mī-ok'lō-nus) (n.)   Sudden, abrupt, shocklike contractions of muscle that are irregular in rhythm and amplitude. Myoclonus is usually asynchronous or asymmetric in distribution.

Myocutaneous Flap (mī-ō"kū-tā'nē-us/flap) (n.)   A flap used for soft tissue defect coverage in which a block of skin is transferred to a new site, using an underlying contiguous muscle as its pedicle. It incorporates the muscle with its overlying fascia, subcutaneous tissue, and skin. Some of the more common skin-muscle units used for grafting include the trapezius, the sternocleidomastoid, the lattissimus, the rectus abdominus, the gracilis, the gluteus maximus, and the biceps femoris muscles.

Myodesis (mī"o-dē'sis) (n.)   The shortening of a muscle; usually secondary to contracture.

Myoelectric Prosthesis (mī"ō-e-lek'trik/pros-thē'sis) (n.)   A device in which electric potentials generated by the contraction of intact muscles move some parts of the prosthesis. Electrodes and microtransmitters carry impulses that are amplified by an electronic device.

Myofascitis (mī"ō-fah-sī'tis) (n.)   An inflammation of a muscle and its fascia.

Myofibril (mī"ō-fi'bril) (n.)   The subdivision of the contractile apparatus of a muscle fiber that contains longitudinally oriented bundles of thick and thin filaments. Each myofibril is made up of many sarcomeres linked end-to-end.

Myofibrosis (mī"ō-fī-brō'sis) (n.)   A condition characterized by the replacement of muscle tissue by fibrous tissue.

Myofibrositis (mī"ō-fī"brō-sī'tis) (n.)   An inflammation of the muscle fiber sheath.

Myofilaments (mī"ō-fil'ah-ments) (n.)   The thick or thin filaments that contain the contractile proteins of muscles and form myofibrils. The thick and thin filaments are arranged to create a regular three-dimensional pattern to the sarcomere. These filaments are linked to each other by cross bridges, which allow the filaments to slide past each other and cause muscle contractions.

Myogenic (mī"ō-jen'ik) (adj.)   Giving rise to, or forming, muscle tissue.

Myogenic Scoliosis (mī"ō-jen'ik/skō"lē-ō'sis) (n.)   A spinal curvature caused by disease or anomalies of the musculature.

Myoglobin (mī"ō-glō'bin) (n.)   An iron-containing pigment found in muscle that resembles hemoglobin. The pigment both contributes to the reddish color of muscle and stores oxygen.

Myoglobinuria (mī"ō-glō"bin-ū'rē-ah) (n.)   The presence of myoglobin in the urine. This usually signifies that muscle breakdown due to disease or trauma has released myoglobin into the circulation, which then is excreted into the urine.

Myogram (mī'ō-gram) (n.)   A recording or tracing of muscle activity. See **Electromyography**.

Myograph (mī'ō-graf) (n.)   An apparatus for recording the activity of muscular tissues. See **Electromyography**.

Myoneural (mī'ō-nū'ral) (adj.)   1. Of or pertaining to

both muscle and nerve. 2. Of or pertaining to the nerve endings in muscle tissue.

Myoneural Junction (mī″ō-nū′ral/jungk′shun) (n.) The junction between a motor neuron and a muscle fiber. Also called a **Neuromuscular Junction**.

Myopathic Scoliosis (mī-ō-path′ik/skō″lē-ō′sis) (n.) A form of scoliosis caused by a muscular disorder. Also known as **Myogenic Scoliosis**.

Myopathy (mī-op′ah-thē) (n.) 1. Any disease, inherited or acquired, that affects the muscles. 2. Disorders are usually characterized by selective involvement of proximal limb musculature before the involvement of the distal muscles; patients therefore show significantly greater weakness early in the course of the disease than the apparent muscle atrophy would suggest.

Myoplasm (mī′ō-plazm) (n.) The contractile part of the muscle cell.

Myoreceptor (mī″ō-rē-sep′tor) (n.) A neural receptor found in skeletal muscle. It is stimulated by muscular contraction to provide information about muscle position to higher nervous centers.

Myosin (mī′ō-sin) (n.) A large contractile protein that is the primary component of the large myofilaments of striated muscle. Each molecule consists of two peptide strands wound around one another in the form of a double helix. At one end of the molecule is a globular, enlarged head of protein that forms cross-bridges between the thick and thin myofilaments. Myosin is restricted to the A band of the sarcomere. See **Actin**.

Myositis (mī″ō-sī′tis) (n.) An inflammation of muscle.

Myositis Ossificans (mī″ō-sī′tis/os″i-fi-kanz) (n.) A condition in which heterotopic ossification occurs in muscles and other soft tissues. This general term applies to all three types of ossification—myositis ossificans progressiva, myositis ossificans circumscripta, and localized traumatic myositis ossificans—but is commonly applied to the latter condition. This posttraumatic form usually follows blunt trauma and hemorrhage and is most often seen in the quadriceps muscle and around the elbow. It may be confused with an osteogenic sarcoma if the history of trauma is obscure. It can be differentiated by a number of factors: its presence over the diaphysis; a decrease in pain and mass over time; radiographically, by an intact underlying cortex; and histologically, by a zonal pattern, with the more differentiated tissues at the periphery of the lesion.

Myositis Ossificans Circumscripta (mī″ō-sī′tis/os″i-fi-kans/ser″kum-skrip′tah) (n.) A localized area of myositis ossificans that occurs without a history of significant trauma.

Myositis Ossificans Progressiva (mī″ō-sī′tis/os″i-fi-kans/prō-gres′iv-ah) (n.) A rare childhood disease of unknown etiology in which progressive ossification of muscles, tendons, ligaments, and aponeuroses occurs. A familial tendency exists, with boys more often affected. Severe functional disability occurs, and it is generally fatal because of the progressive loss of pulmonary function.

Myotatic Reflex (mī″ō-tat′ik/rē′fleks) (n.) See **Muscle Stretch Reflex**.

Myotome (mī′ō-tōm) (n.) 1. In embryos, the muscle part or that part of the somite that gives rise to skeletal muscle. 2. In a formed body, all musculature derived from a given somite and therefore innervated by the same segmental spinal nerve. 3. A knife or knifelike instrument for cutting muscle. Compare **Dermatome** and **Sclerotome**.

Myotomy (mī-ot′ō-mē) (n.) The dissection or surgical division of a muscle.

Myotonia (mī″ō-tō′nē-ah) (n.) Any disorder involving a tonic muscle spasm: a failure of muscle to relax after voluntary contraction is complete. Myotonic disorders include myotonic congenita, paramyotonia congenita, and dystrophia myotonia.

Myotonia Atrophia: See **Myotonia Dystrophia**.

Myotonia Congenita: A rare congenital affliction characterized by myotonia of the entire voluntary musculature. It is present at birth but may not be manifest clinically until after early childhood. These patients appear Herculean because of their generalized muscle hypertrophy. This disease is compatible with a normal life span; in several cases, the myotonia may be decreased by pharmacologic agents. Also known as **Thomsen Disease**.

Myotonia Dystrophia: A rare, slowly progressive, hereditary disease marked by myotonia and muscular atrophy associated with cataracts, hypogonadism, frontal balding, cardiac disorders, and mental defects. The age of onset is usually late adolescence or early adulthood. The electromyographic examination of these patients yields sounds resembling a dive bomber. Also known as **Dystrophia Myotonia** or **Sternet Disease**.

Myotubular Myopathy (mī″ō-tū′bu-lar/mī-op′ah-thē) (n.) A nonprogressive affection of the muscles that may be noted in infancy or may not be apparent until later in childhood. The generalized weakness includes the axial musculature. It is so named because of the resemblance of the striated muscle to the myotubules of fetal life on biopsy.

Myxofibroma (mik′sō-fī-brō′mah) (n.) A benign tumor of fibrous tissue. Myxofibroma contains myxomatous and fibrous elements.

Myxoma (mik-sō′mah) (n.) A benign tumor of uncertain origin that contains the parenchyma of mucinous connective tissue.

Myxomatous Degeneration (mik-sō′mah-tus/dē-jen″er-ā′shun) (n.) Degeneration that involves accumulation of mucus in connective tissues.

Myxosarcoma (mik″sō-sar-kō′mah) (n.) A sarcoma containing mucoid material.

N

N 1. The abbreviation for nerve. 2. The abbreviation for the unit of measure newton.

Nachlas' Knee-Flexion Text (nahk-lahs'/ne-flek'shun/test) (n.) A means of clinical evaluation of low back pain. Have the patient lie prone on an examining table, and rest your hand gently on his or her back. Flex the patient's knee by raising the foot from the table. The test is positive if the patient experiences pain or a feeling of tension that radiates distally in the anterior thigh and the sacroiliac or lumbosacral region. The radiating pain follows the course of the sciatic or the femoral nerve. A positive test indicates that lower back disease and nerve irritation are present.

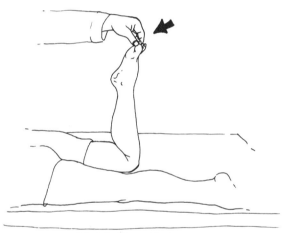

Nachlas' knee-flexion test

Nafcillin (naf-sil'in) (n.) A penicillinase-resistant penicillin.

Naffziger Syndrome (naf'zig-er/sin'drōm) (n.) See **Thoracic Outlet Syndrome**.

Naffziger Test (naf'zig-er/test) (n.) A clinical evaluation of disc herniation. It causes an increase in intrathecal pressure.

With the patient supine, compress both jugular veins with either the index and middle fingers of each hand or with a blood pressure cuff placed around the neck and inflated to about 40 mm Hg. Continue this for a few seconds or until the patient's face begins to flush. Instruct the patient not to hold his or her breath or to strain. By compressing the jugular veins, intraspinal fluid pressure is increased, which results in increased intrathecal pressure. If pain occurs, this suggests that some pathology, such as a herniated disk, is present and is putting pressure on the theca. The patient's sciatic pain is often reproduced or aggravated by this maneuver. Coughing may enhance the results.

Nagele's Pelvis (na'ge-lez/pel'vis) (n.) A pelvic deformity in which the pelvis is distorted, with complete ankylosis of the sacroiliac joint on one side. Nagele's pelvis is associated with imperfect development of the sacrum and its ipsilateral innominate bone.

Nail (nāl) (n.) 1. A flattened, elastic, horny structure found on the dorsal surface of the distal phalanx of the fingers and toes. Each nail is composed of a root, body, and free edge. The nail body, or nail-plate, is the semitransparent, nearly rectangular horny plate. It lies over the highly vascular, pink nail bed. The nail wall is the fold of skin that partially surrounds the plate. The free edge refers to the distal tip of the nail plate. 2. A rod or pin used for the fixation of fractures.

Nail Matrix (nāl/mā'triks) (n.) The proximal part of the nail bed that extends distally as far as the whitened lunula; it is found at the point where the epithelium is very thick. The matrix firmly attaches the body of the nail to the underlying connective tissue. The nail itself develops from this matrix.

Nail-Patella Syndrome (nāl-pah-tel'ah/sin'drōm) (n.) A congenital dysostosis with an autosomal dominant inheritance. It is characterized by rudimentary or absent patellae, radial head dysplasia with variable elbow deformities, and the absence or hypoplasia of the nails. "Iliac horns" sometimes occur, as does a wide spectrum of other abnormalities. Also known as **Osteo-onychodysostosis, Fong's Syndrome, Hereditary Osteo-onychodysplasia, Onychoarthrosis, Turner-Kieser Syndrome, Osterreicher-Fong Syndrome,** or **Touraine Syndrome**.

Nail-Plate Device (nāl/plāt/de-vīs') (n.) Any internal fixation system designed for fixation of proximal or distal femoral fractures in which a nail or compression screw is fixed to or interlocks with a sideplate attached to the shaft with smaller screws. An example of this is the dynamic compression screw or the Neufeld nail.

Nalfon (nal'fon) (n.) The proprietary name for fenoprofen calcium, a nonsteroidal, antiinflammatory drug.

Naprosyn (nah-prō'sin) (n.) The proprietary name for naproxen, a nonsteroidal, antiinflammatory drug.

Naproxen (nah-proks'en) (n.) A nonsteroidal, antiinflammatory drug marketed under the brand name Naprosyn.

Narcotic (nar-kot'ik) (n.) A drug that depresses the central nervous system in order to relieve pain and produce sleep.

Nash-Moe System (nash-mō/sis'tem) (n.) In the evaluation of scoliosis, this system quantifies the degree of vertebral rotation. On an AP radiograph of the spine, divide the vertebral body into six segments, three on either side of the midline. The rotation is then graded from 0 to 4, depending on the segment in which the pedicle is located. See **Pedicle Migration**.

Natatory Ligament (nat-a-torē/lig′ah-ment) (n.) The distal transverse fibers of the palmar fascia that contribute to the stabilization of the metacarpophalangeal joints of the fingers.

Nautilus (naw′ti-lus) (n.) A proprietary name for a system of exercise machines designed to provide variable resistance exercises through a full range of body motion.

Navicular (nah-vik′u-lar) (n.) A small, round bone in the hand or foot that is boat-shaped. The carpal navicular articulates with the radius proximally, the lunate and the capitate medially, and the trapezium and trapezoid distally. The tarsal navicular articulates with the talus posteriorly, the three cuneiforms anteriorly, and, frequently, the cuboid laterally. The carpal navicular is also known as the **Scaphoid**.

Navicular Pad (nah-vik′u-lar/pad) (n.) In shoe terminology, a firm but pliable elliptical pad glued to either an arch support or the insole of a shoe that prevents the navicular bone from sagging. Because of its shape, this is also called a **Cookie**.

Naviculometatarsal Angle (nah-vik″u-lō-met″ah-tar′sal/ang′g′l) (n.) A measurement of the relationship between the tarsal navicular and the metatarsals calculated on a standing AP radiograph of the foot. Define the base of the navicular by drawing a line that joins the extremities of its proximal articular outline. Draw a line through the center of the long axis of the first metatarsal. The lateral angle produced by the junction of these two lines is the naviculometatarsal angle.

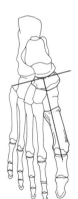

Naviculometatarsal angle

NCV (n.) Abbreviation for nerve conduction velocity.

Nebulizer (neb′u-līz″er) (n.) A device used to reduce a solution to a fine mist or spray.

Neck (nek) (n.) 1. The part of the body between the thorax and the head. 2. In anatomy, any constricted

portion that resembles the neck of an animal. For example, the neck of the femur is the narrowed area of bone that joins the rounded femoral head to the more expanded femoral shaft.

Neck Length (nek/lenth) (n.) 1. In an endoprosthesis, the distance from the center of the prosthetic head to the base of the prosthetic collar or to the top of the widened shaft in a collarless prosthesis. This distance reflects the length of the "neck" in this type of prosthesis.

Neck–Shaft Angle (nek-shaft/ang′g′l) (n.) The angle formed by the axes of the femoral neck and shaft as measured on an AP radiograph of the pelvis. In an adult, the average neck-shaft angle is 135 degrees.

Necrosis (ne-krō′sis) (n.) The death of a cell, groups of cells, or tissues that form part of a living body. Types of necrosis include avascular, coagulative, caseous and gummatous, liquefactive, fibrinoid, enzymatic, and gangrenous. The morphologic changes associated with this dynamic process occur at varying rates of progression.

Necrotizing Fasciitis (nek′rō-tīz″ing/fas″ē-ī′tis) (n.) A rapidly spreading, overwhelming infection caused by a mixed anaerobic flora. This results in separation of the skin from the underlying necrotic fascia and is accompanied by fever and toxicity. Necrotizing fasciitis may follow a seemingly innocuous puncture wound and is more likely to develop in an impaired host, such as a patient with diabetes. Formerly known as **Streptococcal Gangrene**.

Needle Biopsy (nē′d′l/bī′op-sē) (n.) A technique for incisional biopsy in which a hollow needle is inserted into an internal organ to obtain tissue. A variety of needles are available for this procedure, but most consist of a guide, a cannula, and a cuttery needle. Roentgenographic control is usually necessary for biopsy of bone lesions.

Neer Classification (nēr/klas″sĭ-fĭ-kā′shun) (n.) An organization of proximal humerus fractures and fracture dislocations based on the number of displaced segments. Recommendations for treatment of these fractures are based on this four-part classification.

Neer Prosthesis (nēr/pros-the′sis) (n.) A proximal humeral replacement implant. The original umbrella-shaped prosthesis is commonly used for the hemiarthroplasty performed for high-risk fractures

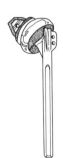

Neer prosthesis

and fracture-dislocations. The newer Neer II prosthesis is generally used in total shoulder replacement.

Neibauer Prosthesis (nī-bow-er/pros-thē′sis) (n.) A silicone and Dacron device used in arthroplasty of the interphalangeal and metacarpophalangeal joints. It features a flexible hinge for flexion and extension.

Neisseria (nīs-se′rē-ah) (n.) A genus of aerobic to facultatively anaerobic bacteria that are gram-negative cocci and usually occur in pairs. Common species pathogenic in man include *N. gonorrhaea*, which causes gonorrhea, and *N. meningitidis*, which causes meningitis.

Nélaton's Dislocation (nā-lah-tawz′/dis″lo-kā′shun) (n.) An ankle injury in which the talus is forced between the ends of the fibula and tibia. A complete diastasis of the distal tibia and fibula must occur to allow this to happen along with other ligamentous and capsular damage.

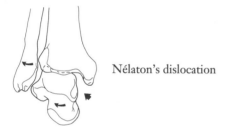

Nélaton's dislocation

Nélaton's Line (nā-lah-tawz′/līn) (n.) A line, based on superficial anatomy, that extends from the anterior superior iliac spine to the ischial tuberosity. Normally, this line passes through the tip of the greater trochanter. In congenital dislocation of the hip, the trochanter is displaced upward, causing it to lie above Nélaton's Line.

Neoplasm (nē′ō-plazm) (n.) Any new and abnormal growth, including both benign and malignant tumors.

Neoplastic Fracture (nē″ō-plas′tik/frak′chur) (n.) Any fracture of a bone containing neoplastic tissue. See **Pathologic Fracture**.

Neostigmine Test (nē″ō-stig′mēn/test) (n.) A pharmacologic diagnostic procedure in myasthenia gravis. The test is positive if a definite increase in muscle strength occurs within 5 to 15 minutes after the administration of neostigmine methylsulfate. See **Tensilon Test**.

Neri's Bowing Sign (nā-rēz/bō′ing/sīn) (n.) A clinical marker noted in lumbar radiculopathy. When a patient with sciatic nerve irritation bends forward with his or her legs extended, the knee flexes on the affected side.

Nerve (nerv) (n.) A group or bundle of nerve fibers along with the accompanying connective tissue and blood vessels. Its various components include a neu-

ron, an axon, and connective tissue sheaths known as the endoneurium, perineurium, and epineurium. The function of nerves is to carry stimuli in both directions between the central nervous system and the periphery.

Nerve Block (nerv/blok) (n.) A type of regional anesthesia that acts by blocking the passage of pain impulses in the sensory nerves supplying a particular region. A local anesthetic is injected directly into or around the nerve or nerves supplying the area involved.

Nerve Cable Graft (nerv/kā′b′l/graft) (n.) See **Cable Graft**.

Nerve Conduction Velocity (nerv/Kon-duk′shun/velo-sity) (n.) An expression of the physiological or pathological state of nerves. It is a test to determine the rate with which a segment of peripheral nerve conducts impulse. By measuring the nerve conduction velocity on different segments of the nerve, one can localize the pathology. There are two kinds of nerve conduction velocity studies: motor nerve and sensory nerve. Conduction velocity is the meters per second traveled by an impulse on the more proximal segment of nerve, that is the conduction time minus the distal latency. This value is compared to normal standards. Abbreviated **NCV**.

Nerve Ending (nerv/end-ing) (n.) The terminal part of a nerve fiber branch. The neuron contacts another neuron or an end-organ, such as a muscle or a gland, through a synaptic junction.

Nerve Entrapment Syndrome (nerv/en′trap′-ment/sin-drōm) (n.) A variety of disorders caused by the mechanical compression of a nerve within a confined anatomic space such as narrow fibrous passages; canals; tunnels; or thick, unyielding tendonous tissue pressing the nerve against bone. See **Carpal Tunnel, Cubital Tunnel, Ulnar Tunnel, Tarsal Tunnel**, and **Radial** and **Pronator Syndromes**.

Nerve Fiber (nerv/fiber) (n.) A filamentous process of a neuron. Although this refers to either a dendrite or an axon, the term usually is applied to the nerve cell axon. Each nerve fiber is composed of one or many axons that are sheathed by a chain of Schwann cells. Nerve fiber classification systems include a numerical system for the sensory fibers and a classification based on a physioanatomic basis, but most commonly the alphabetical classification of fiber type is used. This last classification takes into account function, diameter, conduction velocity, action potential configuration, and refractory period.

Nerve Grafting (nerv/graft′ing) (n.) The transplantation of part or all of a nerve in order to reestablish continuity in another injured nerve.

Nerve Impulse (nerv/im′puls) (n.) A transient, physiochemical excitation that travels from one part of a nerve fiber to another. The membrane of a resting nerve is charged, or polarized, by the different ion concentrations in and out of the cell. When an impulse is triggered, a wave of depolarization spreads, and ions flow across the membrane, which creates an action potential. No further nerve impulses can pass until the nerve repolarizes.

Nerve Plexus (nerv/plek′sus) (n.) A network composed of interjoining nerve fibers. An example of this is the brachial plexus, which is composed of the anterior rami of the C5 through TI nerves.

Nerve Root (nerv/rōōt) (n.) One of the two bundles of nerve fibers that emerge from the spinal cord to join together as a spinal nerve. These bundles are the dorsal and ventral nerve roots.

Nerve Root Canal (nerv/rōōt/kah-nal′) (n.) The region of the spinal canal that encompasses a nerve root. It begins where the nerve root sheath comes off the dural sac and ends where the nerve root emerges from the intervertebral foramen. The roof is formed by the ligamentum flavum, the contiguous borders of the superior articular process and the superior margin of the lamina, and the pars interarticularis. The floor is formed by the posterior surface of the intervertebral disk and the posterior surface of the vertebral body. The medial wall is formed by the dural sac and soft tissues of the epidural space. The lateral wall is formed proximally by the medial aspect and distally by the inferior aspect of the pedicle.

Nerve Stimulator (nerv/stim″u-lā′tor) (n.) Any instrument used to provide an electrical stimulus to a nerve. By recording in vivo nerve action potentials, a stimulator is used to evaluate the presence of viable, functioning nerve tissue.

Nerve Tract (nerv/trakt) (n.) A bundle of nerve fibers of the same area of origin and destination within the nervous system and generally the same or similar functions.

Nervous System (ner′vus/sis′tem) (n.) The receptor-conductor-effector system of the entire nerve apparatus. This includes the brain, spinal cord, nerves, and ganglia.

Neufeld Nail (nū′feld/nāl) (n.) A fixed nail-plate device designed for use in the fixation of intertrochanteric hip fractures. The V-shaped nail is fixed to the plate at an angle of approximately 130 degrees.

Neur Prefix meaning nerve.

Neural Arch (nu′ral/arch) (n.) The posterior portion of a vertebra; it is formed by its laminae and pedicles. Synonym: **Vertebral Arch**.

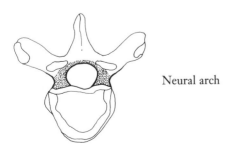

Neural arch

Neural Crest (nu′ral/krest) (n.) A band of cells of ectodermal origin that detach from the forming neural tube to form clusters of cells along its dorsolateral aspect. The peripheral nervous system develops from the neural crest. Also known as **Ganglionic Crest**.

Neural Groove (nu′ral/grōōv) (n.) A dorsal longitudinal groove bordered by two neural folds that forms in the early somite phase in a vertebrate embryo from which the brain and spinal cord develop. This is created by a deepening of the neural plate and forms the neural tube upon tubulation.

Neural Plate (nu′ral/plāt) (n.) A thickened strip of ectoderm that develops in the presomite phase of vertebrate embryos. It forms along the dorsal midline and gives rise to the central nervous system.

Neural Tube (nu′ral/tūb) (n.) The primitive, hollow, dorsal nervous system of the early vertebrate embryo from which the brain and spinal cord develop. It is formed by the fusion of neural folds around the neural groove.

Neuralgia (nu-ral′jē-ah) (n.) A pain in the distribution of a nerve or nerves. Various forms of neuralgia are named according to their etiologic anatomic location or nerve of origin. Example: **Trigeminal Neuralgia**.

Neurapraxia (nŭ″rah-prak-sē-ah) (n.) A type of nerve injury that results in a transient loss of function. It is caused by a minor contusion or compression of a peripheral nerve with no structural damage occurring to the axon. There may, however, be local damage to the myelin sheath. Recovery of function is usually complete. See **Seddon Classification**.

Neurectomy (nu-rek′to-mē) (n.) A surgical procedure in which a segment of a nerve is excised.

Neurilemma (nu″ri-lem′mah) (n.) A cell whose thin membranous sheath forms the myelin layers of myelinated nerve fibers and spirally wraps around the axons of unmyelinated nerve fibers. Synonyms: **Sheath of Schwann**, **Neurolemma**.

Neurilemoma (nu″rĭ-lĕ-mō′mah) (n.) A benign, slow-growing tumor produced by proliferating Schwann cells that is solitary and encapsulated. It often appears as a discrete, soft mass that is movable but remains attached to the nerve sheath from which it originates. The size of the lesion may vary up to several centimeters in diameter. Although the lesion is generally asymptomatic, it may be associated with pain or tenderness. Microscopically, the tumor consists of two tissue types—Antoni A and Antoni B. The Antoni type A tissue is composed of proliferating masses of Schwann cells that are often arranged in pallisading cords. The Antoni type B tissue is mxyomatous and degenerative. The tumor can usually be removed by blunt dissection after the perineurium is incised without causing neurologic dysfunction. Also known as **Schwannoma, Schwann Cell Tumor, Neurinoma, Peripheral Glioma, Perineural Fibroblastoma, Perineural Glioma, Schwannoglioma, Fi-**

broglioma, **False Neuroma**, **Neurilemoblastoma**, and **Neuroma Fibrillare**.

Neuritis (nu-rī′tis) (n.)   An inflammation of a nerve or nerves.

Neuro (nu′ro)   Prefix meaning nerve.

Neuroarthropathy (nu″ro-ar-throp′ah-thē) (n.)   See **Charcot's Disease**.

Neurodynia (nu″ro-dīn′ē-ah) (n.)   A pain in a nerve.

Neurofibroma (nu″rō-fī′brō′mah) (n.)   A benign connective tissue tumor arising from the sheaths of cranial or peripheral nerves that is due to an abnormal proliferation of Schwann cells. The lesions are poorly delineated, and the edges often merge with surrounding fibrious tissues. Except for those of the skin, these may become malignant and should be carefully followed.

Neurofibromatosis (nu″rō-fī″brō-mah-tō′sis) (n.)   An inherited disorder, characterized by disturbed function of cellular elements of neural crest origin. It is considered to be a trait with variable penetrance and a high rate of spontaneous mutation. It results in many congenital abnormalities of the skin, nervous system, bones, endocrine glands, and less commonly, other organs. Schwann cells and endoneurial fibroblasts multiply excessively in multiple foci, resulting in dermal and neural tumors of various sizes and shapes. Abnormal melanocyte function results in café-au-lait, or chocolate-colored, spots on the skin. The most common skeletal manifestations include scoliosis, congenital bowing and pseudoarthrosis, and erosive defects of bone due to contiguous neurogenic tumors. Synonym: **Von Recklinghausen Disease**.

Neurogenic (nu″rō-jen′ik) (adj.)   Originating from any part of the nervous system.

Neurogenic Scoliosis (nu″rō-jen′ik/skō″le-o′sis) (n.)   A lateral spinal curvature caused by either disease or anomalies of nerve tissues.

Neurogenic Shock (nu″rō-jen′ik/shok) (n.)   The clinical state of shock that results primarily from nervous influences. This follows interference with the balance of vasodilator and vasoconstrictor influences to both arterioles and venules so that the patient is normovolemic but peripheral resistance is markedly decreased formerly called **Primary Shock**.

Neuroglia (nu-rog′le-ah) (n.)   The supporting cells of the nervous system that are not neurons. In the central nervous system, these consist of astrocytes, oligodendrocytes, and microglia. They are also known as **Glia**.

Neuroglioma (nu″rō-gli-ō′mah) (n.)   A benign tumor composed of cells of glial origin.

Neurohumor (nu″ro-hū′mor) (n.)   A chemical substance released at the synaptic knob or end-plate of a neuron that either stimulates or inhibits the next neuron or muscle fiber. Acetylcholine and norepinephrine are important neurohumors.

Neurolemma (nu″rō-lem′ah) (n.)   See **Neurilemma**.

Neurologic Deficit (nu″rō-loj′ik/def′i-sit) (n.)   Any dysfunction in motor activity or sensory perception that results from damage to any area of the nervous system.

Neurology (nu-rol′ō-jē) (n.)   The study of the nervous system and its disorders.

Neurolysis (nu-rol′i-sis) (n.)   1. Surgical separation and release of a nerve from any adhering fibrous adhesions and scar tissue. 2. Destruction or disintegration of nerve tissue.

Neuroma (nu-rō′mah) (n.)   1. A term used to designate the nodule of tissue that grows out from the proximal end of a nerve that has been severed. It consists of a tangled mass of Schwann cells. 2. A benign tumor composed of nerve tissue. It is often painful and tender. It usually has a traumatic etiology and is classified by gross pathology and histologic findings as follows:

  I. Neuromas-in-continuity

    A. Spindle neuromas: Lesions with an intact perineurium. A swelling or enlargement in an intact nerve that occurs secondary to chronic irritation, friction, or pressure. Despite their name, these are not true neuromas.

    B. Lateral neuroma: Lesions in which the perineurium of some, but not all, funiculi is broken. These occur when part of the nerve and its perineurium has been injured. They are common following trauma.

    C. Neuromas following nerve repair.

  II. Neuromas in completely severed nerves. These neuromas grow out of the proximal end of severed nerves.

  III. Amputation stump neuromas.

Neuromuscular Disorders (nu″rō-mus′ku-lar/dis-or′derz) (n.)   Any of a large group of disorders in which there is an affection with loss of function of muscles and peripheral nerves. Example: **Muscular Dystrophy**.

Neuromuscular Junction (nu″rō-mus′ku-lar/junk′shun) (n.)   The point where a motor neuron and a muscle fiber meet. Also called a **Myoneural Junction**.

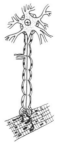

Neuromuscular junction

Neuromyelitis (nu″rō-mī″e-lī′tis) (n.)   An inflammation of nervous tissue and the spinal cord or, simply, myelitis present with neuritis.

Neuromyositis (nu″rō-mī″o-sī′tis) (n.) An inflammation of nerves and the muscles to which the affected nerves are related.

Neuron (nu′ron) (n.) An entire nerve cell, consisting of the cell body, dendrites, and axons. The neuron serves as the unit of structure and function of the nervous system and is both excitable and conductible. The point of contact between two neurons is called a **synapse**.

Neuropathic Fracture (nu″rō-path′ik/frak′chur) (n.) Any pathologic fracture that occurs in a limb or area of a limb that has impaired protective sensation due to a neurologic deficit.

Neuropathic Scoliosis (nu″ro-path′ik/skō″lē-ō′sis) (n.) A form of scoliosis caused by a neurologic disorder.

Neuropathy (nu-rop′ah-the) (n.) A disturbance of function or a pathologic change in a nerve or nerves. If a single nerve is affected, it is called mononeuropathy. If several nerves are affected, it is called mononeuropathy multiplex. If the involvement of several nerves is symmetrical and bilateral, the term **polyneuropathy** is used. **Neuritis** is a special form of neuropathy in which an inflammatory process affects the nerves.

Neurophysiology (nu″rō-fiz″e-ol′ō-jē) (n.) The scientific study of the physiology of the nervous system.

Neuroplasty (nu′rō-plas″tē) (n.) Surgical procedures for the repair and restoration of nerve tissue and function.

Neuropsychologic Disorder (nu″ro-sī-kō-loj′ik/dis-or′der) (n.) Any acute or chronic brain syndrome in which brain pathology causes a disturbance of mental function and behavior. Neuropsychology is that part of psychology that studies the relationship between the brain and behavior and uses psychologic assessment tests to diagnose brain pathologies.

Neuroradiology (nu″rō-rā″dē-ol′ō-jē) (n.) A subspecialty of radiology that uses special procedures to study the central nervous system.

Neurorrhaphy (nu-ror′ah-fē) (n.) The suturing of a divided nerve.

Neurosis (nu-rō′sis) (n.) An emotional illness characterized by errors of thinking and judgment; the patient does not, however, have a marked loss of contact with reality. It is believed that this illness is due to unconscious, unresolved internal conflicts.

Neurosurgeon (nu″rō-sur′jun) (n.) A physician who specializes in neurosurgery.

Neurosurgery (nu″rō-sur′jer-ē) (n.) The surgical treatment for diseases of the brain, spinal cord, and nervous tissue.

Neurotmesis (nu″rot-mē′sis) (n.) A severe type of peripheral nerve injury. A complete severance of the nerve or a severe crushing injury results in the loss of axonal continuity, the disruption of Schwann cells, and the tearing of the perineurial tube. Conduction below the lesion ceases almost immediately. Spontaneous recovery from this type of injury is not expected. Also known as **Neuronotmesis**. See **Seddon Classification**.

Neurotome (nu′rō-tōm) (n.) An instrument used for the division or dissection of a nerve.

Neurotomy (nu′rot′o-mē) (n.) The surgical division of a nerve.

Neurotransmitter (nu″rō-trans′mit-er) (n.) A chemical substance produced by a neuron, usually at the nerve ending, which then reacts with a receptor on a neighboring or distant cell to produce a response in the receptor cells. Examples include **acetylcholine**, **norepinephrine**, and **vasopressin**.

Neurotrophic (nu″rō-trōf′ik) (adj.) Of or pertaining to the influence of nerves on nutrition and the maintenance of normal condition in tissues.

Neurotrophic Arthritis (nu″rō-trōf′ik/ar-thrī′tis) (n.) See **Charcot's Joint**.

Neurotrophic Atrophy (nu″rō-trōf′ik/at′ro-fē) (n.) Atrophy of muscle and overlying tissue due to the separation of these tissues from their nerve supply. Clinically, this is noted in the chronic sensory neuropathies.

Neurotrophic Ulcer (nu″rō-trōf′ik/ul′ser) (n.) The destruction or ulceration of skin and underlying tissue due to the loss of protective sensation in the affected area.

Neurovascular (nu″ro-vas′ku-lar) (adj.) Of or pertaining to both nervous and vascular elements.

Neurovascular Bundle (nu″ro-vas′ku-lar/bun′d′l) (n.) In anatomy, any grouping of nerves with blood vessels that course in juxtaposition and specifically supply a given region.

Neurovascular Pedicle Grafts (nu″ro-vas′ku-lar/ped′i-k′l/grafts) (n.) See **Pedicle Flaps**.

Neutral Axis (nu′tral/ak′sis) (n.) 1. The longitudinal line of a structure, around which torsion occurs. 2. A longitudinal line in a long structure where normal axial stresses are zero when the structure is subjected to bending.

Neutral Plane (nu′tral/plān) (n.) The plane of a structure around which bending occurs.

Neutral Zone Method (nu′tral/zōn/meth′ud) (n.) The method by which all joint motions are measured from a defined zero starting position. The anatomic position of a joint defines the zero position; then motion is measured in degrees of a circle. Example: When a fully extended elbow joint is bent from the anatomic zero position to a right angle, the range of motion is 90 degrees of flexion.

Neutralization Plate (nu′tral-i-zā′shun/plāt) (n.) An internal splinting technique used in conjunction with lag-screw interfragmentary compression in long-bone shaft fractures. A contoured neutralization plate is applied across the fracture site, which protects the lag screw fixation by neutralizing torsional, bending, and shear forces.

Neutrilium (nu-tril-ē-um) (n.) A tradename for a wrought cobalt-chromium-tungsten-nickel alloy (ASTMF90). This metal is used in the production of implant prostheses.

Neutron (nu'tron) (n.) 1. A subatomic or elementary particle that represents a unit of mass. 2. An uncharged or electrically neutral particle of mass found in the nucleus of an atom.

Neviaser Technique (nev-ē-az-er/tek-nēk) (n.) Surgical procedure used for repairing acromioclavicular joint dislocations in which the coracoacromial ligament is used to reconstruct the superior acromioclavicular ligament.

Nevus (nē'vus) (n.) A benign skin lesion that is an area of hyperpigmentation.

Newington Brace (nū-ing-tun/brās) (n.) A fixed abduction weight-bearing orthosis used in the treatment of Legg-Calvé-Perthes disease.

Newton (nu'ton) (n.) A unit of force. One newton equals the amount of force required to accelerate a 1-kg mass at 1 m/s^2 in a vacuum. Abbreviated as **N**.

Newtonian Fluid (nū"ton-ī'an/floo'id) (n.) A fluid that demonstrates constant viscosity over a large range of different rates of shear.

Nicholas-ISMAT Manual Muscle Tester (nik'o-las/man'u-al/mus'el/test'er) (n.) A palm-sized, battery-operated device that uses the break test technique to record the force required to break a muscle contraction while simultaneously testing the linkages to the trunk and spine. Right versus left deficits are easily identifiable. This was developed at the Institute of Sports Medicine and Athletic Trauma.

Nicholas Medial Compartment Reconstruction (nik'o-las / me'de-al / com-part'ment / re"kon-struk'shun) (n.) See **Five-One Procedure**.

Nicola Procedure (nik'ola/pro-sē'jur) (n.) A surgical technique for the repair of recurrent anterior shoulder dislocations in which the long heads of the biceps tendons and the coracohumeral ligament are passed through a long tunnel in the head of the humerus to act as a check-rein on the humerus.

Nicoll Graft (nik'ol'graft) (n.) A technique of cancellous bone grafting. In this technique, gaps in long bones are bridged with solid blocks of cancellous bone that are fixed in place with metal plates.

Nidus (nī'dus) (n.) From the Latin for "nest," this term is used to describe the center or focus of development of a lesion. It is commonly used in reference to the central oval or round sclerotic region seen radiographically in osteoid osteomas.

Niemann-Pick Disease (nē'man-pik/di-zēz) (n.) An intralysosomal storage disease, or lipidosis, in which a deficiency of sphingomyelinase causes an accumulation of sphingomyelin in the histiocytes and reticuloendothelial cells of the spleen, liver, lymph nodes, bone marrow, and central nervous system. The skeletal manifestations result from an accumulation of lipid-bearing foam cells, called **Niemann-Pick Cells**, in the bone marrow. Roentgenographic examination may show an increase in radiolucency and an expansion of the shafts of long bones along with a thinning of the cortex and sparcity of trabecular pattern. Synonym: **Sphingomyelin Lipidosis**.

Nievergett Mesomelic Syndrome (nē-ver-get/mēs"ō-mel'ik/sin'drōm) (n.) A rare, congenital condition characterized by mesomelia. It has an autosomal dominant inheritance pattern. The tibia is often severely deformed, which requires orthopaedic intervention.

Night Bracing (nīt/brās'ing) (n.) Any type of orthosis or bracing intended for a patient's use only at nighttime.

Night Splint (nīt/splint) (n.) A splint applied and used during the nighttime only.

Nightstick Fracture (nīt'stik/frak-chur) (n.) A common name for a fracture of the ulna shaft. This usually results from a blow by a club or stick that strikes the forearm as it is raised in protection.

Ninety-Ninety Method (meth'ud) (n.) To reduce and hold a fracture of the neck of the metacarpal bone, the metacarpal phalangeal and the proximal interphalangeal joints are flexed 90 degrees. Upward pressure is placed on the flexed proximal interphalangeal joint resulting in reduction of the fracture.

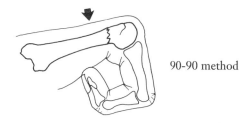

90-90 method

Ninety-Ninety Traction (nīn'tē-nīn'tē/trak'shun) (n.) A type of skeletal traction in proximal femoral

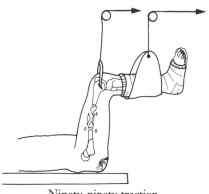

Ninety-ninety traction

fractures that is especially useful for children. A distal femoral pin and a calf sling are used to apply traction to the fracture and maintain hip and knee flexion. "Ninety-ninety" refers to the positioning of the hip and knee at 90 degrees of flexion.

Ninhydrin Test (nin-hī′drin/test) (n.) A print test used to assess sweat patterns in the hand in order to evaluate the integrity of sympathetic fibers in the peripheral nerves. Also known as the **Triketohydrindene Hydrate Print Test.**

Nirschl Procedure (nir-skē/pro-sē′jur) (n.) A surgical operation in resistant chronic tennis elbow. In this technique, the origin of the extensor carpi radialis brevis tendon is released, and the underlying angiofibroblastic pathologic changes are identified and excised. A small arthotomy is also made into the lateral compartment of the elbow.

NMR (n.) Abbreviation for Nuclear Magnetic Resonance.

Nocardia (nō-kar′dē-ah) (n.) A genus of the gram-positive, rodlike bacteria of the family Actinomycetacease. This is the causative agent of nocardiosis, which is primarily a pulmonary disease, although hematogenous spread may occur.

Nociceptor (nō″sē-sep′tor) (n.) A sensory receptor that is preferentially sensitive to a noxious or potentially noxious stimulus.

Node (nōd) (n.) A circumscribed mass of tissue perceived as a swelling or protuberance.

Node of Ranvier (nōd/of/rahn-vē-ā′) (n.) A node that appears in a myelinated nerve at the point of local constriction in the myelin sheath. These constrictions occur at varying intervals on both the central and peripheral axons. At each node of Ranvier, the axis cylinder is also constricted. Electron microscopy reveals that the node is formed by the end of one Schwann cell and the beginning of another. These nodes are important in the conduction of nervous impulses along the axon.

Nodular Fasciitis (nod′u-lar/fas″ē-ī′tis) (n.) A benign soft tissue lesion that consists of proliferating fibroblasts in a myxoid stroma. These lesions are considered pseudosarcomatous in that they are highly cellular and often have bizarre cells and mitotic figures; however, they are not malignant in their behavior.

Nodule (nod′ūl) (n.) A small node.

No-Man's Land (nō-manz/land) (n.) The area of the palm lying between the distal palmar crease and the proximal interphalangeal joint. In this area, the superficialis and profundus flexor tendons run together within the fibro-osseous sheath pulley. The formation of adhesions in this critical area of the pulleys may result in the failure of primary repairs of lacerated tendons at this level, thus the name "no man's land." Also known as the **Critical Zone, Flexor Tendon Zone II**, and the **Critical Area of Pulleys.**

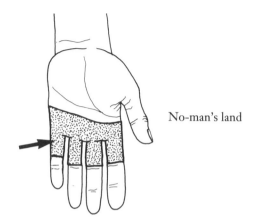

No-man's land

Nomenclature (nō′men-klā″tūr) (n.) Assigned names for classification purposes.

Nomogram (nōm′ō-gram) (n.) A computation chart or diagram on which numerous variables are plotted to solve complex numerical formulae.

Noncemented Arthroplasty (non″sē-ment′ed/ar′thrō-plas″tē) (n.) Any implant prosthesis that does not require methyl methacrylate cement for fixation. These prostheses depend initially for fixation on a press-fit and ultimately on bony ingrowth for permanent fixation.

Nondisjunction (non″dis-junk′shun) (n.) A genetic term that describes an abnormality of cell division in which there is an unequal division of genetic material into the cells.

Non-Hodgkin's Lymphoma (non″hoj′kinz/lim-fō′-mah) (n.) Any lymphomatous conditions other than Hodgkin's disease.

Nonischemic (non″is-kēm′ik) (adj.) Not affected by the mechanical obstruction of blood vessels. Used to describe a limb or digit that has an intact arterial supply.

Noninvasive Technique (non″in-vā′siv/tek′nēk′) (n.) Any method in which equipment or modalities are used on or near the patient's skin, but remain outside the body tissues. Used in contrast to **invasive technique.**

Nonneoplastic (non″nē″ō-plas′tik) (adj.) Any lesion that resembles a tumor but is not neoplastic in origin. In orthopaedics, examples include myositis ossificans and Paget disease.

Nonossifying Fibroma (non″os′i-fī″ing/fī-brō′mah) (n.) A benign, fibrous lesion of bone. It is an eccentric, well-delineated, usually solitary defect in the metaphyseal region of children's long bones. Nonossifying fibromae are common, inconsequential, and usually asymptomatic. Occasionally, a pathologic fracture will occur through a large lesion.

Characteristically, the radiographic finding is a well-demarcated, lucent lesion with densely sclerotic, scalloped margins. The cortex may be thinned, but usually is not expanded. The lesion may appear uniloculated or multiloculated.

Histologically, the lesion consists of benign fibroblastic cells arranged in fascicles and whorls. Benign multinucleated giant cells are distributed irregularly throughout the lesion. A fibrous cortical defect is similar radiographically and histologically, but it is smaller in size.

This lesion is also known as a **Fibrous Cortical Defect**, **Nonosteogenic Fibroma**, or a **Metaphyseal Fibrous Defect**.

Non-Padded Cast (non'paded/kast) (n.) A cast applied either directly to the skin or over a stockinette, without a layer of sheet cotton. Bony prominences may be spot-padded with a small portion of sheet cotton or felt. Also known as a **Skin-Tight** cast.

Nonpathogen (non"path'ō-jen) (n.) A microorganism that does not normally cause disease.

Nonprehensile Movement (non"prē-hen'sīl/m$\overline{oo}$v'ment) (n.) Hand movements that require no grasping or holding. Objects are manipulated by pushing, tapping, or lifting with the hand or fingers. Example: Using a typewriter. This is the opposite of **Prehensile Movement**.

Nonprescription Drugs (non"prē-skrip'shun/drugs) (n.) Drugs available without prescription. These are commonly known as **Over-the-Counter (OTC) Drugs**.

Non–Self-Tapping Screw (non-self-tap'ing/skrū) (n.) A screw with uninterrupted threads from their inception to the tip. Non–self-tapping screws must be inserted into a pilot hole with pre-cut or tapped threads.

Nonsteroidal Anti-inflammatory Drugs (non"ste'roid-al/an"ti-in-flam'ah-to"rē/drugs (n.) Drugs that reduce inflammation but do not have a steroid component. They are generally divided into five groups: indoles, such as indomethacin, sulindac, and tolmetin sodium; pyrazolone derivatives, such as phenylbutazone and oxyphenbutazone; propionic acids, such as fenoprofen, ibuprofen, and naproxen; oxicans, such as piroxicam; and anthranicylic acid derivatives, such as meclofenamate and mefenamic acid. The response to these drugs varies widely in different individuals. Abbreviated **NSAID**.

Nonstructural Curve (non"struk'tūr-al/curv) (n.) A description for a spinal curve or scoliosis that does not have a structural component. A nonstructural curve corrects or overcorrects on recumbent side-bending roentgenograms. Synonym: **Functional Curve**.

Nonunion (non-ūn'yun) (n.) 1. A fracture in which a reparative process has come to a complete standstill. 2. The failure of a fractured bone to unite. Nonunion is diagnosed if it can be determined clinically or radiographically that healing has ceased and union is highly improbable. Nonunions are classified into two general types, hypertrophic or atrophic.

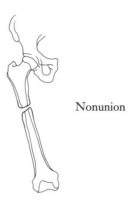

Nonunion

Non–Weight-Bearing (non-wāt-bār'ing) (adj.) A term used to describe an assisted gait in which no weight is placed on the designated lower extremity throughout the gait cycle. It is used in rehabilitation prescriptions and is abbreviated as **N.W.B**.

Noonan Syndrome (noo'nan/sin'drōm) (n.) A congenital abnormality in which a variety of phenotypic abnormalities are seen to affect the skin, the skeleton, and the heart. These patients usually have short stature and decreased intelligence. Male patients are phenotypically similar to females with Turner's syndrome, but they have a normal karyotype.

Normal Foot (nor'mal/foot) (n.) A foot in which the heel is in neutral alignment with the tibia when the forefoot is straight. Five-degree valgus deviation of the heel is the standard deviation from normal. In a normal foot, if you draw one line down the center of the calf in line with the tibia, and another vertical line to bisect the posterior heel, the two lines will be parallel or coincident.

Normal Last Shoes (nor'mal/last/sh$\overline{oo}$z) (n.) Shoes in which there is no excessive curving or straightening of the last.

Normal Saline (nor'mal/sā'lēn) (n.) A physiologic salt solution that contains 0.9% sodium chloride. This concentration is isotonic to cells.

Normal Stress (nor'mal/stres) (n.) A biomechanical term for the intensity of a force applied perpendicularly to a surface on which it acts.

Normal Variant Short Stature (nor'mal/vār'ē-ant/short/stat'ūr) (n.) The presence of short stature with a known, underlying metabolic or endocrine abnormality. It is defined as a current and predicted height below the third percentile, a birth weight greater than 2.5 kg, no apparent organic cause for growth retardation, and a normal serum growth hormone level when tested with pharmacologic provocation.

Nosocomial (nōs"ō-kō'mē-al) (adj.) Relating to a hospital.

Nosocomial Infection (nōs"ō-kō'mē-al/in-fek'shun) (n.) A hospital-acquired infection caused by diagnostic or therapeutic procedures, exposure to the hospital environment, or contact with its staff.

Notch (noch) (n.) 1. An angular cut or indentation; this is usually described on the edge of a flat bone surface. An example of this is the sciatic notch in the pelvis. 2. In knee surgery, an abbreviated reference to the intercondylar notch of the distal femur.

Notchplasty (noch″plas′tē) (n.) Any surgical technique in which a bony notch is modified. Commonly used to refer to a procedure that results in the enlargement of the intercondylar notch of the femur. By widening the intercondylar notch and deepening the anterior roof of the notch, this procedure in conjunction with anterior cruciate ligament reconstructions will prevent impingement in knee extension.

Notochord (nō′tō-kord) (n.) A strip of mesodermal tissue that develops along the dorsal surface of the early embryo, beneath the neural tube. This longitudinal, rodlike structure is solid and elastic, and serves as the internal skeleton in the embryos of all chordates. It becomes almost entirely obliterated by the development of the vertebrae.

No-Touch Technique (no-tuch/tek′nēk) (n.) The use of instruments, instead of fingers, for intraoperative palpation. The instrument ends are never handled.

Notta's Node (nat′-tahz/nōd) (n.) A congenital trigger digit.

Noxious (nok-shus) (adj.) Harmful or injurious to cells, tissues, organs, or organisms.

NPO (n.) Abbreviation for nil per os, or nothing by mouth.

NSAID (n.) Abbreviation for nonsteroidal anti-inflammatory drug.

Nuchal (nū′kal) (adj.) Of or pertaining to the neck.

Nuchal Area (nu′kal/ar′ea) (n.) The surface of the posterior occiput that is below the superior nuchal line. From this surface the neck muscles originate. Also called the **Nuchal Region**.

Nuchal Ligament (nū′kal/lig-ah′ment) (n.) A broad, fibrous, roughly triangular sagittal septum that separates the left and right sides of the base of the neck. It represents the cervical part of the supraspinous ligament and extends from the spines of the cervical vertebrae to the external occipital crest. See **Ligamentation Nuchae**.

Nuchal Lines (nū′kal/līnz) (n.) Any of the paired bony ridges on the distal occiput, including the superior and inferior nuchal lines. The superior nuchal lines arise from the inion.

Nuchal Rigidity (nū′kal/ri-jid′i-tē) (n.) Stiffness of the neck.

Nuclear Magnetic Resonance (nū′klē-ar/mag-net′ik/rez′ō-nans) (n.) A phenomenon in which particular atomic nuclei respond to the application of certain magnetic fields by absorbing or emitting electromagnetic radiation; this is the basis for mag-

netic resonance imaging. Although this term was originally used for the imaging tests that use this principle, public worry about the term "nuclear" led tests to become known as **Magnetic Resonance Imaging**, or **MRI**. Abbreviated as **NMR**. See **MRI**.

Nuclear Scan (nū′kle-ar/skan) (n.) Any imaging technique that uses radioisotopes as tracers. Examples are gallium scans or technetium bone scans. Pathology is evaluated by measuring increase or decrease in activity of nuclear uptake.

Nucleic Acid (nū-klē′ik/as′id) (n.) A long-chain, alternating polymer of ribose sugar rings and phosphate groups that have organic bases, such as adenine, thymine, uracil, guanine, or cytosine, as side-chains. Ribonucleic acid (RNA) and deoxyribonucleic acid (DNA) are the two principal nucleic acids found in the cells of living tissues.

Nucleolus (nū″klē′ō-lus) (n.) An RNA-containing body within the nucleus of a cell.

Nucleoprotein (nū″klē-ō-prō′te-in) (n.) A molecular complex composed of nucleic acid and protein.

Nucleoside (nū″klē-ō-sīd″) (n.) A compound produced by the removal of phosphate from a nucleotide, thereby creating a substance that consists of a five-carbon sugar and a purine or pyrimidine base.

Nucleotide (nū′klē-ō-tīd) (n.) The basic chemical unit that is polymerized in a nucleic acid. The molecule consists of a purine or pyrimidine, a five-carbon sugar, and a phosphate group linked together.

Nucleus (nū′klē-us) (n.) 1. In cytology, a rounded mass in the cytoplasm that consists of an external nuclear membrane and an interior nuclear sap, in which chromosomes and nucleoli are suspended. 2. In neuroanatomy, a group of nerve cells found in the brain or spinal cord that can be clearly demarcated either grossly or histologically from neighboring groups. 3. The central body of an atom.

Nucleus Pulposus (nu′klē-us/pul-pōs′us) (n.) The central, semielastic, spongy zone of the intervertebral disk. It is a hydrodynamic structure that has a greater fluid content than the rest of the disk and is composed of a mucopolysacharride, fine interlaced collagen fibers, and physaliphorous cells.

Nuclide (nu′klīd) (n.) An atomic nucleus composed of any element. See **Isotope**.

Nuprin (nu′prin) (n.) A proprietary name for ibuprofen, a nonsteroidal, anti-inflammatory drug.

Nurse (ners) (n.) A person whose qualifications are obtained at a formal program of an accredited school of nursing. The nurse, under the supervision of a physician, provides nursing services to patients requiring assistance in either recovering or maintaining physical or mental health. These services include assistance in providing medicine and food, wound care, the evaluation of vital signs, help with the toilet, etc.

Nurse, Charge (ners/charj) (n.) A registered nurse who directs and supervises the provision of nursing care in one patient care unit for the duration of one shift.

Nurse, Circulating (ners/ser″ku-la′ting) (n.) A registered nurse responsible for establishing and maintaining a safe, therapeutic environment for patients during surgery. He or she is qualified by specialized training in operating room techniques.

Nurse, Head (ners/hed) (n.) A registered nurse with the ongoing responsibility to direct and manage the nursing care activities of one patient care unit.

Nurse Practitioner (ners/prak-tish′un-er) (n.) A registered nurse who engages in health care evaluation and decision-making related to patient care. He or she is under the supervision of a physician and is qualified by a baccalaureate or formal educational preparation.

Nurse, Primary (ners/pri′mer-ē) (n.) A registered nurse who provides all nursing care to assigned patients throughout their hospitalization.

Nurse, Registered (ners/rej′is-terd) (n.) A person licensed by the state to practice nursing. He or she is qualified by an approved post-secondary program or baccalaureate in nursing.

Nurse, Scrub (ners/skrub) (n.) A registered nurse or operating room technician who assists surgeons during surgery.

Nursemaid's Elbow (ners′māds/el′bō) (n.) Subluxation of the head of the radius seen in young children. There is usually a history of a sudden longitudinal stress across the elbow, often incurred when a child is pulled by its outstretched arm. A snapping sensation is usually appreciated as reduction is accomplished with supination of the forearm and then by flexion of the elbow. This is also known as **Subluxation** of the **Head** of the **Radius** or **Pulled Elbow**.

Nursing Care (ners′ing/kār) (n.) A provision of services by or under the direction of a nurse to patients requiring assistance in recovering or maintaining their physical or mental health.

Nursing Care Institution (ners′ing/kar/in-sti′tu-shun) (n.) See **Nursing Home**.

Nursing Care Plan (ners′ing/kār/plan) (n.) A formal, written plan of nursing care activities con-

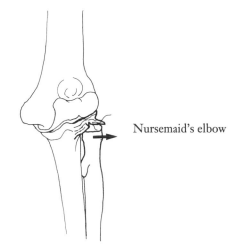

Nursemaid's elbow

ducted on behalf of a given patient. It is used to coordinate the activities of all nursing personnel involved in that patient's care.

Nursing Home (ners′ing/hōm) (n.) A health-provision institution with an organized medical staff and permanent facilities, including inpatient beds, that provides continuous nursing and other health-related services to patients who are not acutely ill yet require continued care on an inpatient basis. Also known as a **Nursing Care Institution**.

Nursing Team (ners′ing/tēm) (n.) A group of registered nurses and auxiliary nursing personnel. A nursing team implements total nursing care programs planned by the team leader for designated patients.

Nutcracker Fracture (nut′krak-er/frak′chur) (n.) A term applied to cuboid bone fractures whose mechanism of injury is thought to be the crushing of the cuboid between the calcaneus and the bases of the fourth and fifth metatarsals in lateral stress injuries of the midtarsal joint.

NWB (n.) Abbreviation for non–weight-bearing.

Nylon (nī′lon) (n.) A type of nonabsorbable monofilament used as suture material.

O

OA Abbreviation for osteoarthritis.

Ober Test (ō′ber/test) (n.) A method used to evaluate contracture of the iliotibial band. Have the patient lie on the side not being tested, with the underlying hip and knee flexed. Fully abduct the leg to be examined, making sure the hip joint is in neutral position and the knee is flexed to 90 degrees. Then allow the leg to fall into maximal adduction. If the test is positive, the thigh will remain abducted when the leg is released; this is due to contracture of the iliotibial band. Normally, the extremity would fall into adduction (below the horizontal axis).

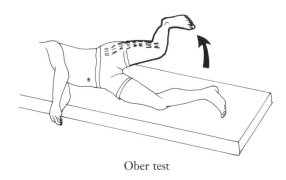

Ober test

Objective Sign (ob-jek′tiv/sīn) (n.) Any sign that can be detected or is otherwise perceptible to the external senses by feel, sight, hearing, smell, measurement, or is clinically elicited. Compare with **Subjective**.

Oblique (o-blēk) (adj.) Slanted, inclined, or sloping.

Oblique Fracture (o-blēk/frak′chur) (n.) Any break in a bone where the direction of the line of fracture is slanted in relation to the long axis of the bone.

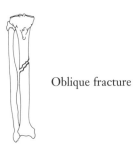

Oblique fracture

Oblique Retinacular Ligament (o-blēk/ret″i-nak′ū-lar/lig′ah-ment) (n.) This ligament is one of Landsmeer's ligaments of the extensor expansion of the fingers. It prevents passive or active flexion of the distal interphalangeal joint when the proximal interphalangeal joint is in extension. It unites the lateral band of the extensor tendon nearest the distal interphalangeal joint to the proximal phalanx, which is proximal to the proximal interphalangeal joint.

Obstetric Paralysis (ob-stet′rik/pah-ral′i-sis) (n.) Birth injuries of the brachial plexus that result in paralysis of the upper extremity. These include Erb's palsy and Klumpke's paralysis.

Obturator Externus Muscle (ob′tū-rā″tor/eks-ter′nus/mus′el) (n.) See **Muscle**.

Obturator Foramen (ob′too-ra″tor/fo-ra′men) (n.) A large, oval-shaped opening in the pelvis between the pubis and the ischium. The obturator vessels and nerves pass out of the pelvis through this opening.

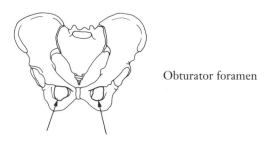

Obturator foramen

Obturator Internus Muscle (ob′tū-rā″tor/in-ter′nus/mus′el) (n.) See **Muscle**.

Obturator Sign (ob′tū-rā″tor/sīn) (n.) A radiographic sign of septic arthritis of the hip in children. Radiographically, a displacement of the obturator fat plane, which lies along the inner wall of the pelvis (adjacent to the hip joint). On an AP roentgenogram of the pelvis this sign may indicate the presence of fluid secondary to an adjacent fracture or a septic arthritis of the hip.

Occipital Bone (ok-sip′i-tal/bōn) (n.) The flat bone that forms the posterior aspect of the head. Also known as **Occiput**.

Occipital Condyles (ok-sip′i-tal/kon′dīlz) (n.) The pair of bony prominences on the external surface of the inferior aspect of the occiput that articulate with the superior atlantal facets.

Occipitoatlantoid Articulations (ok-sip-i-tal/at-lan-toyd/ar-tik″u-la′shunz) (n.) The joints between the occipital condyles and articular facets of the atlas.

Occipitocervical Fusion (ok-sip″ĭ-to-ser′vĭ-kal/fu′zhun) (n.) Arthrodesis of the base of the occiput to the C1 vertebra. It may be attained by a variety of surgical techniques.

Occiput (ok′si-put) (n.) See **Occipital Bone**.

Occiput-to-Wall Distance (ok-si-put/to/wawl/dis′tans) (n.) A measurement used to indicate the degree of fixed flexion and the progressive loss of extension of the cervical spine. Have the patient stand, heels and back against a wall, and then attempt to touch the wall with the occiput, keeping the chin horizontal. Record the distance in centimeters from the occiput to the wall.

Occlusive Dressing (o-klū'siv/dres'ing) (n.) Any bandage that covers a wound completely, protecting it from exposure to the air.

Occult Fracture (o-kult/frak'chur) (n.) A fracture strongly suggested by radiologic signs but whose line is not visible roentgenologically until reparative bone changes have occurred. With bony healing, the decalcification that occurs at the ends of the fracture fragments will make the break more readily visible after a short time. This fracture will be positive by nuclear bone scan, prior to its observation on a radiograph.

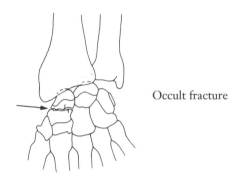

Occult fracture

Occupational Disease (ok'ū-pā'shun-al/di-zēz') (n.) Any disorder caused by job-related factors.

Occupational Medicine (ok'ū-pā'shun-al/med'i-sin) (n.) That branch of medical study and treatment that addresses the relationship of people to their work. The aim of occupational medicine is to identify causes of disease and injury in the work environment and then prevent their development.

Occupational Safety and Health Administration (ok'ū-pā'shun-al / sāf'tē / and / helth / ad-min'is-trā'shun) (n.) An administrative board, created by the Occupational Safety and Health Act of 1970, that encourages employers and employees to reduce hazards in the workplace. It is abbreviated as **OSHA**, and is administered by the United States Department of Labor.

Occupational Therapist (ok'ū-pā'shun-al/ther'ah-pist) (n.) A person trained and licensed to provide instruction and supervision in the activities of occupation therapy.

Occupational Therapy (ok'ā-pū'shun-al/ther'ah-pē) (n.) A system of medically prescribed rehabilitation activities intended to increase coordination, range of motion, power, and function in performing vocational, avocational tasks, or activities of daily living.

Ochronosis (ō-krō-nō'sis) (n.) A metabolic disorder characterized by a blue or blackish blue pigmentation in the connective tissues due to an accumulation of oxidized homogentisic acid. This results from a hereditary deficiency of homogentisic acid oxidase and is associated with alkaptonuria. The deposition of the pigment produces a distinct form of arthritis known as ochronotic arthritis. It usually affects larger joints, while sparing the smaller joints, and classically results in spondylosis. Roentgenographic examination of the spine reveals calcification of the intervertebral disks with marked narrowing of the intervertebral disk space.

Ochsner's Clasping Test (oks'nerz/klasp'ing/test) (n.) A diagnostic procedure used to indicate median nerve paralysis. Have the patient clasp his or her hands together with fingers intertwined. If the index finger fails to flex, the median nerve has been interrupted proximal to its innervation to the flexor digitorium sublimis muscle.

O'Connell's Test (ō-kon-elz/test) (n.) A diagnostic maneuver for lumbar radiculopathy. Using the Lasègue maneuver, test the unaffected leg, recording the angle of flexion and any pain. Next, test the affected limb and again record the findings. Then extend both knees and simultaneously flex the thighs to an angle just short of producing pain. Lower the unaffected limb. In a positive test, this will cause marked exacerbation of pain on the affected side.

O'Connor Operating Scope (ō-kon-or/op'er-ā-ting/skop) (n.) One of the first arthroscope designs to provide an instrument channel that accommodated 3.4-mm surgical instruments.

Ocular Dystrophy (ok'u-lar/dis'trō-fē) (n.) A rare form of muscular dystrophy that affects the extra-ocular and upper facial muscles; it occurs during the teenage years. Also known as **Progressive External Ophthalmoplegia**.

Oculopharyngeal Dystrophy (ok''u-lō-fah-rin'jē-al/dis'trō-fē) (n.) A form of muscular dystrophy that significantly involves the pharyngeal muscles. It occurs during the third decade.

O'Donoghue's Triad (ō-don-ō-hūz/trī'ad) (n.) A simultaneous injury to the medial meniscus, anterior

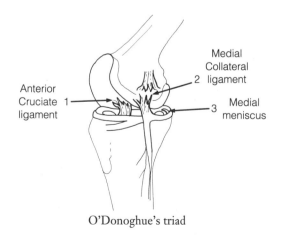

Anterior Cruciate 1 ligament

Medial Collateral 2 ligament

3 Medial meniscus

O'Donoghue's triad

cruciate ligament, and medial collateral ligament. This triad injury results from valgus stress and external rotation at the knee. Also known as the **Terrible Triad**.

Odontoid Process (o-don′toid/pros′es) (n.) A tooth-like, pointed process that arises from the body of the axis (the second cervical vertebra) and articulates anteriorly with the atlas (the first cervical vertebrae). Also known as the **Dens**.

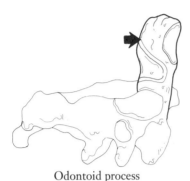

Odontoid process

Offset Cane (of′set/kān) (n.) A cane in which the upper third of the stem is offset so that the vertical handle sits above the lower portion of the stem.

Ogden Classification (og-den/klas″sĭ-fĭ-kā′shun) (n.) A detailed and extensive classification of epiphyseal plate physeal fracture based on roentgenographic appearance.

OI Abbreviation for Osteogenesis Imperfecta.

Ointment (oint′ment) (n.) A semisolid material applied to the skin or mucous membranes as a salve. It usually contains medicinal substances.

Olecranon (o-lek′rah-non) (n.) The large process of the proximal ulna that forms the posterior bony prominence of the elbow.

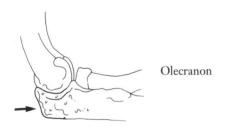

Olecranon

Olecranon Fossa (o-lek′rah-non/fos′ah) (n.) The depression on the posterior surface of the lower humerus into which the olecranon process fits in an extended elbow.

Oligotrophic Nonunion (ol″i-go′trōf′ik/non-ūn′yun) (n.) A type of hypervascular nonunion that contains no callus and is not hypertrophic.

Oliguria (ol″i-gū′rē-ah) (n.) Small amount of urination.

Ollier's Disease (ol″e-āz′/di-zēz′) (n.) A rare developmental abnormality that presents with multiple cartilaginous tumors throughout the skeleton. The lesion occurs on bones that are preformed in cartilage. Bone deformity or malignant transformation may occur. It is also known as **Enchondromatosis** or **Multiple enchondrosis**.

Ollier's Layer (ol″e-āz/lā′er) (n.) The innermost layer of the periosteum. Also known as the **Osteogenetic layer**.

Ollier Skin Graft (ol″e-ā/skin/graft) (n.) A free, split-thickness skin graft that is 0.025 inches in thickness.

Ollier-Thiersch Method (ol″e-ā/tērsh/meth′ud) (n.) A technique of application of very thin skin grafts. This method harvests long, broad strips of epidermis with a portion of the dermis attached and applies them to freshened granulation tissue. Also known as **Dermoepidermic Grafts**.

Ombredanne's Vertical Line (ahm-bra-danz/ver-ti-kal/līn) (n.) A line used in the radiographic evaluation of congenital dislocation of the hip; it is more commonly known as **Perkin's Line**. See **Perkin's Line**.

Omnipaque (om-nē-pāk) (n.) The proprietary name of iohexol, a nonionic, water-soluble, contrast medium used in myelography.

Omovertebral Bone (o″mō-ver′tē-bral/bōn) (n.) An omovertebral process that is ossified. An atavistic bone that attaches the superior medial angle of the scapula to the cervical spine, thus preventing scapula descent, called Sprengel's deformity.

Omovertebral Process (ō″mō-ver′tē-bral/pros′es) (n.) A bony, cartilaginous or fibrous connection that goes from a congenitally elevated scapula to the cervical or thoracic spine.

Oncogenic (ong″ko-jen′ic) (adj.) Cancer causing.

Oncogene (ong′ko-jēn) (n.) A defect in a gene that enhances its ability to initiate cancer. Oncogenes have been described with specific forms of osteogenic sarcoma and Ewing's sarcoma.

One-Plane Instability (wun-plān/in-sta-bil′i-tē) (n.) In the anatomic classification of knee joint instability that results from ligamentous injury, these are simple or straight instabilities—i.e., they go in one direction only. They are subdivided according to the direction of the tibial displacement on the femur: medial, lateral, posterior, or anterior. This classification suggests certain structural deficits but is not defined by these deficits. These instabilities may be seen in combination with a rotatory instability.

Onlay Graft (on-lā/graft) (n.) Any bony graft technique in which large cortical grafts are placed on top of and across the bony defect and held with screw and/or plate fixation. Cancellous bone, usually obtained from the medullary surface of the graft, may be placed around the cortical strips.

Ontogeny (on-toj'e-nē) (n.) The development of the individual organism.

Onych (o-nik) A prefix that means "nail."

Onychectomy (on"i-kek'tō-mē) (n.) Excision of a nail or nail bed.

Onychitis (on"i-kī'tis) (n.) Inflammation of the nail matrix.

Onychoarthrosis (on"nikō-ar-thrō'sis) (n.) See **Nail–Patella Syndrome**.

Onychocryptosis (on"i-kō-krip-tō'sis) (n.) See **Ingrown Toenail**.

Onychogryposis (on"i-kō-gri'pō-sis) (n.) Hypertrophy of a fingernail or toenail that characteristically results in an unusually large and curved nail plate with marked overgrowth. The nail plate becomes discolored, hard, thick, and clawlike. Synonym: **Ram's Horn Nail**.

Onychomycosis (on"i-kō-mī-kō'sis) (n.) A fungal disease in which the nails become opaque, white, thickened, and friable.

Onychopathy (on"i-kop'ah-thē) (n.) Any disease of the nail.

Onychorrhexis (on"i-kō-rek'sis) (n.) A spontaneous splitting or breaking of the nails.

Onychosis (on"i-kō'sis) (n.) A disease or deformity of the nail or nails.

Opacity (ō-pas'i-tē) (n.) The state of being opaque or lacking transparency.

Opaque Media (ō-pāk'/mē'dē-ah) (n.) Any contrast material introduced into a body cavity or structure to render it radiopaque to x-rays.

Open Amputation (ō'pen/am"pu-tā'shun) (n.) 1. An amputation with open wound edges. 2. A guillotine amputation.

Open Anesthesia (ō'pen/an"es-thē'ze-ah) (n.) A form of general inhalation anesthesia in which no rebreathing of the expired gases occurs. This form of anesthesia is rarely used.

Open Fracture (ō'pen/frak'chur) (n.) A fracture in which there is open communication between the bony fragments and the external environment because the skin and soft tissue have been disrupted. These fractures are categorized according to the mechanism of injury, size of the wound, the energy of the soft tissue trauma, degree of skeletal involvement, and the presence or absence of arterial or nerve injury. This used to be called a **compound fracture**. See below for classification of open fractures.

Type I: Small skin wounds, of 1 cm or less; this type is caused by low-velocity trauma.

Type II: Larger skin wounds, greater than 1 cm in length or width, but with little or no devitalized soft tissue and little foreign material present.

Type III: Wounds of moderate or large size with significant soft tissue damage and/or foreign material present; includes traumatic amputation.

Type IIIa: Wounds with extensive soft tissue laceration or flaps, but sufficient soft tissue to cover bone.

Type IIIb: Wounds with extensive soft tissue injury where the bone remains exposed after debridement.

Type IIIc: Any open fracture associated with arterial injuries requiring repair.

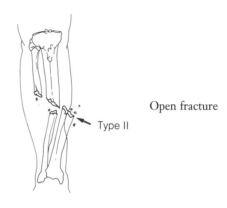

Open fracture

Type II

Open Intramedullary Nailing (ō'pen/in"trah-med'u-lār"ē/nāl'ing) (n.) A technique in which nail placement occurs after the fracture site has been exposed. Compare to **Closed Intramedullary Nailing**.

Open Reduction (o'pen/rē-duk'shun) (n.) A reduction of a fracture or dislocation, or both, performed after a surgical incision has been made through the soft tissues.

Open Reduction and Internal Fixation (ō'pen/re-duk'shun/and/in-ter'nal/fik-sā'shun) (n.) A fracture treatment in which surgery is used to reduce fracture fragments and then hardware is implanted to maintain the reduction. Abbreviated as **ORIF**.

Opening Wedge Osteotomy (ō'pen-ing/wej/os"te-ot'ō-mē) (n.) A procedure used to correct an angular deformity in which a straight cut through bone is wedged open with a pie-shaped bone graft.

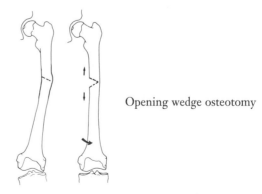

Opening wedge osteotomy

Opera-Glass Hand (op'era/glas/hand) (n.) A descriptive term applied to the characteristic deformities seen in chronic polyarthritis. The joints are eroded and the bones become shortened, osteopenic, and fragile.

Operating Microscope (op′er-ā-ting/mī′kro-skōp) (n.) A microscope designed for use during surgical procedures.

Operating Room (op′er-ā-ting/room) (n.) 1. The properly staffed and equipped hospital area for surgery. 2. A unit to be used for the performance of surgery.

Operating Room Attire (op′er-ā-ting/room/ă-tīr) (n.) The required clothing for scrubbed team members in an operating room. Operating room attire consists of body covers (scrub dress, jumpsuit, pantsuit, or shirt and trouser), head cover, mask, protective eye wear or shield, sterile gown, gloves, and shoe covers. Each article of clothing helps keep external contamination off the patient.

Operating Room Team (op′er-ā-tíng/room tēm) (n.) Personnel necessary to run an operating room. The group may be subdivided by the various functions of its members: (1) The scrubbed, sterile team—operating surgeon, assistants to the surgeon, scrub nurse or technician; (2) The unscrubbed, unsterile team—anesthesiologist or anesthetist, circulating nurse, others, including biomedical engineers or technicians who set up monitoring devices, other people who safeguard patient welfare during the operation.

Operation (op″er-ā′shun) (n.) Any surgical procedure.

Oppenheim's Disease (op′en-hīmz/di-zēz′) (n.) See **Spinal Muscular Atrophy**.

Oppenheim Sign (op′en-hīm/sīn) (n.) One of the extensor reflexes of the toes that suggests upper motor neuron or corticospinal motor paralysis. To elicit this sign, apply heavy pressure with the index finger and thumb to the anterior tibial surface, and stroke from the tibial tubercle to the ankle. In a positive test, the great toe extends and the lesser toes fan. See also **Babinski Sign**.

Opponens (o-pō′nenz) (n.) Any muscle in the hand that brings opposing digits together; the opponens pollicis muscle is an example.

Opponens Bar (o-pō′nenz/bar) (n.) The component of a hand orthosis that keeps the thumb abducted.

Opponens Splint (o-pō′nenz/splint) (n.) A splint used to keep the thumb in abduction at a right angle to the plane of the palm and in opposition to the fingers. Also known as an abduction splint or an opposition splint.

Opponensplasty (o-pō′nenz-plas′tē) (n.) Any surgical technique designed to restore the opposition function of the thumb.

Opportunistic Microorganism (op″or-tū-nis′tik/mī″krō-or′gan-izm) (n.) A generally nonpathologic microorganism that may produce disease in an impaired host. It is usually part of the endogenous flora.

Opposition (op′o-zish′un) (n.) The relationship of the thumb to the other fingers when the thumb is moved toward the palm of the hand.

Opposition Splint (op′ō-zish′un/splint) (n.) See **Opponens Splint**.

Opsonin (op′sō-nin) (n.) Plasma components normally present as part of the immune system. They react with foreign antigens to increase the antigens' susceptibility to phagocytosis.

OR Abbreviation for operating room.

O'Rahilly Classification (ō-ra-hi-lē/klas″sĭ-fĭ-kā′shun) (n.) A system of classification for limb malformations where there has been a failure of formation of part or all of that limb. These deformities are divided into: (1) transverse defects such as amelia; (2) longitudinal defects, such as a lobster-claw hand; (3) interposed transverse defects, such as a phocomelia; and (4) interposed longitudinal defects, such as some radial clubhands.

Organ (or′gan) (n.) A well-formed structure composed of different tissues that are integrated to perform a distinct function for the body as a whole. Examples are the heart, the liver, the brain, and the kidney.

Organelle (or″gah-nel′) (n.) Microscopic, well-formed structures found within the cytoplasm that perform specific cellular functions. Examples are lysosomes, ribosomes, and the endoplasmic reticulum.

Organic Brain Syndrome (or-gan′ik/brān/sin′drōm) (n.) An altered mental function that is a secondary result of organic, metabolic, or pharmacologic causes. The diagnosis should be considered when impaired orientation, memory, or other intellectual dysfunction exist. The diagnostic criteria are:

A clouding of consciousness, accompanied by a reduced capacity to focus and sustain attention to the environment.

The inclusion of at least two of the following: perceptual disturbances, such as misinterpretations, illusions, and hallucinations; incoherent speech; insomnia or daytime drowsiness; and increased or decreased psychomotor activity.

Disorientation and recent memory impairment.

Clinical features that develop over a short period (usually hours to days) and tend to fluctuate over the course of a day.

Evidence found in the medical history, physical examination, or laboratory tests of an organic factor etiologically related to the disturbance.

The syndrome is abbreviated as **OBS**; it is also known as **OMS**, or **Organic Mental Syndrome**.

Organic Disease (or-gan′ik/di-zēz′) (n.) An illness caused or accompanied by structural changes in a body organ or tissue.

Organizations, Orthopaedic See appendix.

O'Riain Wrinkle Test (ō-rī-ān/ringk″l/test) (n.) A clinical evaluation of the innervation of a part of the hand. It is used to objectively evaluate first the interruption and then the regeneration of sensory nerves in the hand. To perform the test, immerse both of the patient's hands in 40°C water for 30 minutes. If the test is positive, the denervated skin remains smooth; the skin of denervated fingers does not shrivel like normal skin. Also known as the **Wrinkle Test**, or **Leukens' Wrinkle Test**.

OREF   Abbreviation for Orthopaedic Research and Education Foundation.

ORIF   Open reduction and internal fixation.

Orthopaedia (or″thō-pē′dik) (adj.)   A term coined in 1741 by Nicholas Andry, who wrote: "As to the title, I have formed it of two greek words, viz. *orthos*, which signified straight, free from deformity, and *pais*, a child, to express in one term the design I propose, which is to teach the different methods of preventing and correcting deformities of children."

Orthopaedic Appliance (or″thō-pē′dik/ah-plī′ans) (n.)   Any prosthetic, orthotic device or brace.

Orthopaedic Heel (or″thō-pē′dik/hēl) (n.)   See **Thomas Heel**.

Orthopaedic Organizations See appendix.

Orthopaedic Oxford (or″thō-pē′dik/oks′ford) (n.) See **Oxford Shoe**.

Orthopaedic Shoe (or″thō-pē′dik/shū) (n.)   A shoe designed with a variety of special features: a wide, high toe-box; a long counter; a large, low heel; a medial half that extends further forward than a regular shoe; and an unusually heavy construction. It is easily adapted to accommodate and support deformed feet, especially when internal and/or external modifications are added.

Orthopaedic Surgeon (or″tho-pē′dik/sur′jun) (n.)   A physician who practices orthopaedic surgery. Also spelled **orthopedic** surgeon.

Orthopaedic Surgery (or″thō-pē′dik/sur′jer-ē) (n.)   1. The medical specialty that includes the investigation, preservation and restoration of the form and function of the extremities, the spine, and associated musculoskeletal structures by medical, surgical and physical means. 2. The medical and surgical specialty concerned with preserving and restoring the functions of the skeletal system, its articulations, and its associated structures. It is also spelled **Orthopedic** surgery and is often referred to as **Orthopedics**.

Orthopaedic Table (or′thō-pē′dik/tā′b′l) (n.)   A table used for many orthopaedic surgical procedures that may require traction, image intensification, conventional x-ray control, and cast application. The many available attachments allow varying body positions and the application of traction. Also known as a **Fracture Table**.

Orthopaedics (or″thō-pē′diks) (n.)   See **Orthopaedic Surgery**.

Orthopedist (or″-thō-pē-dist) (n.)   An orthopaedic surgeon.

Orthoroentgenogram (or″thō-rent″gen′ō-gram) (n.)   A radiographic technique for the measurement of limb length inequality. In this technique, three separate exposures of the limb are used—one centered over the hip, one over the knee, and one over the ankle. This avoids errors of magnification.

Orthosis (or-thōs′sis) (n.)   A mechanical appliance or apparatus that imposes counter forces on a limb in order to support it, to prevent or correct deformities, or to impart active function to a part of the limb. There are four functional classes of orthosis: 1) stabilization or supportive, 2) motorized, 3) functional and corrective, and 4) protective.

Orthotics (or-thot′iks) (n.)   1. The science of orthoses; the designing, creating, and fitting of orthopaedic appliances. 2. In common usage, this refers to simple shoe inserts that may be custom made or prefabricated.

Orthotist (or′tho-tist) (n.)   A person skilled in, and actively practicing, orthotics.

Ortolani Pillow (or-to-lah′nē/pil′ō) (n.)   An abduction device used for treating congenital hip dislocation.

Ortolani Test (or-to-lah′nē/test) (n.)   A diagnostic maneuver used to detect congenital dislocation of the hip in an infant. In a positive test, a click or jolt is appreciated as the dislocated hip is reduced. This maneuver is performed in one hip at a time. To perform the test, stabilize the pelvis with one hand, using the other hand to gently lift the thigh and the trochanter into the acetabulum as the hip is abducted. Also known as **Ortolani Maneuver** or **Reduction Test**.

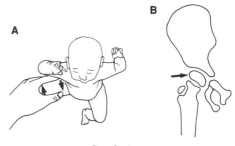

Ortolani test

Orudis (orudis′) (n.)   A proprietary brand of ketoprofen, a nonsteroidal anti-inflammatory drug.

Os Acetabula (os/as″e-tab′ū-la) (n.)   A round or oval accessory ossicle found on the superolateral margin of the acetabulum.

Os Acromiale (os/ah-kro′me-al) (n.)   An accessory bone of the shoulder found adjacent to the tip of the acromion process. It represents a normal secondary ossification center that has failed to undergo complete bony fusion.

Os Calcar Femorale (os/kal′kar/fem′or-al)   See **Calcar**.

Os Calcis (os/kal′sis) (n.)   See **Calcaneus**.

Os Coxae (os/kok′sē) (n.)   The hip bone, which is composed of the ilium, ischium, and pubis.

Os Intermetatarseum (os/in″ter-met″ah-tar′sē-um) (n.)   An accessory bone of the foot located between the proximal ends of the first and second metatarsals.

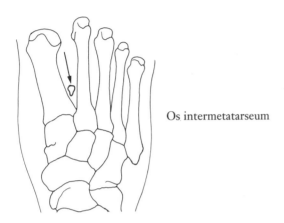

Os intermetatarseum

Os Odontoideum (os/o-don′toid-ē′um) (n.)   An accessory ossicle of the dens that is usually oval or round and has a smooth, dense border of bone. It is of variable size, and may be found either near the normal odontoid tip or near the basio-occipital bone. The presence of this ossicle is almost always associated with hyperplasia of the base of the dens. It may be difficult to distinguish from a nonunion of an odontoid fracture; the etiology may, in fact, be traumatic.

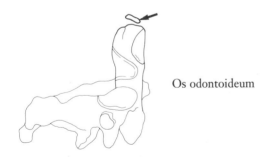

Os odontoideum

Osteoonychodysostosis (os″te-o/on″i-kō-dī-sos-tō-sis) (n.)   See **Nail–Patella Syndrome**.

Os Peroneum (os/per″o-nē′um) (n.)   An accessory bone of the foot found in or adjacent to the peroneus longus tendon; it is inferior and lateral to the os calcis and cuboid.

Os Subfibulare (os/sub″-fib-ū-lahr-e) (n.)   An accessory bone of the ankle found at the distal tip of the lateral malleolus.

Os Subtibiale (os/sub″-tib-ē-al′-e) (n.)   An accessory bone of the ankle found near the distal end of the medial malleolus.

Os Supranaviculare (os/su″-pra-nah-vik-ū-lahr′-e) (n.)   An accessory bone of the foot that occurs as a small, triangular ossicle on the dorsum of the talonavicular joint. Also known as the **Dorsal Talonavicular Ossicle**.

Os Sustentaculi (os/sus″-ten-tahk′-ū-lē) (n.)   An accessory bone of the foot that occurs as a small, pyramidal ossicle at the posterior and medial side of the sustentaculum tali.

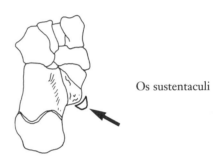

Os sustentaculi

Os Tibiale Externum (os/tib″-ē-ahl′-e/eks-ter′-num) (n.)   An accessory bone of the foot, which is considered a sesamoid bone in the tendon of the tibialis posterior muscle near the point of its insertion. It may fuse to the navicular tuberosity. It may be bipartite and is often bilateral. The bone can also be described as an accessory or secondary navicular or scaphoid. Also called the **Os Tibiale Posterius** or **Os Tibiale Posticum**.

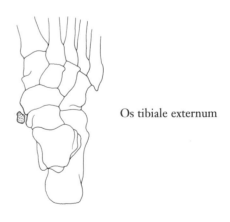

Os tibiale externum

Os Tibiale Posterius (os/tib″-ē-ahl′-e/pōst-ē-rē-us) (n.)   See **Os Tibiale Externum**.

Os Trigonum (os/trī-gōn-um) (n.)   An accessory bone present variably and independently in the tarsus. It usually comprises the posterior talar process. In this process, the flexor hallucis longus tendon passes in the groove of the os trigonum. The posterior tibiotalar and talofibular ligaments, the posterior part of the ankle, and the subtalar capsule then attach to the process. It may be bipartite and often bilateral. Also known as the **Secondary** or **Accessory talus**, or the **Os Intermedium Tarsi**.

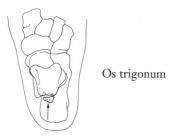

Os trigonum

Os Vesalianum (os/ves-al′-ē-ānum) (n.) An accessory bone of the foot located proximal to the base of the fifth metatarsal.

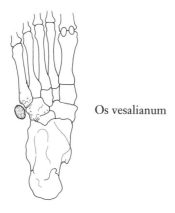

Os vesalianum

Oscilloscope (o-sil′ō-skōp) (n.) An instrument that displays the electrical variations of the fluorescent screen of a cathode-ray tube.

Osgood-Schlatter Disease (oz′gud-shlat′er/di-zēz) (n.) A form of apophysitis that affects the tibial tubercle apophysis. It is usually a self-limiting condition of males between 10 and 16 years of age. It presents with localized pain and tenderness over the tibial tubercle. Lateral radiographs may show irregularity and fragmentation of the apophysis. In some rare instances, an enlarged tibial tubercle or accessory ossicle in the patellar tendon will remain even after skeletal maturity.

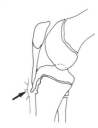

Osgood-Schlatters′ disease

OSHA Abbreviation for Occupational Safety and Health Administration.

Osis (ōs′is) A suffix meaning "condition of."

Osler's Nodes (ōs′lerz/nōdz) (n.) Subcutaneous papules that are pathognomonic of subacute bacterial endocarditis. They are purplish or erythematous areas that are raised, swollen, and tender. They commonly occur in the pads of the fingers or toes, in the palm of the hand, or on the soles of the feet.

Osmolality (oz″mō-lal′i-tē) (n.) The concentration in a solution of solute per kilogram of solvent.

Osmolarity (os-mō-lar′i-tē) (n.) The concentration in a solution of solute per liter of solution.

Osmosis (oz-mō′sis) (n.) The process in which a solvent migrates from an area of lesser concentration of particles to an area of higher concentration while passing through a semipermeable membrane. The migration continues until concentrations are equal on both sides.

Osmotic Pressure (oz-mot′ik/presh′ur) (n.) The pressure that develops when two solutions of different concentrations are separated by a permeable membrane.

Osseous (os′ē-us) (adj.) Being composed of, having the quality of, or resembling bone; bony.

Ossification (os″si-fi′kā′shun) (n.) The formation of or conversion into bone or a bony structure.

Ossifying Fibroma (os″si-fī″ing/fi-brō′mah) (n.) A benign bone tumor that may be locally aggressive. It is most commonly found in the jaw bones, but rarely in long bones. The tibia is the most commonly affected long bone. Radiographically, the lesion is osteolytic and often extensive, involving the diaphysis or metaphysis. Histologically, irregular spicules of trabecular bone are interspersed in a spindle cell that contains collagenous stroma; these spicules are characteristically lined with osteoblasts and a rim of lamellar bone. Also known as **Osteofibrous Dysplasia**, **Osteogenic Fibroma**, or **Fibrous Osteoma**.

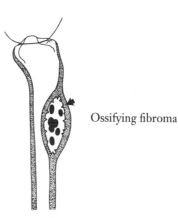

Ossifying fibroma

Osteo, Ost, Oste (os′tē-ō) Prefixes meaning bone.

Ostealgia (os″tē-al′je-ah) (n.) A pain in the bones. Synonym: **Osteodynia**.

Osteitis (os″te-ī′tis) (n.) Bone inflammation.

Osteitis Condensans Ilii (os″tē-ī′tis/kon-dens′sans/il′e-ī) (n.) An inflammatory, often painless disease of unknown etiology that affects the ilium at a point adjacent to the sacroiliac joints. Patients with this disease may present with bilateral lower back pain and tenderness in the area adjacent to the sacroiliac joints. Radiographically, sclerosis is seen in this area of the pelvis.

Osteitis Deformans (os″tē-ī′tis/de-for′mans) (n.) See **Paget's Disease**.

Osteitis Fibrosa Cystica (os″tē-ī′tis/fib-rō′-za/sis-ti-ka) (n.) Bony abnormalities seen in primary or secondary hyperparathyroidism. On radiograph, there may be diffuse osteopenia or well-circumscribed lucent areas. Common sites of resorption are the phalangeal tufts, symphysis pubis, distal clavicles, and vertebral body end-plates. Histologically, there is tunneling resorption, increased woven bone, and marrow fibrosis. Also known as **Von Recklinghausen Disease of Bone**.

Osteitis Fragilitans (os″tē-ī′tis/frah-jil′i-tans) (n.) See **Osteogenesis Imperfecta**.

Osteitis Pubis (os″tē-ī′tis/pū′bis) (n.) An inflammatory condition of unknown etiology that affects the pubic symphysis. The patient usually presents with pain localized over the pubic symphysis; this pain is exacerbated by any activity, especially walking. The pain may also be associated with fever and malaise. Radiographically, sclerosis and rarefaction are noted, and ankylosis of the symphysis may be seen at a later stage. This condition often accompanies genitourinary tract infections, pregnancy, and/or degenerative or rheumatoid arthritis; it can also accompany postpelvic or abdominal surgery. True infections, or osteomyelitis, should be differentiated. One may need to do a needle aspiration and culture for diagnosis.

Osteoarthritis (os″tē-ō-ar-thrī′tis) (n.) A common,

progressive joint disorder characterized by a deterioration of the articular cartilage and reactive new bone formation in the subchondral and juxtaarticular regions. Although the name implies an inflammation, this process is probably not primarily inflammatory; therefore, it can more accurately be called degenerative joint disease. This condition may be a primary one of unclear pathogenesis or a secondary osteoarthritis that may occur post-traumatically. It also may occur as a sequela of bony dysplasia or other arthrides. Also known as **Degenerative Joint Disease**, **Hypertrophic Arthritis**, **Arthritis**, or **Osteoarthrosis**. Abbreviated **OA**.

Osteoarthropathy (os″tē-ō-ar-throp′ah-thē) (n.) A disorder affecting bones and joints in which the new formation of periosteal and periarticular bone causes severe pain and arthritis. An example of this is hypertrophic pulmonary osteoarthropathy.

Osteoarthrosis (os″tē-ō-ar-thrō′sis) (n.) A noninflammatory bone disease. Compare to **Osteoarthritis**.

Osteoblast (os′tē-ō-blast″) (n.) The basic cell that forms all bones; its precursor is unknown. It is approximately 7 microns in diameter and contains a single eccentric nucleus. For these cells to become osteocytes, a scaffolding is required onto which they synthesize bone matrix, or osteoid. They then develop into osteocytes when they become trapped in the mineralized matrix they have generated.

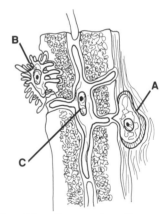

A, Osteoblast; **B**, osteoclast; **C**, osteocyte.

Osteoblastic (os″tē-ō-blas-tik) (adj.) A kind of bone-producing process that occurs in response to metabolic phenomena, tumor, or inflammation. Roentgenographically, osteoblastic activity produces an area of increased bone density.

Osteoblastoma (os″tē-ō-blas-tō′mah) (n.) A benign, osteoid, and bone-forming tumor that has a vascular stroma. It occurs most often in the vertebrae or in the metaphysis or diaphysis of long bones. Radiographically, it is usually a well-defined, lucent defect with some central radiodensity. Microscopically, it is

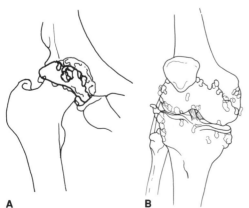

A, Osteoarthritis; **B**, degenerative osteoarthritis.

similar to an osteoid osteoma but is usually larger (>2 cm).

Osteocalcin (os″tē-ō-kal-sin) (n.)   One of the major noncollagenous proteins found only in bone.

Osteocartilaginous (os″tē-ō-kar″ti-laj′i-nus) (adj.) Of, pertaining to, or composed of both bone and cartilage.

Osteochondral (os″tē-ō-kon′dral) (adj.)   1. Of or pertaining to bone and cartilage. 2. A term usually used to describe lesions or fractures near or through the articular surface in which the fractured piece of cartilage remains attached to a piece of the underlying subchondral bone.

Osteochondritis (os″te-o-kon-dri′tis) (n.)   Inflmmation of bones and cartilage.

Osteochondritis Dissecans (os″tē-ō-kon-drī′tis/dis-i-kans) (n.)   An osteonecrotic lesion that affects the subchondral bone and the articular cartilage of the joint that lies over it. These lesions occur most commonly in the knee but also occur in the elbow, the ankle, the hip, and the shoulder. The lesions are seen in both juvenile patients and young adults. The prognosis for spontaneous healing is better for patients with open epiphyseal plates. If the lesion does not heal (either spontaneously or through intervention—including surgery), the necrotic bone and cartilage may separate and create a loose body within the joint. Surface irregularities also may result in degenerative joint changes. Diagnosis for this syndrome is suggested by history and is confirmed radiographically. Treatment depends on the extent of articular and weight-bearing surface involvement and the patient's age.

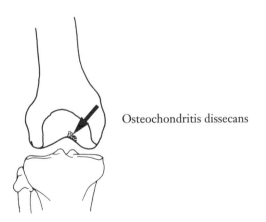

Osteochondritis dissecans

Osteochondrodystrophy   (os″tē-ō-kon″drō-dys′tro-fē) (n.)   See **Morquio's Disease**.

Osteochondroma (os″tē-ō-kon-drō′mah) (n.)   A benign, cartilage-capped bony exostosis that develops on the bone surface. It may be a developmental anomaly that results from growth and endochondral ossification of a cartilage fragment that has separated from the physis (failure of cambrium layer). The le-

sions are juxtaepiphyseal and are usually seen in children or young adults. The presenting symptom is pain or mass effect. The exostosis usually stops growing after the physeal plates close. Also known as **Exostosis**.

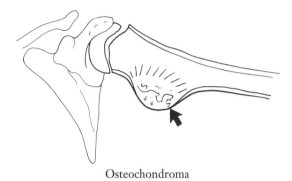

Osteochondroma

Osteochondromatosis (os″tē-ō-kon″drō-mah-tō′sis) (n.)   An inherited condition in which multiple benign exostoses cause shortness of stature and bony deformities. It is inherited as an autosomal dominant condition. Also known as **Hereditary Multiple Exostoses** or **Multiple Osteocartilaginous Exostoses**.

Osteochondritides (os″tē-ō-kon″drid-i-tēz) (n.)   A group of disorders that were formerly believed to share a common pathogenesis. Formerly known as juvenile osteochondroses, these disorders affect the epiphyseal or apophyseal centers in the growing child. Their radiographic appearances—sclerosis and fragmentation of the affected growth center—are similar. Although some of these disorders are due to true osteonecrosis, others probably result from a developmental or post-traumatic abnormality of endochondral ossification. This group of disorders is also known as **Osteochondroses, Epiphysitis**, or **Apophysitis**. See each individual disease. Examples of osteochondroses are true osteonecrosis, such as Legg-Calvé-Perthes disease, Freiberg infraction, osteochondritis dissecans, and Panner disease, and others, such as Osgood-Schlatter disease, Scheurmann disease, Kohler disease, Blount disease, and Sever disease.

Osteochondrosis (os″tē-ō-kon-drō′sis) (n.)   See **Osteochondritis**.

Osteoclasis (os″-tē-ō-klā-sis) (n.)   The deliberate fracturing of a bone to correct a deformity.

Osteoclast (os′tē-ō-klast″) (n.)   A large, multinucleated bone cell that reabsorbs mineralized bone matrix. The osteoclast has a distinctive structure intimately related to its function. Characteristically, it has a plasma membrane specialization, a ruffled border next to the resorptive surface, a high concentration of mitochondria, and many primary and secondary lysosomal vesicles that contain high concentrations of lysosomal enzymes. It is believed that the osteoclast derives from circulating marrow cells in the monocyte-macrophage cell line.

Osteoclastoma (os″tē-ō-klas-tō′mah) (n.) See **Giant Cell Tumor of Bones**.

Osteocyte (os″tē-ō-sīt″) (n.) A mature bone cell derived from an osteoblast. It is found in a lacuna embedded within the mineralized bone matrix; it communicates with other osteocytes through canaliculi or the cellular processes contained within a network of canals.

Osteodynia (os″tē-ō-dīn′ē-ah) (n.) A pain in a bone. Synonym: **Ostealgia**.

Osteodystrophy (os″tē-ō-dis′trō-fē) (n.) Any generalized bone disease that results in abnormal bone development caused by a metabolic disorder. See specific diseases.

Osteofibrous Dysplasia (os″tē-ō-fi′brus/dis-plā′se-ah) (n.) See **Ossifying Fibroma**.

Osteogen (os′tē-ō-jen″) (n.) The inner layer of the periosteum from which bone may be formed.

Osteogenesis (os′tē-ō-jen′e-sis) (n.) The formation, development, and growth of bone.

Osteogenesis Imperfecta (os′tē-ō-jen′e-sis/im-per″fek-tah) (n.) A genetically heterogeneous family of heritable disorders of collagen synthesis. It is characterized by unusually brittle and fragile bones, short stature, scoliosis, impaired dentinogenesis, hypermobility of joints, and blue sclerae. The bones are fragile and osteopenic, have thin cortices, and contain a decreased amount of cancellous elements. Their clinical and radiographic features and their pattern of inheritance are variable. The classification of Sillence is commonly used to categorize affected patients.

Type	Inheritance	Clinical Features
I	Autosomal Dominant	Mild form; bone fractures start after birth: characteristics include bone fragility and blue sclerae.
II	Autosomal Recessive	Lethal in perinatal period. Deformities include fractured bones, beaded ribs, and concertina femora.
III	Autosomal Recessive	Characteristics include severe bone fragility, fractures at birth with progressive deformity. Sclerae are normal.
IV	Autosomal Dominant	Characteristics include bone fragility, with normal sclerae and hearing. The two types of autosomal dominant are: a. Without dentinogenesis imperfecta b. With dentinogenesis imperfecta

Osteogenic (os″tē-ō-jen′ik) (adj.) Derived from or composed of any tissue involved in bone growth or repair.

Osteogenic Sarcoma (os″tē-ō-jen′ik/sar-kō′mah) (n.) A malignant, bone-forming neoplasm in which the bone cells themselves are malignant. Classically, it occurs in children in the second decade, most often at the ends of long bones. It may occur secondary to irradiation or to a pre-existing bone disease, such as Paget's disease. Patients usually present with pain and a mass. Radiographically, the lesions are metaphyseal, a mixture of sclerosis and lysis, and contain significant periosteal new bone formation. Variations in location, such as periosteal tumors, as well as variable cell types, such as telangiectatic osteosarcoma, also occur. Treatment depends on staging; it includes surgery for local control, resection of a limited number of pulmonary metastases, and adjuvant chemotherapy.

Osteogenic Scoliosis (os″tē-ō-jen′ik/skō″le-ō′sis) (n.) An acquired or congenital spinal curvature resulting from an abnormality of the vertebral elements and/or adjacent ribs.

Osteogenic Tumor (os″tē-ō-jen′ik/tū′mor) (n.) Benign or malignant cells that can differentiate into and form bone.

Osteoinduction (os″tē-ō-in-duk′shun) (n.) A process of differentiation of fibroblastlike migratory mesenchymal cells into osteoprogenitor cells. This occurs on calcified tissue matrices.

Osteokinematic Movement (os″tē-ō-kin″e-mat′ik/mo͞ov′ment) (n.) Movement that occurs between two bones. Types of osteokinematic movement include spin, swing, and rotation.

Osteolysis (os″tē-ōl′ī-sis) (n.) The dissolution or loss of bone.

Osteolytic (os″tē-ō-lit′ik) (adj.) A bone destructive process in response to metabolic phenomena, tumors, or inflammation that causes a decreased density of bone.

Osteomalacia (os″tē-ō′mah-la′she-ah) (n.) A disorder in which the protein matrix of bone is inadequately mineralized. Looser's zones are a pathognomonic finding. Histologically, the amount of nonmineralized matrix lining the bone trabeculae and Haversian canals is increased. The serum chemical abnormalities differ with etiology, as does treatment. This disorder is known as rickets when it occurs in a child with a growing skeleton.

Osteoid (os′tē-oid) 1. (n.) The organic matrix formed by the osteoblast that becomes bone when mineralized. 2. (adj.) Of or resembling bone.

Osteoid Osteoma (os′tē-oid/os″tē-ō′mah) (n.) A small, localized, benign bone tumor that usually occurs in the second decade of life. Characteristics include pain of gradually increasing severity, night pain, and pain that is relieved by salicylates. These tumors occur most often in the posterior elements of the vertebral column or the ends of long bones.

They usually arise in membranous bones and present as a painless, slowly enlarging lump. Histologically, these lesions are described as compact (or ivory) or trabecular (or spongy). Roentgenographic findings include a small, relatively radiolucent central zone called a "nidus" (<2 cm) surrounded by bone sclerosis. Histologically, the tumor consists of a network of osteoid trabeculae in a relatively cellular vascular stroma. It is treated successfully with excisional biopsy.

Osteoma (os″tē-ōmah) (n.) A rare, benign tumor composed of compact bone.

Osteomalacia (os″tē-ō-mah-lā′shē-ah) (n.) A disturbance in the metabolism of calcium and phosphorus that results in impaired and decreased mineralization of osteoid (increased osteoid; prolonged mineralization rate, slurred mineralization front). A variety of underlying disorders may result in osteomalacia, including a nutritional deficiency of vitamin D and other vitamin D disturbances, renal disorders, and congenital errors in metabolism. Patients generally present with diffuse bone pain, generalized weakness, and malaise. Radiographically, diffuse osteopenia is seen as noted or angular deformities on long-standing disease.

Osteomyelitis (os″tē-ō-mi″e-lī′tis) (n.) Any infectious process involving bone.

Osteon (os′tē-on) (n.) The basic structural unit of compact bone. An osteon is composed of a Haversian canal and its concentrically arranged lamellae.

Osteonecrosis (os″tē-ō-ne-krō′sis) (n.) The death or necrosis of a bone.

Osteonectin (os″tē-ō-nek-tin) (n.) One of the major noncollagenous proteins unique to bone.

Osteoneuralgia (os′tē-ō-nū-ral′je-ah) (n.) Bone pain.

Osteopath (os′tē-ō-path) (n.) A practitioner of osteopathy.

Osteopathia Condensans Disseminata (os″tē-ō-path′e-ah/kon-den′sanz/dis-sem-i-na′ta) (n.) See **Osteopoikilosis**.

Osteopathia Fibrosa Generalisata (os″tē-ō-path′e-ah/fib-rō′-sa/gen-er-al-i-sa′ta) (n.) See **Von Recklinghausen's Osteitis**.

Osteopathia Hyperostotica Congentia (os″te-o-path′e-ah / hī″-per-ōs-stot′-i-ka / kon-gent-sia) (n.) See **Melorheostosis**.

Osteopathia Striata (os″te-o-path′e-ah/stri-ata) (n.) See **Voorhoeve's Disease**.

Osteopathology (os″te-o-pah-thol′ō-jē) (n.) Any bone disease.

Osteopathy (os″te-op′ah-thē) (n.) A system of medical care with a philosophy that combines the needs of the patient with current practices of medicine, surgery, and obstetrics; an emphasis on the interrelationship between structure and function; and an appreciation of the body's ability to heal itself. See **Osteopath**.

Osteopenia (os″tē-ō-pē′ni-ah) (n.) 1. Any state in which bone mass is reduced below normal. 2. Radiographic finding of decreased bone density.

Osteoperiosteal (os″tē-ō-per″i-os′tē-al) (adj.) Of or pertaining to bone and its periosteum.

Osteoperiostitis (os″tē-ō-per″i-os-tī′tis) (n.) 1. Inflammation of a bone and its periosteum. 2. A disorder in which areas of ossification develop in granulation tissue or they hemorrhage beneath a raised periosteum.

Osteopetrosis (os″tē-ō-pe-trō′sis) (n.) A rare hereditary disease characterized by an increased density of bones. It appears to result from impaired osteoclast function. Radiographically, one sees increased opacity with loss of cortical-medullary differentiation as well as a widening of the diaphysis and metaphysis resulting in an Erlenmeyer flask deformity. Increased brittleness can result in multiple fractures, and loss of marrow space can cause anemia. A severe form of the disease is probably inherited as an autosomal recessive trait; this form results in death in utero or in early childhood. The more moderate form is probably inherited as an autosomal dominant trait. Bone marrow transplantation has recently been used for treatment. Also known as **Albers-Schonberg Disease**.

Osteophage (os′te-ō-fāj) (n.) An osteoclast.

Osteophony (os″te-of′o-nē) (n.) The conduction or transmission of sound through bones.

Osteophyte (os′te-o-fīt″) (n.) A projection or outgrowth of bone. This usually refers to a bony spur in the juxtaarticular regions of arthritic joints. See **Syndesmophytes**.

Osteoplasty (os′tē-ō-plas″tē) (n.) The general term for restorative, reparative, or plastic surgery of the bones.

Osteopoikilosis (os″te-o-poi″kĭ-lo′sis) (n.) A rare, benign bone disease that is inherited and transmitted as an autosomal dominant disorder. It is characterized by many focal sclerotic densities in the epiphyses and metaphyses of the bones; radiographically, these result in a spotted and stippled appearance. Because the disorder is symptomless, it is usually discovered by chance on an x-ray. Also known as **Spotted Bone Disease** or **Osteopathia Condensans Disseminata**.

Osteoporosis (os″te-ō-po-ro′sis) (n.) A common bone disorder characterized by decreased density of normally mineralized osteoid. The etiology includes involutional osteoporosis, known as Type I (or postmenopausal), and Type II (or age-related). Osteoporosis can also have less common causes, e.g., a secondary symptom to disuse, drugs, dietary deficiencies, chronic illness, neoplasm, endocrine abnormalities, genetic disorders, and idiopathic problems found in adolescents and middle-aged males. It is characterized by bone fragility (vertebral fractures, hip fractures, and Colles' fractures).

Osteoporosis Circumscripta (os″te-o-po-ro′sis/ser″kum-skrip′ta) (n.) An early form of Paget disease of the skull that creates a confluent, map-like demineralization and resorption of bone. This gives a striking radiolucent appearance.

Osteoradionecrosis (os″te-o-ra″dē-ō-ne-krō′sis) (n.) Bone necrosis caused by excessive exposure to radiation.

Osteorrhaphy (os″te-or′ah-fē) (n.) The fixing of bone fragments with sutures or wires. This procedure is also called **Osteosuture**.

Osteosarcoma (os″te-o-sar-kō′mah) (n.) See **Osteogenic Sarcoma**.

Osteosclerosis (os″te-o-skle-rō′sis) (n.) An abnormally increased density or hardening of bone that may occur as a result of numerous pathologic states. For example, osteosclerosis is seen in osteopetrosis.

Osteosclerosis Congenita (os″te-o-skle-rō′sis/konjen′i-ta) (n.) See **Achondroplasia**.

Osteosis (os″tē-ō′sis) (n.) The formation of bony tissue.

Osteostixis (os″te-o-stik′-sis) (n.) The surgical puncture of a bone.

Osteosuture (os′te-o-su-tūr) (n.) See **Osteorrhaphy**.

Osteosynthesis (os″te-o-sin′the-sis) (n.) The surgical fixation of fractured bone fragments.

Osteotome (os′te-o-tōm″) (n.) A chisel-like surgical instrument used primarily to cut or shape bone. These instruments may be straight or curved.

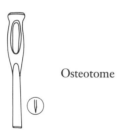

Osteotome

Osteotomy (os″te-ot′o-me) (n.) Any surgical procedure in which bone is transected or cut. The procedures are used to correct rotational or angular deformities by allowing the bone ends to heal in a realigned position.

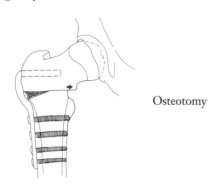

Osteotomy

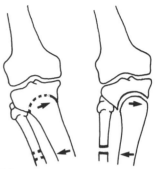

Maquet osteotomy procedure

Osterreicher-Fong Syndrome (ost-rī-ker-fawng/sin′drōm) (n.) See **Nail-Patella Syndrome**.

Otto Pelvis (ot′ō/pel′vis) (n.) An intrapelvic protrusion of the acetabulum that occurs bilaterally. It is determined on an AP radiograph of the pelvis. Also known as **Acetabulum Protrusion, Arthrokatadysis**.

Outerbridge's Ridge (out′-er-brij-ez/rij) (n.) A sign present in chondromalacia patellae. In a normal knee, a minor ridge of varying height crosses the medial femoral condyle at the osteochondral junction. If chondromalacia patellae is present, this ridge, known as Outerbridge's ridge, is composed of a horizontal rim of cartilage, covered bone that lies along the anterior and proximal osteocartilaginous junction of the medial femoral condyle.

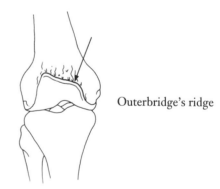

Outerbridge's ridge

Outflare (owt′flār) (n.) In shoe terminology to indicate a swinging out of the forepart of a shoe.

Outpatient Service (owt′pā-shent/ser′vis) (n.) A term used for hospital-provided health services in which the treatment given to patients does not require hospital admission.

Overbone (ō′ver-bōn) (n.) A bony prominence that lies over the dorsum of the foot; it is commonly seen with a high longitudinal and low transverse arch.

Overexposure (ō′ver-ek-spōz′ur) (n.) A term used in radiology to describe an x-ray film that has been subjected to increased exposure time. This results in a significantly lightened radiograph.

Overgrowth (ō'ver-grōth) (n.) Excessive growth of an organ or body part.

Overhead Films (ō'ver-hed/films) (n.) Radiographic films that are made by placing the x-ray tube over the examining table and the film cassette beneath the patient. This is in comparison to spot films, in which a fluoroscopic spot filming device is placed over a specific part of the patient while the x-ray tube is under the examining table.

Overpenetration (ō'ver-pen-e-trā'shun) (n.) A radiologic term indicating excessive kilovoltage. Overpenetration produces a radiograph that is too dense and that lacks contrast.

Over-The-Top (ō'ver/the/top) (n.) A common reference to one position used for sutures that have been placed to repair an anterior cruciate ligament tear or for ligament reconstruction materials that are passed up through the intercondylar notch, then through a hole in the posterior capsule, and finally over the superolateral aspect of the lateral femoral condyle.

Overuse Syndrome (o-ver-ūs/sin'drōm) (n.) A general term applied to disorders that result from repetitive activity and microstresses applied to the musculoskeletal system. This most commonly oc-

curs as a sports or occupationally related disorder. Also known as **Overuse Injury**.

Oxacillin (oks"ah-sil'in) (n.) An oral preparation of a penicillinase-resistant penicillin.

Oxalosis (ok"sah-lō'sis) (n.) A crystal deposition disease in which calcium oxalate crystals are deposited in the connective tissues, which includes the mineralized bone, articular cartilage, and bone marrow. Radiographically, radiodense areas in the metaphyses may be seen. This may occur as a primary, or familial, condition; more commonly, it is secondary to another disorder, such as chronic renal failure.

Oxford Shoe (oks'ford/shoō) (n.) A front-laced, large-heeled shoe that is low to the ground and contains quarters that extend below the malleoli. Named after Oxford University where; in about the year 1715, students changed from high-top shoes to this style of shoe.

Oxidation (ok"se-dā'shun) (n.) A relative loss of electrons in a chemical reaction. Oxidation consists of either the removal of electrons to form an ion or the sharing of electrons with substances that have a greater affinity for them, such as oxygen. Most oxidative reactions, including biologic ones, are associated with the liberation of energy.

Oxyphenbutazone (ok"se-fen-bu'tah-zōn) (n.) A nonsteroidal, antiinflammatory drug.

P

PA (n.) Abbreviation for posteroanterior.

Pachydactyly (pak"ē-dak'ti-lē) (n.) Enlargement of the digits.

Pachyonychia (pak"ē-o-nik'ē-ah) (n.) An abnormal thickening of the nails.

Pacing Gait (pās'ing/gāt) (n.) A walking pattern characterized by slow, measured steps.

Pacinian Corpuscle (pah-sin'ē-an/kor'pus'e) (n.) A pressure-sensitive free sensory nerve ending. Because of its histologic appearance it is also known as a **lamellated corpuscle.**

Pack (pak) (v.) To surround a body part with blankets or wet materials for therapy.

Packing (pak'ing) (n.) Gauze, sponge, or other material used to pack a wound or cavity.

Paget's Disease (paj'ets/di-zēz') Caused by a disturbance in osteoclast and osteoblast activity, this bone disease results in the formation of disorganized bone. Histologically, three phases of this disease are defined. Initially, an osteolytic phase with marked osteoclast activity is seen. This is followed by a phase in which an osteoblastic reaction outweighs the osteoclastic destruction; this results in new bone formation that is disorganized and has a mosaic ap-

pearance and an increased number of cement lines. Finally, a burnt-out phase is seen. Radiographically, the picture varies with the phase of the disease, but an increased radiologic density is most common. The sites of involvement are mostly the lumbar spine, the pelvis, the skull, and the femur. The disease is often seen as an incidental radiographic finding. Symptoms may occur, including bone pain and arthralgias. Complications include stress fractures, arthritis, high output heart failure, and sarcomatous degeneration. Paget disease often leads to varus deformity when the femur or tibia is involved.

Pain (pān) (n.) An unpleasant sensory or emotional experience, associated with actual or potential tissue damage. Pain is always subjective. *Dermatomal* pain is experienced along the cutaneous distribution of a spinal nerve in the limbs and trunk. *Scleratomal* pain is experienced in a region that shares a common embryological origin with the region which is diseased.

Pain Drawing (pān/draw-ing) (n.) A simple screening test used in the initial psychologic evaluation of patients with low back pain. On a standardized drawing of a human form, the patient is asked to indicate location and extent of pain. There is good correlation between the results of this test and the hysteria and hypochondriasis scores on the Minnesota Multiphasic Personality Inventory. Synonyms: **Body Chart, Mooney Body Chart.**

Pain Scale (pān/skāl) (n.) An attempt at a quantitative assessment of the relative amount of pain experienced by an individual patient and the course of such pain during a treatment period. A pain sheet is filled out by an interviewer on the initial treatment day, and the amount of pain suffered by the patient for that day is estimated at 10 points. Thereafter, the patient is asked daily by the interviewer to assess his or her pain quantitatively by comparing it to the pain experienced the day before. The area under the curve is a relative indication of the total amount of pain experienced by the patient during treatment.

Pain Threshold (pān/thresh'old) (n.) The least stimulus intensity at which a subject perceives pain. Variable from subject to subject.

Pain Tolerance Level (pān/tol'er-ans/lev'el) (n.) The greatest stimulus intensity causing pain that a subject is prepared to tolerate.

Painful Arch Syndrome (pān'ful/arch/sin'drōm) (n.) See **Impingement Syndrome.**

Palindromic Rheumatism (pal''in-dro'mic/roo'mah-tizm) (n.) An uncommon type of recurring acute arthritis and periarthritis with sympton-free intervals of from days to months between attacks. Both sexes are equally affected, with the onset usually between the third and sixth decades. Each attach begins suddenly in one or two joints, often in the late afternoon or evening, with pain that may be intense and that reaches a peak within a few hours. Swelling, warmth, and redness over or near the affected joint are noted shortly after the onset of pain. The evidence of inflammation usually disappears in one to three days. The episodes occur irregularly and the extended clinical course is variable.

Palliative (pal'ē-a''tiv) (adj.) Treatment intended to reduce the pain and suffering from a disease without curing the underlying disease process.

Palliative Radiation (pal'ē-a''tiv/ra-dē-ā'shun) (n.) Radiation treatment administered to reduce pain and suffering and possibly to reduce the size of a tumor without hope of a permanent cure. Often used to reduce the chance of local recurrence of tumor after palliative surgical treatment of a pathologic fracture.

Palm (palm) (n.) The volar or anterior surface of the hand; the area between the distal wrist crease and the most proximal digital creases. It is divided into the thenar, the mid-palm, and the hypothenar areas.

Palmar (pal'mar) (adj.) Refers to the volar or anterior side of the hand.

Palmar Fibromatosis (pal'mar/fī''brō-mah-tō'sis) (n.) See **Dupuytren Disease.**

Palmar Spaces (pal'mar/spās'es) (n.) The potential

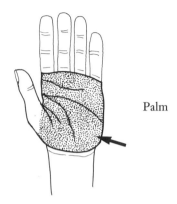

Palm

spaces into which the palm is divided by fascial septa.

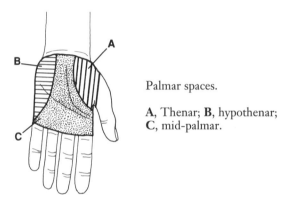

Palmar spaces.

A, Thenar; **B,** hypothenar; **C,** mid-palmar.

Palmaris Brevis Muscle (pal-ma'ris/brev'is/mus'el) (n.) See **Muscle.**

Palmaris Longus Muscle (pal-ma'ris/long'gus/mus'el) (n.) See **Muscle.**

Palpation (pal''pā'shun) (n.) The act and/or process of examining parts of the body by touch.

Palsy (pawl'zē) (n.) Synonymous with paralysis but commonly used to indicate paresis or partial paralysis.

Pan (pan) Prefix indicating all or the entirety.

Panarthritis (pan''ar-thri'tis) (n.) Inflammation of all the joints, or all the structures of a joint.

Pancoast Tumor (pan'kōst/tū'mor) (n.) An apical lung malignancy, usually oat cell tumor, named for an American radiologist. Often causes shoulder pain and hoarseness.

Pandemic (pan-dēm'ik) (n.) A widespread epidemic.

Panner's Disease (pan'erz/di-zēz') (n.) An osteonecrotic osteochondritis of the capitellum of the humerus. Synonyms include: **Capitullum Humeri Epiphyseal Necrosis, Capitullum Humeri Osteochondrosis,** and **Osteochondritis of the Humeral Capitellum.**

Pannus (pan′us) (n.) A vascular granulation tissue composed of proliferating fibroblasts, numerous small blood vessels, and varying numbers of inflammatory cells developing from the vascular synovial membrane of a joint and growing over the joint cartilage. The presence of pannus is characteristic of rheumatoid arthritis.

Pantalar Arthrodesis (pan′tah′lar/ar″thrō′dē′sis) (n.) A surgical fusion of all of the joints surrounding the talus, including the tibiotalar, the subtalar, and the talonavicular. The calcaneocuboid joint is also included in the stabilization, making the procedure a combination of a triple arthrodesis and an ankle fusion.

Pantopaque (pan-tō-pāk′) (n.) The proprietary name for a nonsoluble, highly viscous, iodinated oil used as a radiographic dye in contrast myelography and other diagnostic tests.

Papineau Technique (pap-ē-nō/tek-nēk′) (n.) A surgical procedure for the treatment of varying degrees of bone and soft tissue loss associated with posttraumatic or postoperative infection. The procedure has three stages:

In the first stage, a radical excision of infected and necrotic bone and soft tissue is performed. The resulting wound is packed open until healthy granulation tissue has formed.

In the second stage, the residual cavity is filled in by autogenous cancellous bone grafting. Again, the wound is packed open. Dressing changes are then performed daily, beginning at 5 to 7 days postoperatively and continuing until the graft stabilizes and is covered by granulation tissue.

The third stage consists of soft tissue coverage unless sufficient epithelialization has occurred. Also called **Rhinelander-Papineau Technique**.

Papule (pap′ūl) (n.) A small, solid, elevated skin lesion. Identification of these lesions is based on shape, size, and color variations. The various shapes are rounded, flat, acuminate, or umbilicated.

Paracentesis (par″ah-sen-tē′sis) (n.) The surgical puncture of a cavity for the aspiration of fluid.

Paraffin Bath (par′ah-fin/bath) (n.) A method of applying superficial heat. It is often used in the rehabilitative therapy of arthritic and posttraumatic or postoperative conditions in the hands. The treatment unit consists of a thermal element surrounding a tank filled with a mixture of solid paraffin and mineral oil. When the unit is heated, the paraffin melts and combines with the oil. The unit is then reduced in heat to about 126°F to allow for application of the mixture to the patient.

Parallel Bars (par′ah-lel/barz) (n.) An apparatus used in physical therapy to facilitate a patient's walking after an injury or disease. It consists of two wooden or metal parallel bars that are adjusted to a comfortable height and distance from one another to provide a stable support for the patient while he or she is learning any of the various types of gait.

Paralysis (pah-ral′i-sis) (n.) A complete or partial loss of motor function, in a body part.

Paramedical Personnel (par″ah-med′i-kal/per′sonel′) (n.) Nonphysicians who work in the health field, including but not limited to medical technicians, aides, nutritionists, and physician's assistants.

Paraparesis (par″ah-par′ē′sis) (n.) A partial paralysis affecting both lower extremities.

Paraplegia (par″ah-plē′je-ah) (n.) Paralysis of both lower extremities. The level of trunk and lower extremity paralysis varies according to the spinal level involved. The upper extremities are not involved.

Parapodium (par″ah-pō′dē-um) (n.) A standing frame mounted on a small podium designed to support a paraplegic subject, usually a child. When securely strapped to this frame, the user may be able to progress, either with crutches or by pivoting the whole body along with the device.

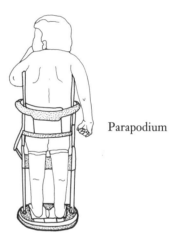

Parapodium

Parasite (par′ah-sīt) (n.) An organism that lives in or on, and at the expense of, another organism, known as the **host.**

Parasympathetic Nervous System (par″ah-sim″pahthet′ik/ner′vus/sis′tem) (n.) A subdivision of the autonomic nervous system, distributed to blood vessels, glands, and the majority of internal organs. Preganglionic nerve fibers are cholinergic and arise in the central nervous system. The autonomic ganglia of this system are usually situated near or in the organs to be innervated. The ganglionic fibers are also cholinergic.

Paratenon (par″ah-ten′on) (n.) The fatty areolar tissue between a tendon and its sheath. It carries vascular supply to the tendon.

Parathormone (par″ah-thor′mōn) (n.) See **Parathyroid Hormone.**

Parathyroid Gland (par″ah-thī′roid/gland) (n.) One of the two pairs of endocrine glands found on the posterior surface of the thyroid gland. It functions in the regulation of extracellular calcium levels by producing parathyroid hormone.

Parathyroid Hormone (par″ah-thī′roid/hor′mōn) (n.) A hormone substance produced by the parathyroid gland. This hormone enhances renal tubular reabsorption of calcium, which decreases urinary calcium excretion and decreases tubular reabsorption of phosphate. It also acts on the kidney indirectly to increase calcium absorption in the gut by increasing the synthesis of 1,25-dihydroxy vitamin D, which is the active form of vitamin D. Finally, it acts on bone to promote reabsorption. Overall, parathyroid hormone thus functions to increase calcium levels in the blood. It is abbreviated PTH. Also known as **Parathormone.**

Paratrooper Fracture (par″ah′troo-per/frak′chur) (n.) A fracture of the distal tibial and fibula shafts.

Paravertebral (par″ah-ver′te-bral) (adj.) Adjacent to a vertebra or the vertebral column.

Paravertebral Line (par″ah-ver′te-bral/līn) (n.) A projected vertical line formed by connecting the tips of the transverse processes of the vertebrae on the AP radiograph of the spine.

Paraxial (par-ak′sē-al) (adj.) Lying on the side of its long axis. An example is the radial portion of the forearm. Used to describe the absent segment of congenital limb loss.

Parenchyma (pah-reng′ki-mah) (n.) The functional part of an organ that is supported by a connective tissue network or stroma.

Parenteral (pah-rent′ter-al) (adj.) The administration of nutrients or drugs into the body by injection, either subcutaneous, intramuscular, or intravenous, or by a route other than through the alimentary canal.

Paresis (pah-rē′sis) (n.) Partial paralysis. Although paresis means a lesser degree of weakness than paralysis, the two words are commonly used interchangeably.

Paresthesia (par″es-thē′ze′ah) (n.) A disturbance of superficial sensation. An abnormal sensation experienced in the absence of specific stimulation, described variously as burning, tingling, creeping, prickling, or "pins and needles."

Parham Band (pahr′am/band) (n.) A wide, flat metallic band that encircles a bone, used in the stabilization of fractures. Bone lysis occurs under the bands.

Parietal Bone (pah-rī′e′tal/bōn) (n.) A large, flat bone that forms the side wall of the skull. It is situated between the frontal and the occipital bones.

Park's Lines (parks/līnz) (n.) See **Harris Growth Arrest Lines.**

Parkinson Disease (par′kin-sun/di-zēz′) (n.) A neurologic disorder of the extrapyramidal cerebral ganglia system. It occurs in middle and late life, with an insidious onset, gradual progression, and a prolonged

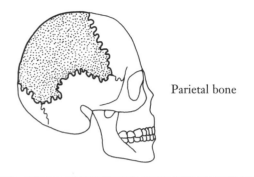

Parietal bone

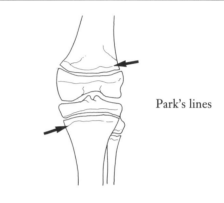

Park's lines

course. It is characterized by a rhythmic tremor, hypokinesia, muscular stiffness, and a festinant gait. Also known as **Paralysis Agitans.**

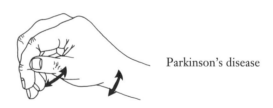

Parkinson's disease

Parkinsonian Gait (par″kin-sōn′e-an/gāt) (n.) A manner of walking associated with Parkinson disease that is characterized by a stooped posture, difficulty initiating the first step, small steps, and shuffling. The upper part of the patient's body tends to stay in front of his or her feet, which results in propulsion or a propensity to run.

Parona's Space (pah-rō′-naz/spās) (n.) An anatomic space in the distal end of the forearm. The space is bounded anteriorly by the deep flexors, posteriorly by the fascia of the pronator quadratus, laterally by the flexor carpi radialis, and medially by the flexor carpi ulnaris. Parona's space can communicate distally with the hand through the carpal canal, but this is normally closed by the contact of the ulnar and the radial bursae. Becomes important in infections of the hand. Also known as **Subtendinous Space.**

Paronychia (par″o-nīk′ē-ah) (n.) A run-around infection involving the folds of tissue surrounding a finger or a toenail. A paronychia usually begins at one corner of the horny nail and travels under the eponychium toward the opposite side. The most common causative organism is *Staphylococcus aureus*.

Parosteal Osteosarcoma (par-os′tē-al/os″te-ō-sarkō′mah) (n.) A histologically low-grade, slow-growing, malignant, bone-forming tumor found on the juxtacortical surface of a bone. The lesion is almost always seen on the posterior cortex of the distal end of the femur. Radiographically, the tumor is a well-circumscribed, radiodense, juxtacortical mass. A lucent line separating the tumor from the cortex may be seen. The prognosis for this lesion is generally better than that of a classic osteosarcoma. Also known as **Juxtacortical Osteogenic Sarcoma.**

Paroxysm (par′ok-sizm) (n.) A sudden attack or recurrence of symptoms of a disease, especially a spasm or convulsion.

Parrot-Beak Tear (n.) A descriptive term for an incomplete radial tear of the meniscus, with posterior or anterior extension toward the periphery of the meniscus. This creates a posteriorly or anteriorly based flap.

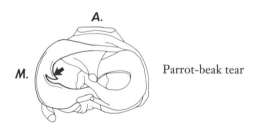

Parrot-beak tear

Pars Interarticularis (parz/in″ter-ar-tik′u-lar″-is) (n.) The part of the posterior arch of a vertebra that lies between the inferior and superior articular facets. See **Spondylolysis** and **Scotty Dog Sign**.

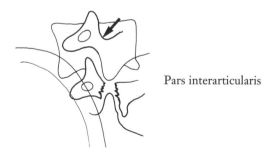

Pars interarticularis

Pars Peronea Metatarsalia Primus (parz/pe-ro′ne-ah/met″ah-tar-sal′e-ah/prī′mus) (n.) An accessory bone of the foot found at the proximal end of the first metatarsal.

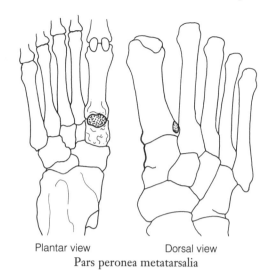

Plantar view   Dorsal view

Pars peronea metatarsalia

Pascal (pas-kal′ or pas′kal) (n.) A unit of measurement of pressure found in the Standard International System. It is expressed as newtons per square meter and abbreviated as **Pa.**

Passive Exercise (pas′iv/ek′ser-sīz) (n.) The moving of parts of the body without the active use of the muscles crossing that segment or joint. It can be self-administered, or it may be administered by a therapist, a machine, or another outside force.

Passive Immunity (pas′iv/i-mu′ni-tē) (n.) Resistance acquired by the transfer of antibodies. This can occur either naturally from the mother or artificially by injection. The resistance is usually temporary and short-lived.

Passive Movement (pas′iv/moov′ment) (n.) A movement of the body or of the extremities performed on a patient by another person or mechanical apparatus without voluntary motion on the part of the patient. See **Continuous Passive Motion.**

Passive Reduction (pas′iv/rēduk′shun) (n.) A form of closed reduction accomplished not with manipulative force but rather by steady traction or the pull of gravity.

Pasteurella (pas″te-rel′ah) (n.) A genus of short gram-negative anaerobic rod-shaped bacteria of the family Brucellae, causing serious infectious diseases. Humans are usually infected with these organisms because of animal contact, e.g., a dog bite.

Patch (pach) (n.) A macule measuring over 1 cm in diameter.

Patch Test (pach/test) (n.) A technique used to test skin for hypersensitivity. The test material is applied via a patch placed on the skin. After a period of exposure, the patch is removed and the skin reaction in this area is compared with the unpatched area surrounding it.

Patella (pah-tel′ah) (n.) 1. The kneecap. 2. A sesamoid bone formed in the quadriceps tendon. Increases the mechanical advantage of the quadriceps muscles across the knee. The undersurface is covered with hyaline cartilage.

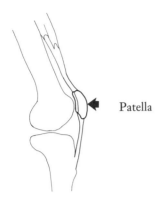

Patella Alta (pah-tel′ah/al-tah) (n.) A high-riding or elevated position of the patella. The position of the patella is evaluated on a lateral radiograph of the knee. The various techniques of measuring this position include Blumensaat's method, the Insall-Salvati method, and the patella index. Compare with **Patella Baja.**

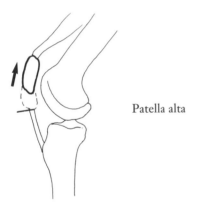

Patella alta

Patella Baja (pah-tel′ah/ba-ha) (n.) A low-riding po-

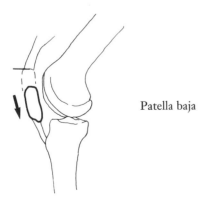

Patella baja

sition of the patella that is evaluated on a lateral radiograph of the knee. It can be measured by the various techniques described for patella alta. Synonym: **Patella Infera.** Compare with **Patella Alta.**

Patella Bursa (pah-tel′ah/ber′sah) (n.) A saclike cavity filled with fluid in various locations around the patella where friction might develop in the tissues. Example: **Pre** and **Suprapatellae Bursae.**

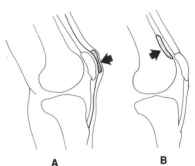

A   **B**

Patella bursa. **A,** Prepatellar bursa; **B,** Suprapatellar bursa

Patella Index (pah-tel′ah/in′deks) (n.) See **Patellar Height, Blackburne and Peel Ratio.**

Patella Infera (pah-tel′ah/in′fer-ah) (n.) See **Patella Baja.**

Patella Femoral Joint (pah-tel′ah/fem′or-al/joynt) (n.) The articulation formed between the femoral groove on the distal femur and the patella.

Patella Femoral Malalignment (pah-tel′ah/fem′or-al/mal″ah-līn′ment) (n.) A disorder in which the patella is too high or laterally subluxated. See **Patella Alta.**

Patella Malalignment Syndrome (pah-tel′ah/mal″ah-līn-ment/sin′drōm) (n.) A disorder characterized by pain in the anterior portion of the knee, often associated with vigorous activity. The pain varies in intensity. The condition is derived from congenital or acquired abnormalities associated with abnormal patellofemoral articulation, deficiencies in the surrounding supporting tissues, or malalignment of the lower extremity.

Patellar Height, Blackburne and Peel Ratio (pah-tel′ar/hīt/blak′burn/and/pēl/ra′she-o) (n.) A technique for measuring patella position on a lateral radiograph of the knee. To calculate, measure the ratio between the perpendicular distance from the lowest articular margin of the patella to the tibial plateau (**A**) and the length of the articular cartilage of the patella (**B**). The normal A/B ratio is 0.80 + 0.14.

Patellar Height, Insall-Salvati Method (pah-tel′ar/hīt in′sla-sol-va-tē′/meth′ud) (n.) A technique for measuring patella position on a lateral radiograph of the knee. The ratio between the length of the patellar tendon, LT, and the length of the patella, LP, is cal-

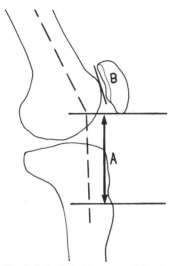

Patellar height, Blackburne and Peel ratio

culated. The accepted normal value of LT:LP is 1.0 + 0.2.

Patellar Lateral Retinaculum (pah-tel′ar/lat′er-al/ ret″i-nak′ū-lum) (n.) A dense ligamentous condensation of capsular tissue on the lateral aspect of the patella, involved in maintaining patellofemoral tracking and stability.

Patellar Ligament (pah-tel′ar/lig′ah-ment) (n.) The central and main portion of the tendon of insertion of the quadriceps femoris muscle, extending from the patella to the tibial tubercle. Also called **Patellar Tendon**.

Patellar Medial Retinaculum (pah-tel′ar/mē′de-al/ ret″i-nak′ū-lum) (n.) A dense ligamentous condensation of capsular tissue on the medial aspect of the patella, involved in maintaining patellofemoral tracking and stability. Balances with lateral retinaculum.

Patellar Reflex (pah-tel′ar/re′fleks) (n.) See **Patellar Tendon Reflex**.

Patellar Retinaculum (pah-tel′ar/ret″i-nak′ū-lum) (n.) The connective tissue fibers that run from the sides of the patella to insert onto the front and sides of the tibial condyles. They are derived from the aponeurotic expansions of the vastus tendons.

Patellar Tendon Bearing (pah-tel′ar/ten′dun/bār-ing) (n.) A design used in plaster cast formation, orthosis production, and lower limb prosthetics that reduces weight transmission through the lower leg. To do this, a specially designed socket or brim allows weight to be supported on the patellar tendon and the tibial flares. Abbreviated **PTB**. See **Sarmiento Cast**.

Patellar Tendonitis (pah-tel′ar/ten″do-ni′tis) (n.) A chronic overload lesion near the insertion of the patellar tendon, especially common in athletes involved in repetitive activity.

Patellar Tendon Reflex (pah-tel′ar/ten′dun/rē′fleks) (n.) The so-called "knee jerk." When the patellar tendon is tapped, it causes a reflex contraction of the quadriceps muscles, so that the leg kicks outward. The reflex arc involves the fourth lumbar nerve root.

Patellar Tilt (pah-tel′ar/til-t) (n.) Refers to the angle of the patella in the horizontal plane with the femur at the beginning of the knee extension, and is a measure of lateral tightness and lateral subluxation.

Patellectomy (pat″e-lek′to-mē) (n.) A surgical procedure in which all or part of the patella is excised.

Pathogen (path′ō-jen) (n.) Any virus, microorganism, or substance that causes disease.

Pathological Calcification (path″o-loj′ĭ-kal/kal″sĭ-fĭ-ka′shun) (n.) A process of calcification that takes place in tissues other than the skeletal structures and teeth. Also called **Dystrophic** or **Metastatic Calcification**.

Pathologic Fracture (path″ō-loj′ik/frak′chur) (n.) A break that occurs in a bone with a preexisting disease that weakens the bone, such as tumor or metabolic bone disease, including osteoporosis. Classically, these will present after minor trauma and often result in unusual fracture patterns, such as transverse subtrochanteric femur fractures.

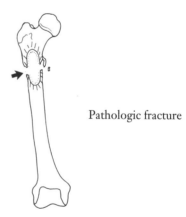

Pathologic fracture

Patient Controlled Analgesia (pa′shent/kon-trōl′d/ an′al-jē′ze-ah) (n.) A method of delivering analgesia in premeasured doses as needed by the patient. The delivery systems include intravenous and epidural routes. Abbreviated **PCA**.

Patrick's Sign (pat′riks/sīn) (n.) A maneuver used in evaluation of disorders of the hip joint. The heel of the affected side is placed on the opposite knee, and the thigh is pressed downward, illiciting pain in the groin with hip disease. See **Fabere Sign**.

Pauwel's Classification (paw′elz/klas″sĭ-fĭ-ka′shun) (n.) A classification of femoral neck fractures that divides them into three types based on the angle of inclination of the fracture line across the neck. Types I, II, III designate the angle of the fracture. Synonym: **Pauwel's Angles**.

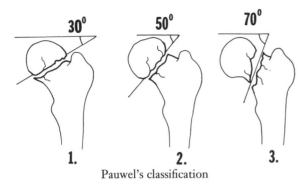

Pauwel's classification

Pauwel Y Osteotomy (paw'el/y/os"te-ot'o-me) (n.) A surgical procedure in the treatment of congenital dislocation of the hip.

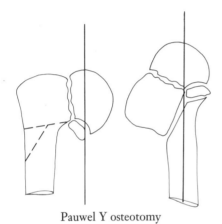

Pauwel Y osteotomy

Pavlik Harness (pahv'lik/har'nes) (n.) A method used in the treatment of a congenitally dislocated or dislocatable hip in the newborn. The harness consists of a chest strap, two shoulder straps, and two stirrups, each with an anteromedial flexion strap and a posterolateral abduction strap. The harness serves as a check rein to maintain the hips in flexion and limit adduction.

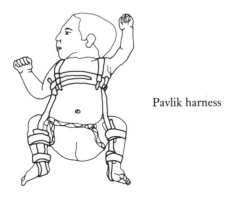

Pavlik harness

PCA 1. Joint replacement systems whose name is derived from their being porous-coated arthroplasties. The components are made of cobalt-chromium alloy and have a porous coating on their nonarticular surfaces and proximal femoral stems; this allows for either cement or bone–ingrowth fixation. These systems are a trademark of Howmedica, Inc. 2. Abbreviation for **Patient Controlled Analgesia**.

PE (n.) Abbreviation for Pulmonary Embolism.

Pearson Traction Attachment (pēr-son/trak'shun/ah-tach'ment) (n.) A metallic frame with a hinge attached to a Thomas splint, to allow knee flexion while in balanced suspension traction for femoral fractures. May be used as a passive knee exerciser.

Pectineal (pek-tin'e-al) (adj.) Of or pertaining to the pubic bone.

Pectineal Ligament (pek-tin'e-al/lig'ah-ment) (n.) A ligament attached to the pubic bone. A triangular expansion from the medial part of the inguinal ligament, attached to the pectineal line of the pubic bone.

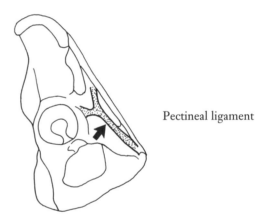

Pectineal ligament

Pectoral Girdle (pek'to-ral/ger'd'l) (n.) The shoulder girdle.

Pectus (pek'tus) (n.) The thorax, chest, or breast.

Pectus Carinatum (pek'tus/kar"i-na-tum) (n.) A congenital anomaly in which the sternum is abnormally prominent, projecting anteriorly in a sharp angle. The anterior posterior diameter of the chest is increased. Synonym: **Pigeon Breast**.

Pectus Excavatum (pek'tus/eks'kah-vā'tum) (n.) A congenital anomaly of the anterior chest wall characterized by a groove or funnel-shaped depression in the sternum. Synonym: **Funnel Chest**.

Pedicle (ped'ĭ-k'l) (n.) 1. A slender stalk or stemlike process, as in the pedicle of a tumor. 2. A bony process projecting backward from the body of a vertebra, which connects with the lamina on either side.

Pedicle Erosion (ped'ĭ-k'l/e'-ro'zhun) A thinning, demineralization, or disappearance of a pedicle visible on plain AP radiographs of a vertebra.

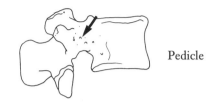

Pedicle

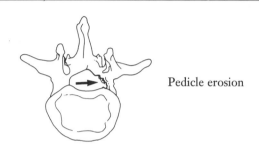

Pedicle erosion

Pedicle Flap (ped'ĭ-k'l/flap) (n.) A type of flap that obtains its blood supply through a narrow base or pedicle. Tissues remain attached at one or both ends of the donor site during transfer to the recipient site. The vascular supply is maintained from the vessels preserved in the pedicle.

Pedicle Migration (ped'i-k'l/mi-gra'shun) The de-

gree of vertebral body rotation is based on the position of the convex pedicle in relationship to the vertebral body, as determined on a standardized AP or PA radiation of a patient with scoliosis. There are five positions:

1. 0 to ¼ of the vertebral body — 0 degrees of rotation
2. ¼ of the vertebral body — 0 to 25 degrees of rotation
3. ¼ to ½ of the vertebral body — 25 to 30 degrees of rotation
4. ½ to ¾ of the vertebral body — 50 to 75 degrees of rotation
5. ¾ to complete — 75 to 100 degrees of rotation

See **Nash-Moe Method**.

Pelkan Spur (pel'kam/spur) (n.) A radiographic sign of scurvy in which a small bony spur protrudes from the lateral border of the epiphyseal line at the junction with the metaphysis.

Pelligrini-Stieda's Disease (pel″a-grē'nē/stē'dahz/di-zēz') (n.) A radiographic finding of heterotopic calcification in the medial collateral ligament of the knee. It usually occurs posttraumatically and may be an incidental finding or symptomatic.

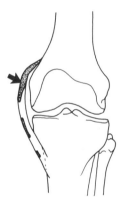

Pelligrini-Stieda's disease

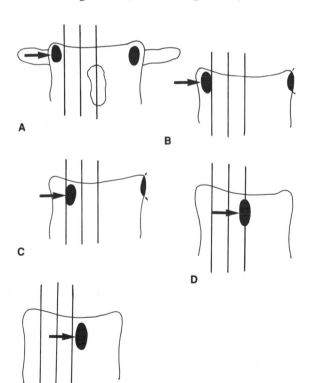

A, B, C, D, E

Pedicle method: *A*, neutral; *B*, grade 1; *C*, grade 2; *D*, grade 3; *E*, grade 4.

Pelvic (pel'vik) (adj.) Of or pertaining to the pelvis.

Pelvic Belt (pel'vik/belt) (n.) A belt that encircles the pelvis and is attached to a lower limb brace or prosthesis.

Pelvic Inlet (pel'vik/in'let) (n.) The superior opening of the pelvis.

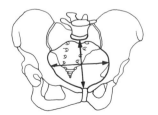

Pelvic inlet

Pelvic Inlet Index (pel'vik/in'let/in'deks) (n.) A radiographic measurement of the pelvis. It is the ratio of the sagittal diameter, or the pelvic inlet, to the transverse diameter.

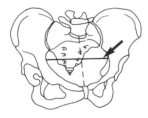

Pelvic inlet index

Pelvic Obliquity (pel'vik/ob-lik'wi-te) (n.) The deviation of the pelvis from the horizontal in the frontal plane. Frequently seen with leg length inequality. The obliquity may be fixed or mobile.

Pelvic Outlet (pel'vik/out'let) (n.) The inferior opening of the pelvis.

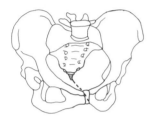

Pelvic outlet

Pelvic Sling (pel'vik/sling) (n.) A type of supportive bandage used in the closed treatment of pelvic fractures. It provides compression across the pelvic ring and thus reduces an open book–type of pelvic fracture or a pubic symphysis diastasis.

Pelvic Traction (pel'vik/trak'shun) (n.) A form of skin traction that provides traction through the lumbosacral spine region and reduces lumbar lordosis. It is used in the management of patients with lumbosacral disc disease.

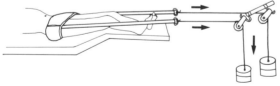

Pelvic traction

Pelvimetry (pel-vim'ĕ-tre) (n.) The radiographic measurement of the dimensions of the bony pelvis, including size, capacity, and diameter.

Pelvis (pel'vis) (n.) The bony basin-shaped ring that provides the weight-bearing for the trunk and lower extremities while protecting the lower abdominal viscera. It consists of two innominate bones that articulate posteriorly with the sacrum. Distally, the pelvis articulates with the proximal end of the fe-

murs at the acetabuli. The pelvic ring is joined posteriorly by the sacroiliac joint and anteriorly by the symphysis pubis.

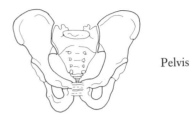

Pelvis

Pemberton Osteotomy (pem'-ber-ton/os-tē-ot-ō-mē) (n.) A type of acetabuloplasty that consists of a pericapsular osteotomy of the ilium. The osteotomy is made through the full thickness of the ilium. The acetabular roof then is rotated anteriorly and laterally, using the triradiate cartilage as the hinge. This osteotomy is used in hip dysplasia and dislocation in which reduction is attained before or at the time of the osteotomy.

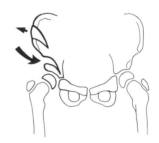

Pemberton osteotomy

PEMFs Abbreviation for Pulsating Electromagnetic Fields.

Pendulum Exercises (pen'du-lum/ek'ser-sizes) (n.) Shoulder exercises using gravity to assist the arm in swinging to achieve a range of shoulder motion.

Penetrating Fracture (pen'ĕ-trāt-ing/frak'chur) (n.) A term used to indicate the type of bone injury that results from penetration of a sharp object such as a bullet or perforation by a sharp piece of metal.

Penicillins (pen"i-sil'inz) (n.) A group of natural or synthetic variants of penicillium, an antibiotic substance that is especially active against many aerobic and anaerobic gram-positive organisms.

Pennate (pen'āt) (adj.) Featherlike; certain muscles have this structure. An example is the lateral portion of the deltoid.

Penrose Drain (pen'rōz/drān) (n.) A thin-walled cylinder of radiopaque latex, used to drain purulent material or fluids from a wound. Also called **Cigarette Drain**.

Per Primam (per pri'mam) (adj.) Healing by first intention. Healing of a wound without the intervention of granulations.

Percutaneous (per″ku-ta′ne-us) (adj.) Used in describing surgical procedures performed without a formal incision; literally, this means "through the skin." An example of this is the placement of percutaneous pins for fracture fixation after a closed reduction.

Percutaneous Discectomy (per″ku-ta′ne-us/dis-kek′to-me) (n.) Removal of disk material through a tube inserted into the disk space via a posterior lateral skin puncture approach.

Perianal Sensation (per″e-ā′nal/sen-sā′shun) (n.) The sensation in the cutaneous regions surrounding the anus provided by the multiple sacral nerve roots. The preservation of sensation in any part of this region is the only indication of an incomplete spinal cord lesion.

Periarteritis Nodosa (per″e-ar″tĕ-ri′tis/no′dōs-a) (n.) A disseminated disease of unknown origin. Characterized by focal inflammatory lesions that chiefly involve medium-sized and small arteries and arterioles. Signs and symptoms occur from infarction and scarring of involved organs and systems. Synonyms: **Polyarteritis**, **Panarteritis**, and **Necrotizing Arteritis**.

Periarticular (per″e-ar-tik′ū-lar) (adj.) Situated around or about a joint.

Perichondrial Ring (per″i-kon′drē-al/ring) (n.) An area of thickened cartilage that forms a fibrocartilaginous ring around the periphery of the epiphyseal plate. It is attached to the groove of Ranvier and to the periosteum at the metaphyseal junction. Believed to play a role in the mechanical integrity of the physis.

Perichondritis (per″i-kon-drī-tis) Inflammation of the perichondrium.

Perichondrium (per″i-kon′drē-um) (n.) The layer of fibrous connective tissue that covers nonarticular cartilage.

Perikaryon (per″i-kar′ē-on) (n.) The cell body of a neuron.

Perimyositis (per″i-mī″ō-sī′tis) (n.) Inflammation of the connective tissue surrounding a muscle.

Perimysium (per″i-mis′ē-um) (n.) The connective tissue enveloping bundles of skeletal muscle fibers.

Perineum (per″i-nē′um) (n.) Area between the root of the thighs extending from the coccyx to the pubis, containing the anus and the external sexual organs.

Perineural (per″i-nū′ral) (adj.) Situated around nervous tissue or a nerve.

Perineurium (per″i-nū′rē-um) (n.) The membrane that forms a sheath around a nerve fascicle, thereby surrounding a collection of axons, their encasing Schwann cells, and the endoneurium.

Periosteal (per″e-os′tē-al) (adj.) Pertaining to or involving the periosteum.

Periosteal Chondroma (per″e-os′tē-al/kon-drō′mah) (n.) A benign cartilaginous lesion that occurs in the cortex of the metaphyses of the tubular bones. Ra-

diographically, the lesion appears as a scalloped cortical defect surrounded by bony sclerosis, often with overhanging edges. Calcification is usually seen. Also known as **Juxtacortical Chondroma**.

Periosteal Desmoid (per″e-os′tē-al/des′moid) (n.) A fibrous lesion seen on the posteromedial surface of the distal femoral metaphysis. Radiographically, this is seen as an irregular area of local bone destruction with a sclerotic base. These are benign lesions that usually present in boys between 10 and 15 years of age. They may be posttraumatic lesions at the insertion of the adductor magnus muscle.

Periosteal Elevator (per″e-os′tē-al/el′e-vā″tor) (n.) A surgical instrument used to strip soft tissue off bone. They come in various sizes and shapes, but all are designed with some type of beveled edge.

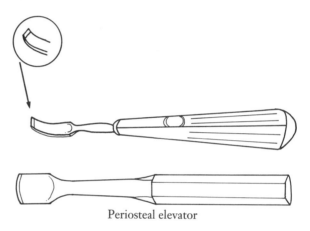

Periosteal elevator

Periosteal Osteosarcoma (per″e-os′tē-al/os″tē-ō-sar-kō′mah) (n.) An uncommon type of osteogenic sarcoma that occurs at the periphery of the bone. On a radiograph, one sees an irregular bone-forming lesion on the surface of the bone along with reactive periosteal new bone. The lesion usually occurs in the second decade, in either the proximal tibia or femoral shaft. Histologically, these tumors tend to be chondroblastic osteogenic sarcomas. Also known as **Peripheral Osteosarcoma**.

Periosteal Reaction (per″e-os′tē-al/rē-ak′shun) (n.) A variety of tissue reactions seen in the periosteum in response to disease in the underlying bone. Usually refers to a linear deposit of new bone by periosteum under elevated periosteum.

Periosteum (per″e-os′tē-um) (n.) A specialized connective tissue membrane that covers bone surfaces except for the points of tendinous and ligamentous attachment and the articular surfaces. The outer layer of the periosteum is dense and vascular. The inner layer is more cellular and contains osteogenic cells, which play a role in the growth of bone width.

Periostitis (per″e-os-tī′tis) (n.) Inflammation of the periosteum.

Peripheral Nerve (pe-rif′er-al/nerv) (n.) A nervous structure that lies outside the central nervous system. The term generally refers to a mixed spinal nerve and its peripheral branches. Each peripheral nerve is composed of a number of axons, each of which is surrounded by a delicate endoneurium. These axons are grouped into fascicles by the perineurium. A denser epineurium encloses groups of fascicles, making the actual mixed spinal or peripheral nerve. Although the cranial nerves are technically "peripheral" nerves, in common usage they are not included in discussions of peripheral nerves and their injuries and repair.

Peripheral Nervous System (pe-rif′er-al/ner′vus/sis′tem) (n.) That part of the nervous system outside the spinal cord, brain, and brainstem in which neurons and their axons are encased by Schwann cells. Used in contrast to the central nervous system, where axons are sheathed by glial cells.

Peripheral Neuropathy (pe-rif′er-al/nu-rop′ah-thē) (n.) A generalized term for a disorder of a peripheral nerve that occurs anywhere along the course of the nerve. This includes the spinal nerve root. The disorder is manifested by weakness, loss of reflex, and sensory loss in the distribution of the affected nerve or nerve root. If this involves only one nerve or root, it is called **Mononeuropathy**. If several nerves or roots are involved, the process is considered a **Polyneuropathy**.

Peripheral Tear (pĕ-rif′er-al/tār) (n.) A vertical tear in the outer margin of the meniscus involving the vascular zone. It has increased potential for healing and therefore are amenable to repair.

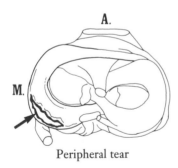
Peripheral tear

Peripheral Vascular Disease (pe-rif′er-al/vas′ku-lar/di-zēz) (n.) A generalized term applied to disease of any of the blood vessels outside the heart.

Periphery (pe-rif′er-ē) (n.) 1. The outer surface. 2. The area farthest from the center of a part.

Peritendineum (per″i-ten-den′ē-um) (n.) See **Peritenon**.

Peritenon (per″i-te-non) (n.) The sheath of a tendon. Also known as a **Peritendineum**.

Perkins Line (per-kins/līn) (n.) A line drawn on an AP radiograph of the pelvis used in the evaluation of congenital dysplasia of the hip. This line is drawn vertically from the most lateral ossified margin of the roof of the acetabulum, perpendicular to and touching Hilgenreiner's horizontal line. The ossific nucleus of the femoral head should lie in the inner lower quadrant formed by the intersection of these two lines. Also called **Ombredanne's Vertical Line**.

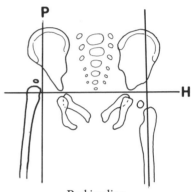
Perkins line

Perkins Traction (per-kins/trak-shun) (n.) A type of skeletal traction used in the treatment of femoral shaft fractures that requires the use of a "split-bed."

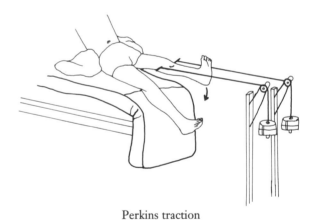
Perkins traction

Permanent Impairment (per-mah′nent/im-pār′ment) (n.) Impairment that either has become static or well stabilized and is not likely to remit, despite medical treatment of the impairing condition.

Permanent Prosthesis (per-mah′nent/pros-thē′sis) (n.) A replacement for a missing member that meets accepted check-out standards for comfort, fit, alignment, function, appearance, and durability. Synonym: **Definitive Prosthesis**.

Permissible Dose (per-mis′i′b′l/dōs) (n.) A term for the amount of radiation that may be received by an individual within a specific period with the expectation of no harmful result. The dose is given in an occupational or therapeutic setting.

Peroneal (per″o-ne′al) (adj.)   Relating to the fibular or lateral side of the lower leg.

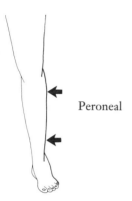

Peroneal

Peroneal Muscles (per″o-ne′al/mus′els) (n.)   One of the muscles of the leg that arises from the lateral aspect of the fibula and runs in the lateral compartment of the lower leg. These muscles function in eversion and dorsiflexion of the foot. See also **Muscle**.

Peroneal Muscular Atrophy (per″o-ne′al/mus′kular/at′ro-fē) (n.)   A progressive, inherited motor and sensory neuropathy. It is inherited as an autosomal dominant disease. The process is slowly progressive, usually beginning in the second decade with initial involvement of the feet and legs, then spreading to the hands and forearms over the next several years. The disorder is characterized by atrophy of certain muscle groups, particularly the peroneals and the intrinsic musculature of the hands and feet. The face, trunk, and proximal limb muscles are usually spared. Also known as **Charcot-Marie-Tooth Disease** and **Progressive Neural Muscular Atrophy**.

Peroneal Nerve (per″-o-ne′al/nerv) (n.)   The lateral portion of the sciatic nerve that separates from it at about the middle of the thigh and ends lateral to the neck of the fibula by dividing into two terminal branches—the deep and superficial nerves.

Peroneal Sign (per″o-ne′al/sīn) (n.)   A sign used in the evaluation of tetany. It is characterized by the inversion and dorsiflexion of the foot that occurs when the region of the leg overlying the peroneal nerve is tapped.

Peroneus Brevis Muscle (pe-ro′ne-us/bre′vis/mus′el) (n.)   See **Muscle**.

Peroneus Longus Muscle (pe-ro′ne-us/long′us/mus′el) (n.)   See **Muscle**.

Peroneus Tertius Muscle (pe-ro′ne-us/tes′ti-us/mus′el) (n.)   See **Muscle**.

Perthes Disease (per-tēz/dĭ-zēz) (n.)   See **Legg-Calvé-Perthes Disease**.

Perthes Sling (per′tēs/sling) (n.)   An orthosis used in the treatment of Legg-Calvé-Perthes disease. It consists of a pelvic belt, from the posterior part of which hangs a strap with a buckle, to which an ankle cuff is attached. This cuff is placed around the ankle of the limb affected by the disease. The strap is tightened to flex the knee sufficiently so that the foot of the affected extremity does not touch the ground.

Pertrochanteric Fracture (per″tro′kan-ter-ik/frak′chur) (n.)   A fracture of the proximal femur that has both intertrochanteric and subtrochanteric components.

Pes (pes) (n.)   1. The foot. 2. A footlike part.

Pes Abductus (pes/ab-duk′tus) (n.)   A foot deformity in which the anterior part of the foot is displaced lateral to the vertical axis of the leg.

Pes Anserinus (pes/an′ser-in-us) (n.)   A goose foot-shaped expansion of the tendons of insertion of the semitendinosis, sartorious, and gracilis muscles along the medial aspect of the proximal tibia.

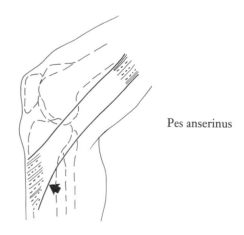

Pes anserinus

Pes Anserinus Bursa (pes/an′ser-in-us/ber′sah) (n.)   A bursa that lies deep to the tendons of the semitendinosis, sartorius, and gracilis muscles along the medial aspect of the proximal tibia, near their insertions.

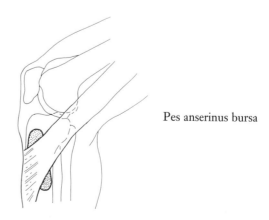

Pes anserinus bursa

Pes Cavus (pes/kāv′us) (n.) A foot with an abnormally high longitudinal arch; this is the result of either a congenital or an acquired deformity. Pes cavus is often seen in various neurologic disorders. The deformity is best assessed radiographically with a weight-bearing lateral view of the foot. An increased angle between the lines drawn through the inferior calcaneal cortex and the inferior cortex of the fifth metatarsal will be noted as will an obtuse angle between the midtalar line and the midline of the first metatarsal.

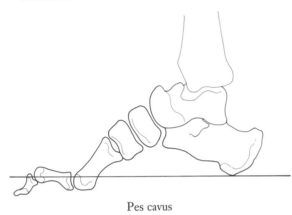

Pes cavus

Pes Planovalgus (pes/plā′no-val′gus) (n.) See **Planovalgus.**

Pes Planus (pes/plā′nus) (n.) A foot with a markedly reduced longitudinal arch height. A flexible or correctible deformity should be differentiated from a fixed pes planus. Commonly known as **Flat Foot.**

Pes Varus (pes/vār′us) (n.) A foot deformity in which the forepart of the foot is deviated inward or medially. Also known as **Pigeon-Toed** or **Talipes Varus.**

Petechia (pe-tē′kē-ah) (n.) A pinpoint-sized, flat, round, purplish red spot on the skin caused by an intradermal or submucous hemorrhage. See **Purpura.**

Petit's Triangle (pe-tēz/tri′ang-g′l) (n.) A small, triangular, anatomic interval located just above the il-ium, between the inferolateral margin of the latissimus dorsi muscle and the external oblique muscle of the abdomen. Synonym: **Lumbar Triangle.**

Petrie Cast (pe′trē/kast) (n.) An abduction, weight-bearing, plaster brace used in the treatment of Perthes disease. Both lower limbs are placed in long leg casts; each hip is then abducted to 30 degrees to 40 degrees and approximately 5 degrees of internal rotation. Cross-bars attached to the foot or back of the casts will secure and maintain the position.

Petrissage (pā″tri-sahzh′) (n.) A massage maneuver. Also known as **Kneading.**

Petrolatum Gauze (pet″ro-lā′tum/gauz) (n.) A nonadherent material produced by saturating sterile absorbent gauze with sterile white petrolatum. It is used to dress wounds.

PFFD Abbreviation for Proximal Femoral Focal Deficiency.

PFT (n.) Abbreviation for Pulmonary Function Tests.

pH A symbol denoting the relative concentration of hydrogen ions in a solution. pH values are measured from 0 to 14 and provide a measure of acidity and alkalinity. The normal blood pH value is 7.40.

Phagocytosis (fāg″ō-sī-tō′sis) (n.) 1. Ingestion and digestion of foreign material. 2. Ingestion and digestion of necrotic tissue by a cell of the body.

Phalangeal Sign (fah-lan′je-al/sīn) (n.) A radiographic sign of peripheral dysostosis. It is present when there is a difference of more than 2 mm between the length of the fourth metacarpal and the combined lengths of the ring (fourth) finger's distal and proximal phalanges.

Phalanges (fah-lan′jēz) (n.) The bones of the fingers and toes (digits). The first digit (thumb/big toe) has two phalanges. Each of the remaining digits has three phalanges.

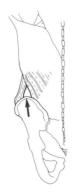

Petit's triangle

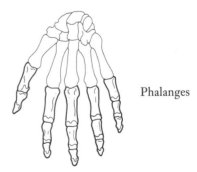

Phalanges

Phalangization (fil″an-ji-za′shun) (n.) A technique for substituting a digital ray for an amputated thumb, or the deepening of the space between the thumb and palm, when there is an amputation of the thumb at or near the metacarpal head.

Phalanx (fā′lanks) (n.)   Any bone of a finger or toe. See **Phalanges**.

Phalen's Sign (fā′lenz/sīn) (n.)   A diagnostic marker of carpal tunnel syndrome. If present, a reproduction or exaggeration of the patient's symptoms will occur after the wrist is held in marked flexion for 30 to 60 seconds. The length of time elapsed until this symptom occurs or worsens should be noted.

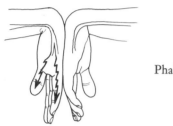

Phalen's sign

Phantom Bone (fan′tom/bōn) (n.)   See **Disappearing Bone Disease**. Synonym: **Gorham's Disease**.

Phantom Limb (fan′tom/lim) (n.)   A type of discomfort experienced by amputees who sense that the distal segments of a lost extremity still exist, as if the limb were still part of the body. The phantom limb is usually described as having a tingling feeling and a definite shape that resembles the actual limb before amputation. If there is a painful sensation, it is referred to as **phantom pain**.

Phase Microscope (fāz/mī′krō-skōp) (n.)   A microscope that alters the phase relationships of the light passing through and around the object being viewed. The contrast produced permits visualization of the object without staining or other special preparation.

Phelps Orthosis (felps/or-thō′sis) (n.)   A single, upright, round, caliper, adjustable ankle–foot orthosis. A stop behind the upright may be used to adjust the degree of plantar flexion of the ankle.

Phelps Test (felps/test) (n.)   A clinical examination used to determine the degree of contracture of the gracilis muscle. Place the patient prone, with the hips in maximum abduction and the knees in 90 degrees of flexion. If the gracilis muscle is shortened, the hip will automatically adduct on passive full extension of the knee. Also called the **Phelps-Baker Test**.

Phemister Graft (fem′is-ter/graft) (n.)   A technique of bone grafting without fixation used for established nonunions. In this technique, onlay grafting is performed by simply placing the graft subperiosteally across the fracture fragments without immobilizing them. In a modification of this technique, the fracture site is exposed, and then the fragments are prepared by using a chisel to elevate the periosteum along with shingles of cortical bone. The graft is then placed between the exposed underlying bone and the osteoperiosteal shingles.

Phenomenon (fe-nom′e-non) (n.)   An observable occurrence, e.g., a clinical sign.

Phenotype (fē′no-tīp) (n.)   The appearance of an organism, which results from the interaction of its genotype and its environment.

Phenylbutazone (fen″il-bū′tah-zōn) (n.)   A nonsteroidal, antiinflammatory drug.

Philips Head (fil′ips/hed) (n.)   A particular slot design in the head of a screw that accepts a screwdriver with a cross-shaped pointed tip.

Philips head

Philipson's Reflex (fil′ip-sons/rē′fleks) (n.)   One of the brainstem reflexes whose persistence after 1 month of age is abnormal and suggests neurologic dysfunction. To obtain the reflex, support the infant by holding one extremity extended at the knee. Then apply firm pressure to the sole of the extended leg by stroking or rubbing it. The opposite free leg will flex, adduct, and then extend. Also known as the **Crossed Extension Reflex**.

Phlebitis (fle-bī′tis) (n.)   Inflammation of the wall of a vein.

Phlebogram (fleb′ō-gram) (n.)   A radiograph obtained during phlebography. Also known as **Venogram**.

Phlebography (fle-bog′rah-fē) (n.)   Radiography of a vein filled with contrast medium. Used in the diagnosis of thrombophlebitis. Also known as **Venography**.

Phlebolith (fleb′ō-lith) (n.)   A stonelike structure that results from the deposition of calcium in a vein. It is usually found incidentally on a radiograph and appears as a small, round opacity in the pelvis. A phlebolith does not produce symptoms and requires no treatment.

Phlebothrombosis (fleb″o-throm-bō′sis) (n.)   See **Thrombophlebitis**.

Phocomelia (fō″kō-mē′le-ah) (n.)   A type of intercalary congenital limb deficiency that results in a limb reminiscent of a seal flipper. Typically, it is characterized by the absence of the arm and the forearm and the attachment of the hand to the shoulder or the attachment of the foot directly to the trunk.

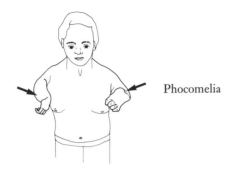

Phocomelia

Phosphatase (fos'fah-tās″) (n.)   An enzyme capable of catalyzing the hydrolysis of phosphoric acid esters.

Phosphate (fos'fāt) (n.)   An ionic compound with the composition PO_4 and a negative ionic charge. It forms a salt with calcium, whose crystalline form accounts for most of the mineral composition of bone.

Phospholipid (fos-fō-lip'id) (n.)   A group of fats that contain phosphate; these include phosphatidic acid and sphingomyelin.

Photon (fō'ton) (n.)   A discrete quantity of energy composed of either visible light or any other electromagnetic radiation.

Physaliphorous Cell (fis″ah-lif'er-us/sel) (n.)   A descriptive name for the large vacuolated cell typically found in chordomas.

Physeal Bar (fiz'ē-al/bar) (n.)   A bridge of bone that forms from the metaphysis to the epiphysis, thereby crossing the physis; this results in a tethering of growth with possible angular deformity. The clinical deformity is determined by the size and location of the bar. It is also known as a bone bridge or a bone bar. This may be removed surgically and replaced with fat or silastic.

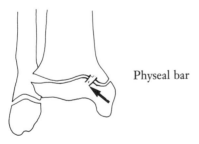

Physeal bar

Physiatrist (fiz″ē-at'rist) (n.)   A physician specializing in physical medicine and rehabilitation.

Physical Sign (fiz'e-kal/sīn) (n.)   An objective clinical sign manifested by a patient or detected by a physician on inspection, palpation, percussion, auscultation, measurement, or some combination of these methods.

Physical Sterilization (fiz'e-kal / ster″i-li-zā'shun) (n.)   The use of heat to achieve sterilization and disinfection.

Physical Therapist (fiz'e-kal/ther'ah-pist) (n.)   A person skilled in the techniques of physical therapy and qualified to administer treatments as prescribed.

Physical Therapy (fiz'e-kal/ther'ah-pē)   The treatment of disease and injury by physical means, such as light, heat, cold, electricity, ultrasound, massage, and exercise.

Physiological Bowing (fiz″e-o-loj'i-kal/bō'ing) (n.)   A normal medial bowing of the lower extremities seen in infants and young children. The bowing involves both the distal femur and the proximal tibia. Spontaneous correction is expected by the time the child is approximately 2 to 2½ years of age. If radiographs are taken, a normal-appearing epiphyseal plate is seen as well as prominence of the tibial and femoral metaphyses and a thickening of the medial tibial cortex. This condition should be differentiated from other causes of bowing. Also known as **Physiologic Genu Varum**.

Physiology (fiz″e-ol'o-jē) (n.)   The scientific study of the functions of living organisms and the individual organs, tissues, and cells of which they are composed.

Physiolysis Colli Femoris (fiz″e-ol'ĭ-sis/ko'lī/fem'or-is) (n.)   See **Slipped Capital Femoral Epiphysis**.

Physis (fi'sis) (n.)   The cartilaginous zone between the epiphysis and the metaphysis responsible for the longitudinal growth of bones formed by endochrondral ossification. Also known as the **Growth Plate** or **Epiphyseal Plate**.

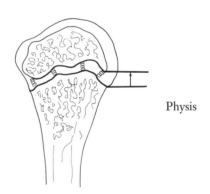

Physis

Piedmont Fracture (pēd'-mont/frak'chur) (n.)   A fracture of the radius at the junction of its distal and middle thirds. This is associated with dislocation of the distal radioulnar joint and is more commonly known as a **Galeazzi Fracture**.

Piezoelectric Effect (pi-e″zo-e-lek'trik/e-fekt) (n.)   1. An electrical current generated when a mechanical stress is applied to certain natural crystals. 2. The induction of a mechanical strain in a crystal by the application of an electrical current. The piezoelec-

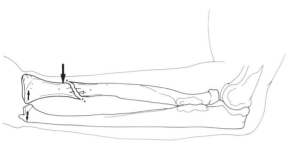

Piedmont fracture

tric effect is seen when bone is mechanically stressed. The areas of compression become electronegative; areas of tension become electropositive.

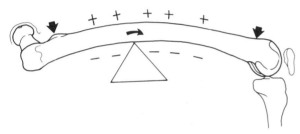

Piezoelectric effect

Pigeon Breast (pij-in/brest) (n.) A deformity of the thoracic cage in which an anterior protrusion of the sternum results in an increased sagittal diameter of the chest. Synonyms: **Congenital Chondrocostal Prominence, Pectus Carinatum.**

Pigeon-Toed (pij-in/tōd) (adj.) A description of an in-toeing position of the feet.

Pigmented Villonodular Synovitis (pig′men-ted/vil″o-nod′u-lar/sīn″o-vī′tis) (n.) A locally invasive but nonmetastasizing synovial lesion that is proliferative and of uncertain etiology. The lesion is usually intraarticular but may also arise from bursae or tendon sheaths. Both forms may show extensive local destruction of bone. Grossly, the lesion consists of a mass of matted reddish brown villous projections and nodules that adhere densely to the capsule and synovium of the joint, occasionally encroaching on the cartilage surfaces or burrowing into the subchondral bone. Histologically, it is characterized by fibrohistiocytic proliferation with deposition of hemosiderin, multinuclear giant cells and foam cells. Aspiration of an involved joint yields dark, serosanguineous synovial fluid. Three forms of pigmented villonodular synovitis are differentiated: (1) a solitary giant cell tumor of tendon sheath; (2) localized nodular synovitis; and (3) a diffuse, pigmented villonodular synovitis of an entire joint.

This disease occurs most frequently in the knee; multiple joint involvement is extremely rare.

Pillion (pil-yon′) (n.) A temporary artificial leg.

Pillion Fracture (pil-yon/frak′chur) (n.) A T-shaped fracture of the lower end of the femur with posterior displacement of the condyle. It typically occurs when a pillion (the British term for the rear seat of a motorcycle) rider's knee is hit in a collision.

Pilon Fracture (pi″lon/frak′chur) (n.) A comminuted fracture of the distal tibia and fibula with severe involvement of the tibial plafond, usually as a result of a fall from a height, driving the talus superiorly into the tibia.

Pilot Hole (pi′lit/hōl) (n.) A relatively small hole that is drilled for either a self-tapping screw or a tap or as a preliminary to a larger drill hole to prevent wandering of the drill or fracture.

Pins (pinz) (n.) A general term for narrow, pointed metallic implants, threaded or unthreaded, used in internal fixation and external fixation of fractures. See also specific pins.

Pin Tract (pin/trakt) (n.) The opening formed when a piece of hardware, such as a pin or screw that is driven into bone and then left exposed externally. It includes the path the transfixing pin or screw makes in the bone and in the overlying skin and soft tissue.

Pinch Graft (pinch/graft) (n.) A small, full-thickness skin graft obtained by elevating the donor area with a needle and then taking off a small area with a knife or razor.

Pinch, Normal (pinch/nor′mal) (n.) The coming together of the tips of the thumb and index fingers, as one would use in picking up a screw. Also called tip pinch, as opposed to lateral or key pinch.

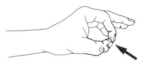

Pinch, normal

Pinched Nerve (pinched/nerv) (n.) A layman's term for a radiculopathy produced by a herniated disk. The herniated disk "pinches" the nerve, ca___g pain.

Pins-in-Plaster (pinz/in/plas′ter) (n.) A___ ___ternal fixation used in the manageme___ ___es. Pins are placed in the proximal and dis___ ___cture fragments and are incorporated into a plaster cast after reduction of the fracture. See **External Fixation**.

PIP Joint (n.) Abbreviation for proximal interphalangeal joint.

Pirie's Bone (pe-rēz/bōn) (n.) An accessory bone of the foot sometimes found anterior to the dorsal edge of the talus.

Piriformis Muscle (pirifor′mis/mus′el (n.) See **Muscle**.

Piriformis Syndrome (pirifor′mis/sin′drōm) (n.) A

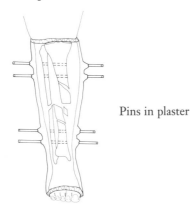

Pins in plaster

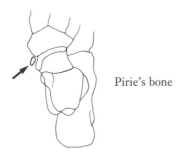

Pirie's bone

disorder that produces sciaticlike symptoms, caused by entrapment of the sciatic nerve by the piriformis muscle. There are no laboratory or diagnostic tests. The diagnosis is entirely clinical and one of exclusion for other causes.

Pirogoff's Amputation (pir″o-gofs′/am″pu-tā′shun) (n.) Removal of the foot in which a portion of the posterior calcaneus is retained and applied to the sawed surface of the distal tibia and fibula.

Piroxicam (pēr-ok′si-kam) (n.) A nonsteroidal, anti-inflammatory drug. It is marketed under the brand name **Feldene.**

PISI (n.) Abbreviation for palmar intercalated segmental instability.

Pisiform (pī′si-form) (n.) 1. A small pea-like carpal bone on the ulnar side of the hand that articulates with the triquetrum. 2. A sesamoid bone within the tendon of the flexor carpi ulnaris.

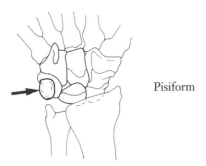

Pisiform

Pistoning (pis′ton-ing) (n.) A sliding movement up and down of a stump in a prosthesis. A form of gait in which there is hip instability, i.e., after girdlestone procedure.

Pitch (pich) (n.) The distance between the crests of two adjacent threads of a screw as measured along the axis of the screw.

Pitch Angle (pich/ang′g'l) (n.) A measurement used to evaluate the orientation of the calcaneus. On a lateral radiograph of the foot, this is the angle formed between the line tangential to the plantar surface of the calcaneus and a horizontal line.

Pitres-Testut Sign (pēt′-re-tes-tō′/sīn) (n.) A diagnostic marker in ulnar nerve paralysis. It is present when a patient is unable to form his or her hand into the shape of a cone because of intrinsic muscle paralysis.

Pittsburgh Triangular Frame (pits′-burg/trī-ang′-ū-lar/frām) (n.) A complex external fixation device intended to control unstable pelvic ring fractures.

Pivot Gait (piv′ut/gāt) (n.) The mode of progression of a paraplegic person in a pivot, ambulating, crutchless orthosis. By rotary motion of the trunk, the subject, together with the support pivot, moves alternately to the right and to the left; this causes him or her to advance or retreat. The axis of rotation is lateral to the feet, which causes both feet to move together with the support.

Pivot Joint (piv′ut/joint) (n.) An articulation between two bones that limits movement to rotation. The movement is uniaxial and is in the longitudinal axis of the bones. For example, the joint between the first and second cervical vertebrae is a pivot joint.

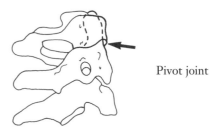

Pivot joint

Pivot Shift Test (piv′ut/shift/test) (n.) A clinical test used to demonstrate anterolateral rotatory instability of the knee. The examiner places one hand over the fibula head and the lateral aspect of the proximal tibia; he or she then grasps the ankle with his or her other hand. The knee is extended, and internal rotation is applied to the leg. As the knee is flexed, a valgus stress is applied to the knee. Initially, the tibial plateau will be anterolaterally subluxed if instability is present. As the knee is flexed, the subluxation will reduce, sometimes with a palpable or audible clunk. The test is positive if the tibia reduces during flexion. Also known as the **Pivot Shift Test of MacIntosh and Galway.**

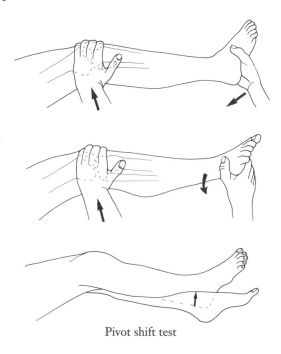

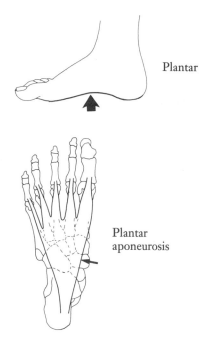

Plantar

Plantar
aponeurosis

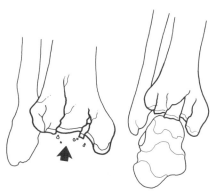

Pivot shift test

Plafond Fracture (plah-fōn/frak′chur) (n.)   A fracture of the distal end of the tibia that extends into the articular surface of the tibiotalar joint. Also known as a **Tibial Plafond Fracture**.

Plafond fracture

Plane Joint (plān/joint) (n.)   A gliding joint.

Planovalgus (plā″no-val′gus) (n.)   A foot deformity in which flattening of the longitudinal arch is associated with lateral deviation of the heel. Also known as **Pes Planovalgus**.

Plantar (plan′tar) (adj.)   Of or concerning the sole of the foot.

Plantar Aponeurosis (plan′tar/ap″o-nu-ro′sis) (n.)   A sheet of dense fibrous connective tissue that helps stabilize the longitudinal arch of the foot. The plantar aponeurosis arises from the tubercle of the calcaneus and passes forward, dividing into five bands that insert into the bases of the proximal phalanges. Also known as **Plantar Fascia** or **Plantar Ligaments**.

Plantar Calcaneonavicular Ligament (plan′tar/kal-ka″nē-ō-nah-vik′ū-lar/lig′ah-ment) (n.)   A supportive ligament in the sole of the foot that extends from the sustentaculum tali and the distal calcaneus to the entire width of the inferior surface of the navicular and on to its medial surface. Also known as the **Spring Ligament**.

Plantar Fasciitis (plan′tar/fas″ē-ī′tis) (n.)   An inflammatory process, usually secondary to trauma or chronic repetitive strain, involving the plantar fascia, most commonly at its attachment to the calcaneus. Commonly known as **Heel Spur Syndrome**.

Plantar Fibromatosis (plan′tar/fī′bro-mah-tō′sis) (n.)   A benign condition in which nodular masses of well-differentiated fibroblastic tissue arise within the plantar fascia, usually on the medial side. The lesion may be aggressive and may invade the bone. Owing to its infiltrative nature, local recurrence is common after excision.

Plantar Flexion (plan′tar/flek′shun) (n.)   1. Flexing or bending of the foot in the direction of the sole so that the angle between the dorsum of the foot and the leg is increased. 2. The opposite of dorsiflexion.

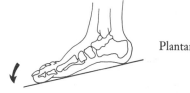

Plantar flexion

Plantar Reflex (plan′tar/re′fleks) (n.) A reflex elicited in response to a stroking of the outer surface of the sole from the heel to the fifth toe. Normally, the response will be flexion of the toes. If the toes extend, this is a sensitive indication of upper motor neuron disease. An extension response, or upgoing toes, is known as a positive **Babinski sign**. This is normal in infants up to approximately 18 months of age.

Plantar Wart (plan′tar/wart) (n.) A common wart that occurs on the sole of the foot. These warts are actually epidermal tumors caused by a virus; usually they are very tender to palpation and sidewards compression. Also known as **Verruca Plantaris**.

Plantaris Muscle (plan-tah′ris/mus′el) (n.) See **Muscle**.

Plantigrade Foot (plan′tī-grād/foot) (n.) The sole of the foot dorsiflexes to neutral (90 degree angle) in relation to the tibia.

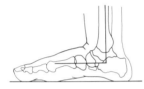

Plantigrade foot

Plantigrade Gait (plan′tī-grād/gait) (n.) A type of gait characterized by walking or running flat on the full sole of the foot.

Plasma (plaz′mah) (n.) The noncellular fluid portion of blood. Plasma is a complex solution and suspension of chemical substances: 90% water, 1% inorganic substances, 6 to 8% protein, and small amounts of glucose, lipids, nitrogenous wastes of metabolism, gases, enzymes, hormones, and other substances.

Plasma Cell Myeloma (plaz′mah/sel/mī-lō′mah) (n.) A malignant neoplastic proliferation of plasma cells of the bone marrow that manifests itself systemically or as a clinically localized osseous lesion. It is differentiated from multiple myeloma by the absence of malignant cells in a distant site, the absence of other radiographic lytic lesions, and the absence of serum or urine protein abnormality. Solitary lesions also tend to occur in patients who are younger than those with multiple myeloma. Also known as **Solitary Myeloma** or **Plasmacytoma**.

Plasmacytoma (plaz″mah-si-to′mah) (n.) See **Plasma Cell Myeloma**.

Plaster Boot (plas′ter/boot) (n.) Usually refers to a short leg cast. See **Cast Shoe**.

Plaster Cast (plas′ter/kast) (n.) An immobilizing, circumferential bandage made from plaster-of-Paris. See related **Cast**.

Plaster Knives (plas′ter/nīves) (n.) Knives with short, slightly curved blades that are used to cut and shape plaster-of-Paris casts before they harden.

Plaster-of-Paris (plas′ter/of/pah′ris) (n.) A chalky white powder made by removing water from gypsum; its chemical composition is anhydrous calcium sulfate. Used to make casts and splints for immobilization; a gauze bandage is stiffened with starch or dextrose and then is impregnated with this powder. The plaster-of-Paris then becomes a homogeneous solid mass after being placed in water owing to an exothermic chemical reaction that occurs when the anhydrous salt is rehydrated.

Plaster Scissors (plas′ter/siz′erz) (n.) Heavy scissors used to cut plaster bandages, often serrated.

Plaster Sore (plas′ter/sōr) (n.) A skin ulceration that occurs beneath a plaster cast. This occurs most often over bony prominences and in areas of altered skin sensibility or where plaster is irregularly applied without proper padding.

Plaster Splint (plas′ter/splint) (n.) A plaster-of-Paris splint used for support or immobilization.

Plastic Behavior (plas′tik/bē-hāv′yor) (n.) A biomechanical term that describes the occurrence of a permanent deformation in a material or tissue after a load is applied and then removed. This deformation occurs when a load is applied beyond the yield point.

Plastic Flow (plas′tik/flō) (n.) The fluidlike behavior a material exhibits when it takes a permanent set.

Plasticity (plas-tis′i-tē) (n.) The property of a material to deform permanently when it is loaded beyond its elastic range.

Plastizote (plas′ti-zōt) (n.) A synthetic, springy, foamlike plastic material used to make padded orthotic devices.

Plasty (plas-tē) (n.) A suffix pertaining to repair of.

Plates (plātz) (n.) A general term for metallic internal fixation implants that have holes through which screws are inserted to affix the plate to bone. See under specific plates.

Platform (plat′form) (n.) In shoe terminology, a thick midsole designed to raise the sole of the shoe.

Platform Crutch (plat′form/kruch) (n.) A crutch with a horizontal support for the forearm and, usually, a peg for the hand. It is used when the elbow is to remain flexed or when the hand is unable to grasp a handle in the usual manner. Synonym: **Shelf Crutch**.

Platybasia (plat″ē-bā′se-ah) (n.) See **Basilar Impression**.

Platypelloid Pelvis (plat′e-pel′oid/pel/vis) (n.) A normal variant of pelvic anatomy. This is a "flat" pelvis, similar to the gynecoid pelvis, except that there is anteroposterior narrowing at all levels. At the pelvic inlet, there is a long transverse diameter and a very short anteroposterior diameter.

Platyspondylia (plat″ē-spon-dil′e-ah) (n.) A broad, flat vertebra.

Playing Surface (pla′ing/sur′fis) (n.) The superficial surface covering of an athletic field or arena.

Pleonosteosis of Leri (ple″on-os″tē-ō′sis/of/leri) (n.) A rare, hereditary syndrome with an autosomal dominant pattern of inheritance that causes abundant and precocious bone formation. The clinical characteristics include shortness of stature; deformity of the hands and toes with broadened, valgus thumbs; general limitation in joint movement; and facial abnormalities.

Plethysmography (pleth″iz-mog′rah-fē) (n.) The measurement of changes in the volume of an extremity or organ caused by either venous or arterial blood flow. This is a useful, noninvasive diagnostic technique for determining the presence of occlusive vascular disease.

Pleurodynia (ploor″o-dīn′e-ah) (n.) Painful affection of the intercostal muscles at their tendinous insertions. Also known as **Pleuralgia.**

Plexus (plek′sus) (n.) A network of interlacing nerves or anastomosing blood vessels.

Plica (plī′kah) (n.) A ridge or fold of tissue. The term is most commonly used to describe a fold of synovial tissue around the knee. A plica here represents persistence of an embryonic synovial septum into adult life. The plicae of the knee are classified according to the membrane from which they arise and their anatomic relationship to the patella; for example, there are suprapatellar or medial patellar plica.

Plica Syndrome (plī′kah/sin′drōm) (n.) A clinical affection of the knee joint in which a plica becomes thickened and inflamed, resulting in painful symptoms. A plica may become symptomatic by any mechanism that converts it into a bowstring. Symptoms usually are preceded by a history of acute blunt or repetitive trauma and are associated with exercise-related pain. On physical examination, patients may have tenderness near the superior pole of the patella or over the femoral condyle. A symptomatic plica is also sometimes palpable as a tender band alongside the patella, and an audible snap may be heard during exercise or flexion and extension of the knee.

PLIF (n.) Abbreviation for Posterior Lumbar Interbody Fusion.

PLRI (n.) Abbreviation for Posterolateral Rotary Instability.

Pluripotential Cell (ploor″i-po-ten′shal/sel) (n.) Any stem cell not yet fixed in terms of development that may still differentiate into various cell types.

Plyometrics (plī′-ō-met-ricks) (n.) An athletic training technique that uses vigorous drills for developing power.

PMMA (n.) Abbreviation for Polymethylmethacrylate.

PM&R (n.) Abbreviation for Physical Medicine and Rehabilitation.

PMRI (n.) Abbreviation for **Posteromedial Rotary Instability**.

Pneumatic Prosthesis (nū-mat′ik/pros-thē′sis) (n.) A temporary prosthesis for the lower limb. It has an air-filled socket, usually in the form of an air sac inserted into a socket.

Pneumatic Tourniquet (nū-mat′ik/toor′ni-ket) (n.) An instrument used to arrest circulation to a limb. It is composed of a rubber bag filled with air or gas above arterial pressure that exerts circumferential pressure on the limb. This instrument is used during extremity surgery to provide a bloodless surgical field.

Pneumoarthrogram (nū-mō-ar′thro-gram) (n.) A roentgenogram of a joint taken after the injection of air or some other gaseous contrast medium.

Pneumoarthrography (nū″mo-ar-throg-rah-fē) (n.) Roentgenography of a joint taken after injection of air or gas as a contrast medium.

Pneumothorax (nū″mo-thō′raks) (n.) A condition in which air or gas is present in a pleural cavity.

Podagra (pō-dag′rah) (n.) Gouty pain in the great toe.

Podalgia (pō-dal′je-ah) (n.) Pain in the foot.

Podiatry (pō-dī′ah-trē) (n.) The specialized field that deals with the study and care of the foot, including its anatomy, pathology, and medical and surgical treatment. Persons trained in podiatry receive degrees as Doctors of Podiatric Medicine (DPM). Synonym: **Chiropody.** Orthopaedic surgeons also specialize in foot surgery.

Poisson's Ratio (pwah-swanz′/rā′she-o) (n.) The ratio of transverse to axial strain. This is generally represented by the Greek letter nu. Because it is a ratio, there is no unit of measurement.

Poker Spine (pōk′er/spīn) (n.) A descriptive term for a spinal deformity in which the vertebral column is relatively rigid and straight owing to the loss of normal kyphosis and/or lordosis. This deformity is seen in certain rheumatologic disorders. Also called **Bamboo Spine.** See **Marie Strumpell Disease**.

Polar Moment of Inertia (pō′lar/mō′ment/of/in-er′she-ah) (n.) A biomechanical quantity that reflects the torsional strength and stiffness of the structure and depends on the size and shape of the structure being evaluated.

Poliomyelitis (pō″lē-ō-mī″e-lī′tis) (n.) An acute, transmissible, infectious disease caused by a group of neurotrophic viruses that initially invade the gastrointestinal and respiratory tracts and subsequently spread to the central nervous system through the circulation. The poliomyelitis virus has a special affinity for the anterior horn cells of the spinal cord and for certain motor nuclei of the brain stem. The afflicted cells undergo necrosis, with subsequent loss of innervation of the motor units they supply; this results in a variable degree of paralysis without sensory loss. Also called **Polio** or **Infantile Paralysis.**

Poliovirus (pō″lē-ō-vī′rus) (n.) The causative agent of poliomyelitis. Poliovirus may be separated into three serotypes, designated as types 1, 2, and 3; these serotypes are divided on the basis of the specificity of neutralizing antibody.

Polio Vaccine (pō″lē-ō/vak′sēn) (n.) A suspension of attenuated or killed viruses administered for the prevention of poliomyelitis.

Pollex (pol′eks) (n.) The thumb.

Pollicization (pol″is-i-za′shun) (n.) The transposition of a finger or toe to replace an absent or amputated thumb.

Polyarteritis (pol″ē-ar″te-rī′tis) (n.) A systemic disease of unknown origin. It is characterized by a segmental inflammatory reaction affecting small and medium-sized arteries. The clinical manifestations vary, depending on the site and extent of arterial involvement. Polyarteritis affects men four to five times more frequently than women and usually appears between the ages of 20 and 40 years. Synonyms: **Periarteritis Nodosa, Disseminated Necrotizing Periarteritis,** and **Polyarteritis Nodosa.**

Polyarthritis (pol″ē-ar-thrī′tis) (n.) Inflammation of multiple joints.

Polyarthritis Rheumatica (pol″ē-ar′thrī′tis/rū-mat′ika) (n.) See **Rheumatic Fever.**

Polyarticular (pol″ē-ar-tik′ular) (adj.) Affecting many joints.

Polychondritis (pol″ē-kon-drī′tis) (n.) The inflammation of many of the cartilages of the body.

Polydactylism (pol″ē-dak′til-izm) (n.) One or more extra digits on the hands or feet. These digits vary from a simple skin tag to developed digits with osseous and neurovascular structures. Treatment usually consists of the removal of the supernumerary part.

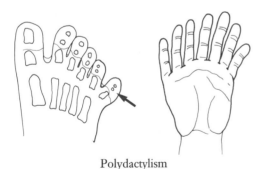

Polydactylism

Polydystrophic Dwarfism (pol″ē-dis-trō′fik) (adj.) See **Marateaux-Lamy Disease.**

Polyethylene (pol″ē-eth′i-lēn) (n.) A type of plastic formed by the polymerization of ethylene. The individual structural properties result from variations in molecular weight, crystallinity, branching, and cross-linkage.

Polyglycolic Acid (pol″ē-glī-kōl-ik/as′id) (n.) A polymer of glycolic acid used as an absorbable surgical material. Classically, this was used as suture material, but currently it is being used to create absorbable pins, tacks, and ligamentous stents.

Polymer (pol′i-mer) (n.) A compound whose molecules consist of many repeating units linked together.

Polymerization (pol″i-mer″i-zā′shun) (n.) The combining of several simpler compounds into a polymer.

Polymethylmethacrylate (pol″e-meth′il-meth′a-crī′lāt) (n.) A self-curing acrylic cement used as a filler or an insoluble grout to fix prosthetic components or other hardware securely into bone. It is a clear liquid with a characteristically penetrating odor. It has a low viscosity and therefore flows readily. The clear liquid is the monomer and starter; the powder component is PMMA. When mixed together they form a low-viscosity liquid that progresses to a doughy consistency. Abbreviated **PMMA.**

Polymyalgia Rheumatica (pol″ē-mī-al′je-ah/rū-mat′ika) (n.) A clinical syndrome of unknown etiology and pathogenesis that afflicts elderly patients. It is characterized by pain and stiffness around the neck, the back, the shoulder, and the pelvic girdles and by marked elevation of the erythrocyte sedimentation rate. Rheumatoid factor generally is not found in the serum or the synovial fluid. It is often associated with temporal arteritis. These patients often show a dramatic clinical response to corticosteroid therapy.

Polymyopathy (pol″ē-mī-op′ah-thē) (n.) Any disease affecting several muscles simultaneously.

Polymyositis (pol″ē-mī″o-sī′tis) (n.) The collective name for a group of diffuse inflammatory disorders of skeletal muscle. These diseases cause symmetric proximal muscle weakness and, to a lesser degree, muscle atrophy. The etiology is unknown.

There are five major criteria for diagnosis: weakness of the proximal muscles, a characteristic rash, elevated serum levels of creatine phosphokinase (CPK), a characteristic triad of findings on electromyography (EMG), and pathologic alterations seen on muscle biopsy. No one criterion alone is diagnostic. A common classification of polymyositis includes five subgroups:

Type I: Primary or idiopathic polymyositis (in adults).

Type II: Primary or idiopathic dermatomyositis (in adults).

Type III: Primary or idiopathic dermatomyositis or polymyositis) with malignancy.

Type IV: Childhood dermatomyositis or polymyositis.

Type V: Polymyositis associated with connective tissue disease.

Polyneuritis (pol″ē-nū-rī′tis) (n.) The simultaneous inflammation of multiple nerves, usually in a symmetrical fashion; this is the type of inflammation seen in leprosy and in Guillain-Barré disease. The term is often used interchangeably with polyneuropathy, although its specific use implies the presence of an inflammatory process as the etiology.

Polyneuropathy (pol″ē-nū-rop′ah-thē) (n.) Any disease involving multiple peripheral nerves. The symptoms are usually symmetrical, initially affecting the distal extremities of the nerve fibers and subsequently spreading toward the trunk. Polyneuropathy may result from metabolic disorders, intoxications, nutritional defects, or a remote effect of carcinoma or myeloma.

Polyneuroradiculitis (pol″ē-nū″rō-rah-dik″ū-lī′tis) (n.) An inflammation of spinal ganglia, nerve roots, and peripheral nerves.

Polynucleate (pol″ē-nū′kle-āt) (adj.) Having many nuclei.

Polyostotic (pol″ē-os-tot′ik) (adj.) Affecting several bones.

Polyp (pol′ip) (n.) Any growth or mass protruding from a mucous membrane.

Polypeptide (pol″ē-pep′tīd) (n.) A compound consisting of two or more amino acids linked together by peptide bonds.

Polypoid (pol′e-poid) (adj.) Resembling a polyp.

Polyradiculitis (pol″ē-rah-dik″u-lī′tis) (n.) See Guillain-Barré Syndrome.

Polysaccharide (pol″ē-sak′ah-rīd) (n.) A carbohydrate composed of many linked monosaccharide units. Examples include glycogen, starch or cellulose.

Polystotic Fibrous Dysplasia (pol″ē-stot-ik/fĭb-rus/dis-plā-sē-ah) (n.) A subtype of fibrous dysplasia in which multiple osseous sites are involved with the disease. See **Fibrous Dysplasia.**

Polytetrafluoroethylene (pol″ē-tet″rah-flū″ro-eth″i-lēn) (n.) See **Teflon.**

Ponseti's Y Coordinate (pon″-sā-tēz)/Y/kō-or-di-nāt) (n.) A radiographic measurement of the pelvis used in the evaluation of congenital dislocation of the hip. It assesses the degree of lateral displacement of the femoral ossific nucleus. It is measured on an AP radiograph of the pelvis by drawing a vertical line through the center of gravity that bisects the sacrum and then drawing a line perpendicular to this that terminates in the center of the ossified nucleus of the femoral head or at the medial tip of the ossified femoral neck. The length of this latter line will be increased as compared with the normal side in a congenital dislocation of the hip. Synonym **Y Coordinate.**

Popcorn Calcification (pop′korn/kal″si-fi-kā′shun) (n.) A descriptive term for stippled calcification. This is seen radiographically in various conditions. Example: **Chondrosarcoma.**

Popliteal (pop-lit″ē-al) (adj.) Pertaining to the area or space behind the knee.

Popliteal Cyst (pop-lit″ē-al/sist) (n.) See **Baker's cyst.**

Popliteal Line (pop-lit′ē-al/līn) (n.) The fold or crease on the posterior surface of the knee joint.

Popliteal Space (pop-lit″ē-al/spās) (n.) A diamond-shaped anatomic space behind the knee joint bounded medially by the medial head of the gastrocnemius muscle, the semitendinosus and semimembranosus muscles, and laterally by the lateral head of the gastrocnemius muscle and the biceps femorus muscle. The roof is the popliteal fascia; the floor is formed by the posterior aspect of the distal end of the femur, the posterior capsule of the knee joint, and the popliteus muscle over the proximal tibia.

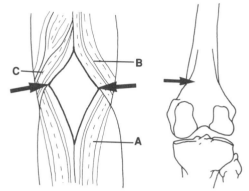

Popliteal space. **A,** Gastrocnemius; **B,** semitendinosus and semimembranosus; **C,** biceps femoris.

Popliteus Muscle (pop-li-tē′us/mus′el) (n.) See **Muscle.**

Porous (po′rus) (adj.) Characterized by pores and open spaces.

Porous-Coated (po′-rus/kō′-ted) (adj.) The design feature of a type of arthroplasty component where the metal has surface openings of 50 to 400 μ in diameter into which bone is intended to grow for permanent stabilization.

Portal (por′tal) (n.) A puncture wound, as in arthroscopic portal. Used as a gateway for the insertion of scopes, probes, inflow, or power and hand equipment.

Porter's Letter Test (por′terz/let′er/test) (n.) A neurologic evaluation of tactile gnosis of the hands. The patient is instructed to close his eyes; he or she is then asked to identify steel type letters by running his or her fingertips over the surfaces. Five letters are used in the test, and the number of letters out of that five that are correctly identified is considered the score.

Position (po-zish′un) (n.) 1. Posture or attitude. 2. The location and alignment of a prosthesis.

Positioning (po-zish′un-ing) (n.) The placing of a patient or a body part into a desired position.

Positive Sharp Wave (poz′i-tiv/sharp/wāv) (n.) A description of an abnormal potential detected by electromyography in which there is a sharp upgoing wave form. It is seen at rest in denervated muscle.

Post- (pōst) A prefix meaning after.

Post-Polio Syndrome (pōst-po′le-o/sin′drom) (n.)

Worsening of muscle weakness during middle age in polio patients.

Postaxial (pōst-ak′sē-al) (adj.)   That portion of the limb that lies distal or caudal to the long axis of a limb. An example is the distal portion of the humerus. Used to describe the absent segment in congenital limb loss.

Posterior (pōs-tēr′ē-or) (adj.)   Rear, back, or dorsal surfaces of the body.

Posterior C1-C2-C3 Cervical Line (pos-tēr′ē-or/C1-C2-C3/ser′vi-kal/līn) (n.)   A technique for the evaluation of subluxation or dislocation of the upper cervical vertebrae on a lateral radiograph of the cervical spine. A line is drawn between the anterior edge of the spinous processes of C1 and C3 on a lateral view in active extension and active flexion; this is the posterior cervical line. The distance between the anterior edge of the spinous process of C2 and this line is then measured. The normal value is 0.7 mm ± 0.5 mm.

Posterior Calcaneal Angle (pos-tēr′e-or/kal-kā′nē-al/ang′g′l) (n.)   On a lateral radiograph of the foot, the angle formed by the intersection of two lines drawn tangential to the posterior and plantar calcaneal surfaces. It is used as a quantitative measurement of calcaneal shape and pitch. A bursal projection is considered prominent if this angle exceeds 75 degrees.

Posterior Cruciate Ligament (pos-tēr′e-or/krū′shē-āt/lig′ah-ment) (n.)   One of the stabilizing ligaments of the knee. It runs from the posterior and upper surface of the tibia into the lateral surface of the medial femoral condyle in the intercondylar notch. Abbreviated as PCL. See **Cruciate Ligament**.

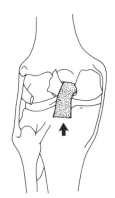

Posterior cruciate ligament

Posterior Drawer Test (pos-tēr′e-or/drawr/test) (n.)   A clinical evaluation of posterior instability of the knee joint. The patient's knee is flexed to 90 degrees, and then the tibia is pushed posteriorly; you should look for any abnormal increased posterior excursion of the tibial condyles. The presence of an initial posterior sag should be noted first. This is evaluated with

the tibia in external rotation, internal rotation, and in a neutral position. See **Anterior Drawer Test**.

Posterior Funiculus (pos-tēr′ē-or/fu-nik′ū-lus) (n.)   The white substance of the spinal cord that lies on either side of the midline between the posterior median sulcus and, laterally, the dorsal root.

Posterior Fusion (pos-tēr′ē-or/fū′zhun) (n.)   A technique of spinal arthodesis of two or more vertebrae performed by decorticating and bone-grafting the neural arches and the zygapophyseal joints. This may be done at one or more vertebral levels.

Posterior Interosseus Nerve (pos-tēr′e-or/in″ter-os′sē-us/nerv) (n.)   One of the terminal branches of the radial nerve that arises from the radial nerve in front of the elbow joint. It winds around the radius in the substance of the supinator muscle. It supplies muscles on the back of the forearm.

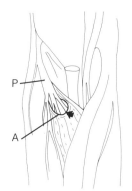

Posterior interosseus nerve

Posterior Longitudinal Ligament (pos-tēr′e-or/lon″ji-tu′di-nal/lig′ah-ment) (n.)   A ligament that runs on the posterior surfaces of the vertebral bodies, extending from the axis down through the entire length of the vertebral column, and fanning out at the vertebral margins to reinforce the intervertebral discs.

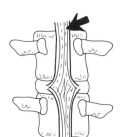

Posterior longitudinal ligament

Posterior Lumbar Interbody Fusion (pos-tēr′e-or/lum′bar/in′ter-bo′dē/fū′zhun) (n.)   A technique of spinal arthrodesis of two or more vertebrae performed by excising the intervertebral disk through the spinal canal posteriorly and then inserting a bone graft into the intervertebral space through the same route. It is abbreviated PLIF. Described by R. Cloward of Hawaii.

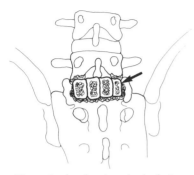

Posterior lumbar interbody fusion

Posterior Oblique Ligament (pos-tēr′ē-or/ō-blēk/ lig′ah-ment) (n.) A thickening of the capsular ligament on the medial side of the knee that is attached proximally to the adductor tubercle of the femur and distally to the tibia and posterior aspect of the capsule. Some consider this to be a portion of the medial collateral ligament instead of a discrete anatomic structure. It has an important role in the stability of the medial side of the knee.

Posterior Splint (pos-tēr′ē-or/splint) (n.) A splint applied to the back of the lower extremity to provide support and immobilization. These may be long or short leg splints.

Posterior Stabilized Knee (pos-tēr′ē-or/stā′bil-īzed/ nē) (n.) A type of semiconstrained total knee arthroplasty that, because of its surface geometry, compensates for the absence of the posterior cruciate ligament.

Posterior Triangle of Neck (pos-tēr′ē-or/tri′ang-g′l/ of/nek) (n.) A triangular anatomic space that is bounded by the sternocleidomastoid and the trapezius muscles and bordered below by the clavicle. The

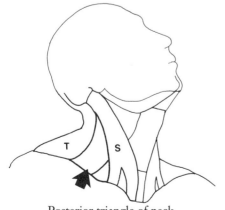

Posterior triangle of neck

posterior triangle is subdivided by the inferior belly of the omohyoid into a larger superior occipital triangle and a small inferior subclavian triangle. The triangle contains the spinal accessory nerve and its inferior portion, the brachial plexus. Compare to **Anterior Triangle of Neck**.

Postero (pos′ter-ō) Prefix meaning posterior to.

Posteroanterior (pos″ter-o-an-tēr′e-or) (adj.) Directed from the back toward the front. Abbreviated **PA**.

Posteroanterior View (pos″ter-ō-an-tēr′e-or/vū) (n.) A radiographic view in which the x-ray tube is placed in front of the body part and the x-ray beam is directed posteriorly to anteriorly. Abbreviated **PA**.

Posterolateral Drawer Test (pos″ter-ō-lat′er-al/ drawr/test) (n.) A clinical test used to evaluate posterolateral instability of the knee joint. Flex the patient's knee to approximately 60 to 90 degrees. Place the tibia into about 15 degrees of external rotation and push posteriorly on the proximal tibia. If there is instability, posterolateral displacement of the tibial plateau will occur, producing a concavity in the contour of the anterior aspect of the knee.

Posterolateral Fusion (pos″ter-ō-lat′er-al/fū′zhun) (n.) A technique of spinal arthrodesis performed by decorticating and bone grafting the zygapophyseal joint, the pars interarticularis, and the transverse processes. This may be done unilaterally or bilaterally at a given vertebral level.

Posterolateral Rotary Instability (pos″ter-ō-lat′er-al/ rō′ter-ē/in-sta′bil-i-tē) (n.) A rotary instability of the knee in which the lateral tibial plateau rotates posteriorly in relation to the femur, with lateral opening of the joint. This is established clinically by the presence of a positive external rotation recurvatum or reverse pivot shift test. It is abbreviated PLRI.

Posteromedial Rotary Instability (pos″ter-o-mē′dē-al/rō′ter-ē/in-sta′bil-i-tē) (n.) A rotary instability of the knee in which the medial tibial plateau rotates posteriorly in relation to the femur, with medial opening of the joint. There is some dispute over the clinical occurrence of this instability pattern. Abbreviated **PMRI**.

Postganglionic (pōst″gang-glē-on′ik) (adj.) A term describing the location of fibers in a nerve pathway. These fibers are distal to a ganglion and complete the neuronal pathway to the effector organ.

Postherpetic Neuralgia (pōst-her-pet′ik/nu-ral′je-ah) (n.) A state of burning pain accompanied by periods of paroxysmally augmented intensity that last a few seconds. It is seen in skin areas previously involved by herpes zoster.

Postoperative (pōst-op′er-ah-tiv) (adj.) After a surgical procedure.

Postoperative Shoe (pōst-op′er-ah-tiv/shoo) (n.) A shoe designed for patient use after surgery that limits foot motion. It is similar to a cast boot but has a wooden sole with a canvas upper, an open toe, and Velcro straps or multiple lacings.

Postphlebitic Syndrome (pōst-fleb-etik/sin-drōm) (n.) A form of chronic venous insufficiency believed to be a residual effect of phlebitis.

Post-traumatic (pōst″traw-mat′ik) (adj.) A term describing the result of an accident or other traumatic event.

Posture (pos′chur) (n.) The positioning of the body. Usual erect posture may be graded as follows:

A: Excellent or almost perfect posture. The head and shoulder are balanced over the pelvis, the hips, and the ankles, with the head erect and the chin held in. The sternum is the part of the body farthest forward, the abdomen is drawn in and flat, and the spinal curves are within normal limits.

B: Good, but not ideal posture.

C: Poor, but not the worst possible posture.

D: Bad and possibly symptom-producing posture. The head is held forward to a marked degree, the chest is depressed, the abdomen is completely relaxed and protuberant; the spinal curves are exaggerated, and the shoulders are held behind the pelvis.

Potential Energy (pō-ten′shal/en′er-jē) (n.) Energy that may be stored within a structure as a result of deformation or displacement of that structure. The unit of measure is newton meters, or joules.

Pott's Disease (pots/di-zēz) (n.) Tuberculosis of the spine.

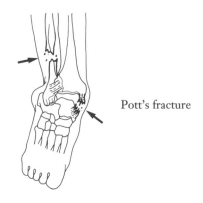

Pott's fracture

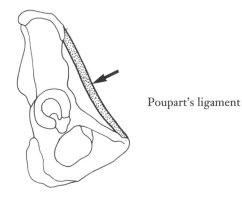

Poupart's ligament

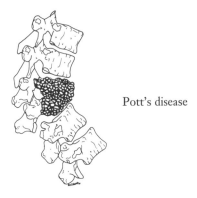

Pott's disease

Pott's Fracture (pots/frak′chur) (n.) An eponym erroneously applied to a bimalleolar fracture of the ankle. The original injury described by Percival Pott in 1765 was a partial dislocation of the ankle, a rupture of the medial ligaments of the ankle, and an associated fracture of the fibula approximately 2 to 3 inches proximal to the lateral malleolus.

Potter-Buckey Diaphragm (pot′er-buk′ē/dī′ah-fram) (n.) A moving grid used to eliminate radiation scatter when radiographs are taken.

Poupart's Ligament (poo-pars′/lig′ah-ment) (n.) The inguinal ligament.

Povidone-Iodine (po′vi-dōn-i′ō-dīn) (n.) A chemical complex produced by the reaction of iodine with the polymer povidone. It is used as a topical antiseptic agent.

Power (pow′er) (n.) The rate of performing work. It is calculated as the derivative of work with respect to time or the product of force and velocity. The unit of measurement is the watt.

Power Grip (pow′er/grip) (n.) A type of hand grip in which a clamping force is produced by the flexed fingers against counterpressure offered by the palm, the thenar eminence, and the distal segment of the thumb. Compare to **Precision Grip**.

Pratt Test (prat/test) (n.) A means of localization of incompetent communicating branches in varicose veins. In order to empty the veins, have the patient lay supine, and elevate his or her leg. Apply a tourniquet around the upper thigh to compress the long saphenous veins. Then, apply an elastic bandage from the toes to the tourniquet. When the patient stands erect, slowly unwind the bandage from the tourniquet downward. An appearance of a bulge or blow out indicates the site of an incompetent communication vein. Mark the site with a pen on the skin. Apply a second elastic bandage from the level of the tourniquet down to the bulging vein, which will compress it. Again, slowly unwind the first bandage downward to the next blow out, which should also be marked and compressed by the second bandage. This procedure is continued until all blow outs are identified while the bandages are applied. If severe pain and swelling occurs in the calf, the deep veins have been occluded.

Pre A prefix meaning before.

Preaxial (prē-ak′se-ăl) (adj.) The portion of a limb that lies proximal or cephalad to the long axis of the limb. An example is the proximal portion of the humerus. Used to describe the absent segment in congenital limb loss.

Precision Grip (pre-sizh′un/grip) (n.) A type of hand grip in which an object is held between the palmar or lateral aspect of the fingers and the opposing thumb. Compare to **Power Grip**.

Predisposition (prē″dis-pō-zish′un) (n.) A susceptibility to a particular disease that may be activated under certain conditions.

Prednisone (pred′ni-sōn) (n.) A synthetic glucocorticoid tht is a dehydrogenated analogue of cortisol. It is frequently used as an antiinflammatory agent.

Preganglionic (prē″gang-glē-on′ik) (adj.) 1. Fibers in a nerve pathway that are proximal to a ganglion. 2. Fibers in the ganglion that form synapses with postganglionic fibers.

Prehallux (prē-hāl′uks) (n.) A supernumerary bone of the foot that is in juxtaposition to the medial border of the tarsal navicular.

Prehensile (prē-hen′sīl) (adj.) Related to the act of grasping.

Prehension (prē-hen′shun) (n.) The act of grasping, seizing, or taking hold.

Preiser's Disease (prī′zerz/di-zēz′) (n.) Osteonecrosis of the carpal navicular bone.

Premature Epiphyseal Closure (prē-mah-tūr/ep″i-fiz′ē-al/klō′shur) (n.) The early closure of physeal plates that may result in deformity, limb shortening, or shortness of stature. This may be caused by an endocrine or metabolic abnormality, or it may occur posttraumatically or after an infectious process. It may be a local or a generalized process, depending on the etiology. Also known as premature plate closure.

Preoperative (prē-op′er-ah′tiv) (adj.) Occurring prior to a surgical procedure.

Preparatory Prosthesis (prep″ah-ra′to-rē/prosthē′sis) (n.) A functional, but not necessarily cosmetic, prosthesis. It is intended to be worn for a limited period during gait training and stump maturation and allows better evaluation of the prosthetic needs and potential of the patient.

Prepatellar Bursa (prē-pah-tel′ar/ber′sah) (n.) The bursa immediately anterior to the patella; it is subcutaneous. See **Patellar Bursitis**.

Prepatellar Bursitis (prē-pah-tel′ar/ber-sī′tis) (n.) An inflammation of the bursa anterior to the patella. Also known as **Housemaid's Knee, Carpet Layer's Knee,** or **Coal Miner's Knee**.

Prescription Drugs (pre-skrip′shun/drugs) (n.) Drugs dispensed only by or on the prescription of a

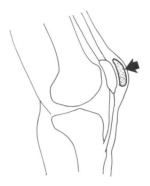

Prepatellar bursitis

licensed medical practitioner, such as a physician or dentist. In general, a drug is restricted to the prescription class if it is not safe for use except under professional supervision. These drugs are also subclassified by law on the basis of dispensing requirements. Compare to over-the-counter and nonprescription drugs.

Presenting Symptoms (pre-zent′ing/simp-tumz) (n.) The symptom or group of symptoms about which the patient complains on initial presentation to a practitioner.

Press-Fit (pres-fit) (n.) A term used to describe the fit at the interface of an implant with the surrounding bone. The prosthesis intended for implantation without cement.

Pressure Bandage (presh′ur/ban′dij) (n.) A bandage used for applying pressure. It is intended to arrest hemorrhage and limit swelling.

Pressure Dressings (presh′ur/dres′ings) (n.) Compressive dressings used to eliminate dead space and to prevent bleeding from a wound, serum accumulation, or hematoma formation.

Pressure Palsy (presh′ur/pawl′ze) (n.) Paralysis resulting from prolonged external pressure on a peripheral nerve. Usually a neuropraxia, temporary palsy, or axonotemesis, a long-lasting injury with the nerve in continuity but nerve fibers injured.

Pressure Point (presh′ur/point) (n.) The point at which an artery lies over a bone. When arresting distal hemorrhaging, it is necessary to compress this point with your finger.

Pressure Sore (presh′ur/sōr) (n.) An ulceration occuring in patients, caused by pressure. Example, patients confined to bed for prolonged periods may develop sacral or heel ulcers. Also called **Decubitus Ulcer** and **Bedsore**.

Pressurization (presh″ur-ī-za-shun) (n.) A technique for the insertion of cement in implant fixation whereby the application of increased pressure directly to less viscous or semifluid cement will result in improved bonding between the bone and the cement by forcing cement into bony interstices.

Pre-Tapping (prē-tap′ing) (n.) The cutting of

threads into a pilot hole before the insertion of a screw. Also known as **Tapping**.

Pretibial (prē-tib′ē-al) (adj.) In front of the tibia.

Prevertebral (pre-ver′te-bral) (adj.) Situated in front of a vertebra or the vertebral column.

Prevertebral Fascia (pre-ver′te-bral/fash′e-ah) (n.) Fascia in front of the vertebral column.

Primary (prī′mer-ē) (adj.) Initial or first.

Primary Curve (pri′mer-e/kurv) (n.) The first or earliest of several spinal curves to appear. It is usually the longest of the curves.

Primary Gout (prī′mer-ē/gowt) (n.) A term applied to those cases of gout in which the underlying hyperuricemia is the result of an inborn error in the intermediary metabolism of purines and related compounds. This results in overproduction and/or retention of uric acid. It is characterized by hyperuricemia, recurrent attacks of acute arthritis, deposition of monosodium urate crystals in and around the joints of the extremities, renal disease, and urolithiasis. See **Gout**.

Primary Nerve Repair (prī′mer-ē/nerv/re-pār′) (n.) The surgical repair of a severed nerve that is undertaken within the first 24 hours after injury. If the repair is performed 2 days to 18 days after injury it is considered a delayed primary repair. Synonym: **Primary Neurorrhaphy**.

Primary Skin Closure (prī′mer-ē/skin/klō′shur) (n.) A technique of skin closure applied to clean lacerations or surgical wounds. The skin edges are apposed within the first several hours after injury, which results in healing by primary intention.

Primary Tendon Repair (prī′mer-ē/ten′dun/rē-pār′) (n.) The repair of severed tendons at the time of primary wound closure. All later tendon repairs are considered delayed primary or secondary repairs.

Primary Tumor (prī′mer-ē/tū′mor) (n.) Tumor from which metastases originate.

Primitive Bone (prim′i-tiv/bōn) (n.) See **Woven Bone**.

Primitive Reflexes (prim′i-tiv/rē′fleks-es) (n.) A group of neonatal reflexes that are outgrown as the normal nervous system matures. In children with cerebral palsy and other nervous system disorders, these reflexes may persist. If these primitive motor activities are present after a certain age, they are then considered to be pathologic. They are also known as infantile reflexes.

Principal Diagnosis (prin′si-pal/di″ag-nō′sis) (n.) The diagnosis of a condition, established after study, that is the chief reason for the admission of the patient to the hospital for care.

Privileges (priv′-i-le-jez) (n.) The commonly used shorthand term for clinical privileges, which is the formal authority granted by a hospital governing board to a physician or health care professional to provide care to patients at that institution within limits based on the physician's or dentist's professional license, experience, and competence.

PRN The abbreviation for "as necessary," from the latin "Pro Re Nata."

Probe (prōb) (n.) A surgical instrument used for exploring body cavities, wounds, fistulas, and other passages. It is a thin rod of pliable metal with a blunt end. May refer to an electronic sensor, such as an ultrasonic probe.

Probenecid (prō-ben′e-sid) (n.) A uricosuric agent that blocks the tubular reabsorption of uric acid and the tubular excretion of penicillin.

Procedure (prō-sējur) (n.) The act or process of treatment, operation, or diagnosis.

Process (pros′es) (n.) A prominence or projection.

Prodrome (prō′drōm) (n.) 1. A symptom indicating the onset of a disease. 2. A premonitory symptom of a disease.

Product Evaluation Committee (prod′ukt/e-val″u-a′shun/kŏ-mit′e) (n.) A hospital committee composed of medical, nursing, purchasing, and administrative staff members whose purpose it is to evaluate products and give advice on their procurement.

Prognosis (prog-nō′sis) (n.) 1. An assessment of the future course and outcome of a patient's disease. This assessment is based on knowledge of the course of the disease in other patients, along with the general health, age, sex, as well as the exercise of clinical judgment of the patient. 2. The expected outcome of surgical procedures.

Progressive Contracture of the Quadriceps Muscle (pro-gres′iv/kon-trak′tūr/of/the/kwod′rĭ-seps/mus′el) (n.) A condition affecting children in which the gradual development of a knee extension contracture occurs secondary to progressive fibrosis of the quadriceps muscle. Idiopathic cases are reported, but more commonly there is a causal relationship with multiple intramuscular injections during infancy or early childhood.

Progressive Diaphyseal Dysplasia (pro-gres′iv/dī″ah-fiz′ē-al/dis-plā′se-ah) (n.) See **Engelmann's Disease**.

Progressive Infantile Idiopathic Scoliosis (pro-gres′iv/in′fan-tīl/id″ē-ō-path′ik/skō″le-ō′sis) (n.) A structural lateral curvature of the spine that develops before 3 years of age and progresses rapidly. The measurement of the Rib-Vertebral Angle Difference (RAVD) is intended to predict the nature of an infantile curve—it will either be progressive or resolve spontaneously.

Progressive Muscular Dystrophy (prō-gres′iv/mus′kū-lar/dis′trō-fē) (n.) A group of inherited, noninflammatory conditions whose common element is a primary progressive degeneration and weakness of the striated musculature. The condition is of unknown etiology. These diseases are classified as myopathies. The following classification by Walton is commonly used.

- I. The "pure" muscular dystrophies:
    - A. Sex-linked muscular dystrophy
        1. Severe (Duchenne type)
        2. Benign (Becker type)
    - B. Autosomal recessive muscular dystrophy
        1. Limb-girdle types
        2. Childhood muscular dystrophy (except Duchenne)
        3. Congenital muscular dystrophies
    - C. Autosomal dominant facioscapulohumeral muscular dystrophy
    - D. Distal muscular dystrophy
    - E. Ocular muscular dystrophy
    - F. Oculopharyngeal muscular dystrophy
- II. Cases with myotonia:
    - A. Myotonia congenita
    - B. Dystrophia myotonia
    - C. Paramyotonia congenita

Progressive Patient Care (prō-gres′iv/pa′shent/kar) (n.) A method of organizing nursing services within a hospital. Patients are grouped into levels of inpatient care units according to degrees of illness—intensive, intermediate, and self-care.

Progressive Resistive Exercise (prō-gres′iv/rē-zis′ tiv/ek′ser-sīz) (n.) See **DeLorme Exercises.**

Progressive Spinal Muscular Atrophy (prō-gres′iv/ spī′nal/mus′kū-lar/at′rō-fē) (n.) See **Spinal Muscular Atrophy.**

Progressive Systemic Sclerosis (prō-gres′iv/sistem′ik/skle-rō′sis) (n.) A generalized disorder of connective tissue characterized by varying degrees of inflammation, fibrosis, degenerative changes, and vascular lesions in the skin and certain internal organs. The etiology is unknown, although an immune mechanism is suggested to play a role in the pathogenesis. The disease course is also extremely variable.

The term "scleroderma" is traditionally used to describe the cutaneous changes of progressive systemic sclerosis, which are a tightening and decreased elasticity of the skin. Although not as accurate a term for the entire spectrum of disease, scleroderma is often used as a synonym of systemic sclerosis. Abbreviated as PSS, it is also known as **Scleroderma, Diffuse Scleroderma,** and **Viscerocutaneous Collagenosis.**

Promontory (prom′on-to″rē) (n.) A projecting process or eminence. An example is **Sacral Promontory.**

Pronation (pro-na′shun) (n.) 1. The turning of the palm downward. 2. A combination of motions, including abduction and eversion of the foot and medial rotation of the ankle. Compare with **Supination.**

Pronator (pro-na′tor) (n.) Any muscle that causes pronation of the hand and forearm.

Pronator Syndrome (pro-na′tor/sin′drōm) (n.) A symptom-complex arising from entrapment of the

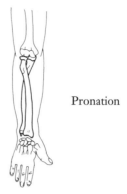

Pronation

median nerve in the proximal forearm. This entrapment can cause pain on the volar surface of the forearm. It is generally increased by activity and associated with reduced sensibility in the radial three-and-one-half digits. The wrist flexion test of Phalen is notably negative in this syndrome, and signs are not limited to the deep volar compartment of the forearm, specifically loss of active flexion of the DIP joint of the index finger or IP joint of the thumb.

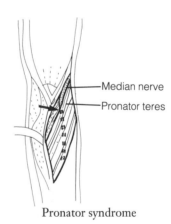

Median nerve
Pronator teres

Pronator syndrome

Prone (prōn) (adj.) 1. A position in which the palm of the hand faces downward. See **Pronation.** 2. A position of a patient lying face down. Compare with **Supine.**

Prophylactic Antibiotics (pro″fi-lak′tik/an″tĭ-biot′iks) (n.) The administration of antibiotics to prevent the development and reduce the development of tissue infection. The goals are to provide adequate antimicrobial concentrations in the tissues at risk and to maintain these levels throughout the period of operative and postoperative contamination.

Prophylaxis (pro″fi-lak′sis) (n.) The prevention of a condition or a disease.

Proportional Limit (prō-por′shun-al/lim′it) (n.) The point on a stress-strain curve before which stress is proportional to strain.

Proprioception (pro″prē-ō-sep′shun) (n.) The sensation of position and change of position of the body and its parts. Proprioception is transmitted through special organs, most of which are muscles, tendons, and joints.

Proprioceptive Reflex (pro″prē-ō-sep′tiv/rē′fleks) (n.) A reflex initiated by stimuli that arise from some function of the reflex mechanism itself. Reflex arising from proprioceptors in a muscle or a tendon.

Pro Re Nata (pro/re/na′tah) (n.) The Latin term "according to circumstances" or as needed, as necessary. Abbreviated **PRN**.

Prosect (prō-sekt′) (v.) Prepare by dissecting a cadaver specimen for later instruction.

Prosector (prō′-sek ter) (n.) A person who prepares the anatomic material for class instruction.

Prostaglandins (pros″tah-glan′dins) (n.) A group of physiologically active substances that are prostanoic acids with side-chains of varying degrees of oxidation and dehydration. The biologic properties vary according to the structure and location and include vasodilatation and constriction, contraction or relaxation of smooth and cardiac muscle, water and salt diuresis, fever production, and wheal and flare skin reactions. Often abbreviated PGE, PGF, PGA, and PGB, with numerical subscripts to describe the structure.

Prosthesis (pros-thē′sis) (n.) The addition to the body of an artificial part, such as a leg, an arm, a denture, or an eye, that substitutes for a missing biologic part. Includes replacements for various joints, ligaments, and sometimes whole or parts of bones.

Prosthetics (pros-thet′iks) (n.) The field of knowledge relating to the design, fabrication, and application of prostheses.

Prosthetist (pros′the-tist) (n.) A person skilled in prosthetics and its application.

Protease (prō′tē-ās) (n.) Enzyme that hydrolyzes peptide bonds in either proteins or peptides. Synonym: **Proteinase**.

Protective Isolation (prō-tek′tiv/ī″sō-lā′shun)(n.) A category established to minimize contact between pathogens and patients whose resistance has been seriously impaired owing to some underlying disease or condition. This also refers to practices used to maintain such isolation.

Protein (pro′tēn) (n.) A complex organic compound of high molecular weight, composed of one or more polypeptide chains, each made up of many amino acids joined by peptide bonds.

Proteoglycan (prō″tē-ō-glī′kan) (n.) A complex macromolecule found in cartilage and bone. These molecules are composed of a core protein to which glycosamino–glycan chains are attached. The proteoglycan monomers then form aggregates by a link protein attachment to a single hyaluronic acid chain.

Proteolytic Enzyme (prō″tē-ō-lit′ik/en′zīm) (n.) An enzyme whose main catalytic function is the cleavage and digestion of a protein or polypeptide chain. The digestive enzymes trypsin, pepsin, and carboxypeptidase are proteolytic enzymes.

Proteus (prō′tē-us) (n.) A genus of gram-negative rods within the family Enterobacteriaceae.

Prothrombin (prō-throm′bin) (n.) A constituent of blood plasma. Prothrombin is converted to thrombin by thrombokinase when calcium ions are present; it is therefore an important factor in the blood clotting mechanism.

Protoplasm (prō′tō-plazm) (n.) The living matter of a cell. This usually refers to the complex of organic and inorganic substances within a cell.

Protrusio Acetabuli (prō-trū′zē-ō/as″e-tab′u-lī) (n.) A radiographic description of an intrapelvic protrusion of the acetabulum by the femoral head A bilateral idiopathic protrusion is called an **Otto Pelvis**. Also known as **Arthrokatadysis**.

Protrusion of Intervertebral Disks (prō-trū′zhun/of/in″ter′ver′tĕ-bral/disks) (n.) See **Herniated Nucleus Pulposus**.

Protuberance (prō-tū″ber-ans) (n.) A projecting part, hump, or prominence.

Provider (prō′vī-der) (n.) A general term for a practitioner, such as a physician or a dentist, who has primary responsibility for assessing the condition of a patient, exercising independent judgment as to the care of this patient, and rendering services to this patient.

Proximal (prok′si-mal) (adj.) Situated near the point of reference. In anatomy, this is usually the main part of the body or the joint of attachment of an extremity. Opposite of **Distal**.

Proximal Femoral Focal Deficiency (prok′si-mal/fem′or-al/fō′kal/dē-fish′en-se) (n.) A congenital limb deficiency in which there is a localized absence of the proximal end of the femur, usually involving the hip joint. The deficiency is classified into four groups based on the radiographic appearance of the femur, the hip, and the acetabulum. Abbreviated **PFFD**.

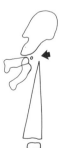

Proximal femoral focal deficiency

Proximal Interlocking Screw (prok′si-mal/in″ter-lok′ing/skrū) (n.) A screw placed through the proximal end of an interlocking intramedullary nail to fix it to the proximal fracture fragment.

Proximal Interphalangeal Joints (prok'si-mal/in″ter-fah-lan'jē-al/joints) (n.)   The diarthrodial joints located between the proximal and middle phalanges of the second through fifth fingers or toes. Abbreviated **PIP**.

Proximal Phalanx (prok'si-mal/fā'lanks) (n.)   A short tubular bone of a digit that articulates proximally with the metacarpal or metatarsal bone and distally with the distal phalanx of the thumb or great toe and the middle phalanx of the other fingers or toes.

Proximal Tibial Osteotomy (prok'si-mal/tib'ē-al/os″te-ot'ō-mē) (n.)   See **High Tibial Osteotomy**.

Proximal Tibiofibular Joint (prok'si-mal/tib″ē-ō/fib'u-lar/joint) (n.)   An arthrodial joint that lies between the fibular head and a posterolateral articular surface on the proximal tibia.

Pruritus (prū-rī'tus) (n.)   An itching sensation that provokes the desire to scratch. It may be localized, migratory, or generalized. The intensity of pruritus ranges from a mild to intermittent pricking or tingling sensation to a severe and constant irritation.

Pseudoarthrosis (sū″dō-ar-thrō'sis) (n.)   A false joint. This may occur as a result of nonunion of a fracture, or it may occur congenitally. The classic radiographic changes include sclerosis of the bone ends, sealing off of the marrow cavity by dense bone, and sclerotic marginal proliferation of bone that fails to bridge the fracture. See **Congenital Pseudoarthrosis**.

Pseudo (sū'dō)   Prefix meaning false.

Pseudobulbar Muscular Paralysis (sū″dō-bul'bar/mus'ku-lar/pah-ral'i-sis) (n.)   See **Duchenne's Dystrophy**.

Pseudofractures (sū″dō-frak'churs) (n.)   The radiographic finding of transverse, fissure-like defects that extend part way or completely through a bone. These defects are frequently seen in patients with osteomalacia. They present with focal collections of osteoid and are also known as **Looser's Zones**, **Milkman's Syndrome**, or **Umbauzonen**.

Pseudogout (sū'dō-gout) (n.)   A type of crystal-induced arthritis associated with the deposition of calcium pyrophosphate crystals in the synovium, fibrocartilage, and articular cartilage. These crystals are radiopaque, and appear on radiographs as a diffuse opacity in the soft tissues or as linear calcifications in the hyaline cartilage. The crystals are usually rhomboid and are weakly birefringent under polarized light. Synonyms: **Articular Chondrocalcinosis**, **Calcium Gout**, and **Calcium Pyrophosphate Deposition Disease**.

Pseudohypertrophic Infantile Muscular Dystrophy (sū″dō-hī″per-trōf'ik/in'fan-tīl/mus'ku-lar/dis'trō-fē) (n.)   See **Duchenne Muscular Dystrophy**.

Pseudohypoparathyroidism (sū″dō-hī″pō-par″ah-thī'roid-izm) (n.)   A metabolic disease in which the kidneys and bones are unresponsive to parathyroid hormone. The clinical picture mimics that of hypoparathyroidism, including hypocalcemia and hyperphosphatemia accompanied by parathyroid gland enlargement.

Pseudometatropic Dwarfism (sū″dō-met-ah-trof'ik/dwarf'izm) (n.)   See **Kniest Syndrome**.

Pseudomonas (sū″dō-mō'nas) (n.)   A genus of gram-negative rods from the family Pseudomonadaceae.

Pseudoparalysis (sū″dō-pah-ral'i-sis) (n.)   The apparent loss of muscular power without actual paralysis.

Pseudopseudohypoparathyroidism (sū″dō-sū″dō-hī″pō-par″ah-thī'roid-izm) (n.)   An incomplete form of pseudohypoparathyroidism. It is marked by the same constitutional features, but normal levels of calcium and phosphorus in the blood serum are present.

Pseudospondylolisthesis (sū″dō-spon″di-lō-lis'thē-sis) (n.)   See **Degenerative Spondylolisthesis**.

Pseudotumor (sū″dō-tū'mor) (n.)   A tumorlike mass that may develop in bone or in the soft tissues. These may be seen in patients with hemophilia as a result of hemorrhaging into the periosteum or bone. The masses also can be a tissue reaction to implanted materials such as polyethylene.

Psoas Abscess (sō'as/ab'ses) (n.)   Extraperitoneal abscess that follows the course of the iliopsoas muscle.

Psoas Muscle (sō'as/mus'el) (n.)   See **Muscle**.

Psoriatic Arthritis (sō″rē-at'ik/ar-thrī'tis) (n.)   An inflammatory joint disease seen in about 7% of patients with psoriasis. Three major groups have been identified. First, patients with an asymmetric peripheral polyarthritis, including those with classic involvement of the distal interphalangeal joints. Second, patients with arthritis mutilans and, often, with sacroiliac involvement. Finally, patients with arthritis that is indistinguishable from rheumatoid arthritis.

Psychologic Testing (sī″kō-loj'ik/test'ing) (n.)   The employment of various standardized techniques in which an individual responds either verbally or behaviorally to various commands. The manner in which he or she responds tends to reveal significant information about him or her not obtained through physical examination or an interview. Numerous tests and models are available.

Psychosomatic (sī″kō-sō-mat'ik) (adj.)   Influence of mind on body functions. Having bodily symptoms of psychic, mental, or emotional origin.

Psychomotor (sī″kō-mō'tor) (adj.)   Of or relating to motor action that directly precedes mental activity.

PTB (n.)   Abbreviation for patellar tendon bearing.

PTB Orthosis (PTB/or-thō'sis) (n.)   See **Patellar Tendon Bearing** and **Sarmiento Cast**.

Pterygium Colli (te-rij'e-um/kō'lī) (n.)   Extreme

webbing of the neck that consists of large skin folds extending from the mastoid to the acromion.

Pterygium Cubitale (te-rij′e-um/kū-bi-ta′lī) (n.) Congenital webbing of the elbow that consists of broad skin folds extending from the mid-arm to the forearm. The elbow is usually flexed to 90 degrees and extension is limited.

Pubic Spine (pū′bik/spīn) (n.) See **Pubic Tubercle**.

Pubic Symphysis (pū′bik/sim′fi-sis) (n.) The fibrocartilaginous junction of the pubic bones at the anterior midline. This is a synchondrosis in which a fibrocartilaginous disk is interposed between the articular surfaces of each pubic bone. Also called **Symphysis Pubis**.

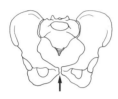

Pubic symphysis

Pubic Tubercle (pū′bik/tū′ber-k′l) (n.) A prominent bony point or spine on the upper border or crest of the body of the pubic bone to which the inguinal ligament is attached.

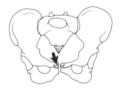

Pubic tubercle

Pubis (pū′bis) (n.) One of the three bones that forms the innominate bone. The pubis is composed of a body and an inferior and superior pubic ramus. Anteriorly, the bodies of the paired pubic bones unite to form the pubic symphysis.

Pugh Sliding Nail (pū/slīd′ing/nāl) (n.) A type of telescoping nail-plate device used in internal fixation of fractures about the hip.

Pulled Elbow (puld/el′bō) (n.) A term for the transient traumatic subluxation of the radial head that occurs in children between the ages of 2 and 6 years. The mechanism of injury is frequently the pulling of the child by an outstretched arm—thus the name. Also called **Nursemaid's Elbow**.

Pulled Muscle (puld/mus′el) (n.) A colloquial expression for a muscular strain.

Pulleys (pul′ēs) (n.) Discrete anatomic thickenings in the flexor tendon sheaths that play a role in preventing bowstinging of the tendons during flexion. The transversely running fibers are called annular pulleys or ligaments and are present over the phalangeal shafts. At the level of the joints, an obliquely criss-crossing fiber arrangement, called the cruciate ligaments or pulleys, is present.

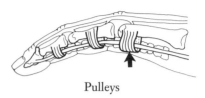

Pulleys

Pullout Suture (pul′out/su′chur) (n.) A technique of soft tissue fixation usually applied in the fixation of tendon or ligament to bone. The transfixing suture is tied over a button or an interposing material on top of the skin. A second wire or suture is placed at the opposite side and is used to pull out the internal suture when the external knot is cut after healing is complete.

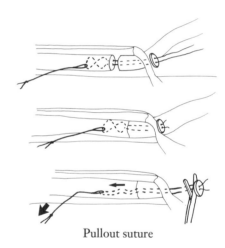

Pullout suture

Pulmonary Embolism (pul′mo-ner″ē/em′bō-lizm) (n.) A pathologic process in which blood clot or clots formed in the deep peripheral veins, usually of the pelvis or legs, break free and migrate to the pulmonary arterial tree. This may result in ventilation perfusion mismatch, hypoxemia, cor pulmonale, and sudden death.

Pulmonary Function Tests (pul′mo-ner″ē/funk′shun/tests) (n.) A series of physiologic tests used in the evaluation of lung capacity and function. Abbreviated **PFT**.

Pulsing Electromagnetic Field Treatment (puls′ing/e′lek″trō-mag′net′ik/fēld/trēt′ment) (n.) A noninvasive method used in delayed or nonunited fractures and failed arthrodeses in which pulsing electromagnetic fields generate weak electric currents in bone. The electromagnetic fields are either created by external coils on the body surface or are incorporated in a cast. The electric current is believed to induce osteogenesis. Abbreviated **PEMF**.

Pulvinar (pul-vī′nar) (n.) A soft, lobulated fibroadipose tissue that covers the nonarticular area of the acetabular socket. This may cushion the femoral head from the floor of the acetabulum.

Pump (pump) (n.) In shoe terminology, any shoe not built above the vamp and quarter lines that is held to the foot without fasteners.

Pump Bumps (pump/bumps) (n.) The tender bumps that develop because of irritation created by the rubbing of the superior tubercle of the os calcis region by a shoe. This is usually associated with pain and local tenderness.

Punch Biopsy (punch/bi′op-sē) (n.) A biopsy in which tissue is obtained by an instrument that directly pierces the body part and "punches out" a piece of tissue.

Punch Test (punch/test) (n.) An evaluation procedure in sciatica in which punching of the buttock produces a referred pain in the back.

Puncture Wound (pungk′chur′wūnd) (n.) 1. A laceration in which the external skin injury is minimal compared to the depth of the wound. The injury may be caused by stepping on a sharp object such as a nail, needle, or thorn. 2. A small surgical portal, as in percutaneous pinning or arthroscopy.

Pure Culture (pūr/kūl′chur) (n.) A culture containing only one species of organism.

Purine (pū′rin) (n.) A chemical compound from which naturally occurring purine bases are formed. Three types of purines exist: aminopurines, oxypurines, and methylpurines. The aminopurines are a component of nucleotides and nucleic acids and are precursors of uric acid.

Purpura (pur′pū-rah) (n.) A condition characterized by the extravasation of blood into skin, mucous membranes, or internal organs that appears as red to dark purple areas. Several types of purpura are recognized: petechiae, hemorrhagic macules less than 3 mm in diameter; ecchymoses, macules larger than 3 mm with deeper, more extensive hemorrhage and a bluish purple color; and hematomata, large, fluctuant hemorrhages.

Purulent (pū′rū-lent) (adj.) Forming or containing pus.

Pus (pus) (n.) The fluid product of an infectious process. It contains serum, bacteria, necrotic cells, and leukocytes.

Pustule (pus′tūl) (n.) A pus-filled vesicle.

Putnam's Sign (put′nams/sīn) (n.) The apparent lengthening of a limb in cases of hysterical hip disease. The patient holds the limb in abduction, which causes the opposite leg to appear relatively longer.

Putrefaction (pū″tre-fak′shun) (n.) The enzymatic decomposition of proteins by microorganisms associated with the production of foul-smelling compounds.

Putti-Platt Procedure (pū′-tē/plat/prō-sē-jur) (n.) Surgical correction of recurrent anterior dislocation of the shoulder. It entails the reefing of the anterior capsule and subscapularis tendon. This repair usually limits external rotation of the shoulder.

Putti's Triad (pū′-tēz/trī-ad) (n.) A term used for the triad of radiographic findings in congenital dislocation of the hip. These include lateral and superior migration of the femoral head; hypoplasia or absence of the proximal femoral ossification center; and increased declivity of the acetabular roof toward the longitudinal axis of the body.

PWB (adj.) Abbreviation for partial weight-bearing.

Pyarthrosis (pī″ar-thrō′sis) (n.) 1. Suppurative arthritis. 2. Infection in a joint. Synonym: **Septic Arthritis**.

Pyknodysostosis (pik″nō-dis″ōs-tō′sis) (n.) A rare and relatively benign osteosclerotic condition characterized by short stature and a peculiar facies, consisting of bossing of the frontal bones and a shallow, obtuse mandibular angle. Radiographically, the bones are sclerotic, without loss of medullarization. There is hypoplasia of the paranasal sinuses, and radiographs of the hand show absent ungual tufts. Laboratory investigations are normal. The disease is inherited in an autosomal recessive manner. Also known as **Osteopetrosis Acroosteolytica**.

Pyle's Disease (pīlz/di-zēz′) (n.) Craniometaphyseal dysplasia. A congenital hyperostosis of the cranial and facial bones that compresses the cranial nerves.

Pylon (pi′lon) (n.) A temporary prosthetic replacement for an amputated lower limb.

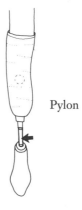

Pylon

Pyo (pī′o) A prefix denoting suppuration.

Pyogenic (pī″o-jen′ik) (adj.) Pus producing.

Pyogenic Granuloma (pī″o-jen′ik/gran″u-lō′mah) (n.) A skin lesion usually found on the dorsum of digits; it is composed of heaped-up granulation tissue and a vascular base that gives it a tendency to bleed easily. There may be a previous history of trauma or infection.

Pyomyositis (pī″ō-mī″ō-sī′tis) (n.)   Purulent infections of skeletal muscle.

Pyramidal Cell (pi-ram′i-dal/sel) (n.)   A type of neuron found in the cerebral cortex.

Pyramidal Tract (pi-ram′i-dal/trakt) (n.)   A bundle of nerve fibers that originate from pyramidal cells in the cerebral motor cortex and travel distally in the dorsal half of the lateral funiculus of the spinal cord. Also known as the **Corticospinal Tract**.

Pyrexia (pī-rek′sē-ah) (n.)   A fever or febrile condition.

Pyridoxine (pēr″i-dok′sēn) (n.)   Vitamin B_6.

Pyriformis Syndrome (pēr′i-form-is/sin′drōm) (n.)   Pain in the buttock that radiates down the lower limb and is caused by sciatic nerve irritation due to spasm in or a contracture of the pyriformis muscle. Tendinitis of the pyriformis muscle.

Pyrimidine (pi-rim′i-dēn) (n.)   A heterocyclic nitrogen-containing substance from which is derived nitrogen bases such as cytosine, thymine, and uracil. These are components of nucleotides and nucleic acids.

Pyrophosphate Arthropathy (pī″rō-fos′fāt/ar′thro-plas″tē) (n.)   See **Pseudogout**.

Pyuria (pī-ū′rē-ah) (n.)   Pus in the urine.

Q

Q Angle (Q/ang′-ğl) (n.)   See **Quadriceps Angle**.

QID   Abbreviation for the Latin, Quarter In Die, i.e., four times a day; used in writing prescriptions. Also written as 4×/day.

Quad Atrophy (kwod/at′-rō-fē) (n.)   Abbreviated term for quadriceps muscle atrophy.

Quad Cane (kwod/Kān) (n.)   Colloquialism for quadripod, four-point, or four-legged cane.

Quadrangular Space (kwod′-drang′-yū-lar/spās) (n.)   An anatomic space in the shoulder region through which the axillary nerve and the posterior humeral circumflex vessels pass around the proximal humeral shaft. This space is bordered by the teres major muscle (inferiorly), the teres minor muscle (superiorly) and the subscapularis muscle (anteriorly) superiorly, the humerus (laterally), and the long head of the triceps muscle (medially).

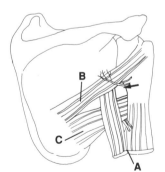

Quadrangular space.
A, Long head of triceps;
B, Teres minor;
C, Teres major.

Quadrate Ligament (kwod′-drāt/lig′-ah-ment) (n.)   A ligamentous structure that extends between the neck of the radius and the inferior border of the radial notch. It reinforces the stability of the proximal radioulnar joint.

Quadriceps (kwod′rĭ-seps) (n.)   Having four heads. Example: **Quadriceps Femoris Muscle**.

Quadriceps Angle (kwod′-dri-seps/ang′-ğ′l) (n.)   The angle formed by the patellar tendon and the axis of the pull of the quadriceps muscle. A clinical measurement describing the plane of the patellar force system; it is measured as the angle formed between a line drawn from the anterior superior iliac spine to the tibial tuberosity. The knee should be flexed less than or equal to 20 degrees. The normal quadriceps angle is approximately 15 degrees. An angle greater than 20 degrees is considered abnormal. Synonym: **Q Angle**.

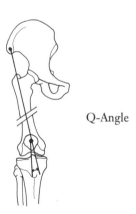

Q-Angle

Quadriceps Contusion (kwod′-dri-seps/kon-too̅′-zhun) (n.)   An injury of the quadriceps muscle produced by an external force sufficient to damage the muscle. It is characterized by a spectrum of symptoms depending on the severity of the blow. This condition may be complicated by the development of traumatic myositis ossificans.

Quadriceps Dysplasia (kwod′-dri-seps/dis-plā′se-ah) (n.)   A clinical term used in the past to describe patellar tracking abnormalities that occurred without obvious patellar malposition. Today, this term is accurately applied in cases of dysplasia of the vastus medialis muscle or abnormal attachments of the vastus lateralis muscle, which do create dynamic patellar maltracking.

Quadriceps Femoris Muscle (kwod'-dri-seps/fem'-or-is/mus'el) (n.) The anterior thigh musculature that is actually four separate muscles grouped together—the rectus femoris, the vastus medialis, the vastus lateralis, and the vastus intermedialis muscles. See **Muscle**.

Quadriceps Reflex (kwod'-dri-seps/rē'-fleks) (n.) A muscle stretch reflex characterized by contraction of the quadriceps femoris muscle, with resulting extension of the leg, in response to a stimulus directed toward the patellar tendon. Synonyms: **Knee jerk**, **patellar tendon reflex**. See **Patellar Tendon Reflex**.

Quadriceps Tendon (kwod'-dri-seps/ten'-dun) (n.) The tendinous common insertion of the quadriceps femoris muscles into the superior pole of the patella.

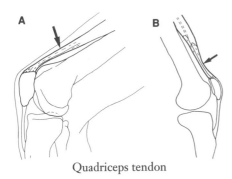

Quadriceps tendon

Quadricepsplasty (kwod-dri-seps'plas-tē) (n.) A surgical procedure intended to release fibrosis or adhesions that have created quadriceps muscle contracture and loss of knee flexion.

Quadriplegia (kwod'-dri-plē-jē-a) (n.) Paralysis affecting all four limbs. Also known as **Tetraplegia**.

Quadripod Cane (kwod'-dri-pŏd/kān) (n.) See **Quad Cane**.

Quadruple Complex (kwod'-roo-pel/kom'-pleks) (n.) A term used by Kaplan to describe four structures that provide stability to the lateral aspect of the knee. This includes the iliotibial tract, the biceps muscle, the lateral collateral ligament, and the popliteus tendon.

Quarter (kwawr'ter) (n.) In shoe terminology, the posterior or back part of the uppers.

Queckenstedt Test (kwek'-en-stet"/test) (n.) An invasive clinical procedure used to evaluate the subarachnoid space. During a lumbar puncture, if the internal jugular vein on one or both sides is compressed, there is normally a rapid rise in cerebrospinal fluid pressure. When digital compression of the vein is released, the rise in pressure disappears. If no pressure change registers on the lumbar manometer upon jugular compression, a subarachnoid block is present between the cerebral ventricles and the lumbar puncture site.

Quengel Cast (kweng'l/kast) (n.) A plaster device designed for correcting severe knee flexion contractures. The cast uses special offset subluxation hinges that correct the tibial subluxation and a toggle stick that permits windlass correction of the flexion deformity.

Quervain's Disease (kār'vanz/dĭ-zez') (n.) See **De Quervain Disease**.

Quigley Traction (kwig'-lē/trak'-shun) (n.) A form of skin traction used in the treatment of ankle injuries. The lower extremity is suspended in a stockinette connected to an overhead pulley system with a thigh sling. The foot will assume a position of internal rotation and adduction, causing ankle inversion. Thus, this traction system will help reduce fractures or fracture-dislocations from eversion injuries. It is also helpful in controlling edema by suspension of the lower extremity in an elevated position.

R

RA Abbreviation for Rheumatoid Arthritis.

RA Factor (RA/fak'tor) (n.) Rheumatoid factor.

Rachi (rā-kē) Prefix pertaining to the spine.

Rachialgia (rā"kē-al'je-ah) (n.) Pain in the spine.

Rachio (rā'kē-ō) (n.) Relation to the spine. Also see **Spondylo**.

Rachiometer (rā"kē-om'e-ter) (n.) An apparatus for measuring spinal curvature.

Rachischisis (rā-kis'ki-sis) (n.) See **Spina Bifida**.

Rachitic (ra-kit'ik) (n.) Pertaining to rickets.

Rad (rad) (n.) Acronym for Radiation Absorbed Dose. It represents a unit of absorbed dose of ionizing radiation equal to 100 ergs per gram of matter. Abbreviated as **R**.

Radial Angle (ra'dē-al/ang'g'l) (n.) A measurement made on a radiograph of the wrist that evaluates the relationship of the distal radial articular surface to the shaft of the radius. On a lateral projection, there is a normal volar or palmar tilt of 12 degrees. To ensure accuracy, a radiograph of the injured wrist should be compared with a radiograph of the normal opposite wrist. Compare to **Dorsal Angle**.

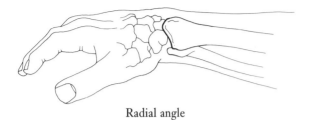

Radial angle

Radial Artery (rā'dē-al/ar'ter-ē) (n.)   A terminal branch of the brachial artery that begins at the elbow.

Radial Bursae (rā'dē-al/ber'sē) (n.)   A common name for the synovial sheath of the flexor pollicis longus tendon, which is found along the lateral aspect of the wrist and palm.

Radial Clubhand (rā'dē-al/klub'hand) (n.)   A congenital anomaly in which there is partial or total absence of the radius. The hand is radially deviated, the forearm is shortened, and usually the wrist is unstable. There may be associated skeletal changes that involve other bones in the upper extremity.

Radial Deviation (rā'dē-al/dē"vē-ā'shun) (n.)   1. Refers to the positioning of the hand relative to the wrist in which the hand is directed radially. Compare to **Ulnar Deviation**. 2. Any abnormal angulation of the carpus or digits in a radial or lateral direction.

Radial Drift (rā'dē-al/drift) (n.)   A condition in which the metacarpals deviate radially. Most commonly seen in rheumatoid arthritis.

Radial Head (rā'dē-al/hed) (n.)   The proximal articular portion of the radius that articulates with the capitulum of the humerus.

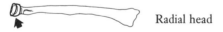

Radial head

Radial Neck (rā'dē-al/nek) (n.)   The constricted area of the proximal radius just distal to the radial head.

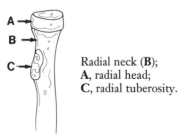

Radial neck (**B**);
A, radial head;
C, radial tuberosity.

Radial Nerve (rā'dē-al/nerv) (n.)   The largest branch of the brachial plexus. It is the main continuation of the posterior cord and is formed by contributors from the C5, C6, C7, C8, and T1 nerve roots.

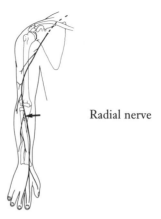

Radial nerve

Radial Reflex (rā'dē-al/rē'fleks) (n.)   A normal muscle stretch reflex elicited by tapping over the distal radius. This tapping causes contraction of the brachioradialis muscle, which results in radial extension of the wrist. Also known as the **Brachioradialis Reflex**.

Radial Shift (ra'de-al/shift) (n.)   An abnormal lateral deviation of the distal radius. The distance between the long axis of the radius and the most radial point of the styloid process is measured on an AP radiograph of the forearm and wrist. This is then compared with an AP radiograph of the normal arm; a radial shift is present if this distance is increased.

Radial Styloid (ra'de-al/sti'loid) (n.)   The terminal bony projection at the distal, lateral end of the radius.

Radial Tear (ra'-de-al/tār) (n.)   See **Meniscal Radial Tear**.

Radial Tubercle (rā'dē-al/too'ber-k'l) (n.)   See **Lister's Tubercle**.

Radial Tuberosity (rā'dē-al/too"br-eos'i-tē) (n.)   An oval prominence just distal to the radial neck that has a roughened area used for the insertion of the biceps brachii tendon. Also known as the **Bicipital Tuberosity**.

Radial Tunnel Syndrome (rā'dē-al/tun'el/sin'drōm) (n.)   A compression neuropathy of the radial nerve in the proximal forearm in which the nerve gets caught between the two heads of supinator muscle.

Radiate Ligament (rā'dē-āt/lig'ah-ment) (n.)   Refers to a fan-shaped ligament that connects the head of a rib with a vertebra and the associated intervertebral disk.

Radiation (rā-dē-ā'shun) (n.)   The process by which the nucleus of an unstable particle emits particles and energy during the process of decay, thereby creating a more stable element.

Radiation Absorbed Dose (rā-dē-ā'shun/ab-sorb'd/dōs) (n.)   See **Rad**.

Radiation Therapy (rā-dē-ā'shun/ther'ah-pē) (n.)   The use of radiation of any type in the treatment of disease.

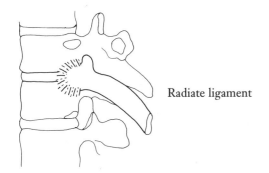

Radiate ligament

Radical Excision (rad′i-kal/ek-sizh′un) (n.) In defining surgical margins for tumor resection a radical excision indicates removal of not just the tumor but the entire compartment involved.

Radicular (rah′dik′ū-lar) (adj.) Pertaining to a root or radicle.

Radicular Pain (rah′dik′ū-lar/pān) (n.) Pain from radiculitis colloquially known as a "pinched nerve."

Radiculitis (rah-dik″ū-lī′tis) (n.) Inflammation of a spinal nerve in the spinal canal or neural canal.

Radiculopathy (rah-dik″ū-lop′ah-thē) (n.) 1. A noninflammatory abnormality of a spinal nerve in the spinal canal or neural foramen, which results in a neurologic deficit. 2. A sensory and/or motor abnormality that follows the distribution of a specific nerve root and is secondary to the irritation of that root. Sensory changes include hyperesthesiae, paraesthesiae (eg, tingling, numbness), or sensory loss. Motor changes include reflex loss, weakness, atrophy, or fasiculation. Factors that further irritate the nerve root (eg, coughing, straining, Valsalva's maneuver, or maneuvers designed to stretch the nerve) may intensify the pain and may be associated with distal radiation of the pain.

Radioactive (rā″dē-ō-ak′tiv) (adj.) The property of disintegration of certain nuclides that emit radiation.

Radioactive Isotope (rā″dē-ō-ak′tiv/i′sō-tōp) (n.) An unstable isotope of an element that decays or disintegrates spontaneously, emitting radiation. Some radioactive elements, such as radium, occur in nature; others are manufactured. In the process of degeneration, a radioactive isotope may either form another radioactive isotope or decompose immediately into a stable atom.

Radioactive Tracers (rā″dē-ō-ak′tiv/trās′erz) (n.) Compounds or cells that contain radioactive isotopes that are injected intravenously and then localized to specific bony sites. These sites can then be detected by external scanning.

Radioactivity (rā″dē-ō-ak-tiv′i-tē) (n.) The spontaneous decay or disintegration of an unstable atomic nucleus. This is usually accompanied by the emission of ionizing radiation.

Radioimmunoassay (rā″dē-ō-im″ū-nō-as′ā) (n.) A laboratory technique used to detect a radioisotope-labeled antigen, hormone, or other substance that may have had an immunologic reaction with the sample being tested.

Radiopharmaceutical (rā″dē-o-fahr″mah-su′tĭ-kal) (n.) A radionuclide or a radioactively tagged drug or compound administered to a patient for diagnostic or therapeutic purposes.

Radioisotope (rā″dē-ō-i′sō-tōp) (n.) See **Radioactive Isotope**.

Radioisotope Scanning (rā″dē-ō-i′sō-tōp/skan′ning) (n.) The production of a two-dimensional record of the emissions of a radioactive isotope that has been concentrated in a specific organ or tissue of the body, e.g., the thyroid gland, the liver, the spleen, or the bone. Radioactive tracers are used for localization. This process is also known as **Scintigraphy**.

Radiologist (rā″dē-ol′ō-jist) (n.) A physician who specializes in radiology.

Radiology (rā″dē-ol′ō-jē) (n.) The branch of medical science that deals with the use of x-rays, radioactive substances, and other forms of radiant energy in the diagnosis and treatment of disease. Also called **Diagnostic Imaging**.

Radiolucent (rā″dē-ō-lū′sent) (adj.) A descriptive term indicating either the permeability or actual passage of an x-ray through a structure on other radiant waves or energy. These areas appear dark on the exposed radiographic film. Compare with **Radiopaque**.

Radionecrosis (rā″dē-ō-ne-krō′sis) (n.) Tissue destruction that is due to exposure to radiation.

Radioneuritis (rā″dē-ō-nu-rī′tis) (n.) Inflammation of a nerve that is due to exposure to radiant energy.

Radiopacity (rā″dē-ō-pas′i-tē) (n.) The degree to which a part is impermeable to x-rays.

Radiopaque (rā″dē-ō-pāk′) (adj.) A descriptive term characterizing the impermeability of a structure to x-rays or other radiant energy or waves. On a radiograph, the opaque areas appear light or white on the exposed films. Radiopaque materials are often used as contrast media in radiologic studies. Compare with **Radiolucent**.

Radiosensitivity (rā″dē-ō-sen″si-tiv′i-tē) (n.) The relative susceptibility of cells, tissues, organs, organisms, or other substances to the injurious action of radiation.

Radiotherapy (rā″dē-ō-ther′ah-pē) (n.) The treatment of cancer and other disease with penetrating radiation. Beams of radiation are directed at a diseased part from a distance, or radioactive material in the form of needles, wires, or pellets is implanted in the body.

Radioulnar Synostosis (rā″dē-ō-ul′nar/sin″os-tō′sis) (n.) A condition in which there is fusion of the radius and the ulna in the forearm. This may be a congenital anomaly, or it may occur posttraumatically or postoperatively. Usually occurs in the proximal portion of the forearm. There is no rotation of the forearm, although there may be full flexion and extension of the elbow.

Ram's Hornnail (ramz/horn-nāl) (n.)   A fingernail or a toenail that is enlarged and increased in curvature. Synonym: **Onychogryposis**.

Ramus (rā′mus) (n.)   1. A branch; often used to refer to a major division of a vessel or a nerve. 2. A slender process of bone that projects from the main part of that bone at an angle. An example of this is the pubic ramus.

Ranawat's Triangle (rahn-a-watz/trī′ang-ǵ′l) (n.)   A method developed to locate the correct anatomic position of the acetabulum in deformed hips. On an AP roentgenogram of the pelvis, parallel horizontal lines are drawn at the level of the iliac crests and the ischial tuberosities. These lines are connected by a perpendicular line passing through a point (A), located 5 mm lateral to the intersection of Köhler's and Shenton's lines. The length of the perpendicular line between the parallel lines is equal to the height of the pelvis; one fifth of the line equals the height of the acetabulum. A second point (B) is located on the perpendicular superior to point (A) at a distance equal to one fifth of the perpendicular line. From B, a perpendicular line is drawn laterally to point C, so that distance B–C equals distance A–B. Joining points A and C completes the isosceles triangle; this indicates the correct position of the acetabulum to be reconstructed. In a normal hip, the superior border of the triangle passes through the superior aspect of the subchondral bone of the acetabulum; the hypotenuse is the roof of the acetabulum. In a deformed hip, the extent of the protrusion deformity can be measured in an axial direction by inward movement of the acetabulum beyond Kohler's line and superiorly by upward movement beyond the superior aspect of the subchondral bone of the acetabulum that was determined by the construction of the triangle.

Range of Motion (rānj/of/mō′shun) (n.)   The area through which a joint may be moved in all planes. This is quantified in degrees and is qualified as either passive or active. The neutral starting position is defined as 0 degrees.

Raphe (rā′fē) (n.)   1. A seam. 2. In anatomic terms, the line of union of the halves of various symmetrical parts.

Rarefaction (rār″e-fak′shun) (n.)   The thinning of bony tissue that can cause a decreased density to x-rays.

Rasp (rasp) (n.)   A file-like surgical instrument used for scraping and smoothing the surface of bone.

Ray (rā) (n.)   The combination of a metatarsal or metacarpal bone and its corresponding phalanges.

Ray Amputation (rā/am″pu-tā′shun) (n.)   An amputation procedure in which the entire metacarpal or metacarpal bone and its corresponding phalanges are ablated.

Raynaud's Phenomenon (rā-nōz/fe-nom′e-non) (n.)   A vasoconstrictive disorder in which lability of the sympathetic nervous system causes episodes of cutaneous cyanosis and coldness felt as numbness and pain in the fingers. The attacks are often precipitated by exposure to cold. The sign of extreme pallor followed by cyanosis can be reproduced by immersion of the hand in cold water. On rewarming, a reactive hyperemia occurs. This phenomenon may occur primarily, in which case it is called **Raynaud Disease**, or it may be associated with other disorders, such as scleroderma.

Razorback Deformity (rā′zer-bak/de-for′mi-tē) (n.)   A severe rib prominence associated with thoracic scoliotic curves.

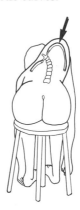

Razorback deformity

Reactive Arthritis (rē-ak′tiv/ar-thrī′tis) (n.)   A sterile, nonspecific synovitis seen in association with an infection distant from the joint, such as a systemic infection. Reactive arthritis usually occurs after a latent period of variable length. Characteristically, rheumatoid factor is absent from serum and synovial fluid. A classic example of reactive arthritis is the polyarthritis seen in patients with rheumatic fever. Other arthropathies usually regarded as reactive are those that follow infection with *Yersinia enterocolitica* (serotypes 3 and 9), *Salmonella enteritidis*, *Shigella flexneri*, *brucella*, *campylobacter*, and *chlamydia*. See **Seronegative Arthropathy**.

Reamer (rē′mer) (n.)   A surgical instrument used to gouge out holes or to enlarge those already made.

Receptor (rē-sep′tor) (n.)   1. A chemical grouping capable of combining specifically with antigen that resides on the surface of an immunologically competent cell. 2. A sensory nerve ending that responds to various stimuli.

Recessive (rē-ses′iv) (n.)   A gene whose phenotypic expression, masked by a dominant allele, is manifest only in the homozygous condition.

Reconstruction (rē″kon-struk′shun) (n.)   In orthopaedics, the surgical recreation of previously damaged structures by incorporating tissues other than those being reconstructed.

Recrudescence (rē″krū-des′ens) (n.)   A recurrence of a disorder after a temporary abatement. A recrudescence occurs after several days or weeks; a relapse, after weeks or months.

Rectus (rek′tus) (adj.)   Straight.

Rectus Abdominus Muscle (rek′tus/ab-dom′i-nus/mus′el) (n.)   See **Muscle**.

Rectus Femoris Muscle (rek′tus/fem′o-ris/mus′el) (n.)   See **Muscle**.

Recumbent Position (rē-kum′bent/po-sizh′un) (n.)   The body position of lying down on a horizontal surface.

Recurrent (rē-kur′ent) (adj.)   1. The return of a disorder or disease after a remission. 2. In anatomic terms, a structure, such as a blood vessel or nerve, that turns back on its course, forming a loop.

Recurvatum (re″kur-va′tum) (n.)   A backward bending or curvature of a joint. This usually describes a position of hyperextension. Recurvatum of the knee refers to hyperextension of the joint.

Reduction (rē-duk′shun) (n.)   In orthopaedics, the correction or restoration of fracture fragments or a joint dislocation or subluxation to normal anatomic relationships.

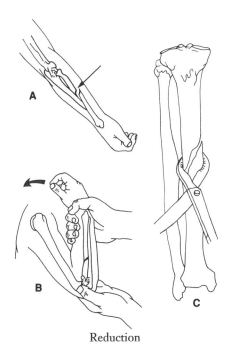

Reduction

Reefing (rēf′ing) (n.)   A surgical technique for the repair of slack or redundant soft tissues in which the tissues are folded and sutured in place.

Reeling Gait (rēl′ing/gāt) (n.)   A walk characterized by staggering or swaying from one side to the other. It is often seen in intoxicated subjects.

Referred Pain (rē′ferd/pān) (n.)   Pain perceived in an area remote from the organ of origin. This usually occurs because the injured or diseased organ and the area to which the pain is referred have a common neural pathway.

Reflex (rē′fleks) (n.)   An involuntary motor response to sensory stimuli. This includes muscle stretch reflexes, superficial reflexes, pyramidal tract responses, reflexes of spinal automatism, and postural and righting reflexes.

Reflex Arc (rē′fleks/ark) (n.)   The simplest functional unit of the nervous system capable of detecting change and causing a response to that change. A reflex arc always has five basic parts: (1) a receptor to detect change, (2) an afferent neuron to conduct the impulse that results from stimulation of the receptor to the central nervous system, (3) a synapse where a junction is made between neurons, (4) an efferent neuron to conduct impulses for appropriate response to an organ, and (5) an effector or organ that demonstrates response to the detected change.

Reflex Sympathetic Dystrophy (rē′fleks/sim″pah-thet′ik/dis′tro-fē) (n.)   A clinical disorder characterized by the presence of pain, hyperesthesia, and tenderness in the affected extremity. The pathogenetic relationship to the autonomic nervous system is unclear. Precipitating factors include trauma, either accidental or surgical, and a variety of disease states. The early changes include constant, burning pain that is out of proportion to the severity of the related injury. In later stages, dystrophic changes in the joints, soft tissues, and skin take place. Finally, progressive atrophic changes of skin, muscle, and joint may occur and may be irreversible. Radiographic changes of diffuse osteoporosis and characteristic areas of spotty rarefaction may be seen in the later stages. Abbreviated as RSD, this disorder is also known as **Posttraumatic Dystrophy**, **Reflex Dystrophy**, and **Sudeck Atrophy**. See the related disorders **Causalgia** and **Shoulder-Hand Syndrome**.

Refractory Period (rē-frak′to-rē/pe′rē-od) (n.)   The brief interval following the response of a neuron or muscle fiber during which it is incapable of a second response.

Refsum's Disease (ref′sūmz/di-zēz′) (n.)   A progressive, hypertrophic neuropathy associated with retinitis pigmentosa, ataxia, and areflexia. It is inherited as an autosomal recessive disorder, begins in childhood or puberty, and has a poor prognosis.

Regeneration (rejen″er-a′shun) (n.)   The regrowth of lost or injured parts of an organism.

Regional Anesthesia (re′jun-al/an″es-thē′zē-ah) (n.)   The anesthesia of a region of the body produced by injection of an anesthetic solution into and around the nerves that supply the area with sensation. Injection may be made at a distance from the site of operation.

Regular Cane (reg'u-lar/kān) (n.) A straight cane with curved handle; the most common type of cane.

Rehabilitation (rē″ha-bil″i-tā′shun) (n.) 1. The restoration of a handicapped individual to the fullest physical, mental, social, vocational, and economic usefulness of which he or she is capable. 2. Through various means and modalities, the process of restoring a person's ability to live and work as normally as possible after a disabling injury or illness.

Reimplantation (rē″im-plan-tā′shun) (n.) Replacement of tissue or a structure into the site from which it was previously lost or removed.

Reinfection (rē″in-fek′shun) (n.) A recurrent infection caused by the same etiologic agent.

Reinforcement (rē″in-fors′ment) (n.) A technique used in neurologic examination that increases the amplitude of a reflex by having the patient perform some related action during elicitation of a reflex. See **Jandrusik Maneuver**.

Reinnervation (rē″in-er-vā′shun) (n.) The restoration of the nerve supply to an organ or muscle by surgical grafting or the regeneration of nerve fibers after injury or repair.

Reiter's Syndrome (rē′terz/sin′drōm) (n.) A rheumatic syndrome that classically consists of the triad of conjunctivitis, nonspecific urethritis, and polyarthritis; other characteristic findings include keratodermia blennorrhagica, balanitis circinata, and mucosal ulceration. This syndrome usually affects young adult males; its etiology is not known, but a genetic predisposition has been suspected. Seventy-five percent of affected patients have a positive HLA-B27 histocompatibility antigen. Synonyms: **Fiessinger-Leroy Syndrome**, **Conjunctivourethrosynovial Syndrome**, **Blennorrheal Idiopathic Arthritis**, **Arthritis Urethritica**, **Venereal Arthritis**, and **Polyarthritis Enterica**.

Relafen (rela′fen) (n.) A proprietary name for Nabumetone, a nonsteroidal, anti-inflammatory drug.

Relaxant (rē-lak′sant) (n.) An agent that causes muscle relaxation.

Release (rē-lēs′) (n.) The setting free of tissues. Most commonly used in reference to the moment when the origins or insertions of soft tissues are surgically freed.

REM (rem) (n.) Acronym for **Roentgen Equivalent Man**. This is the amount of absorbed radiation capable of causing as much damage in human tissue as one roentgen of x-rays.

Remineralization (re-min″er-al-i-zā′shun) (n.) The restoration of mineral elements to a structure; an example is the deposition of calcium salts in bone.

Remission (rē-mish′un) (n.) A period of diminution or abatement of the symptoms of a disease.

Renal Osteodystrophy (rē′nal/os″te-ō-dis′tro-fē) (n.) The skeletal changes seen in and associated with chronic renal failure. One sees a variety of radiographic changes that result from the effects of parathyroid hormone, impairment of vitamin D production, and serum calcium and phosphate abnormalities. The changes include osteitis fibrosa cystica, osteomalacia, osteosclerosis, and generalized osteopenia.

Rennie Sign (ren′ē/sīn) (n.) A radiographic marker indicative of a slipped capital femoral epiphysis. In a lateral radiograph of the hip, there is a relative shortening of the posterior portion of the femoral neck as compared with the anterior portion. An index of this shortening may be obtained by measuring the "angle of tilt." Draw a line passing through the apices of the anterior and posterior corners of the metaphysis. Draw another line perpendicular to the rectilinear shadow cast by the front of the femoral neck. The average angle in normal children is 10 degrees. The average angle in slipped epiphysis is 30 degrees.

Replantation (rē″plan-tā′shun) (n.) The restoration of an organ or other body structure to its original site.

Reposition (rē″pō-zish′un) (n.) The return of an abnormally placed part, organ, or fragment to its proper position.

Res Ipsa Loquitor (res′/ipsa′/lō-kwi-tor′) (n.) The Latin phrase for "the thing speaks for itself." Judicially, in a malpractice suit, this term means that the very occurrence of an injury is itself evidence of the defendant's negligence. There are three requirements for application: (1) The injury or damage must be one that would not ordinarily have occurred if a physician had exercised due skill and care; (2) the action or the conduct that caused the damage must have been that of the defendant physician, or performed under sole control of the physician; (3) the patient must not himself or herself have contributed to the injury.

Resect (rē′sekt) (v.) To surgically remove a portion of a tissue or organ. The operation itself is called a resection.

Reservoir (rez′er/vwar) (n.) In biology, the natural habitat for the growth and multiplication of a microorganism.

Resident Care Facility (rez′i-dent/kār/fah-sil′i-tē) (n.) A facility providing safe, hygienic living arrangements for residents. Regular and emergency health services are available as needed, and appropriate supportive services are provided on a regular basis. Also known as a Resident Care Institution.

Resident Flora or Bacteria (rez′i-dent/flo′rah/or/bak-te′re-ah) (n.) Microorganisms that normally live on the skin, bowel, and oral cavity of an individual.

Resolution (rez″o-lū′shun) (n.) 1. The ability of a system to separate closely related forms or entities to the point where they may be discriminated. 2. The clearing or disappearance of an inflammatory process—pneumonitis, for example.

Resolving Infantile Idiopathic Scoliosis (re′zolv′ing/in′fan-tīl/id′ē-o-path′ik/skō″le-ō′sis) (n.) A type of idiopathic scoliosis in which a structural curve develops before the age of 3 years and resolves spontaneously within a few years with or without treatment. This occurs more commonly in boys, and it is usually a left thoracic curve.

The determination of the rib–vertebral angle difference (Mehta's Angle) is useful in predicting the progressiveness of an infantile scoliosis. If the initial RVAD is less than 20 degrees, the curve is likely to be resolving and not progressive.

Respiratory Isolation (res″pi-ra′to′rē/i″sō-lā′shun) (n.) An isolation category designed to prevent the transmission of infectious disease via droplets and droplet nuclei that are coughed, sneezed, or breathed into the environment. The patient is put into a private room, and all susceptible individuals entering the room are required to wear face masks.

Restraining Harness (re-strān′ing/har′nes) (n.) A vest or combination of straps that holds a person securely in a lying or sitting position. It is used to prevent movements that may result in injuries, such as falling out of bed or chairs.

Resurfacing Hip Arthroplasty (re′sur-fas′ing/hip/ar′thrō-plas″tē) (n.) A type of total hip joint arthroplasty in which only the diseased surfaces of the joint are removed and replaced by a cemented metallic shell and a plastic socket. Owing to the high failure rate of this procedure, it is not presently considered a standard operation. Also known as **Surface Replacement Arthroplasty**.

Reticular Cartilage (re-tik′ū-lar/kar-ti′lij) (n.) Elastic cartilage.

Reticular Connective Tissue (re-tik′ū-lar/ko-nek′tiv/tish′ū) (n.) Connective tissue composed predominantly of small fibers; it forms the internal supporting framework of many body organs (the liver and spleen for example) by providing a three-dimensional support for the cells of these organs.

Reticuloendothelial System (re-tik″u-lō-en″dō-thē′le-al/sis′tem) (n.) A system of tissue phagocytes derived from circulating monocytes found in various organs and tissues, such as the spleen, the liver, and the bone marrow. These cells have an important role in immunity.

Reticuloendothelioses (re-tik″ū-lō-en″dō-thē-le-o′sēz) (n.) A group of diseases characterized by the proliferation of cells of the reticuloendothelial system, leading to hyperplasia and granulomatous lesions of reticuloendothelial tissues.

Reticulum Cell Sarcoma of Bone (re-tik′u-lum/sel/sar-kō′mah/of/bōn) (n.) An antiquated term for a primary non-Hodgkin's lymphoma of bone characterized histologically by the presence of poorly differentiated cells and abundant reticulin fibers.

Retinaculum (ret″i-nak′ū-lum) (n.) A thickened band of restraining tissue.

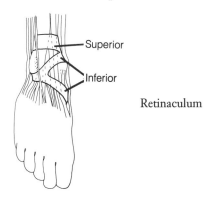

Retinaculum

Retractor (rē-trak′tor) (n.) A surgical instrument that holds tissues out of a surgical field in order to maintain exposure.

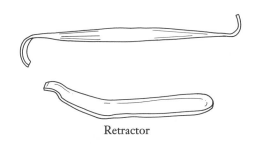

Retractor

Retrocalcaneal Bursitis (ret″ro-kal-kā′nē-al/ber-sī′tis) (n.) An inflammatory disorder of the bursa at the point between the calcaneal tuberosity and the Achilles tendon.

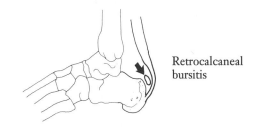

Retrocalcaneal bursitis

Retrolisthesis (re″trō-lis-thē′sis) (n.) The posterior displacement of a vertebra in relation to the one below it.

Retropatellar Pain Syndrome (re″trō-pah-tel′ar/pān/sin′drōm) (n.) A clinical symptom of pain behind the patella most frequently noted with flexion–extension activities during weight-bearing. The underlying pathology is variable. Also called **Patellofemoral Stress Syndrome** or **Anterior Knee Pain Syndrome**.

Retroperitoneal Hemorrhage (re″trō-per″i-tō-ne′al/hem′or-ij) (n.) The extravasation of blood into the retroperitoneal space. This is often seen in association with pelvic fractures, and if significant, it may result in shock, signs that simulate intraperitoneal visceral injury, or a hematoma that can truly rupture into the peritoneal cavity.

Retropulsed (re″trō-pul′sed) (v.) The process of being pushed posteriorly. This term is used in the description of vertebral body fractures to refer to fragments that have fallen back into the spinal canal.

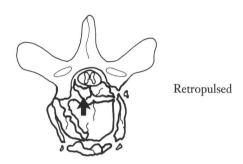

Retropulsed

Retroverted (ret″rō-vert′ed) (v.) Tilted or turned backward without being bent or flexed.

Reunion (rē-ūnyun) (n.) In fractures, the resecuring of union following its interruption by violence or disease.

Reverdin's Graft (ra-ver-danz′/graft) (n.) An epidermal skin graft 0.008 to 0.010 inches in thickness.

Reverses (rē-ver′ses) (n.) A colloquial term for plaster cast reinforcements.

Reverse Isolation (rē-vers′/i″sō-lā′shun) (n.) A synonym for protective isolation.

Reverse Pivot Shift Test (rē-vers′/piv′ut/shift/test) (n.) A clinical evaluation of posterolateral rotary instability of the knee. With the foot in external rotation, extend the flexed knee. There will be sudden reduction as the lateral tibial plateau moves from a position of posterior subluxation to a reduced position. A valgus stress will accentuate this shift of position. See **Pivot Shift Test**.

Reverse Trendelenburg Position (re-vers′/trendel′en-berg/po′zish-un) (n.) An anatomic position of the body in which the head is elevated and the body and the legs are on a declined plane.

Reversed Colles' Fracture (rē-vers′d/kol′ēz/frak′chur) (n.) See **Smith's Fracture**.

Reversed-Last Shoe (re-vers′d-last/shoo) (n.) In shoe terminology, a shoe in which the medial border is convex, not concave. This gives the impression that the shoe was made for the other foot. The shoe may be used in the management of certain foot deformities in children.

Review (re′vū) (n.) In medical terminology, a critical evaluation of data.

Review, Admission (re′vū/ad-mish′un) (n.) Review of the medical necessity of a patient's admission to a hospital. It is conducted prior to, at, or shortly after admission.

Review, Claims (re′vū/klāmz) (n.) The retrospective review by a third-party payer of a request for payment. It determines the liability of the payer, eligibility of the beneficiary and provider, and the appropriateness of the service provided and amount requested under an insurance or prepayment contract.

Review, Concurrent (re′vū/kon-kur′rent) (n.) The evaluation of the medical necessity of a patient's admission to a hospital conducted at or shortly after admission, and the periodic evaluation thereafter of the appropriateness of services provided during the patient's hospitalization. It is used to determine the appropriate payment for services.

Review, Continued Stay (re′vū/kon-tin′ūd/stā) (n.) The review of the appropriateness of the continued hospitalization of a patient.

Review, Peer (re′vū/peer) (n.) The concurrent or retrospective review by practicing physicians or other health professionals of the quality and efficiency of patient care practices or services ordered or performed by other physicians or health professionals.

Review, Prospective (re′vū/prō-spek′tiv) (n.) The evaluation conducted prior to admission of the medical necessity of admission to a hospital.

Review, Rate (re′vū/rāt) (n.) The prospective review by a government or private agency of a hospital's budget and financial data. It is used to determine the reasonableness of the hospital rates and evaluating proposed rate increases.

Review, Utilization (re′vū/ū″til-i-zā′shun) (n.) The concurrent or retrospective review of the appropriateness of hospital admissions, the medical and supportive services rendered, and the length of stay.

Rhabdomyoma (rab″dō-mī-ō′mah) (n.) A rare, benign tumor of striated muscle.

Rhabdomyosarcoma (rab″dō-mī″ō-sar-kō′mah) (n.) A malignant tumor of striated muscle. It is classified according to its clinical and pathologic features into four groups: pleomorphic, alveolar, embryonal, and botryoid. Some tumors are histologically mixed types. Synonyms: **Malignant Rhabdomyoma**, **Myosarcoma**, and **Rhabdomyoblastoma**.

Rheumatic Fever (roo-mat′ik/fē′ver) (n.) An inflammatory disease affecting mainly children and young adults that occurs as a sequela to infection with Group A beta-hemolytic streptococci. The diagnosis of rheumatic heart disease is based on the presence of two major or one major and two minor Jones criteria, as defined by the American Heart Association.

Rheumatism (roo′mah-tizm) (n.) Any of a variety of disorders marked by inflammation, degeneration, or metabolic derangement of connective tissue, especially the joints and related structures. They are characterized by joint pain, stiffness, or limitation of motion.

Rheumatoid Arthritis (roo′mah-toid/ar-thrī′tis) (n.) A chronic inflammatory disease whose joint affections are combined with a variety of extraarticular manifestations. The diagnostic criteria for classic rheumatoid arthritis, clearly defined by the American College of Rheumatology, include joint signs or symptoms present for at least six weeks; the presence of subcutaneous nodules; roentgenographic changes, such as uniform narrowing of joint spaces; juxtaarticular osteopenia and erosions, and a lack of new bone formation; the presence of rheumatoid factor in the serum; and characteristic histologic changes in the synovium or in nodules. Extraarticular manifestations include possible heart, vascular, lung, eye, and nervous system involvement. Systemic complications also occur. Abbreviated **RA** and is also known as **Atrophic Arthritis** or **Arthritis Deformans**.

Rheumatoid Factor (roo′mah-toid/fak′ter) (n.) An antibody present in the serum of 70% to 90% of adult patients with classic rheumatoid arthritis. These antibodies are chiefly in the immunoglobulins M class. Rheumatoid factor may be detected by various techniques; usually these involve agglutination reactions. Rheumatoid factor may be found in a variety of other diseases, such as subacute bacterial endocarditis, leprosy, and sarcoidosis.

Rheumatoid Nodules (roo′mah-toid/nod′ulz) (n.) Firm, nontender, rounded or oval subcutaneous masses seen in association with rheumatoid arthritis. They usually occur over extensor surfaces and in the synovial and periarticular tissues. Less frequently, they occur in internal organs. Histologically, they have a central zone of fibrinoid degeneration or necrosis surrounded by mononuclear cells in a regular palisade arrangement.

Rheumatoid Variants (roo′mah-toid/var′e-ants) (n.) An antiquated term for the seronegative spondyloarthropathies.

Rheumatology (roo″mah-tol′o-je) (n.) 1. The study of rheumatic disease. 2. The medical specialty concerned with the diagnosis and management of diseases involving joints, tendons, muscles, ligaments, and associated structures.

Rhizo (ri′zo) A word element meaning nerve root.

Rhizotomy (ri-zot′o-me) (n.) The surgical transection of a nerve root.

Rhomboid Ligament (rom′boid/lig′ah-ment) (n.) The costoclavicular ligament that connects the first rib to the undersurface of the clavicle.

Rib (rib) (n.) A curved, slightly twisted strip of bone that forms part of the skeleton of the thorax. There are 12 pairs of ribs. The head of each rib articulates with one of the 12 thoracic vertebrae; its other end is attached to a section of cartilage. The first seven pairs, the true ribs, are connected directly to the sternum by their costal cartilages. The next three pairs, the false ribs, are attached indirectly to the sternum—each is connected by its cartilage to the rib above it. The last two pairs, the floating ribs, end

freely in the muscles of the anterior body wall. Anatomic name: **Costa**.

Rib Belt (rib/belt) (n.) An elastic support worn around the thoracic region. It is used to alleviate discomfort from minor painful conditions of the chest wall, including intercostal strains and sprains, pleurisy, and minor rib fractures.

Rib Hump (rib/hump) (n.) The prominence of the ribs on the convexity of a spinal curvature. A rib hump is usually due to vertebral rotation and can best be exhibited by having the patient bend forward.

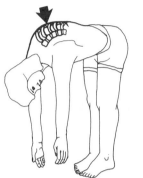

Rib hump

Rib Vertebral Angle Difference (rib/ver′te-bral/ ang′g′l/dif″er-ents) (n.) See **Mehta Angle**.

Ribonucleic Acid (ri″bo-nu-kle′ik/as′id) (n.) A macromolecule composed of ribose, purines, and pyrimidines connected by phosphate linkages. Various ribonucleic acids are involved in protein syntheses and are identified by specific location or form. Abbreviated **RNA**.

Ribosome (ri′bo-som) (n.) A cytoplasmic particle, usually 120 to 150 Å in diameter, composed of ribonucleic acid and protein. It is considered to be the site of protein synthesis.

Rice Bodies (ris/bod′ez) (n.) Loose bodies found in joints that result from excessive fibrinous exudation. These fibrin particulates resemble polished white rice and are seen in the synovial fluid of many types of inflammatory arthritides.

RICE Regimen (ris/rej′i-men) (n.) An acronym for an initial, basic treatment regimen for acute musculoskeletal injuries, including sprains, strain-contusions, and hematomas. RICE stands for Rest, Ice, Immobilization, Compression, and Elevation.

Richards Compression Screw (rich′ardz/kompresh′un/skru) (n.) A compression screw and sideplate appliance used in the treatment of hip fracture. It is a trademark of Richards Manufacturing Company.

Rickets (rik′ets) (n.) A metabolic disorder characterized by a deficiency of calcium, phosphorus, or both. In children, this results in impaired mineralization and growth of the skeleton. The causes of rachitic syndromes are numerous, but most commonly include vitamin D deficiency, renal tubular defects, chronic renal insufficiency, and hypophosphatasia.

Rider's Bone (rī'derz/bōn) (n.)   Ossification of the tendon of the adductor longus muscle of the thigh. This may occur from the pressure of the inner thigh against the saddle during prolonged horseback riding. Synonym: **Cavalryman's Bone.**

Rider's Sprain (rī'derz/sprān) (n.)   A sprain of the adductor longus muscle of the thigh. This may result from a horserider's sudden effort to maintain his or her seat in response to an unexpected movement of the horse.

Ridge (rij) (n.)   A crest, linear projection, or long narrow protuberance, such as those seen on a bone.

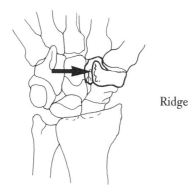

Ridge

Right Angle Test (rīt/ang'g'l/test) (n.)   A radiographic method for assessing the presence of vertebral slip in spondylolisthesis. On a lateral radiograph, a lumbar vertebra normally lies within the right angle formed by the line tangent to the posterior surface of the sacrum and the line perpendicular to the former at the level of the anterosuperior angle of the sacrum.

Rigid Dressing (ri-jid/dres'ing) (n.)   A mildly compressive, total-contact plaster wrap applied immediately following surgery to control edema and pain; it is specifically used to treat amputation stumps.

Rigid Fixation (ri-jid/fik-sa'shun) (n.)   The immobilization of fracture fragments after reduction by using internal or external fixation devices. The goal of rigid fixation is to permit early motion and facilitate a return to normal function.

Rigidity (ri-jid'i-tē) (n.)   1. A biomechanical term that refers to a structure's ability to resist deformation. 2. A type of increased muscle tone in which a steady contraction of both flexors and extensors results in increased resistance to passive motion throughout the range of motion regardless of speed or direction.

Riley-Day Syndrome (ri'lē-dā/sin'drōm) (n.)   See **Familial Dysautonomia.**

Rim Sign (rim/sīn) (n.)   A radiographic sign that strongly suggests the presence of a posterior shoulder dislocation. On a routine AP radiograph of the shoulder, if the humeral head is posteriorly dislocated, the glenoid fossa appears to be partially vacant. A positive rim sign is present if the space between the anterior glenoid rim and the humeral head is greater than 6 mm. Also known as a **Vacant Glenoid Sign.**

Ring Apophysis (ring/ah-pof'i-sis) (n.)   The secondary centers of ossification that develop in the cartilaginous end-plates of the superior and inferior surface of the vertebral bodies. They are peripherally thicker and thus may appear ringlike during early ossification. Often incorrectly referred to as "ring epiphyses."

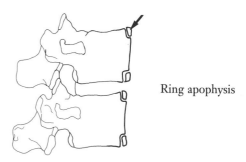

Ring apophysis

Ring Injuries (ring/in'jur-ēz) (n.)   An avulsion injury of the soft tissues of the ring finger. This injury occurs when a part of a finger ring is caught (e.g., on a hook or a nail). This results in separation of the skin and severe damage to the vascularity of the digit distal to the level of the avulsion.

Ringer's Solution (ring'erz/sō-lū'shun) (n.)   An isotonic salt solution used in the replacement of volume deficits. It contains sodium, potassium, and calcium balanced by chloride and lactate. Also known as **Lactated Ringer Solution.**

Risk Management (risk/man-ej'ment) (n.)   The planning, organizing, and directing of a comprehensive program of activities to identify, evaluate, and take corrective action against risks that may lead to patient and employee injury and property loss or damage—all of which resulting in financial loss.

Risser-Ferguson Method (ris'-ser/fer'-gus-on/meth'ud) (n.)   A technique for measuring the angle of a scoliotic curve. On an AP radiograph, place a small dot in the center of the uppermost and lowermost vertebrae in the curve. Place another dot in the center of the apical vertebra. Draw straight lines from the dot in each end vertebra through the dot in the apical vertebra. The intersecting angle is the angle of the curve. Compare **Cobb Method.**

Risser Localizer Cast (ris'-ser/lō'kal-īz''er/kast) (n.)   A type of body cast used for the preoperative correction of a scoliotic curve. Localized pressure is ap-

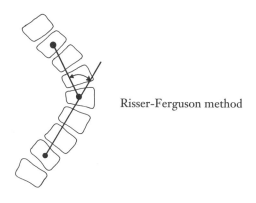

Risser-Ferguson method

On an AP view of the pelvis or spine, the degree of ossification of the iliac crest apophysis is evaluated. The ossification progresses anterolaterally to posteromedially, and the excursion over the iliac crest is divided into thirds. A Risser sign of 0 indicates that the apophysis has not yet appeared; signs of 1, 2, and 3 correlate with the degree of excursion; and a Risser sign of 4 implies fusion of the crest with the remainder of the ilium. Developed by Dr. Joseph Risser of California.

Risser Turnbuckle (ris′-er/turn′buk′l) (n.) A type of casting technique used to correct a scoliotic curve. In this technique, external corrective forces are applied through a turnbuckle welded to the plaster body cast along the concave side of the deformity.

Ritchie Articular Index (ri′chē/ar-tik′u-lar/in′deks) (n.) An index for the numerical measurement of joint tenderness in patients with rheumatoid arthritis. The index is based on the summation of a number of quantitative evaluations of the pain experienced by patients when the joints are subjected either to firm pressure exerted over the articular margin or to movement of the joint. Tenderness of the joints is elicited by applying firm pressure over the joint margin in all joint areas other than the cervical spine, the hip joints, the talocalcaneal, and the midtarsal joints. In these sites, tenderness is elicited by passive movement of the joint.

The four grades of tenderness are:
Grade 0: No tenderness
Grade +1: The patient complains of pain
Grade +2: The patient complains of pain and winces
Grade +3: The patient complains of pain, winces, and withdraws

plied posterolaterally at a point level with the apex of the curve, while traction is exerted on the head and pelvis. A spinal fusion subsequently may be performed through a window in the posterior part of the cast when the desired correction has been obtained. Synomym: **Risser Jacket.**

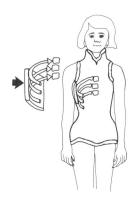

Risser localizer cast

Ritz Stick (rits/stik) (n.) A device used in determining the numerical size of shoes.

Robert Jones Bandage (rob′ert/jōnz/ban-dij′) (n.) See **Jones Bandage.**

Robert's Pelvis (ro-bārz′/pel′vis) (n.) An anomalous pelvis with a rudimentary sacrum and great reduction of the transverse and oblique diameters.

Robin-Aids Hand (ro′bin-ādz/hand) (n.) The proprietary name of a prosthetic hand that is voluntarily opened by a spring-loaded thumb.

Robin-Aids Hand Splint (ro′bin-ādz/hand/splint) (n.) One of several splints produced by Robin-Aids Manufacturing Company of Vallejo, California. Their products include flexor hinge splints and wrist and finger extension splints.

Risser Sign (ris′-ser/sīn) (n.) A radiographic sign using the iliac apophysis as an indicator of the degree of skeletal maturity. It is used in the evaluation of patients with scoliosis because the remaining vertebral growth can be correlated with the Risser Sign.

Robin-Aids Hook (ro′bin-ādz/huk) (n.) The proprietary name of a shoulder-elbow-hand orthosis. It includes a prosthetic hook that, when placed in the patient's paralyzed hand, substitutes for the lost hand function.

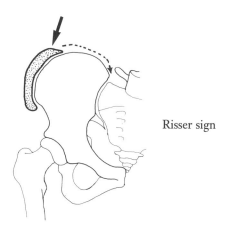

Risser sign

Rocker-Bottom Foot (rok′er/bot′tom/foot) (n.) A congenital deformity of the foot characterized by superior and lateral dislocation of the navicular bone and the rest of the forefoot on the talus, which is locked in plantarflexion. There is associated hindfoot equinus and secondary tendon and ligament deformities. Also known as **Convex Pes Valgus** or **Congenital Vertical Talus**. See **Congenital Vertical Talus**.

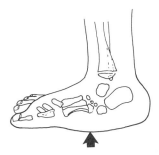

Rocker-Bottom foot

Rocking-Chair Gait (rok'ing/chār/gāt) (n.) A walk with crutches in which the subject advances the crutches minimally and then rocks back and forth to produce the momentum necessary to bring the feet forward, thus overcoming inertia and friction.

Rod (rod) (n.) 1. A bar that is rounded in diameter. 2. In orthopaedics, this commonly refers to intramedullary fixation devices or the connecting rods of external fixation devices. 3. A common reference to rod-shaped bacilli.

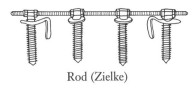

Rod (Zielke)

Roentgen (rent'gen) (n.) The international unit of measurement of x- or gamma-radiation; it is based on the amount of ionization produced in air; abbreviated **R** (formerly r). One R equals the amount of radiation capable of liberating one electrostatic unit of electricity per cubic centimeter of air under standard conditions of temperature and pressure. One R corresponds to the dissipation, in air, of about 83 ergs/g.

Roentgen-Equivalent-Man (rent'gen/ē-kwiv'ah-lent/man) (n.) The unit of dose of ionizing radiation that, when absorbed by man, produces an effect equivalent to the absorption of one roentgen of x or gamma rays. Abbreviated **REM**.

Roentgen Rays (rent'gen/rāz) (n.) See x-rays.

Roentgenogram (rent"gen'o-gram) (n.) A film produced by roentgenography.

Roentgenologist (rent"ge-nol'ō-jist) (n.) A specialist in roentgenology. The person is known familiarly as a **Radiologist**.

Roentgenology (rent"ge-nol'ō-jē) (n.) The study

of the applications of x-rays, or roentgen rays, in medicine.

Roger Anderson Device (roj'er/an'der-son/de-vis') (n.) A system for external fixation of fractures. It uses multiple pins of either the transfixion- or half-pin–type connected to clamps, which are connected to each other by aluminum rods.

Roger Anderson Well Leg Traction (roj'er/an'der-son/wel-leg/trak'shun) (n.) A traction system that uses the "well" leg for countertraction. It was originally described for the treatment of displaced pelvic fractures. After incorporating both legs in plaster casts, the feet are connected by a splinting apparatus that forces the affected leg into full abduction and the well leg into full adduction, thus producing traction on the abducted leg. This apparatus facilitates the simultaneous pulling-down of one leg and the pushing-up of the other.

Rolando Fracture (rō-lan'dō/frak'chur) (n.) An eponym for an intraarticular fracture of the base of the first metacarpal. It has both a volar lip fragment and a large dorsal fragment, which results in a Y- or T-shaped fracture. Compare to **Bennett Fracture**.

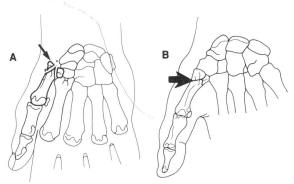

Rolando fracture

Roll Stitch (rōl/stich) (n.) A technique for suturing tendons, usually used to repair extensor tendon lacerations of the hand over or near the head of the metacarpal. In this stitch, the suture is brought through the skin edges medially and laterally, incorporating the margins of both tendon segments. The suture is pulled out at about 4 weeks after repair.

Roller Board (rōl'er/bord) (n.) A device used in rehabilitation therapy that permits abduction and adduction of the hips.

Roller Traction (rōl'er/trak'shun) (n.) A technique of skeletal traction that incorporates suspension from a wheel on an overhead track with normal longitudinal traction. It allows free muscle and joint function while keeping the limb in traction.

ROM Abbreviation for Range of Motion.

Romberg Test (rom'berg/test) (n.) A clinical test for proprioceptive function. The patient stands with his

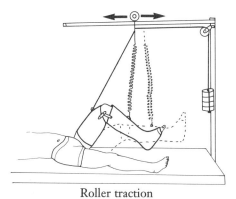

Roller traction

or her feet together and his or her arms held straight in front of him or her. The patient then closes his or her eyes. If he or she sways more with his or her eyes closed than with them opened, the test is positive.

Rongeur Forceps (rawn-zhĕr′/for′seps) (n.) A sharp, biting type of forceps designed to cut bone.

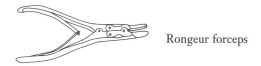

Rongeur forceps

Root (r$\overline{oo}$t) (n.) 1. The origin of any structure; also the point at which it diverges from another suture. The anatomic name is radix. 2. Nerve root. See **Nerve Root.**

Ropes Test (rōps/test) (n.) A test used in joint fluid analysis. The quality of mucin in synovial fluid is assayed by adding a few drops of synovial fluid to 5 to 10 mL of a 5% solution of acetic acid. Four grades of reaction are classified by observation of this mucin precipitate:

Normal: A tight, ropy clump that remains suspended together on top in a clear solution

Fair: A soft mass that strings out and sticks together, remaining loosely intact in a very slightly cloudy solution

Poor: Small, friable masses in a cloudy solution

Very Poor: A few flecks in a cloudy solution

Also known as **Ropes Mucin Precipitation Test.**

Rose-Waaler Test (rōz/vahl′-er/test) (n.) One of several laboratory assays for rheumatoid factor. This assay uses presensitized sheep red cells and evaluates the agglutination reaction with the test sera. A titer of 16 or more is regarded as positive. Also known as **Sheep-Cell Agglutination Test.**

Rose's Gluteal Reflex (ro′zez′/gloo′te-al/re′fleks) (n.) A reflex that indicates the presence of sciatica. The gluteus maximus is percussed at its attachment to the sacrum. The reflex is positive when an exaggerated fascicular contraction of the muscle fibers

occurs at the point of impact; a negative test would show contraction of the entire muscle.

Rose's Position (rō′zez/pō′zish-un) (n.) An anatomic position: the patient is supine, with his or her head over the table edge in full extension.

Rosen Splint (rō′zen/splint) (n.) A splint designed for the treatment of children with congenital dislocation of the hip. The Rosen splint is comprised of one piece of flat metal in the form of the letter H in which the transverse bar extends beyond the longitudinal bars. The bars are bent and molded at their ends to be hooked from the back of an infant over his or her shoulders and thighs to maintain the hips in flexion and abduction. See **Von Rosen Splint.**

Rosenbach's Law (ro′zen-bahks/law) (n.) A law that states that in lesions of the nerve centers and nerve trunks, paralysis appears in the extensor muscles before it occurs in the flexor muscles.

Rossolimo Reflex (ros″ō-lē-mō/re′fleks) (n.) A muscle stretch reflex found in pyramidal tract lesions. To obtain this reflex, tap the plantar surfaces of the toes with a reflex hammer. In the neurologically intact patient, there will be either no movement or a slight dorsiflexion of the toes. If pyramidal tract disease is present, there will be a quick plantar flexion of the toes.

Rotary Click Test of Watson (rō′ter-ē/klik/test/of/waht′son) (n.) An examination for rotary subluxation of the scaphoid. Press your thumb against the distal pole of the scaphoid and rock the wrist back and forth in radial and ulnar deviation. A painful click can sometimes be elicited as the proximal pole of the scaphoid subluxes over the dorsal rim of the radius.

Rotary Instability (rō′ter-ē/in″stah-bil′i-tē) (n.) A term used in the classification of knee ligament instabilities that denotes a rotational component to the direction of tibial displacement. The various types of rotary instability are classified as: Anteromedial Rotary Instability; Anterolateral Rotary Instability—in flexion or near full extension; Posterolateral Rotary Instability; Posteromedial Rotary Instability; and Combined Rotary Instability.

Rotary Subluxation of C1 on C2 (rō′ter-ē/sub″luk-sā′shun/of/C1/on/C2) (n.) A subluxation of the atlantoaxial joint that usually presents with torticollis and restricted neck motion. The diagnosis is suggested by lateral mass asymmetry on an open-mouth radiograph and is confirmed by either cineradiography or computerized tomography. Also known as **Atlantoaxial Rotary Subluxation.**

Rotary Subluxation of the Scaphoid (rō′ter-ē/sub″luk-sā′shun/of/the/skaf′oid) (n.) A subluxation of the carpal scaphoid that results from an insufficient scapholunate interosseous ligament. This is usually a posttraumatic condition. Radiographically, a gap greater than 2 mm is noted between the scaphoid and the lunate on an AP radiograph. The dorsal rotation of the proximal pole of the scaphoid causes it

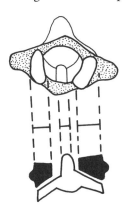

Rotary subluxation of C1 on C2

to appear shortened, producing a so-called "ring sign" on an AP film. On a lateral radiograph, the rotated scaphoid is more vertically oriented. The radiographic findings may be accentuated by taking AP films while the patient is actively making a fist.

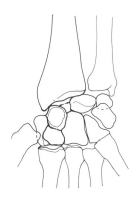

Rotary subluxation of the scaphoid

Rotating Index of the Pelvis (rō′tāt-ing/in′deks/of/ the/pel′vis) (n.) A measurement used in assessing the degree of pelvic rotation on an AP radiograph of the pelvis. The index is obtained by dividing the diameter of the obturator foramen on the right by the diameter on the left. If the pelvis is neutral this index will be 1. If the pelvis is rotated to the right, the index will be less than 1. If the pelvis is rotated to the left, the index will be greater than 1.

Rotation (rō-tā′shun) (n.) The turning or moving of a part around its axis of rotation. The unit of measure is degrees or radiant.

Rotational Deformity (rō-tā′shun-al/dē-for′mi-tē) (n.) A deformity that results from rotation of a particular part. The deformity is described by the direction of malrotation of the distal part. For example, after a long bone fracture, if rotation is not kept in mind in the alignment of the fragments, there may be a resultant internal or external rotational deformity.

Rotator Cuff (rō-tā′ter/kuf) (n.) A group of tendons and muscles surrounding the shoulder joint that in-

cludes the supraspinatus, the infraspinatus, the teres minor, and the subscapularis muscles and tendons. The rotator cuff muscles lock the humeral head into the glenoid and provide active abduction and rotation of the glenohumeral joint.

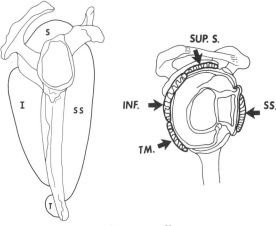

Rotator cuff

Rotator Cuff Arthropathy (rō′tā′ter/kuf/arthrop′ah-the) (n.) An arthritic condition of the glenohumeral joint that results from chronic rotator cuff insufficiency. It is characterized by upward migration of the humeral head, with erosive changes of the underside of the acromion and acromioclavicular joint. Radiographically, due to the upward displacement of the humeral head, a significant reduction of the acromiohumeral distance is noted, along with other degenerative changes. Also known as **Cuff Tear Arthropathy**. See **Geyser Sign**.

Round-Cell Sarcomas of Bone (rownd-sel/sar-kō′ mahs/of/bōn) (n.) A group of malignant tumors involving bone that are histologically similar under examination by light microscopy. These tumors characteristically have sheets of monotonous, small round cells on microscopic examination. This group of tumors includes Ewing's sarcoma, malignant lymphoma, metastatic neuroblastoma, and metastatic oat cell carcinoma of the lung.

Roux-Goldthwait Procedure (roo-gōld′thwāt/prosē′jur) (n.) A surgical technique for the correction of recurrent patellar dislocation. In this procedure, the patellar tendon is split longitudinally and the lateral half is transferred medially.

Roux Sign (roo/sīn) (n.) A diagnostic marker indicating that the hip joint is riding relatively high. This is determined by measuring the distance from the greater trochanter to the pubic spine and then comparing that distance with the normal sign. This distance will be lessened in congenital dislocations of the hip or in lateral compression fractures of the pelvis.

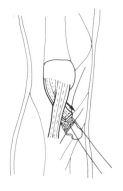

Roux-Goldthwait
procedure

Ruptured Disk (rup'chur'd/disk) (n.)   A colloquial
term for a herniated nucleus pulposus.

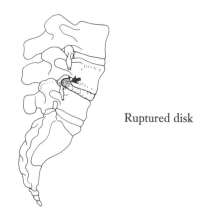

Ruptured disk

Rufen (rū'fen) (n.)   A proprietary name for Ibuprofen, a nonsteroidal, antiinflammatory drug.

Ruffinian Corpuscle (rū-fin'-ē-an/kor'pus'l) (n.)   A
free sensory nerve ending found in the subcutaneous
tissue of the fingers.

Rumpel-Leede Tourniquet Test (rūm'pel-lā'de/
tūr'ni-ket/test) (n.)   A method used in the evaluation of patients with blood dyscrasias or hemorrhagic
tendencies. The presence of spots on the forearm is
noted before beginning the test. A blood pressure
cuff is applied in the usual manner; it is then inflated
to a point midway between the systolic and the di-
astolic pressures. A circle 1 inch in diameter is
marked with ink on the forearm, and the cuff is allowed to remain inflated for 15 minutes. The reference value is less than 10 new pectechiae forming
within this circle. The appearance of more than 10
new pectechiae in the circle is read as a positive test.
Synonym: **Capillary Fragility Test, Tourniquet Test**.

Run-Around Infection of the Nail (run'a-round/in-
fek'shun/of/the/nāl) (n.)   A common name for a
paronychia that has begun at one corner of the nail
and has traveled either under the eponychium or under the nail toward the opposite side. See **Paronychia**.

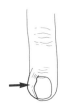

Run-around
infection

Runner's Knee (run'erz/nē) (n.)   A general term denoting peripatellar knee pain caused by a variety of
processes.

Running Traction (run-ing/trak'shun) (n.)   A form
of traction in which the pull is exerted in one plane
only. Running traction may use either skin or skeletal traction and may be either unilateral or bilateral. Example: **Buck's Extension Traction**.

Rupture (rup'chur) (n.)   The act of breaking apart or
separating into parts.

Rush Pins (rush/pinz) (n.)   A type of nonreamed intramedullary fixation device that has a sharp point
for insertion and a blunt hook at the opposite end.
These are available in a variety of widths and lengths.
Also known as **Rush Nails** or **Rush Rods**.

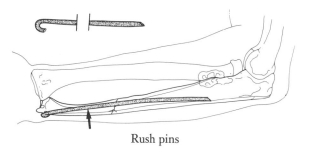

Rush pins

Russe Graft (rūs/graft) (n.)   A surgical procedure for
the treatment of nonunion of the carpal scaphoid.
Through a volar approach to the scaphoid, a cancellous bone peg is placed into a cavity created within
the bone fragments at the nonunion site, to graft and
stabilize the fragments. Also known as a **Matti-Russe
Graft**.

Russell-Taylor Nail (rus'el-tā'ler/nāl) (n.)   A type of
interlocking intramedullary nail manufactured by
the Richards Medical Company. These nails are designed for use in treating both femoral and tibial
shaft fractures.

Russell Traction (rus'el/trak'shun) (n.)   A technique of skin traction for the lower extremity. In this
method, continuous traction pulls anteriorly on a
cuff at the distal thigh; the traction also pulls axially
at the leg through skin traction tape. The resultant
force is in the line of the femoral shaft as the knee
remains flexed. Currently, this technique is used as
a temporary treatment for support of a fractured
limb prior to definitive, usually operative, treatment.
If traction is to be the definitive form of fracture

management, this technique has been largely supplanted by the use of skeletal traction methods.

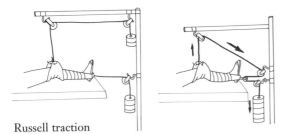

Russell traction

Ryder Method (ri'der/meth'ud) (n.) A radiographic technique for measuring the true anteversion of the femoral neck. This involves making one AP radiograph with the femur in a neutral position and another with the hip and knee flexed to 90 degrees and the thigh abducted 30 degrees. Two projected angles are measured by drawing lines representing the axes of the neck and shaft on the AP film and lines representing the axis of the neck and transcondylar plane or the abduction film. The true anteversion is then determined by reference to a table presented by Ryder and Crane in 1953.

S

S-1 (n.) The first sacral vertebra or nerve root.

S-2 (n.) The second sacral vertebra or nerve root.

S-3 (n.) The third sacral vertebra or nerve root.

S-4 (n.) The fourth sacral vertebra or nerve root.

S-5 (n.) The fifth sacral vertebra or nerve root.

Saber Cut (sā-ber/kut) (n.) A surgical approach to the shoulder. A U-shaped skin incision is made over the top of the shoulder, starting from inferior to the acromioclavicular joint, running posteriorly, and ending inferior to the back of the acromion. Its name is probably derived from its resemblance to injuries incurred by a saber.

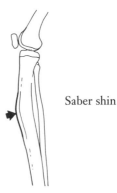

Saber shin

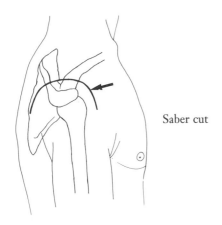

Saber cut

Saber Shin (sā-ber/shin) (n.) A term for a tibial deformity in which an anteriorly convex, sharp-edged ridge is present. This deformity may be seen in congenital syphilis, rickets, or Paget's disease.

Sac (sak) (n.) Any pouch or baglike part of an organ or structure.

SACH Foot (SACH/fut) (n.) A Solid Ankle Cushion Heel prosthetic foot. The SACH foot consists of a

hardwood heel, a compressible cover material around the heel, a short length of belting passing underneath the heel and extending forward into the toe section, a bolt attaching the foot to the shank, and a "cushion heel."

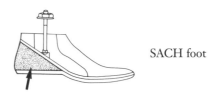

SACH foot

Sacral Agenesis (sa'kral/ah-jen'e-sis) (n.) A rare, congenital anomaly in which all or part of the sacrum is absent.

Sacral Base (sa'kral/bās) (n.) The end plate of the first sacral vertebra. It participates in the formation of the L5–S1 disk space.

Sacral Canal (sa'kral/kah-nal') (n.) The continuation of the spinal canal through the sacrum.

Sacral–Femoral Angle (sa'kral/fem'or-al/ang'g'l) (n.) A radiographic measurement of the degree of

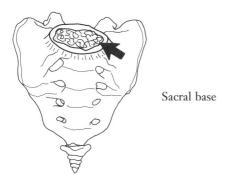

Sacral base

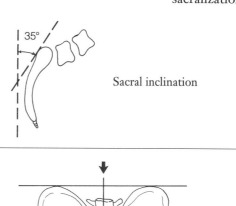

Sacral inclination

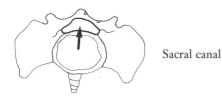

Sacral canal

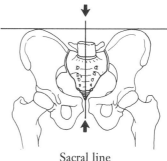

Sacral line

hip flexion deformity in stance. On lateral standing radiographs of the lumbar spine, pelvis, and both hips, draw one line along the superior aspect of the sacrum and another along the femoral shaft. The normal angle in the standing patient ranges from 50 degrees to 65 degrees. If the sacral–femoral angle is under 35 degrees, significant hip flexion deformity is present.

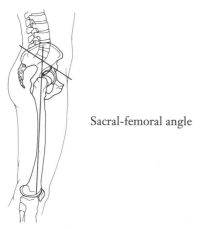

Sacral-femoral angle

Sacral Nerves (sa'kral/nervz) (n.) The five pairs of spinal nerves that emerge from the spinal column in the sacrum. The sacral nerves carry sensory and motor fibers and to and from both the upper and lower leg and from the anal and genital regions.

Sacral Plexus (sa'kral/plek'ses) (n.) A nerve plexus arising from the lumbosacral trunk and ventral branches of the first four sacral spinal nerves.

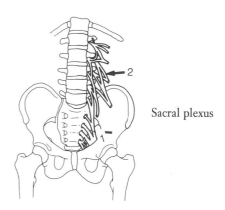

Sacral plexus

Sacral Inclination (sa'kral/in"kli-nā'shun) (n.) In spondylolisthesis, a measure of the degree of vertical orientation of the sacrum. On a standing lateral radiograph of the spine, an angle is formed by a line parallel to the posterior aspect of the first sacral vertebral body and a vertical line is drawn perpendicular to the floor. A completely vertical sacrum therefore has a sacral inclination of 0 degrees.

Sacral Line (sa'kral/līn) (n.) A line drawn perpendicular to the level of the iliac crest and through the center of the sacrum on a radiograph.

Sacral Vertebrae (sa'kral/ver'te-brē) (n.) The five vertebrae that are usually fused together, forming the sacrum.

Sacralization (sa'kral-i-zā'shun (n.) An abnormal fusion of the fifth lumbar vertebra with the sacrum. In this anomaly, one or both of the transverse processes of the fifth lumbar vertebra may be enlarged and fused to or articulated with the sacrum or ilium or a sixth lumbar vertebra, transitional in type, may be almost completely fused with the sacrum. Compare to **Lumbarization**.

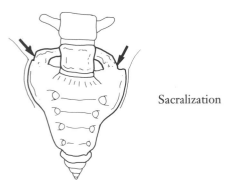

Sacralization

Sacroiliac (sak′rō-il′ē-ak) (adj.)   Of or pertaining to the sacrum and the ilium.

Sacroiliac Joint (sak′rō-il′ē-ak/joint) (n.)   The paired articulations between the sacrum and iliac bone in the pelvis.

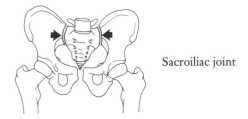

Sacroiliac joint

Sacrosciatic Notch (sa′krō-sī-at′ik/noch) (n.)   The notch formed between the margins of the sacrum and the ilium on the lower margin of the pelvis. More commonly referred to as the **Sciatic Notch**.

Sacrovertebral Angle (sa′kro-ver′tē-bral/ang′g′l) (n.)   The angle formed on a lateral radiograph of the lumbar vertebrae at the intersection of lines drawn through the sacrum and lumbar spine.

Sacrum (sa′krem) (n.)   A curved, triangular element of the backbone consisting of five fused vertebrae known as sacral vertebrae. The sacrum articulates above with the last lumbar vertebra, below with the coccyx, and laterally with the pelvic bones.

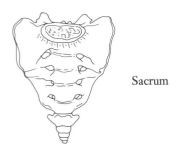

Sacrum

Saddle (sad′l) (n.)   In shoe terminology, a piece of leather extending from the shank, over the throat, and up to the top of the quarters.

Saddle Area (sad′l/a′rē-ah) (n.)   The area including the perineum, the upper inner aspects of the thigh, and the part of the buttocks surrounding the anus.

Saddle Joint (sad′l/joint) (n.)   A form of diarthrosis in which the articulating surfaces of the bones are reciprocally saddle shaped. An example of this is the carpometacarpal joint of the thumb.

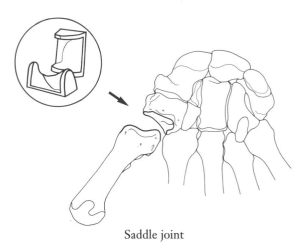

Saddle joint

Safety Factor (saf′tē/fak′tor) (n.)   The factor defining how much stronger a structure is than it needs to be in order to sustain the load for which it is designed.

Sag Sign (sag/sīn) (n.)   A sign of posterior cruciate ligament instability. With the patient supine and the knee flexed to 45 degrees, there is a dropback in the resting position so that there is a concavity beneath the patella on the affected side.

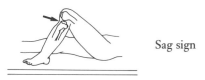

Sag sign

Sage Nail (saj/nāl) (n.)   A solid, reamed rod designed for the intramedullary fixation of the bones of the forearm.

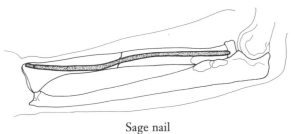

Sage nail

Sagging Rope Sign sag-ging/rōp/sin) (n.) A radiographic marker indicative of Legg-Calvé-Perthes disease of the hip. The sign consists of a thin opaque line in the upper femoral metaphysis. In the AP view, this line extends laterally from the inferior border of the neck for a variable distance, frequently reaching the superior border. It is seen equally well in the lateral view. The line is usually curved, sagging at its center.

Sagittal (saj′ĭ-tal) (adj.) The vertical, anteroposterior plane that runs through the longitudinal axis of the trunk, dividing the body into right and left halves.

Saha's Classification (saha-s/klas″sĭ-ka′shun) (n.) A functional classification of the muscles of the shoulder joint. These are divided into three groups: prime movers, steering group, and depression group.

Saha Procedure (saha/pro-se′jur) (n.) An operative procedure described for the treatment of recurrent anterior shoulder dislocations. In this procedure, the latissimus dorsi muscle is transferred posteriorly into the site of the infraspinatus tendon insertion on the greater tuberosity.

SAID Principle (SAID/prin′sĭ-p′l) (n.) An acronym for the Specific Adaption to Imposed Demand. It states that a reconditioning program must attempt to readapt the athlete to the demands that will be encountered during performance. The intensity, duration, and repetition in the exercises must approximate the actual athletic performance.

Salenius Graph (sa-lē-nē-us/graf) (n.) A graph of normal tibiofemoral angles in growing children.

Salicylates (sal′i-sil′āts) (n.) A group of chemically related compounds with a wide range of pharmacologic properties; it includes salicylic acid and aspirin. Systemic uses are anti-inflammatory and antipyretic; used locally as a keratolytic agent.

Saline Solution (sā′lēn/sō-lū′shun) (n.) A solution containing 0.9% sodium chloride. It is isotonic (ie, of the same osmotic pressure as blood serum).

Salmonella (sal′mo-nel′a) (n.) The genus of non–lactose-fermenting, gram-negative rods, found in the family Enterobacteriaceae.

Salter Fracture (sal′ter/frak′chur) (n.) A commonly used abbreviated reference to fractures through the growth plate. See **Salter-Harris Classification**.

Salter-Harris Classification (sal′ter/har-is/klas″sĭ-fĭ-ka′shun) (n.) A widely used classification system for fractures through the physeal plate.

Type I: The epiphysis separates from the metaphysis without any bony fragment from the metaphysis.

Type II: The line of separation extends along the physis for a variable distance, then through a portion of the metaphyseal bone. On the x-ray, a triangular metaphyseal fragment is visible (see **Thurston Holland's Sign**).

Type III: An intraarticular fracture of the epiphysis, with the plane of cleavage extending from the joint surface to the physis, and then extending parallel with the growth plate to its periphery.

Type IV: The fracture line begins at the articular surface, extending first through the epiphysis, and then through a segment of the metaphysis.

Type V: A crush injury to the epiphysis.

See **Epiphyseal Fracture**.

Salter Osteotomy (sal′-ter/os-tē-ot-o-mē) (n.) An innominate osteotomy used for the management of a congenital dislocated hip (CDH) or a developmental dysplasia of the hip (DDH). The osteotomy forms a horizontal line from just lateral to the anterior inferior spine at a right angle to the vertical axis of the ilium. The entire acetabulum, together with the pubis and the ischium, is rotated and hinged on the symphysis pubis. The roof of the acetabulum is thus shifted laterally and anteriorly. A triangular-shaped bone graft from the anterior iliac crest is used to wedge open the osteotomy site.

Salvage Procedure (sal′vij/pro-se′jur) (n.) 1. A descriptive term for any operation or series of operations intended to maintain attachment of a limb in lieu of amputation. 2. A procedure to save a body part from disaster.

SAM Splint (sam/splint) (n.) An acronym for a Structural Aluminum Malleable splint. This splint is intended for first-aid splinting and consists of soft aluminum strips of variable width coated in polyvinyl that become rigid when folded longitudinally.

Sam Browne Belt (sam/brown/belt) (n.) A synonym for Perthes Sling.

Sampson Nail (samp′sun/nāl) (n.) An intramedullary nail for the treatment of fractures of the femoral shaft. This is a hollow, cylindrical rod with multiple external flutes to improve rotational stability and increase torsional load-carrying capacity. Also known as a **Sampson rod**.

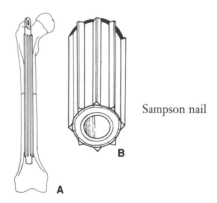

Sampson nail

Sanfilippo's Syndrome (san-fil′-lipōz/sin′drōm) (n.) One of the mucopolysaccharidoses, this has an autosomal recessive pattern of inheritance. On urinalysis, there is increased heparan sulfate excretion. Symptoms are not apparent until past infancy, when the child is noted to have a spastic gait or behavioral problems. By adolescence, these children are usually bedridden, and have no awareness of time or place.

They usually die by early adulthood. Also known as **Mucopolysaccharidosis III** or **Polydystrophia Oligophrenia**.

Saphenous Nerve (sah-fe′nus/nerv) (n.) Sensory terminal branch of the femoral nerve. Supplies the medial border of the foot and the medial side of the proximal tibia via its infrapatellar branch.

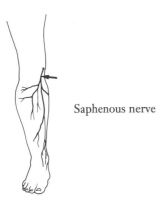

Saphenous nerve

Sarcolemma (sar/kō-lem-a) (n.) The cell membrane of a muscle fiber.

Sarcoma (sar′kō′ma) (n.) Any malignant tumor whose proliferative cells are of mesodermal origin.

Sarcomere (sar′kō-mēr) (n.) One of the basic contractile units of striated muscle fibers. They are bounded at each end by a Z-line.

Sarcoplasm (sar′kō-plazm) (n.) The cytoplasm of muscle cells.

Sarmiento Cast (sarmi-yent′-ō/kast) (n.) A functional, below-knee, patellar, tendon-bearing cast for use in the treatment of tibial fractures. Also known as a **Patellar Tendon Bearing** or **PTB Cast**.

Sartorius Muscle (sar-tor′ē-us/mus′el) (n.) See **Muscle**.

Saturday Night Palsy (sat′ur-dā/nīt/pal-sē) (n.) A nerve compression syndrome in which paralysis results from prolonged compression of a nerve against a hard edge or surface. Classically, Saturday night palsy presents as a wrist-drop in an alcoholic patient. It is noted on awakening after alcohol intoxication and passing out in any position with the arm abducted, e.g., over the edge of a chair or park bench.

Saturn's Ring Sign (sat-urnz/ring/sīn) (n.) Radiologic evidence of a dislocated Charnley-Muller total hip prosthesis consisting of changes in the relationship of the metallic acetabular ring to the "planet" (the femoral head). When normally implanted and assembled, the radiographic appearance of the prosthesis resembles the planet Saturn. Dislocation causes an eccentricity of the ring to the planet, hence the name.

Saucerization (saw″ser-i-zā′shun) (n.) An operative procedure in which tissue is excavated from a wound to form a saucerlike depression. It may be used to facilitate the drainage of infected bone.

Sausage Toe (saw′sij/tō) (n.) In Reiter's syndrome, a characteristic finding in the foot of simultaneous inflammation, with diffuse swelling, of the distal and proximal interphalangeal joints together with swelling of the metartarsophalangeal joints. This gives the toes a sausage-like appearance. Synonym: **Sausage Digit**.

Sayre Jacket (sā′er/jak′et) (n.) A plaster-of-Paris body jacket used to immobilize and support the vertebral column. The Sayre jacket is applied with the help of a Sayre apparatus, which suspends the patient by the head and axillae during application.

SC Joint (es′sē/joint) (n.) Abbreviation for **Sternoclavicular Joint**.

Scab (skab) (n.) A hard crust of dried blood, serum, or pus that develops over a sore, cut, or scratch during the wound-healing process.

Scales (skāls) (n.) A collection of horny material, usually on the skin, that varies in size from small, thin flakes to large sheets. Also called **Squames**.

Scalloped Vertebra (skal′apt/ver′te-bra) (n.) A vertebral body with an exaggeration of the normal concavity of its surface.

Scalpel (skal′pel) (n.) A surgical knife.

Scan (skan) (n.) The record obtained by an imaging technique of the body being examined. Examples include nuclear scans and CAT scans.

Scan Speed (skan/spēd) (n.) The speed at which the detecting system traverses the tissue or organ being scanned.

Scanning (skan′ning) (n.) A diagnostic procedure used in radiology and nuclear medicine used to visualize a structure.

Scaphoid (skāf′oid) (n.) The carpal navicular bone. It is one of the bones in the proximal carpal row that articulates with the distal radius proximally; with the lunate ulnarly; and with the trapezium, trapezoid, and capitate in the distal carpal row.

Scapholunate Dissociation (skāf′-o-lūn-āt/dis-so′-ci-ā′shun) (n.) A traumatic injury to the wrist in which the normal relationship of the scaphoid and lunate bones is altered following ligamentous injury.

Scaphoradial Angle (skāf′o-rā-dial/ang′gl) (n.) On a lateral roentgenogram of the wrist, the angle formed between the longitudinal axis of the carpal scaphoid and the longitudinal axis of the radius.

Scapula (skap′-u-la) (n.) The flat, triangular bone of the shoulder girdle; it is commonly referred to as the shoulder blade. Laterally, it has an acromial process that articulates with the clavicle, and it forms the glenoid fossa with which the humeral head articulates. The undersurface forms parts of the scapulothoracic joint.

Scapula Notch (skap′u-la/noch) (n.) A groove in the upper border of the scapula just medial to the cora-

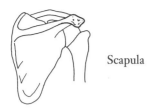

Scapula

coid process. The suprascapular nerve and artery pass through and may be entrapped at this point.

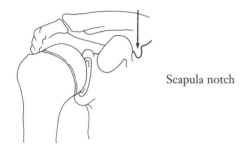

Scapula notch

Scapular Line (skap′-ū-lar/līn) (n.) A vertical line passing through the inferior angle of the scapula that marks the medial edge of the scapula.

Scar (skar) (n.) The connective tissue replacement that follows the loss of dermal tissue. Also called **Cicatrix**.

Scarpa's Fascia (skar′-pahz/fash′-ē-ah) (n.) The deep, membranous layer of the subcutaneous abdominal fascia. It is contiguous with the superficial fascia of the thigh.

Scarpa's Triangle (skar′-pahz/tri′-ang-g l) (n.) An anatomic triangle. It is bounded superiorly by the inguinal ligament, laterally by the sartorius muscle, and medially by the medial border of the adductor longus muscle. The flattened tendon of the adductor longus attaches to the front of the body of the pubis and runs laterally with the pectineus, forming the floor of the triangle. Also known as the **Femoral Triangle**.

Scattered Radiation (skat′erd/rā-dē-ā′shun) (n.) Radiation that, during its passage through a substance, has been diverted, occasionally with an energy loss. This refers to the secondary radiation produced from the deviation in direction.

SCFE Abbreviation for slipped capital femoral epiphysis.

Schaeffer Orthosis (shaf′er/or-thō′sis) (n.) A type of foot orthosis used to increase support at the talonavicular articulation. It features a flange on the medial side from the middle of the heel, flowing first in a modified "S" curve to the middle of the navicular area, then in a straight line to the middle of the first metatarsal head area.

Schaeffer Reflex (shāf′er/rē′fleks) (n.) A pyramidal tract sign elicited by pinching the Achilles tendon. The Schaeffer reflex consists of dorsiflexion of the great toe and fanning of the other toes. See also **Babinski Sign**.

Schanz Screws (shants/skrūz) (n.) Fixation half-pins used in conjunction with a Wagner apparatus for external fixation. The pin sites must be predrilled before screw insertion.

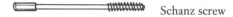

Schanz screw

Scheie's Syndrome (shāz/sin′drōm) (n.) One of the mucopolysaccharidoses, with an autosomal recessive pattern of inheritance. On urinalysis, one sees increased dermatan sulfate excretion. The main clinical features are progressive corneal opacites and joint stiffness and contracture, especially in the fingers. Also known as **Mucopolysaccharidoses**.

Scheuermann Disease (shoi′-er-mānz/di-zēz′) (n.) An eponym for juvenile thoracic kyphosis; it is included in the category of juvenile osteochondroses. The etiology is unknown, but radiographic diagnosis is based on the findings of decreased disk spaces, increased anteroposterior diameter of the involved vertebrae and decreased height of these vertebrae, and plate irregularity. The occurrence of Schmorl's node is also a possibility. Strictly speaking, however, the diagnosis of Scheuermann disease is confined to those patients in whom anterior vertebral body wedging of at least 5 degrees in three consecutive vertebrae is found. Treatment depends on the age of the patient, the degree of kyphosis, the presence or absence of progression of the curve, and the amount of wedging present.

Scheuthauer-Marie Syndrome (shoy′-tow-er/mah-rē/sin′drom) (n.) A cleidocranial dysplasia.

Schmorl's Node (shmorlz/nōd) (n.) A punched-out area in the end-plate of a vertebral body that is surrounded by compact bone. It is due to intraosseous prolapse of the nucleus pulposus into the vertebral body. On a lateral radiograph a Schmorl's node is seen as a radiolucency or hemispherical bone defect in the upper or lower margin of the body of the affected vertebra.

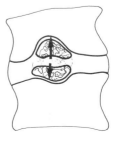

Schmorl's node

Schneider Nail (shnī'der/nal) (n.) A four-flanged, self-broaching, intramedullary nail for fractures of the femoral shaft.

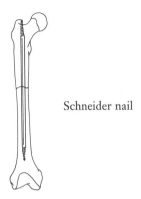

Schneider nail

Schober Test (shō'-ber/test) (n.) A measurement of forward flexion of the lumbar spine. The measurement declines with progressive loss of spinal motion, and this correlates closely with radiologic determinations of the arc of movement of the lumbar spine on the sacrum. With the patient standing erect, make a mark on the skin overlying the lumbosacral junction–this would be at the imaginary line joining the posterosuperior iliac spines. Make another mark 10 cm above this. Ask the patient to bend forward as if to touch his or her toes. With the spine in the fullest flexion, measure the distance between the two marks. Record the final total distance in centimeters to the nearest 0.1 cm (for example, 15.5 cm). A normal measurement is greater than 15 cm.

Schoemaker Line (shō-mah-kerz/līn) (n.) A topographic sign of congenital dislocation of the hip. A line is drawn from the tip of the greater trochanter through the anterior superior spine and toward the midline. Normally, the midline is reached above the umbilicus; in congenital dislocation of the hip, however, the line crosses the midline of the body below the umbilicus.

Schroeder van der Kolk's Law (shrā'der/van/der/kōks/law) (n.) The law stating that the sensory fibers of a mixed nerve are distributed to the parts moved by muscles and that these muscles are stimulated by the motor fibers of the same nerve.

Schwachman-Diamond Syndrome (shwahk'-man/dī-mond/sin-drōm) (n.) Metaphyseal chondrodysplasia with malabsorption and neutropenia.

Schwann Cell (shwon/sel) (n.) A neuroectodermal cell that sheathes the axons of the peripheral nervous system. It is surrounded by an extracellular basement membrane. Nonmyelinated axons are encased in a tunnel within Schwann cells. In myelinated nerves, axons are sheathed by a spiral wrap formed by the Schwann cell itself, with each Schwann cell surrouding only one axon for a longitudinal segment.

Schwannoma (shwon-nō'-mah) (n.) See **Neurofibroma**.

Sciatic Impingement (sī-at'ol/im-pinj'mint) (n.) To strike or hit the sciatic nerve, frequently caused by posterior dislocation of the femoral head from the acetabulum.

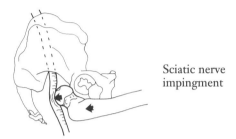

Sciatic nerve impingment

Sciatic Nerve (sī-at'ik/nerv) (n.) The major nerve of the leg that arises from the sacral plexus. It is formed by the confluence of the fourth and fifth lumbars, and the first, second and third sacral nerve roots. It emerges from the pelvis into the gluteal region through the greater sciatic notch. It extends to the distal one-third of the thigh, where it branches into the tibial and common peroneal nerves. It innervates the skin and muscles of both the leg and foot.

Sciatic Notch (sī-at'ik/noch) (n.) See **Sacrosciatic Notch**.

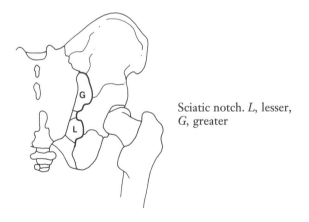

Sciatic notch. *L*, lesser, *G*, greater

Sciatic Stress Test (sī-at'-ik/stres/test) (n.) Any of several clinical tests used in the evaluation of nerve root irritation in the lower extremity. The basic principle of these tests is that extending the knee with the hip flexed will stretch an already inflamed sciatic nerve and cause radicular pain.

Sciatica (sī-at'-i-kah) (n.) A general term applied to the clinical syndrome associated with a herniated lumbar intervertebral disk that causes nerve root irritation, which is characterized by low back pain radiating down the leg. Specific neurologic findings depend on the site of the nerve root involved. See **Radiculopathy**.

Sciatic Foramen (sī-at′-ik/fo-rā′-men) (n.) Either of the two foramina—the greater and the smaller or lesser sciatic foramina—that are formed by the sacrotuberal and sacrospinal ligaments in the sciatic notch of the pelvis.

Scintigram (sin′-ti-gram) (n.) A graphic recording of the distribution of a radioactive tracer in a part of the body. A scintigram is produced by recording the flashes of light given off by a scintillator as it is struck by radiation of different intensities. By scanning the body section by section, a scintiscan, or "map," of the radioactivity in various regions is built up.

Scintillation (sin′-ti-lā′-shun) (n.) A particle emitted in the disintegration of a radioactive element.

Scintillation Scanning (sin′-ti-la′shun/skan′-ning) (n.) A systematic mapping of isotope distribution in an organ system. A detector momentarily records the concentration of isotopes within a particular small area before moving to the next area. This customarily involves rectilinear movement. Also known as **Radioisotope** or **Nuclear Scanning**.

Scintillascope (sin-til′-ah-skōp) (n.) The instrument used to produce a scintigram. The scintillascope incorporates a scintillator, which magnifies the fluorescence produced in it by radiation, and a recording device, which is often aided by a computer.

Scintiphotograph (sin′-ti-fō′-tō-graf) (n.) A photographic record of the isotope distribution in an organ. It is obtained from the oscilloscopic screen of a scintillation camera.

Scintiscan (sin′-ti-skan) (n.) See **Scintigram**.

Scipp Line (ship/līn) (n.) On a lateral radiograph of the pelvis, the line passing from the SacroCoccygeal joint to the Inferior Point of the Pubic bone. Synonym: **Sacrococcygeal Pubic Line**.

Scissoring (siz-or-ing) (n.) The adduction posture of the hips during stance, which is often accentuated by attempted ambulation. It is due to spasm or overpull of the hip adductor muscles. Frequently seen in spastic diplegia or paraplegia.

Scissors Gait (siz′-erz/gāt) (n.) A spastic walk in which the legs are strongly adducted at the hips, crossing alternately in front of one another, with the knees scraping together; this results in short steps and slow progression. A scissors gait is due to a spasticity of the hip adductors and medial hamstrings and is characteristic of patients with spastic diplegia or paraplegia.

Scleroderma (skle″rō-der′mah) (n.) A disease of connective tissue characterized by varying degrees of inflammation, fibrosis, and vascular shunts in the skin and internal organs (skin, lungs, heart, gastrointestinal tract, joints, and kidney). It is more accurately known as progressive systemic sclerosis.

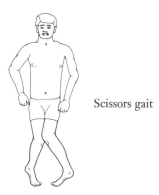

Scissors gait

Scleroderma occurs three times more frequently in women than in men, with peak prevalence during the fourth and fifth decades. Synonym: **Systemic Sclerosis**. See also **Progressive Systemic Sclerosis**.

Sclerosing Osteomyelitis of Garré (skle-rōs′ing/os″te-o-mī′e-lī′tis/of/gar-rā′) (n.) A chronic form of bone infection in which the bone is thickened, sclerotic, and expanded radiographically, but no abscess or sequestrum is identifiable. Cultures are generally negative. The etiology is unclear, but it may result from a low-grade anaerobic infection.

Sclerosis (skle-rō′sis) (n.) 1. Hardening and/or thickening of a tissue or organ, usually due to an increase in fibrous tissue. 2. An abnormal increase in the density of bone, will create a denser, whiter roentgenographic appearance than normal.

Sclerotomal Pain (skle′rō-tomal/pain) (n.) A deep, diffuse, aching, ill-defined pain arising from deep somatic tissues. Contrast to **Dermatomal Pain**.

Sclerotome (skle′rō-tōm) (n.) In the embryo, the ventral mass of the somite that gives rise to the axial skeleton. Compare to **Dermatome** and **Myotome**.

Scoliometer (skō″le-ō-me′ter) (n.) A proprietary name for an inclinometer used in evaluating vertebral body rotation and rib deformity in patients with scoliosis. Developed by Dr. William Bunnell.

Scoliosis (skō″lē-ō′sis) (n.) An appreciable lateral deviation in the normally vertical line of the spine. Sco-

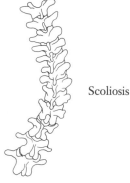

Scoliosis

liosis consists of a lateral curvature of the spine and rotation of the vertebrae around the long axis of the spine. The ribs on the convex side of the curve may become prominent as the vertebral bodies rotate toward the convex side while the spinous processes rotate toward the concave side of the curve. Eventually, the disk spaces are narrowed on the concave side and widened on the convex side. Scoliosis is classified by etiology and described by location, association with other curvature of the spine, and sometimes age of onset. Radiologic evaluation of scoliosis requires upright film of the entire spine in frontal and lateral projection.

Scoliotic Index (skō″lē-ot′ik/in′deks) (n.) A comprehensive representation of a spinal curve, which measures the deviation of each involved vertebral segment from four vertical spinal lines, with multiple points taken along the scoliotic curve. The scoliotic index is calculated by averaging the sums of the linear deviation of the centers of each vertebral body from each vertical line; this figure is then normalized by the length of the vertical line in order to eliminate the influence of magnification. A value of zero is a straight spine; numbers greater than zero will be present in scoliosis.

Scotch Cast (skoch/kast) (n.) A trademark for a synthetic fiberglass casting material.

Scottish-Rite Hospital Orthosis (scot′ish-rīt/hos′pit-'l/or-tho′sis) (n.) A custom-made ambulatory abduction orthosis used in treating Legg-Calvé-Perthes disease. It consists of a pelvic band, free motion single axis hip joints, medial and lateral uprights, thigh lacers, posterior bands, and a telescoping rod to limit adduction while allowing further abduction. The telescoping rod is connected by heavy-duty universal joints, which allow hip flexion and extension as well as abduction.

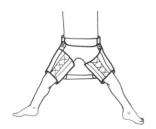

Scottish-Rite hospital orthosis

Scotty Dog Sign (skot′-tē/dog/sīn) (n.) A radiographic sign of spondylolysis. An outline resembling a Scottish terrier can be seen in the normal oblique radiograph of the lumbosacral spine. The nose of the Scotty dog represents the transverse process; the ears, the superior articulating process; the neck, the pars interarticularis; the leg, the inferior articular facet; and the eye, the pedicle. In spondylolysis, the defect in the pars interarticularis shows as a collar

(ie, a break or separation) on the neck of the Scotty dog. See **Pars Interarticularis, Spondylolysis**.

Scotty dog sign

Scout Film (skowt/film) (n.) A preliminary or survey radiographic film of a body part taken prior to either the administration of opaque media or to CT scanning to determine the level of the radiographic cuts.

Screw (skrū) (n.) A mechanical device consisting of a continuous helical thread projecting from a cylindrical shank. It is intended to fix or fasten materials together and is inserted by rotating the device.

Screw–Home Movement (skrū/hōm/mūv′ment) (n.) The terminal medial rotation of the femur that occurs at full extension of the knee during weightbearing. This movement is due to the existence of a larger area of bearing surface on the medial condyle, as compared with the lateral condyle. When the whole articular surface of the lateral condyle has been used, the femur rotates around the tibial spine until the joint is "screwed-home," or closely locked in extension.

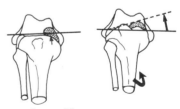

Screw-Home movement

Scrub Nurse (skrub/nurs) (n.) A term used to designate the nursing member of the sterile team. This person may or may not be a nurse; the role of scrub nurse may be filled by a registered nurse, a practical nurse, or an operating room technician. Sometimes called the sterile nurse, instrument nurse, suture nurse, or if this person is not a nurse, the scrub tech.

Scurvy (skur′vē) (n.) The clinical syndrome that results from a vitamin C deficiency.

Seal Fin Deformity (sēl/fin/di-for′mi-tē) (n.) The

appearance of the ulnar deviation of the fingers in patients with rheumatoid arthritis.

Seat Belt Fracture (sēt/belt/frak'chur) (n.) A fracture of the thoracolumbar spine most often described in patients wearing only a lap-type seat belt at the time of a motor-vehicle injury. The body is flexed over the belt, which results in tensile stress to the vertebral body and neural arch, because they are both posterior to the flexion axis. These fractures and dislocations may occur through only bone, bone and soft tissue, or soft tissue only. The all-bone injury is also known as a **Chance Fracture**.

Sebaceous Cyst (se-bā'shus/sist) (n.) A benign cyst of the subcutaneous tissue that contains oily sebum derived from sebaceous glands.

Second Opinion (sek'und/ō-pin'yen) (n.) The examination and evaluation of a patient who has been recommended for surgery by another surgeon.

Second-Opinion Program (sek'und/ō-pin'yen/prō'gram) (n.) The elective or mandatory medical review mechanism established by a health benefit program to encourage the provision of second opinions.

Secondary Astragalus (sek'un-der″ē/ah-strag'ah-lus) (n.) An accessory bone of the foot. The secondary astragalus is a small, rounded bone found just above the head of the astragalus. It is seen only in lateral radiographic views of the foot.

Secondary Closure (sek'un-der″ē/klō'zher) (n.) A technique of wound closure in which a wound that was initially left open is sutured or grafted closed after granulation tissue has appeared.

Secondary Disease (sek'un-der″ē/di-zēz') (n.) A morbid condition subsequent to or consequent to another disease.

Secondary Gain (sek'un-der″ē/gān) (n.) The external, situational gain derived from any illness (e.g., personal attention and service or monetary gains such as disability benefits).

Secondary Gout (sek'un-der″ē/gout) (n.) An identifiable and acquired cause for the clinical manifestations of gout. Unlike primary gout, secondary gout is not due to an inborn error of purine metabolism. Compare to **Primary Gout**.

Secondary Intention (sek'un-der″ē/in-ten'shun) (n.) The healing of a wound by granulation tissue. The wound is allowed to develop good granulation tissue; then epithelialization proceeds from the periphery to the center of the wound to cover the granulation tissue. Compare to **Primary Intention**.

Secondary Ossification Center (sek'un-der″ē/os'si-fi-cā'shun/sen'ter) (n.) The epiphysis.

Secondary Suture Line (sek'un-der″ē/sū'cher/līn) (n.) The sutures reinforcing and supporting the primary suture line, obliterating dead space, and preventing fluid accumulation in the wound during healing by first intention. The secondary suture line exerts tension lateral to the primary suture line, thus contributing to the tensile strength of the wound. Su-

tures used for this purpose are referred to as retention, stay, or tension sutures.

Secretion (sē-krē'shun) (n.) The product of any cell, gland, or tissue that is released through the cell membrane.

Seddon's Classification of Nerve Injury (sed'onz/klas″sĭ-fĭ-ka'shun/ov/nerv/in'ju-re) (n.) A simple classification of traumatic injuries to nerves. The minimal injury is termed **neurapraxia** and may be secondary to localized ischemic demyelination. The moderate injury is termed **axonotmesis** and is characterized by the interruption of the axons and their myelin sheaths while the endoneurial tubes remain intact and guide the regenerating axons to their proper peripheral connections. A severe injury is termed **neurotmesis**, denoting a nerve that has either been completely severed or is so disorganized that spontaneous regeneration is impossible. In summary **neurapraxia** denotes physiologic loss of conduction, **axonotmesis** denotes axonal degeneration with sheaths intact, and **neurotmesis** denotes severence of nerve trunk.

Sedimentation Rate (sed″ĭ-men-ta'shun/rāt) (n.) The rate at which erythrocytes settle out of unclotted blood in one hour. Abbreviated **Sed. Rate** or **ESR**.

Segmental Fracture (seg-men'tal/frak'chur) (n.) A fracture consisting of more than one fracture line at different levels in the same bone, which creates several fracture fragments.

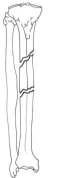

Segmental fracture

Segmental Instability (seg-men'tal/in'stah-bil'i-tē) (n.) An abnormal response to applied loads, characterized by motion in the motor segment beyond normal constraints.

Segmental Spinal Instrumentation (seg-men'tal/spi'nal/in″strū-men-tā'shun) (n.) A variety of techniques of spinal fixation that originally implied the use of sublaminar wires to secure steel rods to the spine. More recently, the term is used to refer to any implant attached by a variety of techniques to multiple vertebrae. Examples include transverse-coupled Luque, Cotrel-Dubousset, Dwyer, L-Rod,

Zielke, Wisconsin, segmented spinal, and augmented Harrington instrumentation. Abbreviated **SSI**.

Segond Fracture (seg-ōnd/frak′chur) (n.) A capsular avulsion fracture at the margin of the lateral tibial plateau seen in association with anterior cruciate ligament tears. It is also called the **Lateral Capsular Sign**.

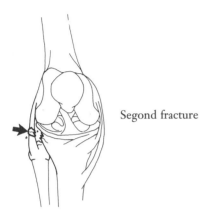

Segond fracture

Seimon's Sign (sī-munz/sīn) (n.) A young child who cries on sitting up from a supine position, but not if his or her head is passively supported during the movement, has a fractured odontoid process until proven otherwise. Described by Leonard Seimon of New York.

Self-Insurance (self/in-shūr′ans) (n.) Means by which hospitals or professionals may, in lieu of commercial insurance, assume financial responsibility for liability.

Self-Limited Disease (self/lim′it-ed/di-zez′) (n.) A disease that, by its very nature, runs a limited and definite course.

Self-Retaining Retractor (self/re-tān-ing/re-trakt′or) (n.) Any one of many surgical instruments having two retractor arms clamped to a bar and adjusted by means of setscrews. The surgical assistant does not have to hold the retractor. See **Charnley Retractor**.

Self-Tapping Screw (self/tap′ping/skrū) (n.) A screw with cutting flutes on the tip. A self-tapping screw cuts its own threads in a pilot hole as it is being inserted.

Sella Turcica (sel′ah/tur′cica) (n.) The saddlelike bone structure at the base of the skull that encloses the pituitary gland.

Semiconstrained Prosthesis (semi/kon-strand/pros-the′sis) (n.) A prosthetic joint that has some inherent stability owing to its geometry but that also relies on native soft-tissue tension.

Semilunar Cartilage (semī-lūnar/kar′ti-lij) (n.) An older name for a knee meniscus. See **Meniscus**.

Semimembranosus Muscle (semī-mem′bra-nō-sus/mus′el) (n.) See **Muscle**.

Semiprivate Room (semī-prī′vit/room) (n.) A hospital room designed and equipped to house two to four inpatients.

Semiprone Position (sem″ē-prōn/pō-zish′un) (n.) A body position in which one side of the body is strictly prone, the head is turned to the other side, and the limbs of that same side are slightly curled up and flexed at the shoulder, elbow, hip, and knee. The body is three-quarters prone.

Semitendinosus Muscle (sem″e-ten′di-nō-sus/mus′el) (n.) See **Muscle**.

Semitubular Plate (sem″e-tū′byu-lar/plāt) (n.) A type of plate used in the internal fixation of bone.

Senile Ankylosing Hyperostosis (se′nīl/ang′ki-lōs-ing/hī′per-os-tō′sis) (n.) See **Forestier's Disease**.

Senile Osteoporosis (sē′nīl/os″te-ō-po-rō′sis) (n.) Osteoporosis in the aged. It is due to deficient bone matrix formation most likely related to reduced gonadal hormones and diminished calcium intake. Blood calcium, phosphorus, and phosphate levels are all normal or low. See **Osteoporosis**.

Sensation (sen-sā′shun) (n.) An awareness or feeling due to stimulation of one of the senses.

Sensheimer Classification (sen-shī-mer/klas″sĭ-fĭ-ka′shun) (n.) An arrangement of subtrochanteric femoral fractures based on the number and the configuration of the fracture lines.

Type I: Nondisplaced fractures (or less than 2-mm displacement).

Type II: Two-part fractures: (1) transverse; (2) spiral, with the lesser trochanter attached to the proximal fragment, and (3) spiral, with the lesser trochanter attached to the distal fragment.

Type III: Three-part fractures: (1) spiral, with the lesser trochanter a part of the third fragment and (2) spiral, with the third part a butterfly fragment.

Type IV: Comminuted, with four or more fragments.

Type V: Subtrochanteric-intertrochanteric.

Sensibility (sen′si-bil′i-tē) (n.) The conscious appreciation and precise interpretation of sensation.

Sensitivity (sen″si-tiv′i-te) (n.) 1. The capacity of an organism to respond to stimulation, as in allergies. 2. The abnormal susceptibility of an organism, eg, that of a microorganism to an antibiotic. 3. In statistics, the ability of a test not to miss a positive result—e.g., a low false-negative rate.

Sensory (sen′so-rē) (adj.) Pertaining to sensation.

Sensory Deficit (sen′so-rē/def′i-sit) (n.) Any decrease or absence in perception of external stimulation of a body sense. This is frequently used to refer to a loss of touch awareness.

Sensory Nerve (sen′so-rē/nerv) (n.) Any nerve that carries impulses only toward the central nervous system or central ganglion and away from the receptor.

Sepsis (sēp′sis) (n.) The presence of pathogenic mi-

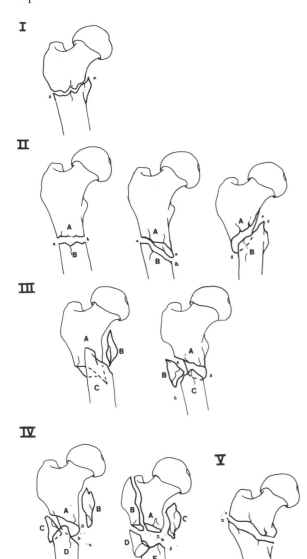

I

II

III

IV

V

Sensheimer classification

croorganisms or their toxins in the blood or other tissues.

Septic (sep′tik) (adj.) Of or pertaining to contamination with microorganisms or their toxins.

Septic Arthritis (sep′tik/ar-thrī′tis) (n.) Any joint infection caused by pyogenic organisms. Synonym: **Pyogenic Arthritis**.

Septic Shock (sep′tik/shok) (n.) A type of shock that results from toxins secreted by an infectious process. In these patients, peripheral vascular resistance and central venous pressure are low, cardiac output may be increased or decreased, and the patient is normovolemic.

Septicemia (sep″ti-sē′mē-ah) (n.) The presence of pathogenic microorganisms or their toxins in the blood. Commonly known as **Blood Poisoning**.

Sequela (se-kwē′lah) (n.) Any disorder or condition subsequent to a disease or injury.

Sequestered Disk (sē″kwes-terd/disk) (n.) See **Disk**.

Sequestration (sē″kwes-trā′shun) (n.) The formation of a fragment of dead bone and its separation from the surrounding tissue. Frequently seen in association with osteomyelitis.

Sequestrectomy (sē″kwes-trek′to-mē) (n.) The surgical removal of a sequestrum.

Sequestrum (sē-kwes′trum) (n.) A piece of detached or necrotic bone within a cavity, abscess, or wound.

Serial Casts (sē′re-al/kasts) (n.) The sequential application of casts for the progressive correction of a deformity.

Serial Films (sē′re-al/filmz) (n.) Radiographs taken in sequence, either during a single study or after longer intervals, to compare or record progressive events.

Seroma (ser-ō′mah) (n.) A benign accumulation of blood serum that produces a tumorlike swelling, usually beneath the skin.

Seronegative (sē″rō-neg′ah-tiv) (adj.) Having a negative serologic test.

Seronegative Spondyloarthropathies (sē″rō-neg′ah-tiv/spon″di-lō-ar-throp′ah-thē) (n.) A diverse group of acute and chronic rheumatic diseases that share certain pathogenic, histologic, morphoradiographic, laboratory, and clinical features; these diseases are so named, however, because of their notable absence of a positive rheumatoid factor in the blood. There is a predilection for spinal and sacroiliac joint involvement and an association with specific human leukocyte antigens (HLA-B27 and others). Ankylosing spondylitis (AS) is the prototype form of this disease group, which includes such other well-defined clinical entities as Reiter syndrome and true psoriatic arthritis.

Seropositive (sē″rō-poz′i-tiv) (adj.) Having a positive serologic test.

Serotonin (sēr″ō-tō′nin) (n.) A peptide hormone that is a powerful smooth-muscle stimulator and vasoconstrictor.

Serous Fluid (sē′rus/flū′id) (n.) The clear, watery fluid secreted by serous membranes of the body, such as the pleural cavity and the peritoneal lining of the abdomen.

Serratia (se-ra′she-ah) (n.) The genus of gram-negative rods found in the family *Enterobacteriaceae*.

Serratus Anterior Muscle (se-ra′tus/an-ter′e-or/mus′el) (n.) See **Muscle**.

Serratus Posterior Muscle (se-ra′tus/pos-ter′e-or/mus′el) (n.) See **Muscle**.

Serum (se′rum) (n.) The fluid portion of blood that remains after the removal of cells, platelets, and fibrin.

Serum Electrophoresis (se'rum/e-lek-trō-for'ē-sis) (n.) A method of separating the main groups of proteins in serum used to locate abnormal proteins and to detect both the presence of abnormal hemoglobins and changes in the relative quantities of proteins.

Sesamoid Bone (ses'ah-moid/bōn) (n.) An ovoid nodule of bone that develops within a tendon. The patella, the fabella, and certain bones in the hand and foot are all sesamoid bones.

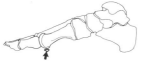

Sesamoid bone

Sesamoid Index (ses'ah-moid/in'deks) (n.) The product of the height and width (both in millimeters) of the medial sesamoid of the metacarpophalangeal joint of the thumb. The normal value for females varies from 12 to 33 and for males from 7.5 to 48.

Sesamoiditis (ses"ah-moi-dī'tis) (n.) A local inflammation of the medial or lateral sesamoid located beneath the head of the first metatarsal.

Sessile Osteochondroma (ses-īl/os-tē-ō-kon-drō-mah) (n.) A benign osteochondral tumor that has a broad-based attachment to the bone of origin.

Sever's Disease (sē-verz/di-zez') (n.) An apophysitis of the calcaneus in which increased density and fragmentation of the apophysis is seen radiographically, and tenderness at this region is found clinically. This disorder used to be considered under the term juvenile osteochondrosis, but no true localized osteonecrosis has been defined.

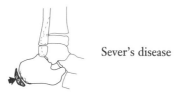

Sever's disease

Sex-Linked (seks/lingk'd) (adj.) Of or pertaining to genetic characteristics determined by genes located on the X or Y chromosomes.

SGPT (n.) An abbreviation for Serum Glutamic Pyruvic Transaminase.

SGOT (n.) An abbreviation for Serum Glutamic Oxaloacetic Transaminase.

Shaft Fracture (shaft/frak'chur) (n.) A fracture that occurs in the diaphyseal portion of a bone.

Shank (shangk) (n.) 1. The long, narrow portion of a screw, extending below the head. It may be fully or partially threaded. 2. In shoe terminology, the portion of the sole between the ball and the anterior border of the heel.

Shank Piece (shangk/pēs) (n.) In shoe terminology, a rigid supportive material that reinforces the shank area of a shoe.

Shank Pitch (shangk/pich) (n.) In shoe terminology, the plane or angle of the shank area that runs from the breast of the heel to the sole contact or ball of the foot.

Shantz Osteotomy (shantz/os"te-ot'o-me) (n.) An osteotomy of the proximal femur to stabilize a congenitally dislocated hip. The distal fragment is placed in abduction.

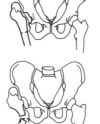

Shantz osteotomy

Sharp Dissection (sharp/dis-sec'tion) (n.) The surgical separation of tissues by means of the sharp edge of a knife or scalpel, or by scissors.

Sharp and Pursor Test (sharp/and/pur'ser/test) (n.) A maneuver used in the evaluation of atlantoaxial instability. With the patient seated, place the palm of one hand on the patient's forehead and the thumb of the other hand on the tip of the spinous process of the axis. Ask the patient to relax the neck in a semiflexed position. By pressing backward with the palm, you can note a sliding motion of the head backward in relation to the spine of the axis. A positive test is indicated by an abrupt shift forward, which is usually accompanied by a palpable clunk.

Sharpey's Fibers (sharp'-ēz/fi'berz) (n.) The thick bundles of collagenous fibers passing from the periosteum into the outer circumferential lamellae. They fix the periosteum firmly to the surface of the bone, particularly the following: at the points of tendon and muscle attachment, at the areas where large blood vessels and nerves enter the bone, and at the epiphyses of long bones.

Sharrard's Procedure (sher-ardz'/prō-se-jur) (n.) A surgical technique for the treatment of paralysis of the gluteus medius and maximus muscles. The iliopsoas tendon and the iliacus muscle are transferred posteriorly through a hole placed in the ilium and reattached to the proximal femur. Named for John Sharrard, M.D., of Sheffield, England.

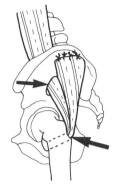

Sharrard's procedure

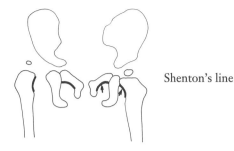

Shenton's line

Shear (shēr) (n.)   In biomechanical terms, a load applied parallel to the surface of a structure. It results in angular deformation.

Shear Modulus (shēr/mod-ū-lus) (n.)   The ratio of shear stress to the shear strain in a material. The unit of measure is either newtons per square meter or pascals (pounds per square foot).

Shear Strain (shēr/strān) (n.)   The amount of angular deformation that occurs from shear loading.

Sheath (shēth) (n.)   The layer or membrane of connective tissue that envelops structures such as tendons, nerves, or arteries.

Sheet Wadding (shēt/wad′ding) (n.)   A glazed cotton bandage used for padding under a cast. It is available in various widths and thicknesses.

Shelf Procedure (shelf/prō-se-jur) (n.)   Surgical treatments of congenital hip dysplasia. A variety of techniques can be used, but all construct an extraarticular bony extensor of the acetabulum. The primary indication is a deficient acetabulum that cannot be corrected by a redirectional pelvic osteotomy.

Shepherd's Crook Deformity (shep-herdz/krook/de-for′mi-tē) (n.)   A deformity of the proximal femur in which lateral bowing of the femoral shaft is associated with marked varus of the femoral neck. This is so named because of the resemblance of the upper end of the femoral shaft to a shepherd's crook. This is classically described in association with fibrous dysplasia.

Shepherd's Fracture (shep-herdz/frak′chur) (n.)   An eponym for an avulsion fracture of the lateral tubercle of the posterior process of the talus. It is sometimes mistaken for a displaced os trigonum.

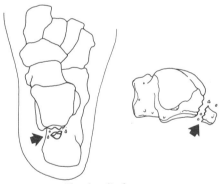

Shepherd's fracture

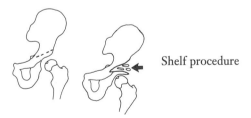

Shelf procedure

Shenton's Line (shen-tonz/līn) (n.)   On an AP radiograph of the pelvis, a line drawn along the medial border of the neck of the femur and the superior border of the obturator foramen. In a normal hip, Shenton's line is an even arc of continuous contour. This line is interrupted in the presence of hip subluxation or dislocation. Less commonly known as **Menard's Line**. Synonym: **Cervico-obturator Line**.

Sherrington's Law (shār-ing-tonz/law) (n.)   The law stating that every posterior spinal nerve root supplies a special region of skin, even though fibers from adjacent spinal segments may invade such a region.

Shielding (shēl-ding) (n.)   1. Any material or obstruction that absorbs radiation, thus protecting personnel from its effects. 2. A bone plate shields the underlying fracture callus from stress.

Shigella (shi-gel′la) (n.)   The genus of pathogenic gram-negative bacilli. It is from the family Enterobacteriaceae.

Shin (shin) (n.)   The colloquial term for the prominent anterior margin of the tibia or the prosthetic leg.

Shin Splints (shin/splints) (n.)   A commonly used term for a syndrome of exercise-induced leg pain more accurately called **medial tibial stress syn-**

drome. The leg pain and tenderness occur along the medial border of the distal third of the tibia. Pain, variable in intensity, is induced by exercise and relieved by rest. Motor, sensory, vascular or radiographic abnormalities are usually not present. This syndrome often occurs in running athletes. It has been previously defined by the AMA Standard Nomenclature as "pain and discomfort in the leg from repetitive running on hard surfaces, or forcible, excessive use of the foot dorsiflexors." Diagnosis should be limited to the musculotendinous inflammations, excluding fracture and ischemic disorders.

Shock (shok) (n.)   A disruption in the effective volume of circulating blood due to various causes. It is characterized by a fall in systolic blood pressure; a rapid, thready pulse; and pale, cool, moist skin. The clinical condition is characterized by signs and symptoms arising from inadequate capillary blood flow to vital organs and tissues. In general, shock may be classified into the following etiologic categories: **hemorrhagic** (or hypovolemic); **neurologic**, **vasogenic** (e.g., septic), and **cardiogenic**.

Shoe (shū) (n.)   An external covering or appliance for the foot. The major components of a shoe are the sole, heel, upper, linings, and reinforcements.

Shoemaker's Line (shoo-māk′erz/līn) (n.)   In the clinical evaluation of hip dislocation, draw a line from the tip of the greater trochanter through the anterior superior iliac spine, and extend it toward the midline. In congenital dislocation of the hip, the line meets the midline of the body below the umbilicus. Normally, the midline is reached at or above the umbilicus.

Short Stature (short/stach′er) (n.)   Lower-than-average body height.

Short Arm Cast (short/arm/kast) (n.)   A cast used for the immobilization of various injuries involving the forearm, wrist, or hand. The short-arm cast extends from below the elbow to the proximal palmar crease. The thumb and the fingers are left free at the metacarpophalangeal joints. After the cast is applied, the patient should be able to use his or her fingers and thumb freely, without any impingement on normal motion. Abbreviated **SAC**.

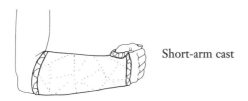

Short-arm cast

Short-Arm Splint (short/arm/splint) (n.)   Any splint extending from below the elbow to the palm. This splint is used to immobilize a number of injuries involving the forearm, the wrist, and the hand.

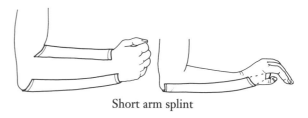

Short arm splint

Short Leg Brace (short/leg/brās) (n.)   An ankle–foot orthosis. Extends below the knee to and including the foot.

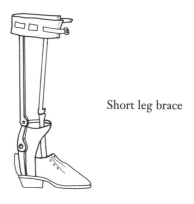

Short leg brace

Short Leg Cast (short/leg/kast) (n.)   A cast extending from below the knee to the base of the toes. After the cast is applied, the patient should be able to move the toes freely.

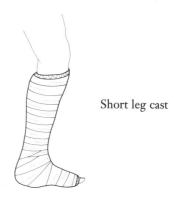

Short leg cast

Short Leg Gait (short/leg/gāt) (n.)   A limp produced by a shortened lower extremity; the severity of the limp depends on the extent of the length discrepancy. Clinically, the patient's head, shoulder, and pelvis dip down as the body weight is borne on the short lower extremity.

Short Leg Walker (short/leg/wok′er) (n.)   A below knee circular reinforced cloth splint attached to a rigid foot plate via ankle hinges.

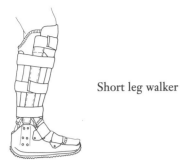

Short leg walker

Shortening (shor'r'n-ing) (n.)   Any loss of length in a body part.

Shortwave Therapy (short'wāve'/ther'e-pē) (n.)   An effective, deep-heating method useful in the treatment of large body segments and deep body parts. Shortwave therapy units produce various high-frequency electromagnetic waves, the most popular being 27 Mc, with wavelengths of 11 m. As the electromagnetic waves pass through living tissue, resistance to their passage is encountered. The electrical component of the electromagnetic wave tends to produce a temperature increase in such tissues as fat, which offer the greatest resistance to electrical currents. Tissues with high electrolyte content, such as muscle, experience vibrational molecular movements owing to the magnetic component and thus sustain a temperature increase.

Shoulder (shōl-der) (n.)   The ball-and-socket joint of the upper extremity, where the humeral head articulates with the glenoid fossa of the scapula. Also called the **Shoulder Girdle** and **Pectoral Girdle**.

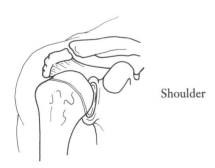

Shoulder

Shoulder-Hand Syndrome (shōl-der/hand/sin' drōm) (n.)   A type of reflex sympathetic dystrophy characterized by pain and stiffness in the shoulder and associated with painful disability of the hand and fingers. The syndrome occurs more frequently in older age groups and after cardiac dysfunction. Shoulder-hand syndrome may follow cervical spondylitis, various types of fractures, a cerebrovascular accident, coronary occlusion, or any visceral, musculoskeletal, vascular, or neural processes involving reflex neurovascular responses.

Shoulder Harness (shōl-der/har'nis) (n.)   A harness applied across both shoulders to provide suspension of an upper-limb prosthesis and to allow for activation of certain mobile parts of the prosthesis. Less commonly, a shoulder harness attaches to an orthosis.

Shoulder Immobilizer (shōl'der/im-mo'bil-īz-er) (n.)   An orthopedic appliance that maintains the arm against the body for shoulder immobilization.

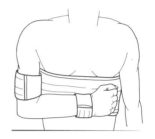

Shoulder immobilizer

Shoulder Periarthritis (shōl-der/per'ē-ar-thrī'tis) (n.)   See **Adhesive Capsulitis**.

Shoulder Roll (shōl-der/rōl) (n.)   A roll of cloth or a preformed foam roll placed under each side of the patient's chest to raise it off the operating table, thus facilitating respiration when the patient is placed in a prone position. Also called a **Bolster**.

Shoulder Spica Cast (shōl-der/spī-ka/kast) (n.)   A body jacket or cast enclosing the trunk, shoulder, and part of the upper extremity.

Shuck Test (shuk/test) (n.)   A means to evaluate the adequacy of the size of the endoprosthesis in total or hemi-hip arthroplasty. After implanting a trial prosthesis, relocate the hip. Look for laxity by pulling on the extended limb and observing the relationship of the components for excessive separation between the head and the acetabulum.

Shuffling Gait (shuf'fling/gāt) (n.)   A walk in which the feet barely leave the ground; often combined with short steps. A shuffling gait is seen in parkinsonism and amyotrophic lateral sclerosis.

SI   International System of Units. From the French, Le Système International d'Unites.

SI Joint (n.)   Abbreviation for Sacroiliac joint.

SI Units (n.)   The International System of Units. Its basic units are meter (m) for length, kilogram (kg) for mass, second (s) for time, and centigrade or Celsius (C) for temperature.

Sicard Sign (sē-karz/sīn) (n.)   A diagnostic marker in sciatica. In a modification of the Lasègue test, have the patient lie supine and raise his or her extended leg to a point just short of producing pain. Dorsiflexion of the big toe elicits the sciatic pain.

Sicca Syndrome (sē-ka/sin-drōm) (n.)   See **Sjögren's Syndrome**.

Side Effect (sīd/ē-fekt) (n.) A secondary, usually adverse effect of a drug or other form of therapy.

Sideswipe Fractures (sīd′-swīp/frak′-churz) (n.) Any of a variety of injuries resulting when an elbow protruding from a car window is hit by a car passing in the opposite direction.

Sign (sīn) (n.) 1. Any objective evidence of disease or dysfunction. 2. An observable physical phenomenon so frequently associated with a given condition as to be considered indicative of its presence.

Significance (sig-nif′i-kens) (n.) In statistics, a relationship between two groups of observations that indicates that the difference between them is unlikely to have occurred by chance alone.

Significant Difference (sig-nif′e-kant/dif′er-ens) (n.) A difference between two statistical constants calculated from two separate samples and of such magnitude that it is unlikely to have occurred by chance alone. This probability must usually be less than 0.05 (5%) before a difference is accepted as significant. The smaller the probability, the more significant the difference.

Silastic (sī-las′tik) (n.) The trademark for polymeric silicone substances that have some of the properties of rubber. Silastic is biologically inert and is used in surgical prostheses.

Silastic Rods (sī-las′tik/rods) (n.) As described by Hunter, a narrow, cylindrical piece of polymerized silicone used in a two-stage flexor tendon reconstruction. The rod is intended to preserve a tunnel in the area of the absent flexor tendons into which a tendon graft can be inserted when the rod is removed. See **Hunter Rod**.

Silesian Bandage (sī-lē-zhun/ban′dig) (n.) A device used in prosthetics that either helps keep a lower limb prosthesis attached to its body part or controls the motion of the prosthesis. A Silesian bandage consists of a light webbing band attached to the socket that does not restrict action.

Silfreskiold Test (sil-fer-shōld/test) (n.) A test used in the evaluation of the etiology of an ankle equinus contracture. Test the affected leg for passive contracture first with the knee fully extended, then with the knee flexed to 90 degrees. If the ankle can be passively dorsiflexed with the knee flexed, the deformity is caused chiefly by contracture of the gastrocnemius muscle. If the deformity cannot be corrected, regardless of the position of the knee, the deformity is caused by contracture of both the gastrocnemius and soleus muscles.

Silver Fork Deformity (sil′ver/fork/de-for′mi-tē) (n.) A descriptive term for a deformity of the wrist due to the dorsal displacement of the distal radial fragment. This is characteristic of Colles' fracture.

Silver Procedure (sil′ver/pro-se′jur) (n.) A surgical procedure for the correction of a hallux valgus deformity. In this operation, the medial eminence is excised, the lateral capsule and conjoined tendon are incised, and then the medial capsule is imbricated by advancing the distally based U-shaped capsular flap proximally.

Sim's Position (simz/pō-zish′shun) (n.) A lateral position with the left side of the body down. The patient's left shoulder and buttocks are positioned at the edge of the table, the left arm is positioned and supported behind the patient, and the right arm is positioned in front of him or her. The left leg may be straight or slightly flexed; the right knee is flexed over the left, with the lower leg supported on the table.

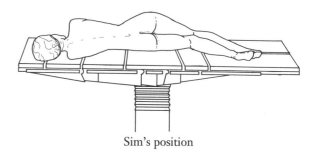

Sim's position

Simmonds Sign (sim′onds/sīn) (n.) See **Thompson Squeeze Test**.

Simmons' Procedure (sim′-monz/pro-sē′jur) (n.) A technique for anterior cervical discectomy and fusion in which a keystone square or rectangular trough is created into which an iliac crest bone graft is placed.

Simon's Line (sī′monz/līn) (n.) On an AP radiograph of the pelvis, the arching iliofemoral line along the lateral margin of the ilium to the outer edge of the acetabulum, continuing downward and outward along the upper margin of the femoral neck. An interruption in the usual concavity occurs in congenital dislocation of the hip.

Simple Bone Cyst (sim′pl/bōn/sist) (n.) See **Unicameral Bone Cyst**.

Simple Fracture (sim′pl/frak′chur) (n.) 1. A fracture with only one fracture line in which two fragments are created. 2. A closed fracture. See **Fracture Classification**.

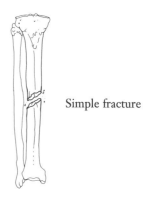

Simple fracture

Simplex Cement (sim′-plex/se-ment) (n.) A proprietary name for a brand of polymethylmethacrylate cement.

Sinding-Larsen-Johansson Syndrome (sin′-ding/lar′-sen/yō-hahn-son/sin-drōm) (n.) An inflammatory process of the patellar tendon associated with the radiographic finding of calcification or ossification adjacent to the distal pole of the patella.

Singh Index (sing/in′deks) (n.) A roentgenographic method for grading osteoporosis based on the trabecular pattern of the proximal femur:

Grade 6: Normal trabecular pattern with primary compression and tension trabeculae and secondary compression and tension trabeculae.

Grade 5: Decrease in secondary trabecular pattern. Ward's triangle becomes prominent.

Grade 4: Secondary trabecular pattern is absent. The primary trabecular pattern is decreased.

Grade 3: A break occurs in the tension trabeculae.

Grade 2: Loss of primary tension trabeculae is complete. There is marked reduction in the compression trabeculae.

Grade 1: Only a few compression trabeculae are seen.

Single Energy Photon Absorptiometry (sing′g′l/en′er-je/fo′ton/ab-sorp″she-om′ĕ-trē) (n.) A technique that provides measurements of the total mass of bone present in the scan path. The technique is applicable only to peripheral sites, which primarily contain cortical bone. See **Dual Energy Photon Absorptiometry**.

Single-Point Cane (sing′g′l/point/kān) (n.) A cane so named to emphasize its single tip, distinguishing it from tripods and other canes.

Sinogram (sī′-nō-gram) (n.) A radiographic image of a natural or acquired sinus tract after the introduction of contrast material into that tract.

Sinography (sī-nog′ra-fē) (n.) The injection of contrast medium into a sinus and the subsequent radiographic imaging.

Sinus (sī′nes) (n.) 1. A hollow or cavity. 2. A large channel containing blood, especially venous blood.

Sinus Tarsi (sī′nes/tar′sī) (n.) On the lateral aspect of the dorsum of the hindfoot, a cavity between the neck of the talus and the calcaneus containing the interosseous talocalcaneal ligament.

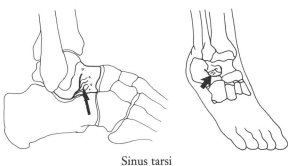

Sinus tarsi

Sinus Tarsi Syndrome (sī′nes/tar′sī/sin-drōm) (n.) A post-traumatic foot disorder characterized by pain over the lateral aspect of the sinus tarsi. In this syndrome, pain persists in the area for a prolonged period after acute or recurrent lateral ankle sprains. The findings include pain at the lateral side of the foot (which is increased by firm pressure over the lateral opening of the sinus tarsi), a sense of hindfoot instability on uneven ground, and decreased symptoms after injection of local anesthetic into the sinus tarsi.

Sinus Tract (sī′nes/trakt) (n.) The channel through which a sinus cavity communicates with the external surface.

Sitz Bath (sits/bath) (n.) A therapeutic bath in which the patient sits with buttocks and perineal region immersed in warm water. The term originates from the German word sitz, meaning seat.

Sjögren's Syndrome (shō-grenz/sin-drōm) (n.) A chronic inflammatory disorder characterized by diminished salivary and lacrimal gland secretion. Primary Sjögren's syndrome, also known as the **Sicca Syndrome**, is defined as xerostomia (dry mouth) and xerophthalmia (dry eyes) in the absence of connective tissue disease. Secondary Sjögren's syndrome is diagnosed when a connective tissue disease, including rheumatoid arthritis, occurs in conjunction with one or both of the other two symptoms, even though the causal link between the glandular condition and the connective tissue disease may be uncertain. Also known as **Mikulicz Disease**, **Gougerot-Houwer-Sjögren Syndrome**, **Keratoconjunctivitis Sicca**, and **Chronic Sialoadenitis**.

Sjovall Epiphyseal Quotient (shō-val/ep″i-fiz′ē-al/kwō′shent) (n.) A radiographic determination of the degree of collapse of the proximal femoral epiphysis in Legg-Calvé-Perthes disease. The epiphyseal index is calculated as the ratio of the height of the epiphysis to its width at the epiphyseal line, which is then multiplied by 100 to obtain a percentage. The epiphyseal index is converted into an epiphyseal quotient by dividing the epiphyseal index of the affected side by that of the uninvolved side. Again, it is expressed as a percentage.

Skeletal (skel-e-tal) (adj.) Of or pertaining to the skeleton or bony framework of the body.

Skeletal Age (skel-e-tal/aj) (n.) A determination of age based on an analysis of the degree of epiphyseal ossification seen on an AP roentgenogram of the hands and wrists, using the standards of the **Atlas** of Greulich and Pyle. This is also called **bone age**. The degree of skeletal maturity may vary from the true chronologic age.

Skeletal Traction (skel-e-tal/trak′shun) (n.) Traction using wires, pins, or tongs placed through bones.

Skeleton (skel′e-t′n) (n.) In vertebrates, the bony framework of the body.

Skew Foot (skyoo/foot) (n.) See **Metatarsus Adductus**.

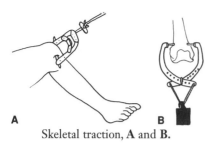

Skeletal traction, **A** and **B**.

Skiameter (ski-am′e-ter) (n.) An instrument for measuring the intensity of x-rays.

Skier's Thumb (ski-erz/thum) (n.) A condition characterized by injuries to the thumb, especially the ulnar collateral ligament. See **Gamekeeper's Thumb**.

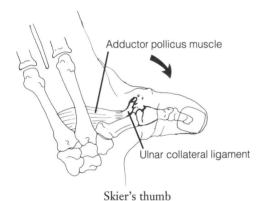

Adductor pollicus muscle

Ulnar collateral ligament

Skier's thumb

Skilled Nursing Facility (skild/nurs′ing/fa-sil′i-tē) (n.) Medical facility with an organized professional staff and a transfer agreement with one or more hospitals. Such a facility provides medical, health, and social services, as well as continuous nursing, to patients not in an acute phase of illness who still primarily require restorative or skilled nursing care on an inpatient basis. Abbreviated **SNF**.

Skilled Nursing Unit (skild/nurs′ing/ū′nit) (n.) Unit that provides physician services and continuous professional nursing supervision for patients not in an acute phase of illness but who still primarily require restorative or skilled nursing care.

Skin (skin) (n.) The membranous protective covering of the body. It is composed of an outer layer (epidermis) and an inner layer (dermis). Also known as the **Cutis**.

Skin Flap (skin/flap) (n.) A full-thickness mass or flap of tissue containing epidermis, dermis, and subcutaneous tissue.

Skin-Fold Assessment (skin/fold/a-ses′-ment) (n.) A method for estimating body fat composition. An estimate of body density is obtained from predictive equations using caliper measurements from a few se-

lected skin folds. The percentage of fat may then be ascertained from a formula that uses the resulting estimate of density.

Skin Graft (skin/graft) (n.) A piece or portion of skin removed from one area of the body to replace a lost portion of skin in another area. The thickness of skin taken for a graft depends on the condition and size of the damaged area.

Skin Testing (skin/testing) (n.) The introduction of an antigen (bacterial, fungal, or chemical) to the skin surface or directly beneath the skin to determine body sensitivity and reaction.

Skin Traction (skin/trak′shun) (n.) A type of traction accomplished by a weight pulling on tape, a sponge rubber, or plastic materials attached to the skin. The pull of the weights is transmitted indirectly to the involved bone. See **Bucks Traction**.

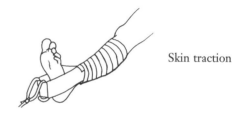

Skin traction

Skinner's Line (skin-erz/līn) (n.) On the radiograph of the pelvis, a horizontal line drawn perpendicular to the axis of the shaft of the femur and then through the uppermost margin of the greater trochanter to the top of the obturator foramen of the pelvis, passing through or below the fovea centralis of the femoral head. A perpendicular line is then dropped through the axis of the shaft of the femur to this line. In fractures with shortening of the femur, the greater trochanter will be displaced above this line.

Skive (skīv) (v.) 1. To cut off in thin layers or pieces. 2. To incise skin during a surgical procedure at a nonperpendicular angle.

Skull Tongs (skul/tongz) (n.) A metallic grasping device whose pronged ends are inserted into the bones of the skull to provide skeletal traction for the cervical spine. See **Barton Tongs**.

Skyline View (skī′-līn/vū) (n.) In radiography, a tangential view of the patella. Also known as a **Sunset** or **Sunrise View**. See **Merchant's View**.

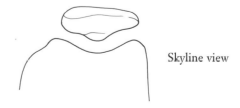

Skyline view

SLAP Lesions (slap/le′zhunz) (n.)   An acronym for lesions to the Superior Labrum of the glenoid fossa of the scapula from Anterior to Posterior. These are classified as follows:

Type I: The superior labrum is frayed and degenerative but is firmly attached to the glenoid.

Type II: The superior labrum and the biceps tendon are stripped off the underlying glenoid.

Type III: Bucket-handle tear of the superior labrum without involvement of the biceps tendon or its point of anchor.

Type IV: A bucket-handle tear that extends across the superior labrum and into the biceps tendon.

Slatis Frame (slat′-is/frām) (n.)   A type of external fixation frame for the pelvis. This is a trapezoidal frame useful in the treatment of lateral compression-type pelvic disruptions.

Slice Fracture (slīs/frak′chur) (n.)   A term applied to an unstable fracture-dislocation of the lumbar spine produced by a flexion and rotation injury. It is characterized by a fracture of the upper border of the lower vertebra and dislocation of the articular processes of the upper vertebra.

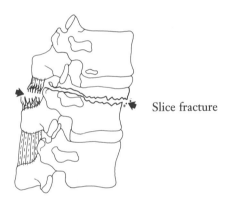

Slice fracture

Sliding Nail-Plate Device (slīd′ing/nāl/plāt/de-vīs) (n.)   Any implants designed for the internal fixation of proximal femur fractures (intertrochanteric and femoral neck fractures) in which a screw or parallel pins are placed across the femoral neck into the fem-

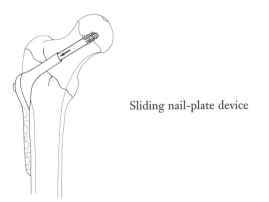

Sliding nail-plate device

oral head and then attached to a side-plate. The screw or pins can slide proximally through the side-plate to allow for impaction at the fracture site.

Sling (sling) (n.)   A bandage arranged to support and rest an injured limb. The limb is then suspended from an external frame (such as with a thigh sling used in traction set-ups) or another body part (such as an arm sling suspended from around the neck).

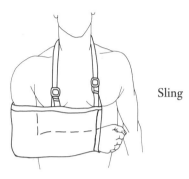

Sling

Sling and Swathe (sling/and/swath) (n.)   A type of immobilization for the upper extremity in which the forearm is suspended in a sling and then secured to the anterior chest wall with a swathe wrapped around the trunk.

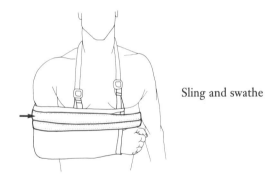

Sling and swathe

Slip Angle (slip/ang′g′l) (n.)   In spondylolisthesis, the degree of forward tilting of the vertebral body at the level of the slipping. The angle is formed on a radiograph by a line drawn parallel to the inferior aspect of the proximal vertebral body and a line drawn perpendicular to the posterior aspect of the body of the distally involved vertebra.

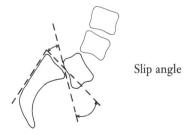

Slip angle

Slip Angle Percentage (slip/ang′g′l/per-sent′ij) (n.) A modification of the method of Taillard used for measuring the amount of displacement in spondylolisthesis. The percentage of "slip" is determined by comparing the distance the vertebra is displaced with the width of the subjacent vertebral body.

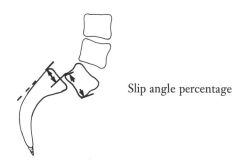

Slip angle percentage

Slipped Capital Femoral Epiphysis (slip′t/cap-i-tal/fem′or-al/e-pif′i-sis) (n.) An affection of the proximal femoral epiphysis seen in late childhood or early adolescence in which a transepiphyseal separation occurs. The pathogenesis remains unclear. Commonly referred to as "slips," these may be classified according to their severity (mild, moderate, severe) and their status (acute, chronic, or acute-on-chronic). Abbreviated **SCFE**.

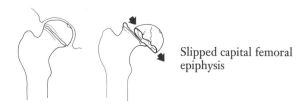

Slipped capital femoral epiphysis

Slipped Disk (slip′t/disk) (n.) A term commonly applied to a herniated nucleus pulposus.

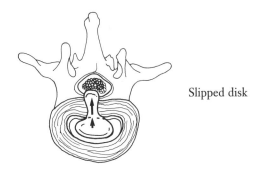

Slipped disk

Slipper Cast (slip′er/kast) (n.) A cast incorporating the foot up to the ankle

Slipsole (slip′sōl) (n.) In shoe terminology, a half-sole extending from toe to shank, between the outersoles and innersoles.

Slocum Procedure (slō-kum/pro-sē′jur) (n.) A surgical reconstruction of the medial compartment of the knee when valgus laxity is present. In this complex procedure, the posterior capsule is repaired; then the posteromedial corner is repaired and reinforced by advancement of the semimembranosus tendon. Reinforcement of the medial collateral ligament and anterior capsule is also needed.

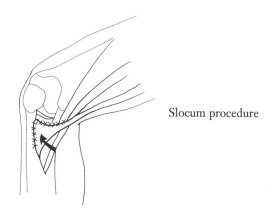

Slocum procedure

Slocum Test (slō-kum/test) (n.) A method used to evaluate the integrity of the anterior cruciate ligament of the knee and the possible presence of rotatory instability. In this test, the examiner performs an anterior drawer test with the leg held in neutral position, then rotated 30 degrees internally, and finally 15 degrees externally. Anterolateral rotary instability is present if the anterior drawer is accentuated with internal tibial rotation and reduced with external tibial rotation. The opposite is true for anteromedial rotary instability.

SLR (n.) Abbreviation for straight leg raising.

SMA (n.) Abbreviation for Sequential Multiple Analysis. A sequence of tests is performed on an automated instrument in the laboratory for the chemical analysis of serum. This instrument is designed with multiple channels to be used for a corresponding number of tests. Examples SMA 12.

Smear (smēr) (n.) A specimen smeared on a microscope slide for examination.

Smillie Knife (smil′-ē/nīf) (n.) A surgical scalpel designed for excision of a meniscus.

Smith Fracture (smith/frak′chur) (n.) A fracture of the distal aspect of the radius in which there is volar displacement of the distal fragment and dorsal angulation at the fracture site. Sometimes referred to as a **Reverse Colles' Fracture**.

Smith-Petersen Approach (smith/pē-ter-son/ap-prōch) (n.) An anterolateral surgical approach to the hip joint.

Smith-Petersen Cup (smith-pē′ter-son/kup) (n.)

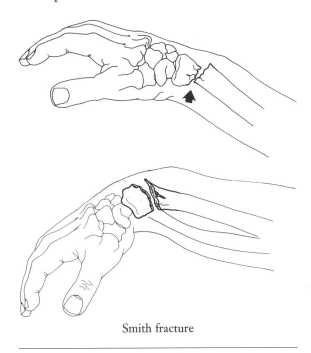

Smith fracture

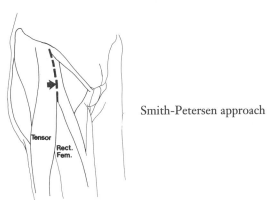

Smith-Petersen approach

An outdated type of prosthesis that was used for mold arthroplasty of the hip.

Smith-Petersen Nail (smith-pē'ter-son/nål) (n.) A type of hardware, no longer used, for fixation of femoral neck fractures.

Smith-Petersen Test (smith-pē'ter-son/test) (n.) A method of evaluation of diseases of the sacroiliac joint. With the patient supine, place your hand under the lower part of the patient's spine, and slowly raise the outstretched leg. As the hamstrings tighten, gradually apply leverage to the affected side of the pelvis. If pain is brought on before the lumbar spine begins to move, either sacroiliac or lumbosacral disease may be present. The leg on the side opposite the pain site can be brought to a higher level than the other without pain. If sacroiliac disease is present in lumbosacral conditions, pain comes on when both legs are brought to the same level.

Smooth Muscle (smūth/mus-el) (n.) Muscle controlled by the autonomic nervous system. Histologically, it lacks the characteristic striations seen in voluntary or cardiac muscle. It consists of spindle-shaped fibers 2 to 5 μm in diameter and 50 to 100 μm in length. Each fiber has a single nucleus located near its center, in the widest portion of the cell. A sarcolemma surrounds the fiber. The fibers are capable of maintaining relatively constant tone regardless of length. Smooth muscle is usually said to be involuntary, although its activity may be modified. This type of muscle lines the walls of the gastrointestinal tract and blood vessels. Two types of smooth muscle are distinguished:

1. **Unitary Smooth Muscle**: This exhibits spontaneous activity and conducts impulses from one muscle cell to another, as though the entire muscle mass were a single cell. This type of muscle is found in the alimentary tract, uterus, ureters, and small blood vessels.

2. **Multiunit Smooth Muscle**: This does not exhibit spontaneous contraction, usually requires stimulation by nerves, and can grade its strength of contraction. This type of muscle is found in the ciliary muscles and the iris of the eye and in larger blood vessels.

Snapping Hip (snap'ping/hip) (n.) A descriptive name of a disorder caused by the presence of a tendinous band on the surface of the gluteus maximus muscle. It is characterized by an audible, palpable, yet invisible snap on the lateral aspect of the hip as the tight fascia band slips and slides over the prominence of the greater trochanter. The snapping generally gives rise to little inconvenience unless the underlying trochanteric bursa becomes inflamed, or if the patient is unable to tolerate the sensation. The patient can usually reproduce the snap by actively flexing the hip with the thigh internally rotated.

Snapping Tendon (snap'ping/ten'don) (n.) A condition, often asymptomatic, in which the slipping of a tendon over a bony prominence or exostosis may produce a well-marked snap or stimulation of locking.

Snuff-box (snuf-boks) (n.) A shortened reference to the anatomic snuff-box, that depression noted along the dorsoradial aspect of the thumb with the thumb extended, which is bounded radially by the extensor pollicis brevis and the abductor pollicis longus ten-

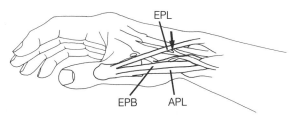

Snuffbox. *EPL*, Extensor pollicis longus; *EPB*, extensor pollicis brevis; *APL*, abductor pollicis longus.

dons (first extensor compartment) and ulnarly by the extensor pollicis longus tendon (third extensor compartment). The radial artery passes through the snuff-box, and the scaphoid bone is palpable at its base. See **Anatomic Snuff-box**.

Snyder Sling (snī′der/sling) (n.) A non–weight-bearing orthosis for the treatment of Legg-Calvé-Perthes disease. A sling is supported on one shoulder opposite the involved hip and is attached to the involved limb just above the ankle, with the length adjusted to hold the knee in flexion and prevent weight-bearing during ambulation.

SOAP (n.) Acronym for Subjective, Objective, Assessment Plan; a system used in problem-oriented medical recordkeeping.

Sock Lining (sok/līn′ing) (n.) In shoe terminology, a piece of leather or coated fabric pasted over the whole insole on the inside of the shoe to cover stitches and staples.

Socket (sok′et) (n.) The part of a prosthesis containing the amputation stump.

Sofield Osteotomy (sō-fēld/os″te-ot′ō-mē) (n.) A technique used in the treatment of bony deformities in osteogenesis imperfecta. The entire shaft of the bone is exposed subperiosteally, and then multiple osteotomies are performed. The bone fragments are shifted and rotated so as to align them straight and fix them with a medullary nail.

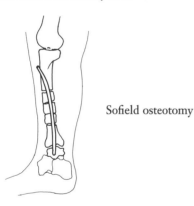

Sofield osteotomy

Soft Cervical Collar (soft/ser′vi-kal/kol-er) (n.) A type of cervical orthosis, typically made of foam rubber, that is covered with a cotton stockinette. It is fastened behind the neck with Velcro. Most wearers consider it comfortable, but it does not provide rigid immobilization.

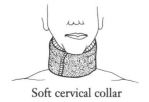

Soft cervical collar

Soft Corn (soft/korn) (n.) A painful hyperkeratotic lesion that occurs between the toes. It is usually caused by the pressure of one condyle against a contiguous condyle of the opposing toe. The lesion is soft, and the skin is often eroded due to moisture between the toes. Also called a **Heloma Molle**, **Clavus Mollus**, or **Tyloma Molle**. Compare to **Hard Corn**.

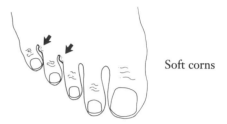

Soft corns

Soft Disk (soft/disk) (n.) A discarded term applied to an intervertebral disk disorder caused by herniation of soft disk material such as the nucleus pulposus; this is in contrast to nerve root impingement due to spondylosis or a hard disk.

Soft Tissue (soft/tish′ū) (n.) The nonosseous and noncartilaginous connective tissue of the body.

Soft Tissue Shadow (soft/tish′ū/shad′ō) (n.) On a roentgenogram, the record of density of soft tissue as compared with bone.

Sole (sōl) (n.) In shoe terminology, that part of the shoe between the upper and the floor. In a well-constructed shoe, there are two soles—the outer and the inner. The outer sole contacts the floor; the inner sole lies directly under the foot. The space separating the inner from outer sole is occupied by a compressible filler. Above the inner sole is stitched a welt, which is a narrow strip of leather attached to the upper portion of the shoe.

Sole Wedge (sōl/wej) (n.) Shoe modifications intended to shift the body weight from the medial to the lateral side of the foot, or vice versa.

Soleal Line (sō′lēl/līn) (n.) A line on the upper third of the posterior surface of the tibia, marking the origin of the soleus muscle. Also called **Popliteal Line** or **Line** of the **Soleus Muscle**.

Soleus Muscle (sō-lē-us/mus′el) (n.) See **Muscle**.

Solitary Enchondroma (sol′ĭ-ter″e/en″kon-dro′mah) (n.) See **Enchondroma**.

Solute (so′lūt) (n.) A dissolved substance in a solution.

Solution (so-lū′shun) (n.) A mixture consisting of molecules or ions less than 1 mm in diameter suspended in a fluid medium (water, in most biologic systems).

Solvent (sol′vent) (n.) The dissolving medium in a solution.

Somatosensory Evoked Potentials (sō-ma-tō-sen′

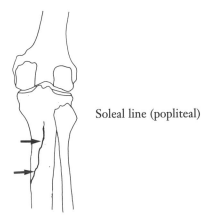

Soleal line (popliteal)

so-rē/ev-oked/pō-ten′shulz) (n.)   The electric potentials generated by stimulation of peripheral
nerves and recorded by transcutaneous electrodes
placed over the cerebral cortex. The monitoring of
these potentials is useful during spine surgery procedures to prevent neurologic injury because, even
though the findings are nonspecific as to level,
changes in the shape or size latency or amplitude of
the recorded potentials will indicate a problem between the cerebral cortex and the end-organs. Abbreviated SSEP.

Somatotype (sō-mat′ō-tīp) (n.)   The body type of an
individual.

SOMI Collar (SOMI/kol′lar) (n.)   An acronym for
Sternal-Occipital-Mandibular-Immobilizer. A type of
head-cervical-thoracic orthosis that is named according to its attachment points.

Sonography (so-nog′rah-fē) (n.)   The application of
sound waves to produce a radiologic image called a
sonogram. It is frequently used to provide images of
a baby in utero.

Sontag's Table (sōn-tahgz/ta′b′l) (n.)   A reference
table based on roentgenograms of the entire left side
of the skeleton that lists the total number of ossification centers normally present from 1 to 60
months.

Soto-Hall Test (sō′tō/hawl/test) (n.)   A clinical evaluation of vertebral disease and spinal injuries. With
the patient supine, depress the sternum with one
hand and raise the patient's head with the other
hand. Pain is elicited at the site of the spine disorder.

Southwick Osteotomy (sowth-wick/os″te-ot′ō-mē)
(n.)   A biplane, wedge osteotomy of the intertrochanteric region of the femur. This osteotomy is prescribed for the treatment of a malunited slipped capital femoral epiphysis after the cessation of growth.

Space Available for the Cord (spās/a-vāl′e-b′l/for/
the/kord) (n.)   In the evaluation of atlantoaxial instability, a radiographic measurement of the potential space available for the spinal cord to pass. This
is the distance from the posterior aspect of the odon-

toid to the anterior edge of the posterior arch of the
atlas.

Space of Poirer (spas/of/pwah-rā′) (n.)   A relatively
bare area between the capitate and lunate volarly.

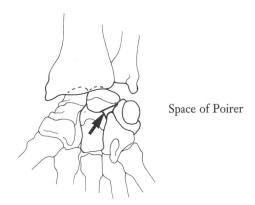

Space of Poirer

Space Shoe (spās/shū) (n.)   See **Custom-Molded
Shoe.**

Spasm (spazm) (n.)   A sudden, involuntary muscular
contraction.

Spastic (spas′tik) (adj.)   Contracted; a state of continuous muscular contraction.

Spastic Crouch (spas′tik/krouch) (n.)   An attitude
noted in cerebral palsy patients with spastic diplegia
or total involvement in which the patient stands and
ambultates with excessive hip and knee flexion, ankle dorsiflexion, and extension of the lumbar spine.

Spastic Diplegia (spas′tik/di-plē′je-ah) (n.)   A disorder characterized clinically by spasticity of the
lower extremities, choreiform movements, and occasionally, mental deficiency due to central neuronal degeneration. Grossly, the brain is usually
small and shrunken, with patches of microgyri; there
may be gross defects in the cerebellum and pons as
well. Although the cause is thought to be a defect in
development, some diffuse active process may also
be at work, inducing the symptomatology. The syndrome is duplicated in infantile encephalomyelitides
and in toxic reactions. Microscopically, the atro-
phied areas show gliosis. Synonym: **Little's Disease.**

Spastic Gait (spas′tik/gāt) (n.)   In spasticity, a walk
that is characterized by abrupt, uncoordinated motions of one or several parts of the body.

Spastic Paralysis (spas′tik/pa-ral-a-sis) (n.)   Immobility accompanied by increased muscle tone and
heightened deep muscle reflexes. It results from an
upper motor neuron disorder.

Spasticity (spas-tis′i-tē) (n.)   A state of increase in
muscle tone when the muscle is passively lengthened. No objective means for accurate measurement
of the degree of spasticity are available.

Special Care Unit (spesh′el/kar/ū′nit) (n.)   A medical care unit in which there is appropriate equip-

ment and a concentration of physicians, nurses, and others with the skills and experience necessary to provide both optimal medical care for critically ill patients and continuous care of patients in special, diagnostic categories.

Species (spē'sēz) (n.)   A narrow taxonomic category consisting of a group of actually or potentially inter-breeding natural populations. One or more species constitute a genus. A species may be further divided into subspecies.

Specific Gravity (spĕ-sif'ik/grav'ĭ-tē) (n.)   The density of a substance, defined as its weight compared with an equal volume of another substance, which is assigned a unit density. The term is usually applied to the weight of a liquid as compared with that of distilled water. Abbreviated **Sp.g.**

Spenco Insole (spen-ko/in'sōl) (n.)   A commercially available insole made of Neoprene, which has nitrogen air cells. It is used to prevent heel and sole blistering and to offer mild arch support.

Spheroidal Joint (sfe-roi'dal/joint) (n.)   A ball-and-socket joint.

Sphincter (sfingk'ter) (n.)   A ring-shaped muscle capable of closing a tubular opening or orifice by constriction.

Sphingomyelin (sfing″gō-mī'e-lin) (n.)   A phospholipid containing sphingosine, which is composed of a fatty acid, phosphoric acid, and choline. Sphingomyelins are found in large amounts in brain and nerve tissue. Also known as **Phosphosphingosides**.

Spica Bandage (spī'kah/ban'dij) (n.)   A figure-8 bandage that incorporates the trunk and an extremity, the hand and a finger, or the foot and a toe.

Spica Cast (spī'kah/kast) (n.)   A cast that incorporates the trunk and an entire extremity, or a part. See **Hip Spica**.

Spicule (spīk'ūl) (n.)   A small, sharp fragment, as of bone.

Spina Bifida (spī'nah/bif'ida) (n.)   A developmental defect of the spinal column characterized by a failure of fusion between the vertebral arches (with or without protrusion) and dysplasia of the spinal cord or its membranes. Also known as **Spinal Dysraphism**. The defect is classified as **Spina Bifida Occulta, Meningocoele, Myelomeningocoele,** or **Rachischisis**.

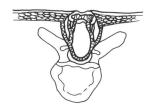

Spina bifida

Spina Bifida Occulta (spī'nah/bif'ida/okul'ta) (n.) Incomplete closure of the laminae of one or more vertebrae without protrusion of intraspinal contents

to the surface and the absence of a discernible external cyst. There may or may not be overlying cutaneous defects, neurologic deficit, or dysplastic changes in the spinal cord. Spina bifida occulta is usually asymptomatic and demonstrated by radiograph examination only. An overlying subcutaneous fat pad, a portwine hemangioma, and a skin dimple or tuft of silky hair are occasional findings.

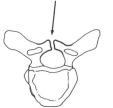

Spina bifida occulta

Spina Ventosa (spī'nah/ventō'sa) (n.)   A radiographic finding in bones in which there is absorption of the bone in the medulla, with new periosteal bone; this gives the appearance that the bone was inflated with air. Occasionally seen in tuberculosis or neoplasms of bone.

Spinal (spī'nal) (adj.)   Of or pertaining to the spine or vertebral column.

Spinal Accessory Nerve (spī'nal/ak-ses'o-rē/nerv) (n.)   The eleventh cranial nerve.

Spinal Anesthesia (spīnal/an'esthē'zhēa) (n.)   Regional anesthesia produced by the injection of a local anesthetic into the subarachnoid space of the spinal cord, with resultant anesthetization of the spinal ganglia and nerve roots.

Spinal Canal (spī'nal/ka-nal') (n.)   The hollow canal formed by the sequence of vertebral foramina that enclose the spinal cord and meninges. The articulated vertebral bodies form the floor of the canal; the posterior elements of the vertebral column form the roof and the sides. The normal lumbar spinal canal varies in shape at different levels; normally, it is circular in a cross-section in the upper part of the lumbar spine and trefoil in shape at the lower part. Also called the **Vertebral Canal**.

Spinal Column (spī'nal/kol'-um) (n.)   The spine or vertebral column.

Spinal Cord (spīnal/kord) (n.)   The portion of the central nervous system enclosed in the vertebral column. It consists of nerve cells and bundles of nerves connecting all parts of the body to the brain.

The spinal cord contains a core of gray matter surrounded by white matter; it extends from the medulla oblongata at the upper border of the atlas to the level of the second lumbar vertebra. Below the first lumbar vertebra, the canal is occupied by a leash of lumbar, sacral, and coccygeal nerve roots termed the **cauda equina**. The spinal nerves emerge from the spinal cord in pairs: eight cervical, twelve

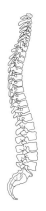

Spinal column

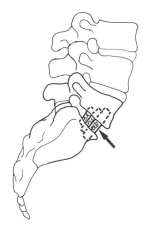

Spinal anterior fusion

thoracic, five lumbar, five sacral, and one pair of coccygeal nerves. The cord has two enlargements, cervical and lumbar, that correspond to the nerve supply of the upper and lower limbs. The spinal cord is enveloped by three membranes—the dura, the arachnoid, and the pia mater; these are direct continuations of those surrounding the brain.

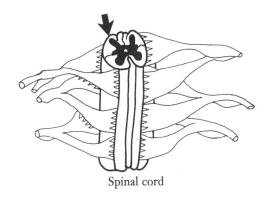

Spinal cord

Spinal Cord Syndrome (spī′nal/kord/sin-drōm) (n.) Any clinical entity that results from incomplete trauma to the spinal cord, as distinguished from complete sectioning of the spinal cord. These syndromes include the central cord syndrome, the anterior cervical cord syndrome, the posterior cervical cord syndrome, and the Brown-Séquard syndrome. See also individual syndromes.

Spinal Fusion (spī′nal/fū′zhun) (n.) The surgical creation of ankylosis or fusion of contiguous vertebrae.

Spinal Index (spī′nal/in′deks) (n.) A method of assessing the size of a lumbar spinal canal on plain radiographs. Measure the anteroposterior diameter of the spinal canal on the lateral radiograph from the middle of the back of the vertebral body to the base of the opposing spinous process, which can be recognized by tracing forward along its inferior margin a distance marked B in the radiograph. Also measure the interpedicular distance on the AP radiograph, which is marked A. Multiply these two values to get

a product, AB. This product is then compared as a ratio with the product of the anteroposterior and transverse diameters of the middle of the adjacent vertebral body, marked D and C respectively, so that AB is related to CD.

Spinal Manipulative Therapy (spī′nal/me-nip′ū-la′tiv/ther′ah-pē) (n.) Any procedure in which the hands are used to immobilize, adjust, stimulate, or otherwise influence the spinal and paraspinal tissues, with the aim of influencing the patient's health.

Spinal Nerve (spī′nal/nerv) (n.) Any of the 31 pairs of nerves that arise from the spinal cord, passing out from the vertebral canal through the spaces between the arches of the vertebrae. Each nerve has two roots: an *anterior*, carrying motor nerve fibers, and a *posterior*, carrying sensory fibers. Immediately after leaving the spinal cord, the roots merge to form a mixed spinal nerve on each side. There are eight cervical nerves, twelve thoracic nerves, five lumbar nerves, five sacral nerves, and one coccygeal spinal nerve on each side of the spinal cord.

Spinal Nerve Root (spī′nal/nerv/rūt) (n.) Neural structures that exit the spinal cord anteriorly and posteriorly, combining to form a single spinal nerve.

Spinal Puncture (spī′nal/pungk′chur) (n.) The introduction of a hollow needle into the subarachnoid space of the spinal canal. This is usually performed at the level of the lumbar spine. Also called **Lumbar Puncture**.

Spinal Reflex (spī′nal/rē′fleks) (n.) Any reflex mediated through the spinal cord without the necessary participation of more cephalad central nervous system structures.

Spinal Rotatory Manipulation (spi′nal/ro″tah-to′re/mah-nip″u-la′shun) (n.) A controlled twisting of the spine in the plane of the vertebral facet joints.

Spinal Shock (spī′nal/shok) (n.) A condition of flaccid paralysis and suppression of all reflex activity that immediately follows injury to the spinal cord and involves all segments below the lesion. It is necessary for spinal shock to pass in order to determine

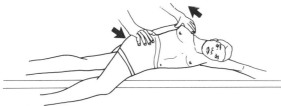

Spinal rotatory manipulation

whether neurologic deficit following injury is complete or incomplete.

Spinal Stenosis (spī′nal/sten-ō-sis) (n.) A condition in which the cross-sectional area of the spinal canal is sufficiently reduced to cause cord or spinal nerve compression.
Classification:
I. Congenital developmental stenosis
 A. Idiopathic
 B. Achondroplastic
II. Acquired stenosis
 A. Degenerative
  1. Affecting central spinal canal
  2. Affecting lateral canals, recesses, and foramina
  3. Degenerative spondylolisthesis
 B. Combined (all conditions of congenital/developmental stenosis, degenerative stenosis, and herniations of the nucleus pulposus)
 C. Spondylolisthetic
 D. Iatrogenic
  1. Following laminectomy
  2. Following anterior or posterior spine fusion
  3. Following chemonucleolysis
 E. Late changes after trauma
 F. Miscellaneous
  1. Paget's disease
  2. Fluorosis

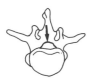

Spinal stenosis

Spine (spīn) (n.) 1. The backbone or vertebral column. 2. A sharp process of a bone. See **Spinal Column.**

Spine of the Ischium (spīn/of/the/is′kē-um) (n.) A pointed eminence on the posterior border of the body of the ischium that forms that lower border of the greater sciatic notch.

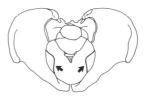

Spine of the ischium

Spine of the Scapula (spīn/of/the/skap′ū-la) (n.) The triangular bony process attached obliquely to the dorsum of the scapula, projecting upward and outward; it divides the scapula into two unequal parts—the supraspinous and the infraspinous fossae.

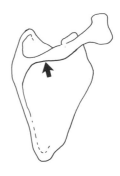

Spine of the scapula

Spine of the Tibia (spīn/of/the/tib-e-a) (n.) See **Tibial Eminence**.

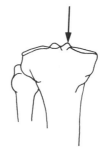

Spine of the tibia

Spinous (spi′nus) (adj.) 1. Of or pertaining to a spine or spinelike process. 2. Having spines or sharp processes.

Spinous Process (spī′nus/pros′es) (n.) That part of a vertebra that projects backward from the arch, giving attachment to muscles of the back.

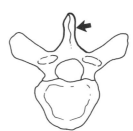

Spinous process

Spiral Fracture (spī'ral/frak'chur) (n.) A type of fracture in which a torsional stress produces a winding fracture line relative to the long axis of the broken bone.

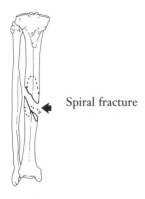

Spiral fracture

Spiral Groove (spi'ral/grūv) (n.) A shallow sulcus along the posterior aspect of the humerus through which the radial nerve courses. Also known as the **Radial Nerve Groove**.

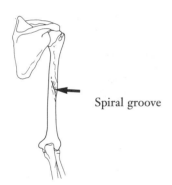

Spiral groove

Splayfoot (splā'fut) (n.) A foot with a flattened transverse arch. In this deformity, the metatarsal bones abduct from one another at their heads mediolaterally and compress at the closely mated articular margins of the tarsometatarsal joints, thus depressing the anterior metatarsal arch. The degree of abduction and depression is dependent on the laxity of the intrinsic muscles of the foot.

Splint (splint) 1. (n.) An orthosis. An appliance or support used to maintain a part of the body in a set position. 2. (v.) To support.

Split a Cast (split/a/kast) (n.) See **Bivalve a Cast**.

Split-Russell Traction (split/rus'-l/trak-shun) (n.) A type of balanced suspension skeletal traction for the treatment of femur fracture in which traction is applied through both a supracondylar and an os calcis pin, both of which are attached to separate weights. See **Russell Traction**.

Split-Thickness Graft (split-thik'nes/graft) (n.) A skin graft consisting of only a portion of the total skin thickness—the epidermis and part of the dermis (to a depth of 0.010 to 0.035 in, or 0.3 to 1 mm). Split-thickness grafts are widely used to cover large, denuded areas on body surfaces, such as the back, the trunk, and the legs.

Spondylitis (spon-de'lī-tis) (n.) An inflammatory disease of the spine.

Spondylo (spon-dē-lō) Prefix meaning vertebral.

Spondyloarthritis (spon-dē-lō-ar-thrī-tis) (n.) Arthritis of the spine.

Spondyloepiphyseal Dysplasia (spon'dēlō-ep-i-fiz'ē-al/dis-plā'ze-a) (n.) Any of the bone dysplasias that involve abnormalities in both the vertebrae and the epiphyses. This includes spondyloepiphyseal dysplasia congenita, spondyloepiphyseal dysplasia tarda, and pseudoachondroplastic spondyloepiphyseal dysplasia.

Spondylolisthesis (spon'dē-lō-lis-thē'sis) (n.) Anterior displacement of a vertebra on the adjacent lower vertebra. It may be classified by etiology as follows:

A. *Dysplastic:* The orientation of the facets of the zygapophyseal joint is sufficiently horizontal to permit slipping, or the superior facet of the lower vertebra is hypoplastic, thus allowing displacement of the upper vertebrae.

B. *Isthmic:* Fibrous defects are present in the pars interarticularis, permitting forward displacement of the upper vertebrae and separation of the anterior aspects of that vertebra from its neural arch.

C. *Degenerative:* Anterior displacement of a vertebra, which arises from erosive degenerative changes in the zygapophyseal joints.

D. *Traumatic:* Anterior displacement of a vertebra due to traumatic injury to its restraining structures.

E. *Pathologic:* Anterior displacement of a vertebra due to elongation of the pedicles from a disease process in the bone. Spondylolisthesis is graded by various systems to indicate degree of slippage. For example, see **Meyerding Classification**.

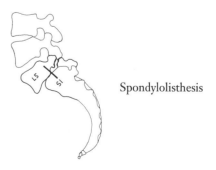

Spondylolisthesis

Spondylolisthesis Dysplasia (spon'dē-lō-lis-thē'sis/dis-plā'ze-a) (n.) A congenital dysplasia of the upper portion of the sacrum or neural arch of L5 that results in a structural deficiency unable to withstand the forward thrust of the last lumbar vertebra, which gradually slips forward on the sacrum.

Spondylolysis (spon-de-lŏl′ĭ-sis) (n.)   1. A unilateral or bilateral defect in the pars interarticularis. The defect may or may not be associated with spondylolisthesis. Oblique radiographic views of the lumbar spine are often necessary to view the defect in this area clearly. See **Scotty Dog Sign.**

Spondylopathy (spon-dē-lop′a-thē) (n.)   Any disease of the vertebrae.

Spondylosis (spon-dē-lō′sis) (n.)   Degenerative disease of both the disk and the zygapophyseal joints of the spine. Symptoms include pain and restriction of movement. Spondylosis produces a characteristic appearance on x-ray that includes narrowing of both the disk space and the neural foramina, and the presence of osteophytes.

Sponge (spunj) (n.)   Any piece of porous material used for the absorption of liquids, especially during surgery.

Spongiosa (spon″je-ō′sah) (n.)   The osseous tissue in the metaphysis of growing bones.

Primary Spongiosa—That part of the metaphysis just distal to the last intact transverse cartilage septum in the hypertrophic zone. The longitudinal septa are partially or completely calcified, and osteoblasts are lined up along the calcified bars.

Secondary Spongiosa—That region of the metaphysis a short distance down the calcified longitudinal septa in which bone is laid down by osteoblasts within or on the cartilage.

Spontaneous Fracture (spon-tā′nē-us/frak′chur) (n.)   A fracture occurring with little or no apparent trauma and usually as a result of intrinsic bone disease. Synonym: **Pathologic Fracture.**

Sporadic (spo-rad′ik) (adj.)   Occurring only occasionally, at a low level of incidence or in a few isolated places.

Spot Film (spot/film) (n.)   A small radiographic film of a limited area made with a spot-filming device.

Spot-Film Radiography (spot/film/ra-dē-og′ra-fē) (n.)   The process of making radiographic exposures of a limited area at the instant a part is visualized on the image intensifier (fluoroscopic) screen.

Spotted Bone Disease (spot′ed/bōn/di-zēz′) (n.)   The descriptive name for osteopoikilosis.

Sprain (sprān) (n.)   A soft tissue injury limited to the ligaments. It is graded by severity as follows:

First Degree: A tear of a minimum number of ligamentous fibers that results in localized tenderness without instability.

Second Degree: A tear of a greater number of ligamentous fibers that results in a greater loss of function and joint reaction but is still without instability.

Third Degree: A complete tear of the ligament with resultant joint instability.

Sprain Fracture (sprān/frak′chur) (n.)   An uncommon term for an avulsion fracture.

Spreader Bar (spred′er/bar) (n.)   A metallic bar used in traction set-ups. It has a hook at each end that is attached to a suspension sling in order to separate

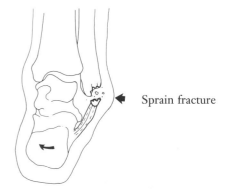

Sprain fracture

its ends and a loop in the middle to which traction rope is attached.

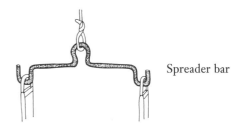

Spreader bar

Sprengel's Deformity (spreng′-lz/de-for′-mi-tē) (n.)   A congenital anomaly characterized by elevation and medial rotation of the scapula. The affected scapula is usually small, and there may be an associated absence or hypoplasia of the surrounding musculature. There also may be a bony, cartilaginous or fibrous attachment to the cervical or upper thoracic spine. This is a nonprogressive deformity that will not improve with conservative treatment. Numerous surgical procedures have been described. Also known as congenital elevation of the scapular. See **Omovertebral Bone.**

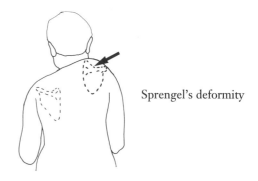

Sprengel's deformity

Spring Ligament (spring/lig′ah-ment) (n.)   The plantar calcaneonavicular ligament. It is attached to the anterior margin of the sustentaculum tali and to the plantar surface of the navicular. Broad and thick, the spring ligament supports the head of the talus, and the deltoid ligament is attached to its medial edge.

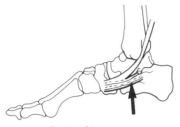

Spring ligament

Sprinter's Fracture (sprin'-terz/frak'chur) (n.) An avulsion fracture of the anterosuperior or, more commonly, the anteroinferior spine of the ilium. It is so-named because of its frequent occurrence in sprinters; it is caused by a sudden, forcible muscular pull of the sartorius or rectus femoris muscles.

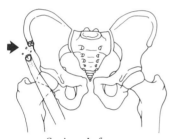

Sprinter's fracture

Spur (sper) (n.) 1. A sharp projection. 2. An osteophyte, beak, or lip on the articular margin of a bone. Example: Heel spur.

Spurling's Test (sper'-lingz/test) (n.) A clinical evaluation of cervical radiculopathy. Exert pressure downward on the top of the patient's head. The test is positive if the pain is intensified or the previous radiation of pain to the shoulder or arm is reproduced, or both.

Spurring (spur'ing) (n.) The development of a bony spur.

Squamous Cell Carcinoma (skwā'mus/sel/kar-si-nō'ma) (n.) A malignant neoplasm arising from epithelial cells. These tumors can occur in the sinus tract of a long-standing, chronic osteomyelitis.

Squared Foot (skwārd/fut) (n.) A foot in which the big toe is the same length as the second toe.

Squatting Position (squat'ting/po-zish'en) (n.) A position in which the feet are flat on the ground and the knees and hips are in complete flexion.

Squeeze-Film Lubrication (skwēz/film/lū'bri-cā' shun) (n.) A form of fluid lubrication in which the approaching surfaces generate pressure on the lubricant while squeezing it out of the area of impending contact between them. The resulting pressure keeps the surfaces apart.

SSEP Abbreviation for Somato Sensory Evoked Potentials.

SSI Abbreviation for Segmental Spinal Instrumentation.

Stabilization (sta"bil-i-zā'shun) (n.) The process of making something firm and steady.

Stable Zone of Harrington (stā'bl/zōn/of/hār-ing-ton) (n.) 1. A radiographic determination, when parallel lines are drawn through the lumbrosacral facets and perpendicular to the iliac crests, those vertebral bodies within the lines are in the stable zone. Harrington stated that the lower level of hook placement for spinal instrumentation and fusion should fall within this zone. 2. A more accurate determination of the stable zone is gained by a single line drawn through the center of the sacrum perpendicular to the iliac crests, which is designated the central sacral line. When a limb-length discrepancy is present, the pelvis should be leveled with an appropriate lift under the short limb. The central vertical line must always be based on a horizontal pelvis. The vertebra that is bisected or most closely bisected by this line is determined and is recorded as being the stable vertebra.

Stage (stāj) (n.) A definite period or distinct phase, e.g., as in the development of a disease or organism.

Staggering Gait (stag'er-ing/gāt) (n.) A gait due to lack of coordination of the lower limbs. It manifests itself as unsteadiness. It may be suggestive of a brain lesion.

Staging (stā'jing) (n.) 1. A way of grouping malignant neoplasms so that a prediction of the necessary surgical procedure as well as a comparison of treatment results can be accurately made. The groupings are based on physical examination, roentgenographic findings, and biopsy. For musculoskeletal tumors, the **Ennekings Staging System** is commonly used. It is as follows: **IA**, low-grade intracompartmental; **IB**, low-grade extracompartmental; **IIA**, high-grade intracompartmental; **IIB**, high-grade extracompartmental; and **III**, high or low grade, either extra- or intracompartmental, with either regional or distal metastases. 2. A sequential approach to the treatment of a disease or disorder.

Stagnara's Wake-up Test (sta-nya-raz/wāk-up/test) (n.) A test used to ascertain neurologic status during spinal surgery, especially spinal instrumentation procedures. In the middle of the procedure, the patient is awakened from anesthesia and asked to move his or her toes or fingers to ensure that there is no neurologic injury. Compare to **Ankle Clonus Test of Hoppenfeld.**

Stainless Steel (stān'lis/stēl) (n.) An iron-based metal alloy often used as an orthopaedic implant ma-

terial. Type 316 stainless steel is used most frequently in the human body.

Stance Phase (stans/fāz) (n.) A component of the
gait cycle that encompasses the period during which
weight is being borne by the extremity. It begins
when the heel of the shoe of the leading limb touches
the floor and ends when the toe of the same foot
leaves the ground. It is subdivided as follows:

Heel strike: The instant the heel of the shoe of the leading
extremity touches the floor.

Foot-flat: Shortly after heel strike, when the sole of the shoe
of the same foot touches the floor.

Mid-stance: After foot-flat, when the body weight is brought
forward directly over the supporting extremity.

Heel-off: The heel leaves the floor.

Push-off: The time interval between heel-off and toe-off positions of the same foot. Finally, the foot loses all contact
with the floor.

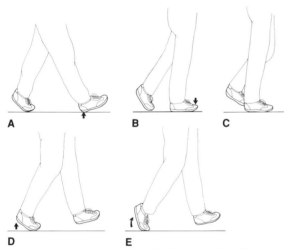

Stance phase. **A**, Heel strike; **B**, foot flat; **C**, mid-stance;
D, heel off; **E**, push off.

Standard Crutch (stand′ard/kruch) (n.) A traditional axillary crutch made of wood. See **Crutch**.

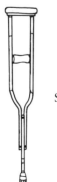

Standard crutch

Standard Deviation (stan′dard/dē′vē-ā′shun) (n.)
In statistics, the standard deviation is a derived expression of variation in a set of measurements. It is
a useful descriptive term reflecting the degree of
scatter among the measurements. Abbreviated SD
and is often symbolized by the Greek letter sigma.

The standard deviation is calculated as follows:
Determine the arithmetic mean in the set of observations. Find the algebraic difference between each
observation and this mean. The resulting figure is the
deviation or variance of the individual observation.
Then square each deviation and divide the sum of
the squared deviations by one less than the total
number of observations. The standard deviation is
the square root of this number.

Standard Error (stan′dard/er′or) (n.) In statistics,
when taking repeated random samples of a given size
from the same population, this is a measure of the
variability any statistical constant would be expected to show. Differences between means are said
to have statistical significance when they are greater
than twice the standard error of those means. This
is also known as the **Standard Error of the Mean**.

Standard Position (stan′dard/po-zish′un) (n.) The
usual and accepted position for the radiographic examination of any body part.

Staphylococcus (staf-i-lō-kok′us) (n.) A genus of
gram-positive cocci. It is from the family Micrococ-
caceae.

Staple (stā′p′l) (n.) A U-shaped metal wire or hook
used as an orthopaedic implant for the internal fixation of bone to bone or soft tissue to bone. Staples
are available in a wide range of sizes and shapes.

Staple Capsulorraphy (stā′p′l/kap-su-lor′a-fē) (n.)
A surgical technique for the treatment of recurrent
anterior shoulder dislocations in which staples are
used to attach the labrum and capsule to the anterior
glenoid rim. This technique may be done openly, as
described by du Toit and Roux, or it may be arthroscopically assisted.

Stapling (stā′pling) 1. (n.) Any procedure that uses a
bone staple for internal fixation. 2. (v.) Using a staple. See **Magnuson Stack Procedure**.

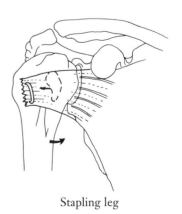

Stapling leg

Starch (starch) (n.) A complex carbohydrate or polysaccharide.

Starling's Law (star'lings/law) (n.) A physiologic law stating that the force of a muscular contraction is proportional to the resting length of that muscle.

Startle Reflex (star't'l/rē'fleks) (n.) One of the brain stem reflexes that usually disappear by 3 months of age. It is more commonly known as the **Moro Reflex**. Make a loud noise to startle the baby; his or her arms and legs will suddenly shoot out to the side.

Stasis (stā'sis) (n.) The stoppage of fluid flow; equilibrium.

Static (stat'ik) (n.) The branch of mechanics dealing with the equilibrium of bodies at rest or in motion with zero acceleration.

Stature (stach'er) (n.) Height.

Steel Osteotomy (stēl/os"te-ot'ō-me) (n.) A surgical procedure for repositioning the acetabulum in hip dysplasia in which the ischium, the superior pubic ramus, and the ilium are all divided. Also known as **Triple Innominate Osteotomy**.

Steel's Rule of Thirds (stēlz/rūl/of/thirdz) (n.) An anatomical and mechanical consideration of the **Atlantoaxial articulation**. At the first cervical vertebra one third of the space is for the odontoid, one third is for the spinal cord, and one-third is space.

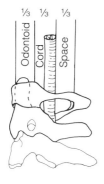

Steel's Rule of Thirds

Steffensen's Angle (stef'-en-senz/ang'g'l) (n.) A radiographic measurement in the foot that may represent predisposition to developing Achilles bursitis if it is increased. On a lateral radiograph, a line is drawn from the most proximal point on the tuber calcanei to the lowest point of the sinus tarsi. Another line is drawn from the posterosuperior edge of the calcaneus body to the first point. Normally, these intersect at an angle of 60 degrees. If this angle exceeds 65 degrees; it is considered abnormally elevated.

Steinbroker Scale (stīn-brō-ker/skāl) (n.) A four-stage grading system for the radiographic evaluation of rheumatoid arthritis:
Stage I: Osteoporosis may exist; no erosions.
Stage II: Osteoporosis; slight cartilage or subchondral bone destruction may be present.

Stage III: Osteoporosis; cartilage and bone destruction.
Stage IV: Same as Stage III, with bony ankylosis.

Steinbroker Syndrome (stīn-brō-ker/sin-drōm) (n.) See **Shoulder–Hand Syndrome**.

Steindler's Test (stīnd-lerz/test) (n.) A technique used to differentiate low back strain from disk disease. A local anesthetic agent is injected into the area of tenderness. The diagnosis of strain instead of disk disease is indicated if contact of the needle aggravates the local pain and/or the radiating pain; if injection of the anesthetic abolishes the local pain and/or the radiating pain; and if normal straight leg raising is restored after injection.

Steinmann Pin (stīn'man/pin) (n.) Rigid, stainless steel pins used for internal fixation of bones. These pins come in varying lengths and diameters and may be smooth or threaded.

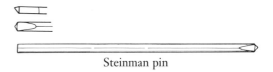

Steinman pin

Steinmann Test (stīn'man/test) (n.) A clinical test used in the evaluation of meniscal injuries. Place the knee in at least 90 degrees of flexion and gently stabilize the foot. Grasp the calf firmly and internally and externally rotate the tibia. Sharp pain will be repeated along the joint line of the affected meniscus if a tear is present.

Stellate Block (stel'-āt/blok) (n.) A type of regional anesthesia in which the anesthetic agent is injected into the region of the stellate ganglion in the neck.

Stellate Fracture (stel'āt/frak'chur) (n.) A fracture with a central point of injury, from which radiate numerous fissures.

Stellate Ganglion (stel'āt/gang'lē-on) (n.) A star-shaped collection of sympathetic nerve cell bodies in the root of the neck, from which sympathetic nerve fibers are distributed to the region of the face and neck and the blood vessels and organs of the thorax. The stellate ganglion is formed by the complete or partial fusion of the inferior cervical and first thoracic sympathetic ganglia; it is situated between the base of the transverse process of the last cervical vertebra (the seventh) and the neck of the first rib.

Stem Length (stem/lenth) (n.) In the femoral component of a hip prosthesis, the distance from the medial base of the collar or neck to the tip of the stem.

Stener Lesion (stēner/le'zhen) (n.) A finding associated with ruptures of the ulnar collateral ligament of the thumb. In this lesion, the adductor aponeurosis becomes interposed between the ends of the torn ligament, thereby preventing healing of the ligament without operative intervention.

Stenosis (sti-nō′sis) (n.) A narrowing of an opening or passage. Example: spinal stenosis.

Step Length (step/lenth) (n.) The perpendicular distance in meters from the heel strike of one foot to the heel strike of the opposite foot.

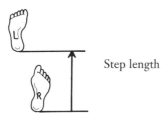

Step length

Step-Time Differential (step/tīm/dif′-er-en′shul) (n.) The absolute value of average step time for one limb minus average step time for the opposite limb. The average step time, in seconds, is derived from step-length data by dividing average step length by velocity.

Steppage Gait (step′aj/gāt) (n.) The high-stepping walk seen in patients with a footdrop. There is footdrop during the entire gait cycle as well as excessive knee and hip flexion, which allows clearance of the involved extremity during the swing phase. Steppage gait is caused by the weakness or paralysis of the dorsiflexors of the foot. Also known as **Footdrop Gait**.

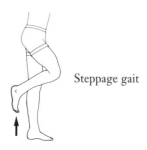

Steppage gait

Sterile (ster′l) (adj.) 1. Free from all living microorganisms; aseptic. 2. Unable to reproduce sexually.

Sterile Field (ster′l/fēld) (n.) The area around the site of incision into tissue, or the introduction of any instrumentation into a body orifice that has been prepared for the use of sterile supplies and equipment. The sterile field includes all equipment covered with sterile drapes and all properly attired personnel.

Sterile Technique (ster′l/tek-nēk) (n.) The method by which contamination with microorganisms is prevented to maintain sterility throughout the operative procedure. Synonym: **Surgical Asepsis**.

Sterilization (ster′i-li-zā′shun) (n.) The process by which all microorganisms, including spores, are destroyed to produce sterility.

Sterilizer (ster′il-īz′er) (n.) The chamber or equipment used to attain either physical or chemical sterilization. The agent used must be capable of killing all forms of microorganisms and their spores.

Sternal (ster′nal) (adj.) Of or pertaining to the sternum.

Sternal Angle (ster′nal/ang′gl′) (n.) The angle formed between the manubrium and the body of the sternum. Also known as the **Angle of Louis**.

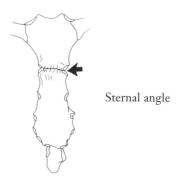

Sternal angle

Sternal Line (ster′nal/līn) (n.) A vertical line corresponding to the lateral margin of the sternum.

Sternal Puncture (ster′nal/pungk′cher) (n.) The insertion of a hollow needle into the manubrium of the sternum for the purpose of obtaining a sample of bone marrow.

Sternert Disease (stern-ert/di-zēz) (n.) See **Myotonic Dystrophy**.

Sternoclavicular (ster′nō-kla-vik′ū-lar) (adj.) Of or pertaining to the joint between the sternum and the clavicle.

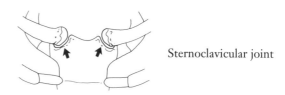

Sternoclavicular joint

Sternocleiodomastoid Muscle (ster′nō-klī-dō-mas′toyd/mus′el) (n.) See **Muscle**.

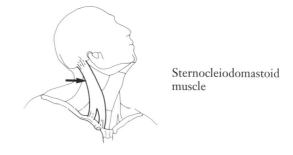

Sternocleiodomastoid muscle

Sternum (ster′num) (n.) A flat bone, 15 to 20 cm long, that extends from the base of the neck to just below the diaphragm, forming the anterior arch of the skeleton of the thorax. The sternum articulates with the clavicles and the costal cartilages of the first seven pairs of ribs. It consists of three sections: the **body**, or middle section, that is attached to the **manubrium** at the top, and the **xiphoid process** at the bottom. Also called **Breastbone**.

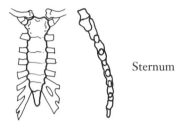

Sternum

Steroid (ster′oid) (n.) One of many fat-soluble, complex, biologically active compounds whose molecules contain a system of four rings made up of 17 carbon atoms.

Steroid Flare (ster′oid/flār) (n.) An acute, self-limited synovitis that follows intra-articular corticosteroid injection. Joint swelling, sometimes disproportionately greater than accompanying pain, generally begins 6 to 12 hours after the injection, and resolves spontaneously within 12 to 24 hours. The demonstration of steroid crystals within polymorphonuclear leukocytes suggests that this phenomenon represents a true crystal-induced arthritis.

Stickler Disease (stik′ler/di-zēz) (n.) Hereditary arthro-ophthalmopathy, an osteochondral dysplasia inherited as an autosomal dominant trait that is manifest in later life. The most characteristic finding is severe hip joint arthropathy, which is often associated with vertebral body flattening and narrowed intervertebral disk spaces. The ophthalmopathy may be as simple as myopia.

Stieda Fracture (stē′dah/frak′chur) (n.) An avulsion fracture of the medial femoral epicondyle found at the level of origin of the medial collateral ligament

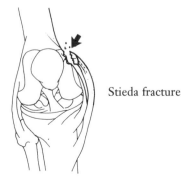

Stieda fracture

of the knee. See related term: **Pelligrini-Stieda Disease**.

Stiffness (stif′nes) (n.) A measure of resistance offered to external loads by a specimen or structure as it deforms. The stiffness of a material is represented by the slope of the stress-strain curve in the elastic region or Young's modulus.

Still's Disease (stilz/di-zēz) (n.) An eponym applied to all forms of juvenile rheumatoid arthritis but originally intended to describe systemic-onset JRA. In this presentation, in addition to the polyarthritis, there are characteristic systemic manifestations that include high fever, an evanescent salmon-colored rash, lymphadenopathy, hepatosplenomegaly, cardiac involvement, and pneumonitis or pleuritis. Laboratory tests for rheumatoid factor and ANA are usually negative. Synonyms: **Juvenile Rheumatoid Arthritis, Chauffard-Still, Dreie's Syndrome, Acute Polyarthritis.**

Stimson Dressing (stim′son/dres′ing) (n.) An adhesive strapping for nonoperative treatment of subluxation of the acromioclavicular joint.

Stimson Maneuver (stim′son/ma-nū′ver) (n.) A technique for the reduction of a posterior dislocation of the hip. The patient is placed prone, with the injured hip flexed at 90 degrees or more over the end of the table. Keeping the patient's thigh and knee both flexed at 90 degrees, apply firm downward pressure to the flexed leg while an assistant stabilizes the pelvis. A gentle rocking or rotational motion may be helpful. By gradually increasing the downward traction on the leg, and with slight increase in internal rotation, flexion, and adduction, reduction will be achieved.

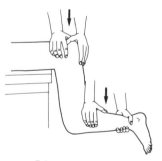

Stimson maneuver

Stimson Method (stim′son/meth′ud) (n.) A technique for the reduction of an anterior dislocation of the shoulder. Place the patient prone with the arm hanging off the side of the table and a pillow or folded sheet placed under the shoulder. Attach a strap to the wrist or distal forearm, and suspend weights (from 10 to 15 pounds) from the strap for a period of 20 to 30 minutes. During this time, gentle spontaneous reduction will occur.

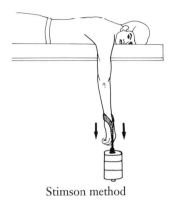

Stimson method

Stimulus (stim′ū-lus) (n.) Any internal or external change in the environment that evokes a response from a tissue, an organ, or another body part.

Stingers (sting′erz) (n.) A colloquial term for a transient brachial plexopathy experienced by athletes. The common mechanism of injury is a fall or blow that depresses the shoulder and deviates the head backward or toward the opposite shoulder. Clinically, the player experiences a sudden, burning pain in the shoulder, radiating into the arm, forearm, and hand. These usually last only several seconds, and no objective neurologic abnormalities are found. Also known as **Burners**.

Stippled Epiphysis (stip′ld/ē-pif-i-sis) (n.) A rare congenital condition characterized by discrete spots of calcification affecting cartilaginous structures, especially the epiphysis. The long bones are shortened. It is not hereditary. See **Dysplasia Epiphysial Punctata**.

Stirrup Brace (stur′ep/brās) (n.) An orthosis for the lower limb in which two upright bars articulate at the level of the ankle, with a stirrup-like shoe attachment designed to receive two uprights.

Stirrups (stur′eps) (n.) Metal positioning devices used to support the legs and feet in a lithotomy position.

Stockinet (stok-i′net) (n.) A knitted, seamless tubing of cotton 1 to 12 inches (2.5 to 30.4 cm) wide and woven like a stocking, but of uniform caliber. The stockinet stretches to fit any contour. It is used as a padding under a cast, splint, or as a covering for a stump when a prosthesis is worn. Also spelled stockinette.

Stone Heel (stōn/hēl) (n.) In shoe terminology, an oblique-shaped Thomas heel.

Stoop Test (stūp/test) (n.) A test used in the evaluation of low back pain. After a conventional neurologic examination, the patient stands upright and begins a brisk walk, preferably down a straight corridor. If during ambulation compression of part or all of the cauda equina occurs, pain in the buttock and radiating limb pain will result. As the activity is continued, the limb pain intensifies, and sensory symp-

toms begin—then motor weakness may occur. The patient then assumes a stooped posture, even while continuing to walk, and pain and neurologic symptoms begin to subside. Have the patient stop walking and stand upright again; the symptoms frequently return. Symptoms are abrogated when the patient sits in a chair and leans forward. These events represent a positive stoop test. A positive test suggests a diagnosis of spinal stenosis.

Storage Disease (stor′ij/di-zēz) (n.) Any metabolic disorder in which some substance, such as lipids, iron, or carbohydrate, accumulates in certain cells in abnormal amounts.

Straddle Fracture (strad′l/frak′chur) (n.) A term applied to pelvic fractures in which bilateral fractures of the superior and inferior pubic rami have occurred.

Straight Last Shoes (strāt/last/shūz) (n.) Shoes made over a last that eliminates the inward flares of the medial border of the shoes, resulting in a straight medial border of the forepart of the shoes.

Straight Leg Raising (strāt/leg/rās′ing) (n.) The lifting of the leg with the knee extended.

Straight Leg Raising Test (strāt/leg/ras′ing/test) (n.) A qualitative test to determine if nerve root impingement is the cause of back pain. Nerve root motion occurs from 30 degrees to 80 degrees of straight leg raising above the horizontal. No movement occurs at any vertebral level in the first 30 degrees of straight leg raising. The maximal angle achieved in the straight leg raising test is limited by tightness of the hamstrings and may also be influenced by hip joint dysfunction. With the knee held in full extension, raise the leg gradually from the table until limiting symptoms occur or the maximal angle is reached. A positive test is one that causes radiating pain down the leg that is relieved by flexing the knee and aggravated by forceful dorsiflexion at the ankle. The opposite leg is then moved in a similar fashion. See **Lasègue Straight Leg Raising Test**. Abbreviated **SLR**.

Strain (strān) (n.) 1. In biomechanics, the change in unit length (normal strain) or angle (sheer strain) in a material subjected to load. 2. A stretching or tearing of a musculotendinous unit. A strain can be arbitrarily classified as first, second, or third degree. A first-degree strain consists of minimal stretching of the musculotendinous unit without permanent injury. A second-degree strain indicates partial tearing of the musculotendinous unit. A third-degree strain indicates complete disruption of a portion of this unit. Swelling, bleeding, and localized discomfort also accompany a third-degree strain, possibly producing temporary disability. Initial treatment following an acute strain should consist of ice application, immobilization of the musculotendinous unit, and subsequent rehabilitation. Occasionally, surgical intervention may be indicated.

Strain Energy (strān/en′er-ji) (n.) In biomechanical

terms, the energy stored in a structure by virtue of its being deformed under the application of load.

Strain Gauge (strān/gāj) (n.)   A device that measures strain.

Strain Rate (strān/rāt) (n.)   The rate of change of deformation per unit length with time. The unit of measure is per second.

Strap Muscles (strap/mus′els) (n.)   A term applied to the ribbon-like muscles in the anterior neck. This includes the thyrohyoid, the omohyoid, the sternohyoid, and the sternothyroid muscles. See **Muscle**.

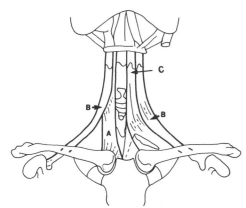

Strap muscles. **A**, Sterno-thyroid; **B**, omo-hyoid; **C**, sterno-hyoid.

Street Nail (strēt/nāl) (n.)   A diamond-shaped intramedullary nail used in the treatment of fractures of the femoral shaft. See **Hansen Street Nail**.

Strength (strenth) (n.)   In biomechanical terms, the property of materials by which the application of force is endured without the material yielding or breaking. A structure's strength is determined by three parameters: the load to failure, the deformation to failure, and the energy stored before failure. The strength of a structure is affected by its size and shape and the type of load applied—compressive or tensile.

Streptococcus (strep-tō-kok′us) (n.)   A genus of gram-positive cocci, from the family Streptococcaceae, that tend to be arranged in chains.

Stress (stres) (n.)   In biomechanics, the force per unit area of a structure in response to externally applied loads. The unit of stress is newtons per meter squared, or Pascal (N/M^2 or Pa).

Stress Concentration (stres/kon′sen-trā′shun) (n.)   Any localized stress peak that cannot be predicted.

Stress Fracture (stres/frak′chur) (n.)   A break in the continuity of presumably normal bone caused by recurring and repetitive subthreshold trauma. Also called a **March**, **Fatigue**, or **Insufficiency Fracture**.

Stress Rate (stres/rāt) (n.)   The rate of change of load per unit area with time. The unit of measure is newtons per square meter per second (or pound force per square foot per second).

Stress Riser (stres/rī′zer) (n.)   A small defect in a structure (usually bone) that reduces the strength of that structure by preventing the stresses applied by loading from being distributed evenly throughout the structure. Instead, a local concentration of stress around the defect occurs.

Stress-Strain Curve (stres-strān/kurv) (n.)   A graphic representation of the mechanical behavior of a material. This plots stress, usually on the ordinate or Y-axis, versus strain, usually on the abscissa or X-axis.

Stress Test (stres/test) (n.)   A clinical evaluation of ligamentous injury in which force is applied across a joint that would normally tighten that ligament in order to assess its integrity. For example, the medial collateral ligament (MCL) of the knee is examined with a valgus stress test. These stresses may be applied manually or with the assistance of an instrument that will quantify the stress applied.

Stress X-Rays (stres/eks′raz) (n.)   Radiographs obtained during the application of stress across a joint.

Stretch Receptor (strech/ri-sep′tor) (n.)   A cell or group of cells found between muscle fibers that respond to a stretching of the muscle by transmitting impulses to the central nervous system through sensory nerves. Stretch receptors are part of the proprioceptor system necessary for the performance of coordinated muscular activity.

Stretch Reflex (strech/re′fleks) (n.)   The reflex contraction of a muscle in response to passive longitudinal stretching. Also known as the **Myotatic Reflex**, **the Muscle Stretch Reflex**, or the **Deep Tendon Reflex**.

Stretching Exercise (streching/ek′ser-sīz) (n.)   An exercise intended to increase the resting length of a musculotendinous unit or ligament. Stretching exercises involve the use of as much force as the patient can tolerate within pain limits or as is felt safe at that stage of fracture or soft tissue healing.

Striated Muscle (strī-āt-id/mus′el) (n.)   A contractile tissue that constitutes the bulk of the body's musculature. Also known as a **skeletal muscle** (it is attached to the skeleton) or **voluntary muscle** (it is under voluntary nervous system control). Striated muscle is composed of parallel bundles of multinucleate fibers, which reveal cross-banding when viewed under the microscope. This effect is due to the alternation of actin and myosin protein filaments within each myofibril.

Strict Isolation (strikt/ī-sō-lā′shun) (n.)   A form of patient separation used to prevent the transmission of highly communicable bacteria and viruses that are spread by both the contact and airborne routes. The patient should be kept in a private room at all times. Gown and mask must be worn by every individual entering the room, and gloves should be worn by all persons coming in contact with the patient or with any article touched by him or her.

Stride Length (strīd/lenth) (n.)   The perpendicular distance in meters from the heel strike of one foot to the next heel strike of the same foot.

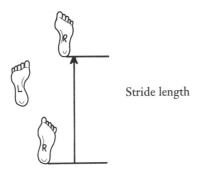

Stride length

Stride-Time Differential (strīd/tīme/dif′er-en′shul) (n.)   The absolute value of average stride time for one limb minus average stride time for the opposite limb. Average stride time in seconds is first derived from stride length data by dividing the average stride length by the velocity.

Striding Gait (strīd′ing/gāt) (n.)   A type of walking characterized by taking long steps.

Strip (strip)   1. (v.) To remove a covering or the contents of a structure, such as the periosteum covering bone. 2. (v.) To break or damage either the thread on a screw or the threads on bone formed by a tap so that a screw will not be firmly securable. 3. (n.) A narrow, elongated piece of material.

Stroke Test (strōk/test) (n.)   An examination to determine if there is fluid in the knee joint. Also called **Wipe Test**.

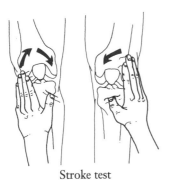

Stroke test

Stroma (strō′ma) (n.)   The supportive tissue of the framework of an organ, as contrasted to the functional tissue. Contrast to **Parenchyma**.

Structural Curve (struk′chural/kurv) (n.)   A segment of the spine that has a fixed lateral curvature. Radiographically, a structural curve is identified in

supine, lateral, and side bending films by its failure to correct.

Strumpell Confusion Test (strum′pel/kon-fū′zhun/ test) (n.)   In cerebral palsy, a test of the function of anterior tibial muscle. Have the child dorsiflex the ankle with the knee in extension and in flexion. The gastrocnemius portion of the triceps surae relaxes when the knee is flexed. If the anterior tibial muscle does not contract with the knee flexed, ask the child to flex the hip and knee against resistance. This maneuver, called synkinesia, will cause the anterior tibial muscle to contract, bringing the ankle and foot into dorsiflexion.

Strunsky Sign (strun′skē/sīn) (n.)   A means used to detect lesions of the anterior arch of the foot. Grasp the patient's toes and flex them suddenly. This procedure is painless in the normal foot but painful in the presence of inflammation of the anterior arch.

Stryker Frame (strī-ker/fram) (n.)   The proprietary name of an apparatus with a mattress that can be turned around on its longitudinal axis with the patient on it. It provides a means of pivoting an immobilized patient, allowing positional and postural changes. This was developed in 1939 by Homer H. Stryker for the care of patients with injuries of the spinal cord or paralysis. Also known as a **Stryker Bed**.

Stryker Notch View (strī-ker/noch/vū) (n.)   A radiographic view of the shoulder used to demonstrate defects in the posterolateral aspect of the humeral head in recurrent anterior shoulder dislocators. The patient is placed supine with the x-ray cassette under the shoulder. The elbow is flexed and pointed upward, and the palm of the hand is placed on top of the head. The x-ray beam is then tilted 10 degrees toward the head.

Student's T Test (stood′nts/T/test) (n.)   A test for determining statistical significance.

Stump (stump) (n.)   1. The termination of a limb that remains after amputation. 2. Any pedicle or piece of tissue remaining after removal or amputation of its distal aspect.

Stump revision (stump/rē-vizh′un) (n.)   A surgical procedure to alter an amputation stump.

Stump Shrinker (stump/shringk′r) (n.)   A compressive, elastic band worn on an amputation stump to reduce its size.

Stump Sock (stump/sok) (n.)   A sock worn over an amputation stump to protect and cushion the skin.

Stylet (stī′lit) (n.)   1. A wire inserted through the lumen of a catheter or cannula, rendering it stiff. It is used to either maintain patency or remove debris and reestablish patency. 2. A slender probe.

Styloid Process (stī′loid/pros′-es) (n.)   1. Any long, slender, spiny projection of bone. 2. Specifically, the bony projection occurring at the distal aspect of the ulna and the radius or from the lower surface of the temporal bone of the skull.

Sub A prefix meaning below or beneath; refers to quantity or location.

Subacromial (sub-a-krō'mē-al) (adj.) Below the acromion.

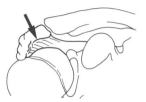

Subacromial

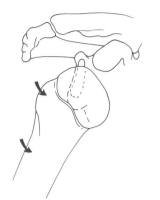

Subcoracoid

ɔccur-

Subaponeurotic (sub-ap-ō-nu-rot ik) (adj.) Below an aponeurosis.

Subarachnoid (sub-a-rak'noyd) (adj.) Between the arachnoid and the pia matter.

Subarachnoid Space (sub-a-rak'noyd/spās) (n.) The space between the arachnoid and pia meninges of the brain and spinal cord. It contains circulating cerebrospinal fluid and large blood vessels. Several large spaces formed within it are known as cisternae.

Subcapital Hip Fracture (sub-kap'it'l/hip/frak'chur) (n.) A femoral neck fracture that occurs just below the femoral head.

Subchondral Bone (sub-kon'dral/bōn) (n.) The bone immediately beneath the articular cartilage of a joint surface.

Subclavian Steal Syndrome (sub-klā'vē-an/stēl/sin' drom) (n.) A syndrome that results from blockage of one of the subclavian vessels proximal to the origin of the vertebral artery so that blood is transferred from the contralateral vertebral artery through the basilar artery into the ipsilateral vertebral artery. This "steals" blood from the cerebral circulation, causing the development of neurologic symptoms.

Subclavius Muscle (sub-klā'vē-us/mus'el) (n.) See **Muscle**.

Subclinical (sub-klin'i-kal) (adj.) A disease process that is suspected but not sufficiently developed to produce definite signs and symptoms.

Subcoracoid (sub-kor'a-koyd) (adj.) Situated below the coracoid process, e.g., a subcoracoid dislocation of the humeral head.

Subcutaneous (sub-kū-tā'nē-us) (adj.) Beneath the dermis.

Subcutaneous Tissue (sub'kū-tā'nē-us/tish'ū) (n.) The layer of loose connective tissue under the dermis.

Subcuticular (sub-kū-lik'ū-lar) (adj.) Beneath the epidermis.

Subdural (sub-du'ral) (adj.) 1. Below the dura mater. 2. Of or related to the space between the dura mater and the arachnoid.

Subjective (sub-jek'tiv) (adj.) Perceived by the patient but not apparent to the examiner. This describes the symptoms (pain, puritus, dizziness, and so forth) that the patient experiences, in contrast to objective signs elicited by the examiner.

Subjective Symptom (sub-jek'tiv/simp'tom) (n.) Any symptom perceptible only to the patient.

Subluxability (n.) The state of being subluxable.

Subluxable (adj.) Capable of being subluxed.

Subluxate (sub-luks'āt) (v.) To alter the relationship between joint surfaces by translation. Some contact between the articular surfaces remains, as compared with a dislocation.

Subluxation (sub-luk-sa'shun) (n.) 1. A malalignment of opposing joint surfaces with a partial loss of joint congruity or contact. 2. A partial dislocation.

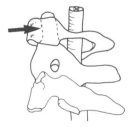

Subluxation

Submental Triangle (sub-men'tal/trī'ang'gl) (n.) A small area beneath the central part of the mandible.

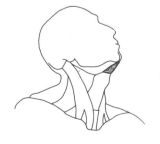

Submental triangle

Subperiosteal New Bone (sub-per-ē-os'tē-al/nū/bōn) (n.) Any bone that is newly formed beneath the periosteum or in the juxtacortical region. Also known as **reactive periosteal bone**, it is seen in association with trauma, infection, neoplasm, nutritional deficiency, and other disease states.

Subscapular Fossa (sub-skap'u-lar/fos'ah) (n.) The slightly concave, costal surface of the scapula.

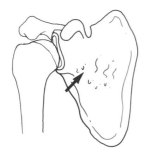

Subscapula fossa

Subscapularis Muscle (sub-skap-yu-la'is/mus'el) (n.) See **Muscle**.

Subsidence (sub-sī'dens) (n.) The settling of a prosthetic component. It is determined by a radiographic change in position when a comparison is made with the radiographs taken at the time of the original implantation. More sophisticated methods for determining subsidence include stereophotogrametric techniques. Subsidence is considered an absolute sign of loosening of the prosthesis.

Substrate (sub'strāt) (n.) The molecule or molecules on which an enzyme exerts catalytic action.

Subtalar (sub'tā'lar) (adj.) Below the talus.

Subtalar Joint (sub'tā'lar/joint) (n.) A complex joint of the hindfoot in which the talus articulates with the calcaneus. The term subtalar complex is a collective term for the talocalcaneal, talonavicular, and calcaneocuboid joints.

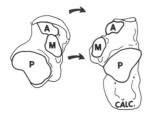

Subtalar joint. **A**, Anterior facet; **M**, middle facet; **P**, posterior facet.

Subtrochanteric (sub-trō-kan-ter'ik) (adj.) Below the lesser trochanter of the proximal femur.

Subtrochanteric Fracture (sub-trō-kan-ter'ik/frak'chur) (n.) A fracture of the proximal end of the femur below the lesser trochanter. See **Sensheimer Classification**.

Subungual (sub-ung'wal) (adj.) Beneath the nail.

Subungual Exostosis (sub-ung'wal/ek"sos-to'sis) (n.) A small, benign, bony outgrowth that is found on the dorsal aspect of a distal phalanx, beneath the nail.

Subungual Hematoma (sub-ung'wal/hē'ma-tō'ma) (n.) A localized mass of extravasated blood found beneath a toe or fingernail. It usually occurs post-traumatically.

Sucrose (sū'krōs) (n.) A common sugar. It is a disaccharide composed of fructose and glucose.

Suction (suk'shun) (n.) The application of less than atmospheric pressure through a drainage device, either continuously or intermittently, to aspirate blood and tissue fluids from an operative field.

Suction Suspension (suk'shun/sus-pen-shun) (n.) A form of prosthesis attachment that relies on a vacuumlike form fit to maintain suspension.

Sudeck's Atrophy (soo'deks/at'ro-fē) (n.) A minor form of reflex sympathetic dystrophy characterized by the radiographic finding of severe, regional osteoporosis. See **Reflex Sympathetic Dystrophy**.

Sugar (shu-ger) (n.) Any monosaccharide or disaccharide.

Sugar Tong Splint (shu'ger/tung/splint) (n.) An immobilizing splint applied to the humerus or forearm as a U-shaped coaptation splint. It is so named for its resemblance to the arms of the tongs used to pick up sugar cubes. Also known as **Coaptation Splint**.

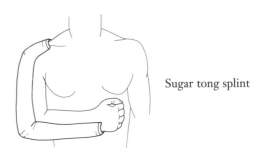

Sugar tong splint

Sulcus (sul'kus) (n.) 1. A groove or furrow used in anatomic nomenclature to designate a linear depression. 2. Specifically, the depressions that separate the gyri of the brain.

Sulcus Angle (sul'kus/ang'g'l) (n.) The angle reflecting the depth of the patellar sulcus and the steepness of the distal femoral condyles. It is determined on a tangential radiographic view of the patellofemoral joint. Draw lines from the depth of the sulcus to the peaks of each of the femoral condyles, and measure the angle between the two lines. The greater the angle, the more shallow the sulcus, which means there is a greater potential for patellar instability. Discrepancies in radiographic technique may alter the normal values. See **Merchant's Angle**.

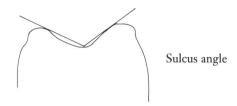

Sulcus angle

Sulindac (sul-in′dak) (n.)   A nonsteroidal, anti-inflammatory drug marketed under the brand name Clinoril.

Sulkowitch Test (sul-kō-wich/test) (n.)   A test used for the estimation of calcium in urine. It uses Sulkowitch's reagent, which is composed of specific concentrations of oxalic acid, ammonium oxalate, and glacial acetic acid. Random urine specimens are tested. The density of the precipitate formed is noted and reported as 0 to 4 plus. A zero test indicates hypocalcemia (serum calcium less than 75 mg/100 mL). A 3 to 4 plus suggests hypercalcemia (serum calcium greater than 105 mg/100 mL).

Sunderland's Classification (sun-der-landz/klas″si-fi-kā′shun) (n.)   A classification scheme of the degree or grade of peripheral nerve injury based on electromyographic and nerve conduction velocity studies.

1A—Mild   Rest Silence
Effort—Normal or slight decrease in number of potentials
Chronaxy less than 1 msec. No Reaction Degeneration (RD)

1B—Moderate   Rest—Very few fibrillations
Effort—Few Motor Unit Potential (MUP) Chronaxy 1 to 10 msec. No RD.

1C—Severe   Rest—Few fibrillations
Effort—No MUP. Chronaxy 10 to 20 msec after 7 days. No RD.

2A—Partial   Rest—Fibrillations in many samples
Effort—Few MUP. Occasional polyphasics. Chronaxy over 20 msec.

2B—Complete   Rest—Fibrillations in all samples
Effort—No MUP after 5 days. Chronaxy over 30 msec after 5 to 7 days.

3—Severance   Rest—Abundant continuous fibrillations
Effort—No MUP. Chronaxy 30 to 60 msec. RD from injury on.

Sunrise View (sun′rīz′/vū) (n.)   See **Skyline View**.

Sunset View (sun′set/vū) (n.)   See **Skyline View**.

Super   Prefix for above or on top of.

Superficial (sū-per-fish′al) (adj.)   Near or close to the surface.

Superficial Infrapatella Bursa (sū-per-fish′al/in″frah-pah-tel′a/ber′sah) (n.)   See **Infrapatella Bursa Superficial**.

Superficial Fascia (sū-per-fish′al/fash′ē-ah) (n.)   1. A fascial sheet lying directly beneath the skin. 2. Subcutaneous tissue.

Superimpose (sū-per-im-pōz) (v.)   To place one object on top of another. A term used in radiology to describe an overlying structure that obscures the view of the primary structure.

Superinfection (sū′per-in-fex′shun) (n.)   A secondary, subsequent infection following antibiotic therapy or chemotherapy; caused by different microorganisms.

Superior Mesenteric Artery Syndrome (sū-per′ē-or/me′sen′ter-ik/ar′ter-ē/sin′drōm) (n.)   A syndrome that results from compression of the duodenum in its third portion by the superior mesenteric artery. The cast syndrome is an acute form of this syndrome that may occur after the application of a body jacket. Vascular compression of the duodenum causes acute duodenal obstruction and gastric dilatation, which results in abdominal pain, distention, and vomiting, often projectile. See also **Cast Syndrome**.

Superior Vena Cava (sū-per′ē-or/ven′a/ca-va) (n.)   The large vein that returns blood from the head, neck, upper extremities, and chest to the right atrium of the heart.

Supernumerary (sū-per-nū′mer-ar-ē) (adj.)   More than the normal or expected number. For example, a supernumerary digit is a congenital anomaly in which more than five digits are present on one hand or foot.

Supination (sū′pi-nā′shun) (n.)   1. In the upper extremity, rotation of the forearm so that the palm faces up, or anteriorly, in the anatomic position. Compare to **Pronation**. 2. In the foot, the use of a combination of motions, including adduction and inversion of the foot and lateral rotation of the ankle, to rotate the medial aspect of the plantar surface away from the ground.

Supinator (sū′pi-nā-ter) (n.)   Any muscle that functions to produce supination of a body part.

Supinator Muscle (sū′pi-nā′ter/mus′el) (n.)   See **Muscle**.

Supine (sū-pīn′) (adj.)   Lying on the dorsal surface, with the face upward. Compare to **Prone**.

Supine Position (sū-pīn/pō-zi-shun) (n.)   The position in which the patient lies flat on his or her back, with arms at his or her side, palms down, fingers extended and freely resting on the table, and legs straight, with feet slightly separated. Synonym: **Horizontal Position**.

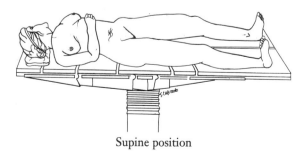

Supine position

Support (su-port) (n.)   A reinforcement or arch used to control the stress of weight-bearing areas.

Suppuration (sūp′yū-rā′shun) (n.)   The formation of pus.

Supraclavicular (soo″-prah-klah-vik′ū-lar) (adj.)   Of or pertaining to the anatomic region above the clavicle.

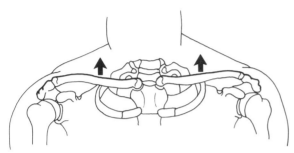

Supraclavicular

Supraclavicular Fossa (soo″prah-klah-vik′u-lar/fos′ ah)   The space immediately posterior to the clavicle.

Supracondylar (soo′-prah-kon′dī-lar) (adj.)   Of or related to an area above the condyle. Used in reference to the anatomic area immediately proximal to the condyles of the distal humerus or distal femur.

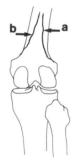

Supracondylar

Supracondylar Fracture of Humerus (soo″prah-kon′dī-lar/frak′chur/of/hu′mer-us) (n.)   A fracture situated above the humeral condyle.

Supracondylar Process (soo″-prah-kon′dī-lar/ pros′es) (n.)   An inconstant, small, vestigial, beak-like projection arising from the distal humerus several centimeters above the medial epicondyle. The supracondylar process may be joined to the medial epicondyle by a band of fibrous tissue known as the ligament of Struthers.

Supraglenoid Tuberosity (soo″prah-ĝle′noid/too″bë-ros′ĭ-te) (n.)   A small bony prominence on the upper border of the glenoid cavity.

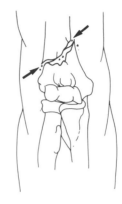

Supracondylar fracture of humerus

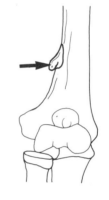

Supracondylar process

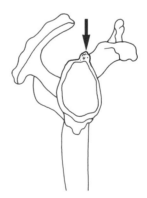

Supraglenoid tuberosity

Supranavicular Bone (soo″-prah-na-vic′u-lar/bōn) (n.)   An accessory bone of the foot. It is a small, triangular bone occurring at the proximal superior edge of the navicular, and articulating with the talus and the navicular. The supranavicular bone is relatively common, and may easily be mistaken for a fracture. Also known as **Pirie's Bone**.

Suprapatellar Pouch (soo″-prah-pa-tel′ar/pouch) (n.)   That part of the articular cavity of the knee that extends between the quadriceps tendon and the distal femur, proximal to the patella.

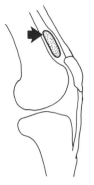

Suprapatellar pouch

Suprapubic (soo″-prah-pu′bik) (adj.)   Referring to the anatomic region situated immediately above the symphysis pubis.

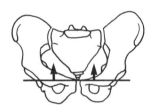

Suprapubic

Supraspinatus Muscle (soo″-prah-spī-na′tus/mus′el) (n.)   See **Muscle**.

Supraspinatus Test (su-pra-spī-na′tus/test) (n.)   A clinical test used in the evaluation of rotator cuff lesions. With the patient's arm at 90 degrees of abduction and neutral rotation, assess the strength in resisted abduction. Then, internally rotate the shoulder and flex it forward to 30 degrees. This position will isolate supraspinatus tendon function; if resisted abduction in this position is weakened or painful, a lesion of the supraspinatus tendon, such as a tear or inflammation, is indicated.

Supraspinous (soo″-prah-spī′nus) (adj.)   Above the spinous process of the scapula or a vertebra.

Supraspinous Ligament (soo″-prah-spi′nus/lig′ah-ment) (n.)   See **Ligament**.

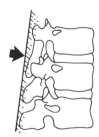

Supraspinous ligament

Suprasternal Notch (soo″prah-ster′nal/noch) (n.)   An excavation or notch in the proximal end of the sternum.

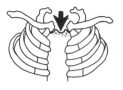

Suprasternal notch

Supratentorial (su′pra-ten-tor′ē-al) (adj.)   1. Structures situated above the tentorium cerebelli, the fold of dura mater separating the posterior cranial fossa from the remainder of the cranium. 2. Commonly used to refer to a psychologic or functional disorder.

Surcingle Cast (ser-singl′/kast) (n.)   An ambulatory body cast used to correct scoliosis.

Surgery (ser′jer-ē) (n.)   The field of medicine dedicated to the treatment of disease or injury by operation.

Surgical Asepsis (ser′ji-kal/a′sēp′sis) (n.)   Practices that render and keep objects and areas free from all microorganisms.

Surgical Drape (ser′ji-kal/drāp) (n.)   A sterile covering positioned over nonsterile surfaces to maintain aseptic conditions during surgery.

Surgical Neck of Humerus (ser′ji-kal/nek/of/hū′mer-us) (n.)   A narrowed area of the proximal humeral shaft lying just distal to the tubercles (anatomic neck). Fractures frequently occur here. Compare to **Anatomic Neck of Humerus**.

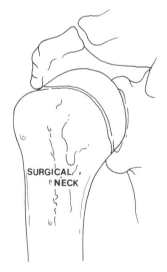

Surgical neck of humerus

Surgical Procedure (ser′ji-kal/prō-se′jur) (n.)   Any single, separate, systematic manipulation on or within the body that can be complete therapy in itself. Also known as an **Operation**.

Surgical Scrub (ser′ji-kal/skrub) (n.)   The process of removing as many microorganisms as possible from the hands and arms by mechanical washing and chemical antisepsis. This is done before participating in an operative procedure.

Surgical Shoe (ser'ji-kal/shū) (n.)   A type of orthopaedic shoe that is usually high-topped and laced to the toes.

Surgical Suite (ser'ji-kal/swēt) (n.)   The operating theater, which includes one or more operating rooms and necessary adjunct facilities, such as scrub room(s), recovery room(s), and a sterile storage area.

Surgically Clean (ser'ji-kal-ly/klēn) (adj.)   Mechanically cleansed but unsterile. Items are rendered surgically clean by the use of chemical, physical, or mechanical means that markedly reduce the number of microorganisms on them.

Surgivac (ser'-je-vak) (n.)   A wound drainage device. It is a trademark of Zimmer Co.

Susceptibility (sus'cep'ti-bil'itē) (n.)   1. The state of being open to disease; the capability of being infected. 2. The degree of resistance of a host to a pathogen.

Suspension Traction (sus-pen'shun/trak'shen) (n.)   Any form of skeletal traction to which slings are added beneath the extremity to keep it hanging in the air. This may be useful for a wound or for proper alignment of the fracture.

Sustentaculum (sus'ten-tak'yu-lum) (n.)   Any anatomic structure that supports another structure.

Sustentaculum Tali (sus'ten-tak'yu-lum/ta'lī) (n.)   The bony eminence on the medial aspect of the calcaneus that supports the middle articular facet of the talocaneal joint. Insertion of the tendon of the posterior tibialis muscle.

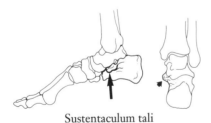

Sustentaculum tali

Sutherland Osteotomy (suth'er-land/os"te-ot'ō-mē) (n.)   A double innominate osteotomy for the treatment of congenital hip dysplasia by acetabulum repositioning. In this technique, the ilium is cut superior to the acetabulum, and the pubic rami are osteotomized lateral to the symphysis pubis. The acetabulum is then repositioned and stabilized with a bone graft and smooth wires.

Suture (su'chur) (n.)   1. In anatomy, the line of union of adjoining bones of the skull. The cranial sutures include the coronal suture, which lies between the frontal and parietal bones; the lamboidal suture, which lies between the parietal and occipital bones; and the sagittal suture, which lies between the two parietal bones. 2. In surgery, a strand of material used for ligating or approximating tissue, as for wound closure.

Swage (swāj) (v.)   To fuse, as suture material to the end of a suture needle.

Swan-Neck Deformity (swon-nek/di-for'mi-tē) (n.)   A finger deformity involving flexion of the distal interphalangeal joint and hyperextension of the proximal interphalangeal joint. This may begin as a mallet deformity associated with a disruption of the extensor tendon, with secondary overpull of the central tendon, which causes hyperextension of the proximal interphalangeal joint.

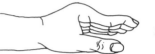

Swan-neck deformity

Swanson Prosthesis (swan-son/pros'thē-sis) (n.)   A silicone-type prosthesis for arthroplasty of the interphalangeal and metacarpophalangeal joints. The Swanson design is a nonfixed, flexible, hinged, intramedullary, and stemmed spacer that improves the stability of resection arthroplasties.

Sweat Test (swet/test) (n.)   The application of iodine and starch to specific areas of the body to demonstrate the distribution and degree of perspiration. The sweat test is used to determine the location and extent of lesions in the sympathetic nervous system and to evaluate the results of sympathectomy.

Swedish Knee Cage (swē'dish/nē/kāj) (n.)   An orthosis designed to control genu recurvatum. It consists of two aluminum uprights connected posteriorly by a semicircular transverse bar, two webbing straps, above and below the knee, and an adjustable fluid-filled pad in the popliteal space.

Swedish Massage (swē'dish/ma-sahj') (n.)   The traditional massage, as practiced today in nearly all countries, but originally taught in conjunction with therapeutic exercises at the Central Institute of Gymnastics in Stockholm. Its name emphasizes its medical nature and traditional origin.

Swimmer's Shoulder (swim'erz/shōl'der) (n.)   An overuse syndrome causing pain in the anterior portion of the shoulder in swimmer's doing the crawl, butterfly, and backstrokes. The etiology is variable and includes adverse tendinitis of the rotator cuff or anterior shoulder subluxation, which causes secondary impingement of the surrounding tendons as well as subluxation of the long head of the biceps from the longitudinal groove in the humerus.

Swimmer's View (swim'erz/vū) (n.)   A radiographic view of the cervical spine that is often used to visualize the lower cervical spine and the cervicothoracic junction. In this view, one arm is abducted to 180 degrees, and the other arm is pulled down at the patient's side. The x-ray beam is then angled obliquely at 60 degrees. Overlapping bony structures may make this view difficult to evaluate.

Swimming Pool Granuloma (swim′ing/pool/gran″u-lō′mah) (n.)   A term applied to mycobacterial infections of the hand that is so named because the infecting organism, *Mycobacterium marinum*, is found in swimming areas and other bodies of water.

Swing Phase (swing/fāz) (n.)   A component of the gait cycle, between toe-off and heel strike. It may be subdivided as follows:
  Acceleration: This initial part begins the instant the toe leaves the ground. At this point, the leg must accelerate in order to catch up to and get in front of the body in preparation for the next heel strike.
  Mid-Swing: Occurs when the leg has caught up to and passes directly beneath the body. At this point, the extremity must be shortened sufficiently to clear the ground.
  Deceleration: Occurs after mid-swing, when the forward motion of the leg is restrained to control the position of the foot immediately before heel strike.

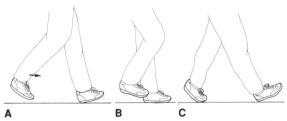

Swing phase. **A,** Acceleration, swing phase; **B,** mid-swing phase; **C,** deceleration swing phase.

Swing-Through Gait (swing/throo/gāt) (n.)   A gait in which the crutches are first advanced, and then both lower limbs are simultaneously swung through and beyond them.

Swing-To Gait (swing-to/gat) (n.)   A gait in which crutches or a walker are first advanced, and then both lower limbs are simultaneously swung to the same point.

Swivel Gait (swiv′el/gat) (n.)   The mode of progression with a swivel walk prosthesis designed for children without functional lower limbs. The trunk, with the help of the upper limbs, is rotated alternatively to the left and the right. One foot piece leaves the floor slightly and moves in a small arc around the other. The swivel gait resembles the pivot gait, except its arc of progression is smaller.

Syme's Amputation (sīmz/am′pu-tā′shun) (n.)   An amputation performed just proximal to the ankle joint. Both malleoli are removed, and a flap is made of the skin of the heel, to provide an end-bearing well-controlled stump.

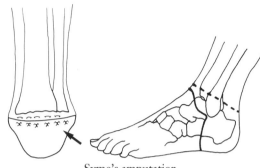

Syme's amputation

Syme Prosthesis (sīm/pros-thē-sis) (n.)   A below-the-knee total contact socket prosthesis.

Symmetry (sim′e-trē) (n.)   In anatomy, the state of opposite parts of an organ or parts at opposite sides of the body corresponding to one another.

Sympathetic Nervous System (sim′pe-thet′ik/ner′vus/sis′tem) (n.)   A subdivision of the autonomic nervous system. The sympathetic nervous system slows digestion but has a general excitatory effect on other functions. Centers are located in the midportion of the spinal cord.

Symphysis (sim′fe-sis) (n.)   A joint in which two bones are united by fibrocartilage. There is minimal motion of the joint. An example is the symphysis pubis.

Symphysis-Os Ischium Angle (sim′fe-sis-os/is′ke-um/ang′g′l) (n.)   A radiographic angle used in the evaluation of the degree of inclination of the pelvis. Lines are drawn on each side of the pelvis from the most prominent to the symphysis, then to the inside of the pelvis, and finally to the highest inside point of the os ischium. Inclination of the pelvis is determined by the angle formed.

Symptom (simp′tom) (n.)   Any indication of disease perceived by the patient.

Synapse (si-naps) (n.)   The functional junction between the axonal termination of one neuron (the presynaptic neuron) and the dendrites, cell body, or axon of another neuron (the postsynaptic neuron). This is the region of nerve impulse transfer between two neurons.

Synarthrodial Joint (sin″ar-thrō′de-al/joint) (n.)   Fibrous joint.

Synarthrosis (sin′ar-thrō′sis) (n.)   A form of joint in which the bones are united by fibrous tissue; the cranial sutures are one example.

Synchondrosis (sin″kon-drō′sis) (n.)   A joint in which two bones are united by hyaline cartilage. An example of this is the articulation between the ribs and sternum.

Syncytium (sin-sish′e-um) (n.)   Cells that run together anatomically or functionally, behaving as a single, multinucleated mass.

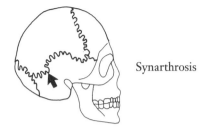

Synarthrosis

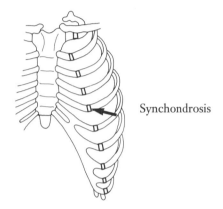

Synchondrosis

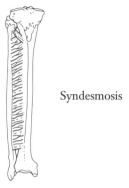

Syndesmosis

Syndrome (sin′drōm) (n.) A combination of signs and symptoms that forms a distinct clinical picture indicative of a disorder.

Synergist (sin′er-jist) (n.) 1. A muscle that helps another muscle perform its job. 2. An agent that interacts with or enhances the action of another agent.

Synostosis (sin-os-tō′sis) (n.) The joining or union of two bones by osseous material.

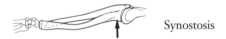

Synostosis

Synovectomy (sin-o-vek′to-mē) (n.) Excision of the synovial membrane of a joint.

Synovial (si-nō′vē-al) (adj.) 1. Of or pertaining to synovia. 2. Secreting synovial fluid.

Synovial Chondromatosis (si-nō′vē-al/kon″dro-mah-tō′sis) (n.) A rare condition in which cartilage is formed in the synovial membrane of joints, tendon sheaths, or bursae. The cartilage may become detached, producing a number of loose bodies that may or may not be radiopaque.

Synovial Cyst (si-nō′vē-al/sist) (n.) Cavities occurring near joints that are filled with synovial fluid and lined by either synovial membrane or reactive fibrous tissue that communicates with the adjacent synovial spaces.

Synovial Fluid (si-nō′vē-al/flū′id) (n.) A dialysate of plasma containing a sulfate-free mucopolysaccharide called hyaluronic acid that is secreted by the synthesizing cells of the synovium that lines joints, bursae, and tendon sheaths. Normally, this is a clear, straw-colored fluid.

Synovial Hemangioma (si-nō′vē-al/he-man″je-ō′mah) (n.) A benign, soft-tissue lesion seen mostly in children and adolescents. It most commonly occurs in the knee. Grossly, these tumors are brown and soft, with overlying villous synovium. On x-ray, a soft tissue mass may be seen in severe cases, and a periosteal reaction or lucency in the adjacent bones may be noted.

Syndactyly (sin-dak′til-ē) (n.) A congenital anomaly of the hand or foot marked by the persistence of webbing between adjacent digits. Syndactyly varies in severity from simple webbing of the skin and subcutaneous tissues to complete bony fusion of adjacent digits. Also called **Mitten-Hand** or **Sock Foot**.

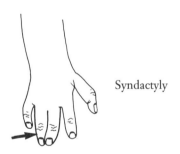

Syndactyly

Syndesmophyte (sin-des′mō-fīt) (n.) A vertically oriented calcification or ossification adjacent to a vertebra or intervertebral disk. These may bridge across adjacent vertebrae to reduce spine mobility. Their vertical orientation differentiates them from the more horizontal osteophytes seen in degenerative diseases of the spine.

Syndesmosis (sin′des-mō′sis) (n.) A joint in which the bones are united by fibrous connective tissue, forming an interosseous membrane or ligament. An example is the distal tibiofibular joint.

Synovial Fluid Findings in Normal and Diseased Joints

Parameter Evaluated	Type of Joint Fluid Examined			
	Normal	Noninflammatory	Inflammatory	Septic
Clarity	Transparent	Transparent	Translucent to opaque	Opaque
Color	Clear	Yellow	Yellow to Green	Yellow to Green
Viscosity	High	High	Low	Variable
WBC/mm^3	< 200	200–2,000	2,000–150,000	15,000–200,000
Polys	< 25%	< 25%	> 50%	> 75%
Culture	Negative	Negative	Negative	Usually positive
Protein (gm%)	< 2.5	< 2.5	> 2.5	> 2.5
Example Diseases		Deg. jt. disease, osteochondritis dissecans, early or subsiding inflammation, SLE, hypertrophic osteoarthropathy	Rheumatoid arthritis, gout, pseudogout, Reiter's syndrome, ankylosing spondylitis, rheumatic fever, arthritis, inflammatory bowel disease	Bacterial infection, acute T.B. cocci

Benson DR, et al: Synovial fluid analysis in the diagnosis of joint diseases. Contemp Orthop 3(5):430–439, 1981.

Synovial Membrane (si-nō'vē-al/mem'brān) (n.) A specially adapted, highly vascularized connective tissue lining a synovial bursa, a synovial sheath, or the capsule of a synovial joint. It secretes synovial fluid, glycoproteins, and other macromolecules for joint lubrication and nutrition. Also known as **Synovium**.

Synovial Plica (si-nō'vē-al/plī'kah) (n.) In the knee, an embryonic remnant of synovial membrane that may persist into adulthood as a partial or complete intra-articular membranous shelf. These occur most commonly in the suprapatellar, mediopatellar, and infrapatellar regions. They may cause symptoms (especially pain with activity) if they become inflamed and thickened.

Synovial Sarcoma (si-nō'vē-al/sar-kō'mah) (n.) A rare malignant neoplasm that occurs in soft tissues around joints and rarely directly involves the synovium. Histologically, these tumors usually have a biphasic pattern of pleomorphic spindle cells and columnar cells forming a glandlike space. They often show calcifications. The histogenesis of these tumors is unclear.

Synovial Sheath (si-nō'vē-al/sheath) (n.) The synovial membrane lining the cavity through which a tendon glides.

Synovial Villi (si-nō'vē-al/villē) (n.) Slender projections from the surface of the synovial membrane into the cavity of a joint.

Synovio- (si-no've-o) Prefix meaning synovial.

Synovioma (si-nō-vē-ō'ma) (n.) Any tumor, benign or malignant, whose parenchyma is composed of cells similar to those comprising the synovial membranes.

Synovitis (sīn"ō-vī'tis) (n.) A usually painful inflammation of a synovial membrane. It is characterized by swelling due to hypertrophy of the synovium and overproduction of synovial fluid.

Synovium (si-nō'vē-um) (n.) See **Synovial Membrane**.

Synthesis (sin'the-sis) (n.) The formation of a more complex substance from simpler ones.

Synthetic (sin-thet'ik) (adj.) Of or pertaining to non-biologic or man-made materials.

Syringomyelia (si-ring'go-mī-e'le-a) (n.) A chronic, slowly progressive disease of the spinal cord in which a cyst or gliosis occurs within the cord. This cavity, known as a syrinx, may be focal and round, fusiform, or linear. Neurologic damage is due to its location in the center of the cord. This affects the more central nerve traits, such as pain and temperature, but not touch and the motor nerve cells to the upper extremities. Partial sensation is therefore maintained, and there is greater motor loss in the upper extremities.

Systemic Lupus Erythematosus (sys'tē-mik/lū'pus/er"i-thēm'at'ō-sus) (n.) A chronic disease characterized by autoimmune reactions affecting the cell constituents and tissues of one or more organ systems. The varied clinical manifestations include fever; any erythematous rash, especially a butterfly rash of the face; polyarthralgia; polyarthritis; polyserositis; anemia; thrombocytopenia; and renal, neurologic, and cardiac disorders. The intensity of the disease also varies widely. The cause of SLE is unknown, although many factors, including infections and exposure to sunlight or drugs, have been associated with exacerbations of the disease. Females are affected six to eight times more commonly than males, the peak incidence occurring between the ages of 20 to 40 years. Numerous serum protein and serologic abnormalities, including a variety of auto-antibodies, may be found. The most important are the distinctive LE cell found in blood or other body fluids, the extracellular rosettes that form due to the

presence of a specific antibody, and the presence of antinuclear antibodies. Treatment depends on the severity of the illness but relies on the use of corti-costeroids, other anti-inflammatory medications, and immunosuppressive drugs. Abbreviated **SLE**.

T

T-Cane (t-kān) (n.) A cane whose handle sits at a right angle to the shaft, resembling the letter T.

T-Fracture (t-frak′chur) (n.) A descriptive term for the lines of a fracture relative to the long axis of the broken bone that form the shape of the letter T. It usually occurs near a joint, with a transverse fracture extending through the level of the bony condyles and a vertical component extending into the joint and separating the condyles. For example, it is seen at the distal aspect of the femur and humerus or the proximal end of the tibia.

T-Handle (t-hand″l) (n.) A handle attached to an instrument, such as an extractor or a reamer, that is shaped like the letter T.

Tabes Dorsalis (tā′bēz/dor-sa′lis) (n.) A slowly pro-gressive form of neurosyphilis, developing in approx-imately 5% of patients with untreated syphilis. It is characterized by a selective degeneration of the pos-terior roots of the spinal nerves and the posterior columns of the spinal cord. Symptoms usually ap-pear 5 to 20 years after the initial infection, resulting in disturbances of sensation and interference with reflexes. Synonym: **Locomotor Ataxia**.

Table Top Test (tā′b′l/top/test) (n.) A useful clin-ical guide to the timing of surgery for Dupuytren's contracture. Ask the patient to place his or her hand flat on a table top. The test is positive if the patient is unable to do this. Surgery following a positive test should prevent the progression of the deformity to uncorrectable proximal interphalangeal flexion contracture.

Tachdjian Orthosis (tahj-yun/or-thō′sis) (n.) A de-vice used for treatment of unilateral Legg-Calvé-Per-thes disease. A jointed medial steel bar connects a thigh socket to a support that prevents contact of the shoe to the ground while keeping the limb in abduc-tion and internal rotation, allowing ambulation. A lift is required under the opposite shoe. Also known as **Trilateral Socket Hip Abduction Orthosis**.

Tackler's Exostosis (tak′lerz/ek″sos-tō′sis) (n.) A bony mass resulting from traumatic myositis ossifi-cans in the lateral aspect of the midhumerus. Oc-casionally, a patient may require excision of the mass following complete maturation of the process.

Tagged Compound (tăgd/kom′pound) (n.) A com-pound to which a radioactive nuclide or other readily identifiable entity has been attached. Also known as a **Labeled Compound** or **Tracer**.

Tailor's Bottom (tāl′erz/bot′m) (n.) A common name for ischiogluteal bursitis that refers to its prev-alence in tailors owing to their professional posture.

Tailor's Bunion (tāl′erz/bun′yun) (n.) A common name for a painful area resulting from an exostosis on the lateral aspect of the head of the fifth metatar-sal, causing a bunionlike prominence with an over-lying callus bursa. Formally known as a **Bunionette**.

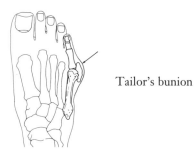

Tailor's bunion

TAL Abbreviation for Tendon Achilles Lengthening.

Talar Tilt (ta′lar/tilt) (n.) Any abnormal tilting of the superior aspect of the talus from its usually hor-izontal level with the distal tibia. It is evaluated on a mortise view or stress view of the ankle. The pres-ence of a talar tilt of more than 5 degrees indicates ligamentous injury to the ankle, or can be normal in an extremely loose-jointed patient.

Talectomy (tāl′ek-tō′mē) (n.) Surgical removal of all or part of the talus.

Talipes (tāl′i-pēz) (n.) Any congenital or acquired deformity in which the foot is twisted out of shape or position. Examples:

Talipes Arcuatus: A foot deformity in which there is an abnormal elevated arch. See **Cavus**.

Talipes Calcaneovalgus: A calcaneus deformity of the foot in which there is an increased valgus position of the heel in addition to dorsiflexion of the foot. In newborns it is usually a flexible and correctable deformity. As an ac-quired deformity associated with paralytic disorders, it appears as a flatfoot clinically and often requires surgical intervention.

Talipes Calcaneovarus: A calcaneus deformity of the foot also associated with a varus deformity of the heel. It is usually seen in association with paralytic disorders.

Talipes Calcaneus: A foot deformity in which there is ex-cessive dorsiflexion or calcaneus of the foot. It usually

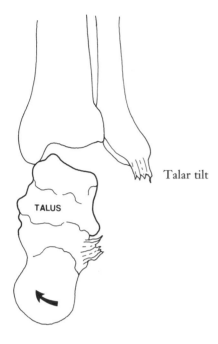

Talar tilt

TALUS

results from insufficiency or paralysis of the triceps surae muscle causing unopposed ankle dorsiflexion by intact musculature.

Talipes Equinovarus: A foot deformity in which there is excessive plantar flexion and supination of the foot and varus of the heel. More commonly known as **Clubfoot.** See **Congenital Talipes Equinovarus** or **Clubfoot.**

Talipes Equinus: Any foot deformity in which there is excessive plantarflexion of the foot, including plantarflexion of the calcaneus.

Talipes Planovalgus: A foot deformity in which there is flattening of the longitudinal arch and valgus of the heel. More commonly known as **Flatfoot.**

Talipes Plantaris: A foot deformity in which the os calcis

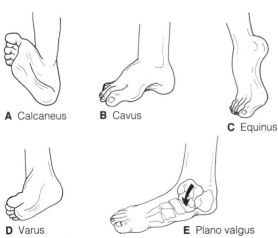

A Calcaneus   **B** Cavus   **C** Equinus

D Varus   **E** Plano valgus

Talipes. **A,** Calcaneus; **B,** Cavus; **C,** Equinus; **D,** Varus; **E,** Plano Valgus.

is parallel to the ground but the forefoot is pulled into plantarflexion by contracture of the sole fascia and musculature.

Talocalcaneal (tā″lō-kal′kā-nē′al) (adj.)   Of or pertaining to the articulation between the talus and the calcaneus.

Talocalcaneal Angle (tā″lō-kal′kā-nē′al/ang′g′l) (n.) An angle determined on an AP radiograph of the foot formed by a line passing through the long axis of the talus and a line passing parallel to the lateral border of the calcaneus. The normal angle is 20 degrees to 35 degrees. A greater angle indicates valgus of the hindfoot and a lesser angle implies varus. Also known as **Kite's Angle.**

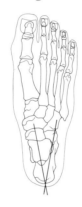

Talocalcaneal angle

Talocalcaneal Coalition (tā″lō-kal-kā-nē′-al/kō′a-lish′un) (n.)   A type of tarsal coalition in which the congenital synostoses occur between the talus and the calcaneus. Clinically, it may be associated with foot fatigue and pain. There is usually loss of the longitudinal arch and peroneal muscle spasm, but there is always decreased subtalar motion. Radiographically, the use of Harris views, or posterior superior oblique projections, is most helpful. Plain and, especially, computerized tomography or magnetic imaging is very useful in making the diagnosis.

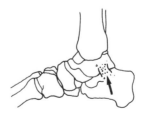

Talocalcaneal coalition

Talocrural Angle (tā″lō-krū′ral/ang′g′l) (n.)   Angle measured at the intersection of a line connecting the tips of the malleoli and another parallel to the plafond. Normally, this intersection forms an angle of approximately 13 degrees. A 2 degrees or greater difference between the talocrural angles of the patient's injured and unaffected ankle indicates that the lateral malleolus has been shortened.

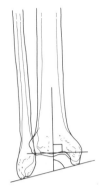

Talocrural angle

Talofibular Ligament (tā″lō-fib′u-lar/lig′ah-ment) (n.) One of two ligaments, either anterior or posterior, that provides lateral ankle stability by running from the distal fibula to insert onto the talus. Functions and is injured with the calcaneal fibular ligament.

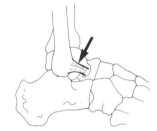

Talofibular ligament, anterior

Talometatarsal Angle (tā″-lō-met″ah-tar′sal/ang′g′l) (n.) An angle determined on an AP radiograph of the foot by a line through the longitudinal talar axis and a line passing through the long axis of the first metatarsal. The normal angle is 0 degrees to −20 degrees. Measurement in a positive direction is abnormal and indicates medial deviation of the foot. Abbreviated **TMT Angle**.

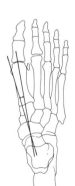

Talometatarsal angle

Talonavicular (tā″lō-nah-vik′u-lar) (adj.) Of or pertaining to the articulation between the talus and the tarsal navicular bones.

Talonavicular Ossicle (tā″lō-nah-vik′u-lar/os′sĭ-k′l) (n.) An accessory bone on the dorsum of the foot overlying the talonavicular joint.

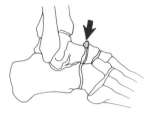

Talonavicular ossicle, dorsal

Talus (tā′lus) (n.) One of the tarsal bones consisting of a head, neck, and body. Its head articulates with the navicular and calcaneus anteriorly and inferiorly. The body forms the posterior talocalcaneal joint inferiorly and articulates with the tibia and fibula superiorly to form the ankle joint.

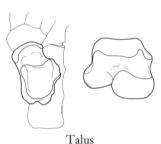

Talus

TAMBA An acronym for the talar axis, first metatarsal base angle. It is measured on a weight-bearing lateral radiograph of the foot, along with the calcaneal axis, first metatarsal base angle (CAMBA), if it is used to describe the obliquity of the talus and calcaneus.

Tandem Gait (tan′dem/gāt) (n.) A walk in which the feet advance alternately, in a straight line. The facility with which a patient can ambulate in this fashion is used as a test of coordination.

Tap (tap) (n.) 1. A tool used to cut threads for the placement of screws on the inner surface of a pilot hole. 2. The metal part of a shoe heel or tip of a sole repair.

Tape (tāp) (n.) 1. A flat, long strip of material, either natural or synthetic, used as a tie or suture. 2. Commonly used reference to adhesive tape.

Tapotement (tah-pōt-maw′) (n.) A maneuver of massage. Synonym: **Percussion**.

Tapping (tap′ing) (n.) The process of cutting threads into a pilot hole before inserting a screw. Also known as **Pretapping**.

Tapping Fracture (tap′ing/frak′chur) (n.) Any break in bone resulting from a force of dying mo-

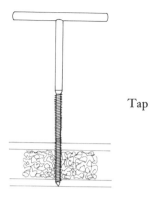

Tap

talonavicular. CT scanning and MRI have made diagnosis easier to document radiographically.

Tarsal Tunnel (tahr'sal/tun'el) (n.) The fibro-osseous passage for the posterior tibial vessels, tibial nerve, and flexor tendons formed by the flexor retinaculum and the tarsal bones.

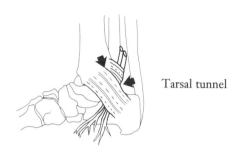

Tarsal tunnel

mentum applied over a small area. The resulting fracture line is usually transverse.

TAR Syndrome (TAR/sin'drōm) (n.) Abbreviation for **T**hrombocytopenia-**A**bsent **R**adius Syndrome. A rare congenital syndrome that combines orthopaedic and hematologic abnormalities. The most common bony abnormality is bilateral radial club hand.

TARA Acronym for Total Articular Replacement Arthroplasty, a trademark of De Puy for a surface arthoplasty system involving the proximal femur and acetabulum.

Tardy Median Nerve Palsy (tahr'dē/mn'de-an/nerv/pawl'zē) (n.) See **Carpal Tunnel Syndrome**.

Tardy Ulnar Nerve Palsy (tahr'dē/ul'nar/nerv/pawl'zē) (n.) A compression neuropathy of the ulnar nerve at the cubital tunnel. Most specifically, the term is applied to those cases of neuropathy that occur as a later sequela of trauma, for example, after a supracondylar fracture of the distal humerus.

Target-Film Distance (tahr'get/film/dis'tans) (n.) The distance between the x-ray tube anode and the x-ray film. Abbreviated **TFD**.

Target-Scan Distance (tahr'get/skan/dis'tans) (n.) The distance between a detector device (i.e., stationary camera or moving detector scanner and its crystal) and the organ being investigated by the scan after radionuclide injection.

Target-Skin Distance (tahr'get/skin/dis'tans) (n.) The distance between the x-ray tube anode and the patient's skin. It is a term used more frequently in radiation therapy than in radiography.

Tarsal (tahr'sal) (adj.) 1. Of or relating to the bones of the ankle and foot forming the tarsus. 2. Most often used to delineate the seven bones of the middle and hind foot: calcaneus, talus, navicular, three cuneiform, and cuboid bones.

Tarsal Coalition (tahr'sal/kō'a-lish-un) (n.) A failure of segmentation of two or more tarsal bones. It may be cartilaginous, fibrous, or bony. Patients may have foot pain and fatigue, peroneal muscle spasm, and decreased subtalar motion. The most common coalitions are calcaneonavicular, talocalcaneal, and

Tarsal Tunnel Syndrome (tahr'sal/tun'el/sin'drōm) (n.) An entrapment neuropathy of the posterior tibial nerve due to compression beneath the flexor retinaculum in the foot. Symptoms include pain and paresthesias and may be confined to the medial plantar nerve, the lateral plantar nerve, or the medial calcaneal nerve. Diagnosis is confirmed by electromyographic testing.

Tarsometatarsal (tahr"so-met"ah-tahr'sal) (adj.) Of or pertaining to the area between the tarsus and the metatarsals of the foot.

Tarsus (tahr'sus) (n.) The seven bones—talus, calcaneus, navicular, medial, intermediate and lateral cuneiform, and cuboid—composing the articulation between the forefoot and leg.

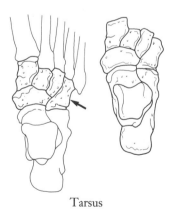

Tarsus

Taylor Spinal Brace (tā'ler/spī'nal/brās) (n.) A thoracolumbar hyperextension orthosis with two paraspinal steel bars reaching to the scapular spines. The bars' upper ends are prolonged by shoulder straps; their lower ends are attached to a pelvic band. A corset or full-front abdominal support reaching to the inguinal area and covering the lower ribs is attached to the metal frame and may come with peroneal straps. This brace tends to restrict both trunk flexion and hyperextension in the thoracolumbar area while assisting the abdominal musculature to increase intraabdominal pressure. Synonyms: **Thoracolumbar A-P Orthosis, Spinal Assistant.**

TC[99] Abbreviation for Technetium[99].

Team Nursing (tēm/ners'ing) (n.) Method of organizing nursing services within an inpatient care unit. Groups of registered nurses and auxiliary nursing personnel implement a planned program for designated patients during a shift.

Teardrop (tēr'drop) (n.) On an AP radiograph of the pelvis, the radiographic U formed by the parasagittal surface of the ilium medially and the wall of the acetabular fossa laterally and inferiorly. See **U-Figure.**

Teardrop Fracture (tēr'drop/frak'chur) (n.) A compression fracture of the anterior portion of the cervical vertebral body. The classic teardrop fracture involves the anteroinferior corner of the vertebral body in association with an acute flexion injury, as described by Schneider and Kahn: "In most cases, the fragment resembled a drop of water dripping from the vertebral body, and it has been associated with dire circumstances (paralysis) so frequently that . . . 'tear-drop' . . . seemed to describe the lesion." Currently, the term teardrop has been used indiscriminately to designate any triangular fragments or fractures of the cervical spine, thereby detracting from the precise nature of the original description.

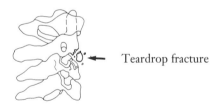

Teardrop fracture

Teardrop Sign (tēr'drop/sīn) (n.) 1. Sign composed laterally by the posterior part of the acetabular fossa

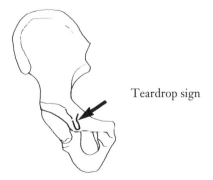

Teardrop sign

and medially by the anterior part of the quadrilateral surface of the iliac bones on the AP radiograph of the pelvis. See **Köehler's Teardrop Figure, U-Fracture.** 2. An ankle effusion, recognized on a lateral radiograph as a teardrop-shaped density displacing the normal pretalar fat pad and sometimes the posterior juxtaarticular fat pad.

Technetium [99](tek-nē'shum/99) (n.) Radionuclide used as a tracer for scanning techniques. It has a physical half-life of 6 hours.

Technetium Scan (tek-ne'shum/skan) (n.) A scintigraphic examination that uses Technetium [99]as a tracer. Commonly used in bone scanning in a chelated form with diphosphonates. Its localization in bone depends on blood flow and osteoblastic activity.

Teevan's Law (tē-vanz/law) (n.) A principle that states fractures of bone occur in the line of extension, not in the line of compression.

Telangiectasia (tel-an"je-ek-tā'ze-ah) (n.) A focal red-blue lesion created by the abnormal dilation of preexisting small vessels, characterized by a localized, dilated, cutaneous venule, capillary, or arteriole. Telangiectases range from fine, bright-red lines to heavy cords 0.5 mm in diameter. They may occur in normal skin at any age, especially in persons chronically exposed to wind and sun. Telangiectasia also may occur in association with a variety of systemic disorders.

Telangiectatic Osteosarcoma (tel-an"je-ek-tat'ik/os" te-ō-sar-kō'mah) (n.) A type of osteosarcoma characterized histologically by dilated vascular channels lined by multinucleated giant cells, a sarcomatous stroma, and bone formation. Radiologically, these tumors appear as large lytic defects.

Teleoroentgenogram (tel"e-ō-rent-gen'ō-gram) (n.) A radiographic technique to determine leg lengths in which the entire length of both limbs is exposed on one film. This technique has the disadvantages of magnification and inconvenience owing to the large film necessary.

Telfa Dressing (tel-fah/dres'ing) (n.) A proprietary, sterile, nonadherent wound dressing.

Telophase (tel'o-fāz) (n.) The final phase of mitosis or meiosis, during which chromosomes become diffuse, nuclear membrane reforms, and nucleoli begin to appear in the daughter nuclei.

Template (tem'plāt) (n.) 1. A pattern or mold guiding the formation of a duplicate. 2. An outline used to trace bones in order to standardize its form.

Temporal Arteritis (tem'po-ral/ar"te-rī'tis) (n.) An inflammatory and granulomatous disease of elderly persons, largely involving the carotid arterial system and temporal arteries. It is marked by headache, constitutional symptoms, and ocular involvement. Histologically, it is characterized by focal necrosis of the arterial wall and granulomas containing many giant cells. It is treated with steroids; it can be fatal. Synonyms: **Cranial Arteritis, Giant Cell Arteritis.**

Temporary Prosthesis (tem-po-ra′rē/pros-thē′sis) (n.) A device used to assess an amputee's physical and psychologic ability to accept an artificial limb to help accustom the patient to a prosthesis and to hasten the shrinkage of the stump that must precede the choosing of a permanent prosthesis.

Temporomandibular Joint Syndrome (tem″po-rō-man-dib′ū-lar/sin′drōm) (n.) A pain–dysfunction phenomenon, characterized by severe to excruciating pain in the temporomandibular joint and craniofacial–cervical areas; frequently associated with clicking, popping, tinnitus, vertigo, headache, and neck pain. Treated by balancing the bite or bite plates. Described by Dr. N. A. Shore.

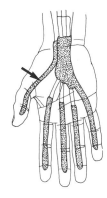

Tendon sheath

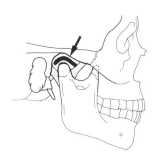

Temporomandibular joint

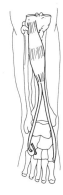

Tendon transfer

Tender Points (ten′der/pointz) (n.) Discretely palpable areas in muscle or soft tissue that respond to stimulation with local pain, brief local or general contraction of muscle (jump response), involuntary starting or wincing by the subject (jump sign), or pain surrounding the point of palpation (trigger point).

Tendinitis (ten″di-nī′tis) (n.) See **Tendonitis**.

Tendo (ten′do) Prefix meaning tendon.

Tendon (ten′dun) (n.) A band of dense fibrous tissue that forms the termination of a muscle and attaches it to a bone. When the muscle contracts, it pulls on the tendon, which moves the bone.

Tendon Organ (ten′dun/or′gan) (n.) A sensory receptor found within a tendon that responds to the tendon's movements and relays impulses to the central nervous system. Tendon organs are part of the proprioceptor system. Synonym: **Golgi Tendon Organ**.

Tendon Reflex (ten′dun/rē′fleks) (n.) Contraction of a muscle following its sudden stretching that is elicited by tapping against its tendon. See **Deep Tendon Reflex**, **Stretch Reflex**.

Tendon Sheath (ten′dun/shēth) (n.) The synovial cover surrounding a tendon; it provides increased lubrication.

Tendon Transfer (ten′dun/trans′fer) (n.) Any surgical procedure used to restore function and reestablish strength and balance in an extremity by transferring the insertion of a functioning musculo-

tendinous unit to substitute for a nonfunctioning unit.

Tendonitis (ten″do-nī′tis) (n.) Inflammation of a tendon, usually at the point of its attachment to bone. Sometimes spelled **Tendinitis**.

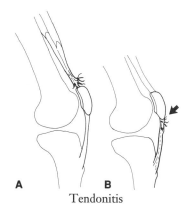

A   **B**

Tendonitis

Tendovaginal (ten″dō-vaj′i-nal) (adj.) Pertaining to a tendon and its sheath.

Tendovaginitis (ten″dō-vaj″i-nī′tis) (n.) Inflammatory thickening of the fibrous synovial sheath containing one or more tendons. Synonyms: **Tenovaginitis** or **Tenosynovitis**.

Tenectomy (te-nek′tō-mē) (n.) Excision of a lesion of a tendon or its sheath, or both.

Tennis Elbow (ten′is/el′bō) (n.) A common name for lateral epicondylitis at the distal humerus, a disorder prevalent in tennis players. Clinically, patients complain of pain over the lateral aspect of the elbow. This is associated with point tenderness over the lateral epicondyle and exacerbation of pain with resisted wrist extension and forearm supination. See **Lateral Epicondylitis**.

Tennis Leg (ten′is/leg) (n.) A common name for injuries of the medial head of the gastrocnemius muscle near its musculotendinous junction, including strain and partial or complete tearing of the muscle belly. It is usually caused by overstretching of the muscle by sudden knee extension and ankle dorsiflexion (i.e., going in for a drop shot near the net), often associated with underlying muscle fatigue and/or degenerative changes. Pain is often acute and sharp, giving the patient the sensation that he or she has been "shot in the calf." The area becomes swollen, tender, and ecchymotic. Conservative, symptomatic treatment is usually effective. Important to differentiate from a torn Achilles tendon. It also may be a tear of the plantaris muscle.

Tennis Shoulder (ten′is/shōl′der) (n.) See **Impingement Syndrome**.

Tennis Toe (ten′is/toe) (n.) See **Jogger's Toe**.

Tenodesis (ten-od′e-sis) (n.) Suture of a tendon to a bone or another tendon or shortening the excursion of a tendon.

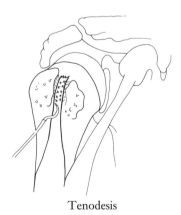

Tenodesis

Tenolysis (ten-ol′i-sis) (n.) The surgical release of a tendon from adhesions. Also called **Tendolysis**.

Tenomyotomy (ten″o-mī-ot′ō-mē) (n.) Surgical division of tendons and muscles.

Tenoplasty (ten′ō-plas″tē) (n.) Surgical repair of a ruptured or severed tendon.

Tenoreceptor (ten″ō-rē-sep′tor) (n.) A nerve receptor in a tendon.

Tenorrhaphy (ten-or′ah-fē) (n.) The suture of a divided tendon.

Tenostosis (ten-os-tō′sis) (n.) Ossification of a tendon.

Tenosynovectomy (ten″o-sin″o-vek′tō-mē) (n.) Excision or resection of a tendon sheath and synovium surrounding a tendon.

Tenosynovial (ten″o-sin″o-vi′al) (adj.) Of or relating to a tendon and its synovial covering.

Tenosynovitis (ten″ō-sīn″ō-vī′tis) (n.) Inflammation of a tendon and/or its sheath, producing pain and swelling. It may be associated with crepitus on movement.

Tenotomy (ten-ot′ō-mē) (n.) Surgical transection of a tendon. Example: Origin of the **Adductor Brevis Muscle**.

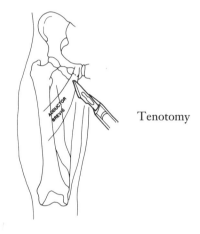

Tenotomy

Tenovaginitis (ten″ō-vaj″i-nī′tis) (n.) See **Tendovaginitis**.

TENS Abbreviation for transcutaneous electric nerve stimulation.

Tensconer (ten′-skō-ner) (n.) A device used to pretension plates and compress bone ends in the internal fixation of bone. The device is attached by a cortical screw to bone, then by a hook into a slot in the plate that is being applied. The tension device is re-

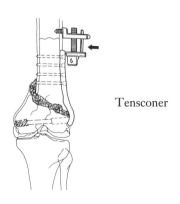

Tensconer

moved after the plate is secured. Also known as **Tension Device**.

Tensor Fascia Lata Muscle (ten′sar/fash′e-ah/la′ta/mus′el) (n.) See **Muscle**.

Tensile Strength (ten′sīl/strenth) (n.) A measurement of the amount of stress required to cause a given material to fail.

Tensilon Test (ten′sil-on/test) (n.) A provocative pharmacologic test for myasthenia gravis. See **Neostigmine Test**.

Tension (ten′shun) (n.) A force that tends to elongate the fibers of a material. The unit of measure is newtons (pound force).

Tension Band Fixation (ten′shun/band/fik-sā′shun) (n.) A principle of mechanics that has been applied to the internal fixation of fractures. The intent is that the implant absorb tension and that the bone absorb compression when loaded. This results in interfragmentary compression that is dynamically increased with loading.

Tension Band Plate (ten′shun/band/plāt) (n.) The application of the tension band principle to bone fixation using a plate applied to the tension side of a bone.

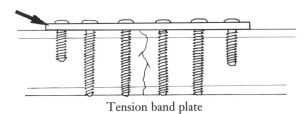

Tension band plate

Tension Band Wire (ten′shun/band/wīr) (n.) The use of wires to apply the tension band principle to bone fixation. This results in dynamic compression. For example, in the tension band wiring of a transverse patella fracture, the circular wire is inserted over the front of the patella, through the quadriceps

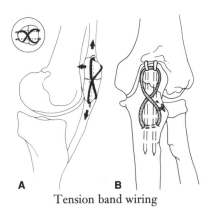

A   B
Tension band wiring

and patellar tendons very close to the bone. With active motion, the wire absorbs all the tensile forces and the bone absorbs pure compressive stresses.

Tension Device (ten′shun/dĕ-vīs) (n.) See **Tensioner**.

Tension Fracture (ten′shun/frak′chur) (n.) A fracture that occurs when bone fibers fail at right angles to the direction of the tensile force applied, resulting in a transverse fracture. Also known as **Traction Fracture**.

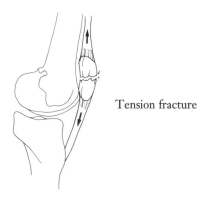

Tension fracture

Tensor (ten′sor) (n.) Any muscle that causes stretching or tensing of a body part. Example: **Tensor Fascia Lata Muscle**.

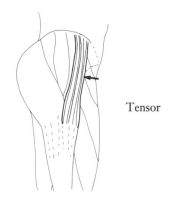

Tensor

Teres Major Muscle (te′rēz/mā′jor/mus′el) (n.) See **Muscle**.

Teres Minor Muscle (te′rēz/mī′ner/mus′el) (n.) See **Muscle**.

Terminal Device (ter′mi-nal/de-vīs′) (n.) The hook or artificial hand on the end of an upper extremity prosthesis.

Terminal Disinfection (ter′mi-nal/dis″in-fek′shun) (n.) The process of disinfection of a patient's environment and belongings after his or her illness is no longer communicable.

Terry Thomas Sign (ter-ē′/tom-as/sīn) (n.) An excessive scapholunate gap, suggestive of rotary sub-luxation of the scaphoid, secondary to rupture of the scapholunate ligaments. Frankel calls it the "Terry Thomas sign," after the dental diastema of the British comedian. It may be seen on standard AP roentgenograms of the hand. Dynamic views, including supination and radial and ulnar deviation views, and a clenched-fist view may be necessary to obviate the diastasis.

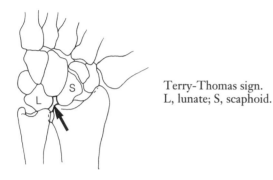

Terry-Thomas sign.
L, lunate; S, scaphoid.

Tertiary Care (ter′shē-er-ē/kār) (n.)   Highly specialized medical and surgical care for unusual and complex medical problems. The patients given this care have been referred for clarification of diagnosis and/or treatment by a primary or secondary care giver.

Testut's Ligament (tes-tūz/lig′ah-ment) (n.)   Eponym for the volar radioscapholunate ligament of the wrist.

Tetanus (tet′ah-nus) (n.)   1. An acute and potentially fatal infectious disease caused by the toxin of the anerobic organism *Clostridium tetani*. It affects the nervous system and is characterized by local convulsive spasm of the voluntary muscles and a tendency toward episodes of respiratory arrest. It may occur as a complication in lacerations, open fractures, burns, and abrasions. 2. A single smooth response to repeated stimuli of a certain critical frequency. This phenomenon allows motions to occur smoothly and not in jerky fashion.

Tetany (tet′ah-nē) (n.)   Continuous and sustained tonic spasm of a muscle.

Tethered Cord Syndrome (teth′er′d/kord/sin′drōm) (n.)   A progressive, often asymmetric, neurologic deficit of the lower extremities seen in a growing child with spinal dysraphism. In these patients, the spinal cord or filum terminale is transfixed by an osseous or fibrocartilaginous septum, and thus excessive traction is placed on it during growth. Also known as **Filum Terminale Syndrome** or **Cord-Traction Syndrome**.

Tetracycline (tet″rah-sī′klēn) (n.)   An antibiotic with a broad spectrum of activity against many gram-positive and gram-negative organisms as well as my-coplasma, Rickettsia, and Chlamydia. Available in oral and parenteral forms.

Tetracycline Labeling (tet″rah-si′klēn/lā′bel-ing) (n.)   A technique of labeling active surfaces of bone with the antibiotic tetracycline. Owing to its autofluorescence, the labeled areas can be studied by fluorescence microscopy. This technique is used in the histomorphometric analysis of bone.

Tetraplegia (tet″rah-plē′je-ah) (n.)   See **Quadriplegia**.

Tevdek (tev′dek) (n.)   A brand name of a commercially available nonabsorbable suture material.

TFD   Abbreviation for Target-film distance.

THA   Abbreviation for Total Hip Arthroplasty.

Thalassemia (thal″ah-sē′mē-ah) (n.)   One of the hemoglobinopathies. It is a hereditary disease characterized by a defect in hemoglobin synthesis causing the formation of morphologically altered erythrocytes that are destroyed at an abnormally rapid rate. Severity of the disease varies from asymptomatic with mild anemia, thalassemia minor, to extremely severe thalassemia major. Moderate to severe cases feature pallor, mild icterus, progressive splenomegaly, mongoloid facies, and growth retardation. Radiologic changes, secondary to marked hyperplasia of the bone marrow, include coarse trabecular patterns in bones of the extremities and vertebrae and striations in the calvarium, giving a characteristic hair-on-end appearance. It is most frequently seen in individuals of Northern Mediterranean extraction.

Thalidomide (tha-lid′ō-mīd) (n.)   A teratogenic drug that causes phocomelia if ingested during early pregnancy.

Thanatophoric Dwarfism (than″ah-tō-fōr′ik/dwarf′izm) (n.)   A lethal short-limbed, disproportionate dwarfism, clinically apparent at birth.

THARIES   Abbreviation for Total Hip Articular Replacement by Internal Eccentric Shells; used by the UCLA group to describe its surface replacement arthroplasty system. The prosthesis is seldom used.

Theater Sign (thē-ah-ter/sīn) (n.)   A descriptive term for a complaint of patients with chondromalacia patella. They describe dull, aching, anterior knee pain, especially after sitting in one position for a prolonged period, such as occurs at a movie theater.

Theca (thē′kah) (n.)   A tissue sheath or covering. Usually associated with the brain and the spinal cord.

Thecal Sac (thē′kal/sak) (n.)   A common name for the space surrounded by the theca vertebralis or dura mater.

Thenar (thē′nar) (adj.)   1. Of or pertaining to the thenar eminence of the thumb. 2. The muscles that particularly control the thumb, found on the palmar side of the first metacarpal of the hand.

Thenar Abscess (thē′nar/ab′ses) (n.)   A deep palmar space abscess occurring in the thenar space.

Thenar Eminence (thē'nar/em'i-nens) (n.)   The prominent fleshy area of the palm of the hand, overlying the first metacarpal, whose bulk is formed by the thenar muscles.

Thenar Flap (thē'nar/flap) (n.)   A type of local coverage procedure for fingertip amputations that require replacement of both deeper tissues and skin to cover exposed bone. This procedure requires two stages and a split-thickness skin graft to the donor site on the thenar eminence.

Thenar Muscles (thē'nar/mus'els) (n.)   The intrinsic muscles of the thumb that give prominence to the thenar eminence. They are the abductor pollicis brevis, the opponens pollicis, and the flexor pollicis brevis muscles. See **Muscles**.

Thenar Space (thē'nar/spās) (n.)   A potential space in the palm of the hand that lies on the radial side of the septum to the third metacarpal. It contains the radial bursa, flexor pollicis longus tendon, lumbrical muscle to the index finger, thenar muscles, and adductor pollicis muscle.

Theory (the'o-rē) (n.)   A formulated scientific statement based on experiments that verify a hypothesis.

Therapeutic Exercise (ther″ah-pū'tik/ek'ser-sīz) (n.)   A bodily movement to correct an impairment, improve musculoskeletal function, or maintain a state of well-being.

Therapeutic Index (ther″ah-pu'tik/in'deks) (n.)   The ratio of the toxic dose of a substance to its therapeutic dose. It is intended to serve as an estimate of the safety of a drug.

Thermocautery (ther″mō-kaw'ter-e) (n.)   Cauterization by a heated wire or point.

Thermocoagulation (ther″mo-kō-ag″u-lā'shun) (n.)   Coagulation of tissue by means of high-frequency currents.

Thermography (ther-mog'rah-fē) (n.)   The technique of measuring variations in the body's radiant heat-emission patterns and transferring them into electronic signals and color, which can then be visualized, computer-analyzed, and recorded photographically. The resulting picture is a thermogram and is examined for abnormalities in the normally symmetrical radiant-heat-emission pattern.

Thermoplastics (ther″mō-plas'tiks) (n.)   Plastics that will soften repeatedly at high temperatures, then re-harden at lower temperatures.

Thick-Split Graft (thik-split/graft) (n.)   See **Split-Thickness Graft**.

Thiersch Skin Graft (tēr'sh/skin/graft) (n.)   A medium split-thickness skin graft (0.012 to 0.015 inches in thickness).

Thigh (thī) (n.)   Familiar name for the proximal part of the lower extremity between the hip and the knee.

Thigh-Foot Angle (thī-foot/ang'g'l) (n.)   A measurement used in the evaluation of tibial torsion. Place the prone child's knees together and flex them to 90

degrees; gently place the foot at a right angle to the tibia. The angle between the thigh and the long axis of the foot indicates the degree of tibial torsion. Normally, this measures 0 degrees to +15 degrees. A negative angle means there is internal tibial torsion.

Third-Degree Sprain (therd-de'grē'/sprān) (n.)   The most severe degree of ligamentous injury in which there is a complete disruption with resultant instability. See **Sprain**.

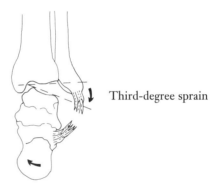

Third-degree sprain

Third Space (therd/spās) (n.)   A term to indicate the extracellular and extravascular spaces of the body where extravasated fluid collects.

Thomas Collar (tom'as/col'er) (n.)   An eponym used for a variety of semirigid cervical collars. The original, described by Hugh Owens Thomas, was made of sheet metal covered with felt and sheepskin. The metal, whose edges were flared, reached from the chin to the sternum anteriorly and from the base of the neck to the occiput posteriorly, encircling the neck. Today, a thick plastic sheet usually replaces the metal. "Ready-made" collars are supplied in different sizes or are adjustable.

Thomas Heel (tom'as/hēl) (n.)   A medially extended, corrective heel. Unlike a normal heel, whose front surface is slightly concave and runs transversely across the sole, the medial part of a Thomas heel's breastline is extended forward at least 1 inch (2.5 cm). This causes the front of the heel to lie under the navicular bone, giving support to the medial longitudinal arch. Synonym: **Orthopaedic Heel**.

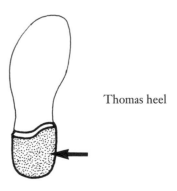

Thomas heel

Thomas Position (tom′as/pō-zish′un) (n.) 1. A supine position in which one lower limb is in complete extension and the other is flexed at the hip and the knee, with the thigh pressed against the trunk. This position is used in the Thomas test and for stretching tight hip flexors. 2. A supine position in which both lower limbs are flexed with the hips and knees at right angles and the legs resting on a stool or other support. This position is used for muscle relaxation, especially of the lower back, and for pelvic traction.

Thomas Splint (tom′as/splint) (n.) A knee-ankle-foot orthosis consisting of two straight steel bars, connected distally by a crossbar beyond the foot and proximally by a padded ring fitting tightly to the perineum and ischium. It is used for emergency splinting, transportation, and traction in acute fractures of the thigh or leg. Its side-bars are of unequal length, and the padded ring is set at an angle of 120 degrees to the inner bar. The half-ring Thomas splint is most commonly used, and a variety of sizes and lengths are available.

Thomas Test (tom′as/test) (n.) A method to assess flexion contracture of the hip. With the patient supine, completely flex the limb not being tested until the knee touches the chest, the lumbar spine is flattened, and the pelvis is rotated. Measure the angle of the tested hip relative to the table to determine the degree of flexion deformity.

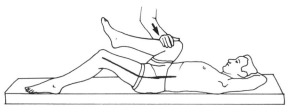

Thomas test

Thompson Hip Endoprosthesis (tom′son/hip/en″do-pros-thē′sis) (n.) A metallic femoral head endoprosthesis used in the treatment of subcapital hip fractures. It closely approximates the normal femoral head and neck in design and is available in different head diameters. Also called the **F.R. Thompson Femoral Head Prosthesis**.

Thompson Squeeze Test (tom′son/skwēz/test) (n.) A method to assess continuity of the Achilles tendon. In suspected rupture of the Achilles tendon, place the patient prone, with his or her feet hanging over the edge of the table. Squeeze the calf musculature of the leg just below its widest part. Normally, this causes plantar flexion of the foot. If the Achilles tendon is ruptured, the foot will not plantarflex. Also called **Simmond's Sign**.

Thomsen's Disease (tom′sens/di-zēz′) (n.) **Myotonia Congenita**.

Thoracic (tho-ras′ik) (adj.) Of or pertaining to the chest or midback.

Thoracic Curve (tho-ras′ik/kurv) (n.) Any spinal curvature in which the apex of the curvature is between T2 and T11. Most commonly used to describe a lateral thoracic or scoliosis curve.

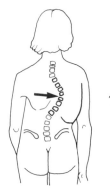

Thoracic curve

Thoracic Outlet Syndrome (tho-ras′ik/owt′let/sin′drōm) (n.) A syndrome caused by lesions that reduce the cervicothoracic outlet aperture and cause symptoms due to compression of the brachial plexus or the subclavian artery or vein at the base of the neck. Symptoms are varied and may include radicular pain, paresthesias, muscular atrophy, hypothermia, pallor, and venous distention. The etiology is also varied, including cervical ribs, hypertrophic scalenus anticus muscle, spasm of scalenus medius muscle, and many others. Treatment depends on the patient's symptoms and the underlying cause. Also known as **Neurovascular Compression Syndrome**.

Thoracic Pelvic Phalangeal Dystrophy (tho-ras′ik/pel′vik/fah-lan′jē-al/dis′trō-fē) (n.) See **Jeume Syndrome**.

Thoracic Scoliosis (tho-ras′ik/skō″lē-ō′sis) (n.) A lateral curvature of the spine with an apex T2 to T11.

Thoracic Vertebra (tho-ras′ik/ver′te-brah) (n.) Any of the 12 bony elements of the spine between the cervical and the lumbar regions, numbered 1 through 12. Also called **Dorsal Vertebra**.

Thoracogenic Scoliosis (tho-rak′-ō-jenik/skō″le-ō′sis) (n.) A lateral spinal curvature secondary to disease or operative trauma in or on the thoracic cage.

Thoracolumbar Curve (tho″rak′-ō-lum′bar/kurv) (n.) Any spinal curvature that has its apex at T12 or L1.

Thoracolumbosacral Orthosis (tho″rah-ko-lum′bo-sa′kral/or-tho′sis) (n.) A type of appliance or brace incorporating the thoracic and lumbar spine. Abbreviated **TLSO**.

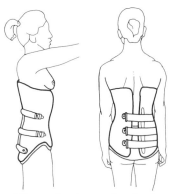

Thoracolumbosacral orthosis

Thoracotomy (tho″rah-kot′ō-me) (n.) Any surgical procedure that involves cutting through the thorax or chest wall.

THR Abbreviation for Total Hip Replacement.

Thread (thred) (n.) The spiraling, nearly transverse extensions of a screw that gain purchase in bone. The diameter of the thread defines the diameter of the screw.

Three-Column Spine Concept (thrē-kolum-spīn-kon′-sept) (n.) The concept that introduced the middle column as a key to spinal stability. It is composed of the posterior vertebral body, the posterior annulus fibrosus, and the posterior longitudinal ligament. The anterior column is composed of the anterior vertebral body, the anterior annulus fibrosus, and the anterior longitudinal ligament. The posterior column includes the supraspinous ligament, the interspinous ligament, the ligamentum flavum, and the posterior joint capsules as well as the bony arch. Loss of stability is based on the loss of one, two, or three columns, inducing progressively greater instabilities. The main nuance resides in the preservation of one of the columns as a hinge or stabilizer, particularly the anterior or middle columns. Potential for neurologic loss occurs as a failure of either the middle column under axial load (burst fracture) or all three columns in the fracture dislocation. Described by Francis Denis.

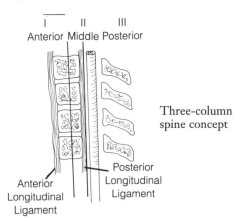

Three-column spine concept

Three-Legged Cane (thrē-leg′ed/kān) (n.) A cane with three relatively long tips.

Three-Point Cane (thre-point/kān) (n.) A cane with three tips. Synonym: **Tripod Cane**.

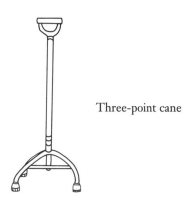

Three-point cane

Three-Point Gait (thrē-point/gāt) (n.) A walk in which two crutches or one cane and the affected leg advance together, followed by the unaffected leg.

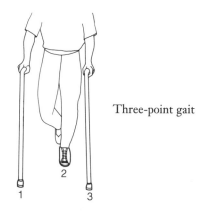

Three-point gait

Threshold (thresh′hōld) (n.) Minimum intensity of a stimulus that causes a given structure to respond.

Throat (thrōt) (n.) In shoe terminology, the entrance for the foot into the shoe, usually at the waist or where the vamp and quarters meet at the base of the tongue.

Throckmorton's Sign (throk′mortons/sin) (n.) A facetious sign in which it is said that when a penis is seen on an AP radiograph of the pelvis, it points to the side of the lesion.

Thrombin (throm′bin) (n.) An enzyme resulting from activation of prothrombin that catalyzes the conversion of fibrinogen to fibrin.

Thromboangiitis Obliterans (throm″bō-an″je-ī′tis/ob-lit″er-ans) (n.) A segmental, inflammatory obliterative disease affecting primarily small and medium-sized arteries and veins in the extremities. It results in vascular claudication and ischemia. Also known as **Buerger's Disease**.

Thrombocytes (throm'bo-sītz) (n.) Platelets, originating from megakaryocytes located primarily in bone marrow. Their components are necessary for the normal process of blood coagulation and clot retraction. The normal quantity in peripheral blood ranges from 200,000 to 400,000/mm.

Thrombocytopenia (throm″bo-sī″to-pē'ne-ah) (n.) A decrease in the number of platelets in the circulating blood.

Thromboembolism (throm″bo-em'bo-lizm) (n.) The condition in which a blood clot, i.e., a thrombus, formed in one area becomes detached and lodges in another.

Thromboendarterectomy (throm″bo-end″ar-ter-ek'to-mē) (n.) Procedure in which an incision is made into an obstructed artery, and the thrombus, intima, any atheromatous plaques, the internal elastic lamina, and the inner part of the tunica media are removed.

Thrombogenesis (throm″bo-jen'e-sis) (n.) Formation of a clot.

Thrombokinase (throm″bo-kin'ās) (n.) An enzyme released from platelets during clotting that converts prothrombin into thrombin in the presence of calcium ions. Synonym: **Thromboplastin**.

Thrombolysis (throm″bol'ī-sis) (n.) Dissolution of a thrombus.

Thrombophlebitis (throm″bo-fle-bī'tis) (n.) Inflammation of a vein. This inflammation may be associated with venous thrombus formation.

Thromboplastin (throm″bo-plas'tin) (n.) See **Thrombokinase**.

Thrombosis (throm-bo'sis) (n.) The formation of a blood clot, i.e., a thrombus, in the intact cardiovascular system.

Thrombostat (throm-bo'stat) (n.) An enzyme preparation, extracted from dried beef blood, that unites with fibrinogen to accelerate the coagulation of blood and contain capillary bleeding. Supplied as a powder, it may be applied on the surface of bleeding tissue in either solution or powder form. Marketed under the name Thrombin, USP.

Thrombus (throm'bus) (n.) A blood clot within a vessel.

Thrust (thrust) (v.) 1. A force to move an object in any direction. (n.) 2. An abnormal medial or lateral movement of the knee during gait. It may be seen in association with advanced degenerative joint disease of the knee or in poorly aligned lower extremity prostheses.

Thumb (thum) (n.) Common name for the first digit of the hand.

Thumb-In-Palm Deformity (thum-in-palm/de-for'mi-tē) (n.) A descriptive term for an adduction-contraction of the thumb. It blocks entry of objects into the palm and prevents the thumb from assisting the fingers in grasp or pinch. Frequently found in patients with cerebral palsy or following a stroke. Synonym: **Adducted Thumb**, **Clutched Thumb Deformity**.

Thumb Spica Cast (thum/spi'kah/kast) (n.) A type of cast, splint, or orthotic device that encircles and immobilizes the thumb in addition to the wrist.

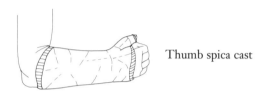

Thumb spica cast

Thurston Holland Fragment (thur'-ston/hol'-and/frag'ment) (n.) On radiograph the triangular metaphyseal fragment of the bone that remains attached to the epiphysis in a Salter-Harris type II fracture of the epiphyseal plate. See **Salter Classification**.

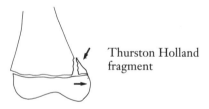

Thurston Holland fragment

Thymidine (thī'mid-en) (n.) A nucleotide of DNA.

Thymine (thī'min) (n.) A pyrimidine component of nucleotides and nucleic acids.

TIA Abbreviation for Transient Ischemic Attacks.

Tibia (tib'ē-ah) (n.) The medial and larger bone of the lower leg, commonly called the shin bone. It articulates with the femur superiorly, with the talus inferiorly, and the fibula laterally at both its proximal and distal aspects.

Tibia Vara (tib'ē-ah/vā'ra) (n.) See **Blount's Disease**.

Tibial Collateral Ligament (tibē-al/ko-lat'er-al/lig'ah-ment) (n.) The ligament that connects the medial side of the tibia to the femur. Consists of a superficial and deep portion. See **Collateral Ligament**.

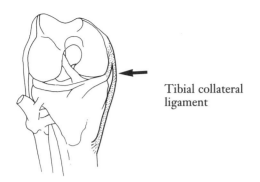

Tibial collateral ligament

Tibial Condyle (tib′ē-al/kon′dīl) (n.)   See **Tibial Plateau**.

Tibial Eminence (tib′ē-al/em′i-nens) (n.)   An elevated area on the superior surface of the proximal tibia found between the medial and lateral articular facets. The **intercondylar eminences**, or **tibial spines**, mark its medial and lateral extents.

Tibial Plateau (tib′e-al/plah-to′) (n.)   The flattened, most proximal part of the tibia. The medial or lateral buttress of the proximal aspect of the tibia that supports the superior articular surface that is widened to receive the femoral condyles. Synonym: **Tibial Condyle**.

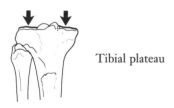

Tibial plateau

Tibial Plateau Fracture (tib′ē-al/plah-tō′/frak′chur) (n.)   Any fracture through the medial and/or lateral tibal plateau. Also called **Bumper Fracture**.

Tibial Spine Fracture (tib′ē-al/spīn/frak′chur) (n.)   Any fracture through the tibial eminence or tibial spines.

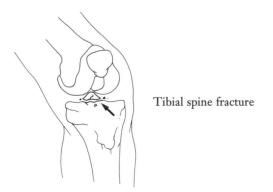

Tibial spine fracture

Tibial Spines (tib′ē-al/spīnz) (n.)   The two bony projections on the proximal aspect of the tibia that border the intercondylar eminence medially and laterally. Also known as **Intercondylar Eminences**.

Tibial Tray (tib′ē-al/trā) (n.)   The flat, metallic, tibial resurfacing component of a total knee prosthesis.

Tibial Tuberosity (tib′ē-al/tū″be-ros′i-tē) (n.)   A bony projection on the anterior aspect of the proximal tibia to which the patellar tendon attaches.

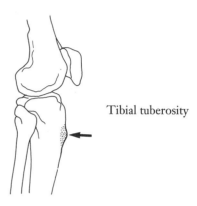

Tibial tuberosity

Tibialis Anterior Muscle (tib″ē-a′lis/an-ter′ē-or/mus′el) (n.)   See **Muscle**.

Tibialis Posterior Muscle (tib″ē-a′lis/pos-tēr′ē-or/mus′el) (n.)   See **Muscle**.

Tibiofibular (tib″ē-ō-fib′ū-lar) (adj.)   Of or pertaining to the tibia and fibula.

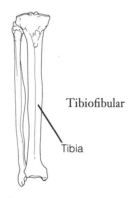

Tibiofibular

Tibia

Tibiofibular Ligament (tib″ē-ōfib′ūlar/lig′ah-ment) (n.)   Ligaments connecting the tibia to the fibula at either end of the bones.

TID   Abbreviation for the Latin ter in dié, 3 times a day.

Tidemark (tīd′mark) (n.)   In the structure of hyaline, articular cartilage, the demarcation between the deep vertical zone and the zone of calcified cartilage. It appears as an undulating line on light microscopy.

Tidy Hand Injury (ti′dē/hand/in′ju-rē) (n.)   A hand

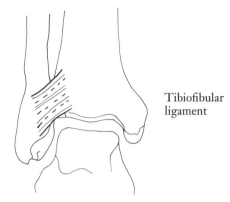

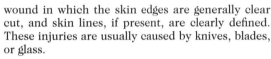

Tibiofibular ligament

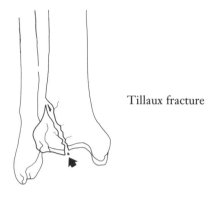

Tillaux fracture

wound in which the skin edges are generally clear cut, and skin lines, if present, are clearly defined. These injuries are usually caused by knives, blades, or glass.

Tie (tī) (n.) Colloquial term for suture material used to occlude the lumen of a blood vessel. A free tie is a single strand of suture. A strand attached to a needle before use is referred to as a stick tie or suture/ligature. The needle is used to anchor the strand in tissue before occluding a deep or large vessel. Synonym: **Ligature**.

Tietze's Syndrome (tēt'sez/sin'drōm) (n.) A benign inflammation of the costal cartilage. Symptoms include pain in one or more costal cartilages, enhanced by motion, coughing, and sneezing. The pain may radiate to the neck, the shoulder, and the arm. On examination, there may be swelling of the affected costal cartilage and tenderness and mild hyperemia of the overlying skin. The second rib is most frequently affected. Also known as **Costochondritis** and **Chondropathia Tuberosa**.

Tikhoff-Linberg Procedure (tik-hōf/lin-berg/pro-sē'jur) (n.) A surgical technique for resection of the shoulder girdle (including the scapula, the humerus, and the clavicle) with preservation of the distal aspect of the upper extremity.

Tillaux Fracture (tē-yōz'/frak'chur) (n.) An avulsion fracture of the anterolateral articular surface of the distal tibia due to the pull of the anterior tibiofibular ligament. The mechanism of injury is forced external rotation of the foot. Also known as **Fracture of Kleiger**.

   Adult Tillaux Fracture (ah-dult/tē-yōz'/frak'chur) (n.) A Tillaux fracture occurring in a skeletally mature patient.

   Juvenile Tillaux Fracture (jū've-nīl/tē-yōz'/frak'chur) (n.) A Tillaux fracture occurring in a skeletally immature patient. This is a physeal injury, classified as **Salter-Harris type III**.

Tillman Hip Resurfacing Prosthesis (til-man/hip/rē-ser'-fa-sing/pros-thē'sis) (n.) A cemented cobalt-chromium alloy-UHMW polyethylene replacement for the articulating surfaces of the hip joint.

Tilt Table (tilt/tā'b'l) (n.) A table used for the rehabilitation of a patient who has been recumbent for a prolonged period and must be brought to an upright position progressively. A mechanism allows the table to tilt gradually toward the vertical. Transfer the patient from bed to litter, then strap him or her to the tilt table. Tilt the table gradually toward the vertical, allowing the patient to become adjusted to an increasingly upright position. This procedure decreases the problem of syncopal episodes from postural hypotension caused by abrupt assumption of the vertical position.

Time to Walk 50 Feet (tīm/to/wok/50/fēt) (n.) A clinical measurement of neuromuscular and articular function of the lower back and lower extremities. Any disturbance of function will increase the time required to traverse a 50-foot distance. The test may be employed to serially evaluate improvement or worsening due to disease but is highly dependent on patient cooperation. Note whether aids or devices are used.

Tincture (tink'tūr) (n.) An alcoholic or hydroalcoholic solution prepared from an animal, vegetable, or chemical substance.

Tine Test (tīn/test) (n.) A skin test for tuberculosis, using a multiple-puncture, disposable device. Results are reported within 48 to 72 hours.

Tinea (tin'ē-ah) (n.) A fungus infection of the skin. The specific type, depending on characteristic appearance, etiologic agent, and site is usually designated by a modifying term. For example, **Tinea pedis**, more commonly known as athlete's foot. Also known as **Ringworm**.

Tinel Sign (tin-el/sīn) (n.) 1. A test used to assess and diagnose nerve injury. It indicates the presence of axons in the process of regeneration. It is elicited by gentle percussion by a finger or percussion hammer along the course of an injured nerve. A transient tingling sensation is experienced by the patient in the distribution of the injured nerve rather than at the area percussed and may persist for several seconds. An advancing Tinel Sign, found on serial examinations over time, indicates that the nerve is regenerating. Synonym: **Formication Sign**. 2. A diagnostic test that indicates possible entrapment neuropathy at a specific site. It is elicited by percussing over the suspected level of compression. For example, at the level of the carpal tunnel or Guyon's canal.

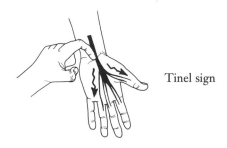

Tinel sign

Tissue (tishū) (n.) A collection of cells specialized to perform a particular function.

Tissue Dose (tish'u/dōs) (n.) Amount of radiation received by tissue in a specific area during radiation therapy.

Titanium (ti-tā'nē-um) (n.) A metal used in the production of orthopaedic implants. It has high corrosion resistance, good fatigue resistance, and a low modulus of elasticity compared with other commonly used metals. Titanium-based alloys, unlike cobalt-chrome alloys, are advantageous in their machinability.

TKA Abbreviation for Total Knee Arthroplasty.

TKR Abbreviation for Total Knee Replacement.

TMT Angle Abbreviation for Talometatarsal angle.

TNS Abbreviation for Transcutaneous nerve stimulator.

Tobruk Splint (tō-bruk'/splint) (n.) A modification of a Thomas splint in which plaster-of-Paris is added to the device.

Todd's Standards (todz/stan'dardz) (n.) An atlas of skeletal maturation prepared by Todd and associates, showing the normal epiphyseal development in the male and female wrist and hand at varying ages.

Toddling Gait (tod'ling/gāt) (n.) Gait characterized by instability, such as that seen in small children learning to walk.

Toe (tō) (n.) A digit of the foot. See **Claw**, **Hammer**, **Jogger's**, **Mallet**, **Sausage**, and **Tennis Toes**.

Toe Box (tō/boks) (n.) In shoe terminology, the upper part of the shoe above the sole, from tip to laces. The reinforcement used to retain the original contour of the toe and guard against trauma or abrasion.

Toe Cap (tō/kap) (n.) In shoe terminology, an extra piece sewed to the vamp, covering the toe area.

Toe Gait (tō/gāt) (n.) A walk characterized by weight-bearing on the forefoot, without the usual heel-toe pattern. It may be intentional, as in exercise or dancing, or pathologic owing to shortened calf muscles; it also may be used as a test of balance or strength. Also known as **Toe Walking**.

Toe-off (tō-off) (n.) In normal gait, the stage that follows heel-off and precedes heel strike. As the center of mass moves forward, weight-bearing moves laterally from the proximal phalanx of the great toe to the proximal phalanx of the fifth toe. The tibia externally rotates, and the foot goes into supination. As the toes dorsiflex, the plantar tissues tighten and shorten the arch and then push off the ground.

Toe Point (tō/point) (n.) In shoe terminology, the foremost point of a last.

Toe Spring (tō/spring) (n.) In shoe terminology, the space between the anterior portion of the sole and the floor.

Toeing-in (tō'ing-in) (adj.) Pertaining to a stance or gait in which the feet or toes are rotated inward.

Toeing-out (tō'ing-out) (adj.) Pertaining to a stance or gait in which the feet or toes are rotated outward.

Tolectin (tol'ek-tin) (n.) The proprietary name for tolmetin, a nonsteroidal anti-inflammatory drug.

Tolmetin (tol'met-in) (n.) A nonsteroidal, antiinflammatory drug marketed under the name Tolectin.

Tomography (tō-mog'rah-fē) (n.) A radiographic technique that reveals detailed images of objects in a specific plane by layers while blurring or eliminating details of objects in other planes and layers. Also known as **Body-Section Tomography**, **Laminography**, **Planography**, and **Stratiography**.

Tone (tōn) (n.) 1. A continuous submaximal contraction that maintains a small degree of tension in a muscle. It apparently keeps the muscle in a state of readiness for contraction. Also known as **Resting Tone**. 2. The resistance offered by muscles to passive stretch.

Tongue (tung) (n.) In shoe terminology, the strip of material lying under the laces.

Tonus (tō'nus) (n.) Sustained partial contraction of a muscle. See **Tone**.

Too Many Toes Sign (too/mĕ'ne/tōz/sīn) (n.) Rupture of the tendon of the tibialis posticus results in a planovalgus position of the midfoot. When viewed from the back of the foot, more toes are shown laterally than on the uninvolved foot.

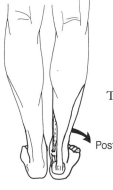

Too many toes sign

Posterior tibial tendon rupture

Top Angle (top/ang′g′l) (n.) A method of determining whether motion occurring at a segment of the cervical spine is principally sliding or tilting, measured on a lateral radiograph. Select a point on the anterior margin of a vertebral body and a second point on the posterior margin. Connect the positions taken by each of these points in flexion and in extension with a line, then follow these two lines in a cranial direction until they cross. The angle they form is the top angle. The larger the angle, the greater the slide of the vertebral bodies; the smaller the angle, the greater the tilt of the vertebral body. At C2-C3, the normal top angle approaches 100 degrees, indicating considerable sliding motion. At C7-T1, the top angle of 80 degrees shows tilting predominant.

Tophaceous (tō-fā′shus) (adj.) Gritty or sandy.

Tophus (tō′fus) (n.) A collection of sodium urate crystals, characteristically appearing as a hard, yellowish white, subcutaneous, irregular nodule that is sharply circumscribed from surrounding tissues. Tophi may be found anywhere in the body, but are most commonly seen in the foot, the olecranon, the pinna, the Achilles tendon, and the dorsum of the hands. They must be distinguished from rheumatoid and other nodules and nodular vasculitis. Chalky material consisting of negatively birefringent monosodium urate crystals may be aspirated from tophi; this constitutes proof of its nature.

Topical Anesthesia (top′i-kal/an″es-thē′ze-ah) (n.) Local anesthesia produced by application of an anesthetic to the surface of a specific area.

Toplift (top′lift) (n.) In shoe terminology, the layer of material forming the plantar-wearing surface of the heel.

Toronto Brace (tō-ron′-to/brās) (n.) A dynamic abduction orthosis allowing full weight-bearing of an involved hip for children with Legg-Perthes disease. It consists of bilateral proximal thigh cuffs, center tubular column with universal multiaxial joints at the base, and outriggers with angled mounting blocks at either end for shoe attachment. The brace holds the lower limbs of the child in abduction and slight internal rotation, while allowing sitting as well as ambulation with crutches.

Torque (tork) (n.) The force that acts to produce rotation. It is equal to the load multiplied by the perpendicular distance between the line of action of the load and the center of the object being rotated. The unit of measure is newton meter (inch pounds).

Torque Wrench (tork/rench) (n.) An instrument that measures the amount of torque as it is being applied by the wrench. The wrench can be preset to apply a given torque.

Torsion (tor′shun) (n.) A load applied by two forces around the long axis of a structure that are parallel but opposite in direction. This results in a twisting force.

Torsional Rigidity (tor′shun-al/ri-jid′i-tē) (n.) The torque per unit of angular deformation. The unit of measure is newton meters per radian (foot pound–force per degree).

Torso Decompensation (tor′so/dē″kom-pen-sā′shun) (n.) A measurement used to evaluate the erectness of the torso, especially in patients with scoliosis. On a standing AP roentgenogram, draw a line between the most proximal points on the iliac crests. From the midpoint of this line, draw a perpendicular line in a cephalad direction to the level of the first thoracic vertebra. The horizontal distance from a point on the center of the vertebral body to the perpendicular line, measured in centimeters, represents the degree of torso decompensation. In a fully compensated scoliosis, this distance should be negligible.

Torticollis (tor″ti-kōl′is) (n.) Stiff neck, or wry neck, caused by spasmodic contractions of neck muscles drawing the head to one side with the chin pointing to the other side. Most often involving the sternocleidomastoid muscle unilaterally. It can be congenital or acquired. Synonym: **Wry Neck**. See **Congenital Torticollis**.

Torus Fracture (to′rus/frak′chur) (n.) A buckling type of fracture in which one cortex of the bone wrinkles but does not break through. It is an impaction injury of childhood, primarily affecting developing metaphyseal bone. The buckling of the cortex occurs outwardly, producing a bump on the surface of the bone without displacement of the fracture fragments. From the Greek word meaning "to buckle." Also known as **Buckle Fracture**.

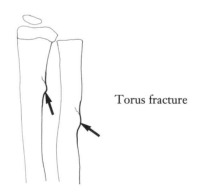

Torus fracture

Total Active Motion (tō′tal/ak′tiv/mō′shun) (n.) Sum of angles formed by the metacarpophalangeal, proximal interphalangeal, and distal interphalangeal joints of a finger in maximum active flexion minus the total extension deficit across these joints with active finger extension.

Total Articular Replacement Arthroplasty (tō′tal/ar-tik′u-lar/re-plās′ment/ar′thro-plas″tē) (n.) See TARA.

Total Body Scanning (tō′tal/bod′ē/skan′ing) (n.) A

survey of the total body by traversing it with an active or passive sensing device. 1. Commonly used to refer to computerized axial tomographic cross-section of the entire body. 2. A scintinographic technique in which imaging of the entire body is performed following injection of a radionuclide instead of limiting the scan to a body part or region.

Total Condylar (tō'tal/kon'di-lar) (n.) A type of semiconstrained total knee prosthesis.

Total Hip Arthoplasty (tō'tal/hip/ar'thrō-plas"tē) (n.) An implant arthroplasty of the hip in which the femoral head is replaced by a type of endoprosthesis and the acetabulum is resurfaced.

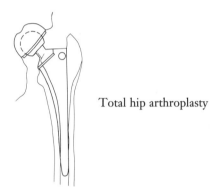

Total hip arthroplasty

Total Hip Articular Replacement by Internal Eccentric Shells (tō'tal/hip/ar-tik'ū-lar/re-plās'ment/by/in-ter'nal/ek-sen'trik/shelz) (n.) See **THARIES**.

Total Hip Prosthesis (tō'tal/hip/pros-thē'sis) (n.) The prosthesis used in total hip arthroplasty.

Total Hip Replacement (tō'tal/hip/re-plās'ment) (n.) See **Total Hip Arthoplasty**.

Total Knee Arthoplasty (tō'tal/nē/ar'thrō-plas"tē) (n.) An implant arthroplasty of the knee in which both the distal femoral and proximal tibial surfaces are replaced. The prosthesis may be confined to one compartment (unicompartmental) or both compartments (bicompartmental). A patella resurfacing is usually performed, creating a tricompartmental arthroplasty. Also, the prosthesis may be described by the degree of mechanical restraint provided by the prosthetic design or by the type of fixation to bone.

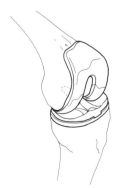

Total knee arthoplasty

Tottering Gait (tot'er-ing/gāt) (n.) An unsteady walk, similar to the ataxic gait, seen in very weak patients.

Toughness (tuf'nes) (n.) The ability of a material to absorb energy by bending without breaking, usually expressed as the energy required to fracture a material (feet pounds, ergs).

Tourniquet (toor'ni-ket) (n.) Any circumference device applied to a limb or digit that exerts sufficient pressure to occlude blood flow. These may be useful in trauma patients to maintain central pressure or prevent excessive blood loss. Commonly used in orthopaedic surgery to create a bloodless field during operative procedures.

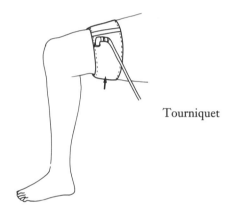

Tourniquet

Tourniquet Paralysis (toor'ni-ket/pah-ral'i-sis) (n.) A loss of motor function seen following prolonged tourniquet application due to nerve compression. The paralysis is usually transient.

Tourniquet Test (toor'ni-ket/test) (n.) 1. A test for capillary fragility. 2. A test for venous insufficiency. See **Trendelenburg Test**. 3. A test for carpal tunnel syndrome. See **Gilliat Test**.

Townley Prosthesis (town'le/pros-thē'sis) (n.) A total knee arthroplasty implant system.

Toxigenicity (tok-si-gen-i'-sitē) (n.) The ability of a microorganism to produce toxic substances (exotoxins, endotoxins, etc.)

Toxin (tok'sin) (n.) Metabolic product of an organism, usually a protein, that is poisonous to another organism (e.g., toxin produced by bacteria).

Toxoid (tok'soid) (n.) Toxin treated to destroy its poisonous quality while leaving it capable of stimulating the production of antibodies (e.g., tetanus toxoid used to maintain immunity).

Trabecula (trah-bek'ū-lah) (n.) 1. One of the variously shaped spicules of bone in cancellous bone. 2. Any one of the fibrous bands extending from the capsule into the interior of an organ. 3. A small line or beam visible on radiographs of bones.

Trabecular Bone (trah-bek′u-lar/bōn) (n.) A type of mature bone composed of a three-dimensional latticework of osseous plates and columns. It is found in both the developing skeleton and the adult skeleton. Trabecular bone is typically located at the ends of a bone. It seems to change its pattern with time, usually reflecting the direction of principal mechanical stresses. As a general observation, trabecular bone is progressively oriented, organized and transformed to provide maximum strength whie using minimal osseous material. Compare with **Cortical Bone**.

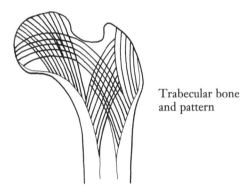

Trabecular bone and pattern

Trabecular Pattern (trah-bek′u-lar/pat′ern) (n.) The arrangement and orientation of bone trabeculae into a pattern of arches, as seen on radiographs.

Tracer (trās′er) (n.) Common name for a radioactive compound in scintigraphy.

Tracer Element (trās′er/el′e-ment) (n.) The radioactive isotope contained in a tracer.

Tract (trakt) (n.) A bundle of nerve fibers in the central nervous system that carries motor or sensory impulses.

Traction (trak′shun) (n.) A treatment using pulling forces applied to the extremities, the neck, the trunk, and other areas in an attempt to relieve pain and promote healing by obtaining reduction and regaining normal length and alignment. It also relieves pain by breaking muscle spasm. To apply the force needed to overcome the natural force or pull of muscle groups, a system of ropes, pulleys, and weights is used. Traction may be static or dynamic and may be applied to the skin or through the skeletal system. Continuous traction is used to reduce and immobilize fractures, overcome muscle spasm, stretch adhesions, and correct certain deformities.

Traction Bow (trak′shun/bō) (n.) A U-shaped metal device incorporating a Steinmann pin or K-wire for use in skeletal traction to which the traction rope is attached.

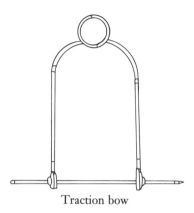

Traction bow

Traction Fracture (trak′shun/frak′chur) (n.) See **Tension Fracture**.

Traction Knot (trak′shun/not) (n.) The rope tie that connects the traction apparatus to the weights. The knot tightens as weight is applied.

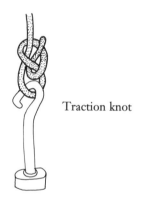

Traction knot

Traction Rope (trak′shun/rōp) (n.) The sturdy rope or cord used to interconnect pulleys, weights, and bows in traction.

Traction Splint (trak′shun/splint) (n.) A splint designed so that traction can be applied to it.

Traction Spur (trak′shun/sper) (n.) Any bony ex-

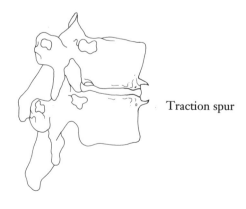

Traction spur

crescence occurring on or near the attachment of a ligament or fascia to bone. The term is most commonly applied to the spurs seen on the anterolateral margin of vertebral body in association with degenerative disk disease. A spur also is found frequently on the plantar surface of the distal calcaneus (e.g., heel spur).

Traction Suture (trak'shun/su'chur) (n.) A suture, usually nonabsorbable, used to retract a structure to the side of the operative field.

Tranquilizer (tran″kwi-līz'er) (n.) A drug used to reduce anxiety or other emotional disturbance.

Trans A prefix meaning across or through.

Transaxial (trans-ak'se-al) (adj.) Directed at right angles to the long axis of the body or a part.

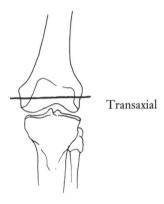

Transaxial

Transcaphoid-Perilunate Fracture Dislocation (trans-skaf'oid-per-ē-lū'-nāt / frak'chur / dis″lō-kā'shun) (n.) A traumatic injury to the wrist in which there is a fracture through the scaphoid and a dislocation of the carpus around the lunate.

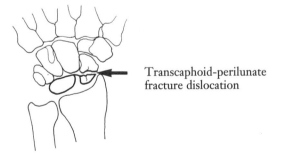

Transcaphoid-perilunate fracture dislocation

Transcervical Fracture (trans-ser'vi-kal/frak'chur) (n.) A fracture through the neck of the femur.

Transchondral Fracture (trans-kon'dral/frak'chur) (n.) A break that occurs through cartilage, usually articular cartilage. These fractures may not be apparent on plain radiography because there is no true osseous injury.

Transcondylar Fracture (trans-kon'dĭ-lar/frak'chur)

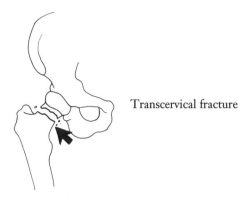

Transcervical fracture

(n.) A transverse fracture through the condyles of a bone.

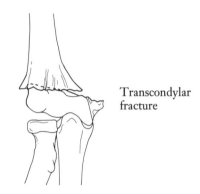

Transcondylar fracture

Transcutaneous Electrical Nerve Stimulation (trans″kū-tā'nē-us/e-lek″tri-k'l/nerv/stim″ū-lā'shun) (n.) The application of a low amperage, faradic (AC) electrical current through the skin as a noninvasive, distinct modality for treating acute and chronic pain. Stimulation of the large myelinated sensory fibers has been shown to promote local anesthesia and eventual pain relief by inhibiting activation of the A-delta and C-delta fibers, which transmit pain. The stimulator is a battery-powered electrical device that creates either a spike or square wave variable by standard electrical parameters. It generates 0 to 50 volts with pulse of 50 to 500 milliseconds and frequencies of from 0 to 200 hertz. To use, electrodes are applied to the skin and a transmission gel is used to conduct the electrical current and prevent skin irritation. Abbreviated by the acronym **TENS**.

Transfemoral Line (trans-fem'or-al/līn) (n.) A line joining the most inferior aspects of the medial and lateral femoral condyles. It intersects the anatomic axis of the femur at approximately 99 degrees.

Transfer (trans'fer) (n.) 1. A pattern of movements by which the patient moves his or her body from one surface to another. 2. A change in a hospital inpatient's medical care unit, medical staff unit, or responsible physician.

Transfer Belt (trans'fer/belt) (n.) A strap placed

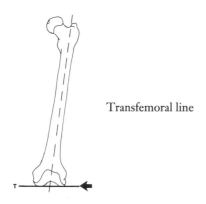

Transfemoral line

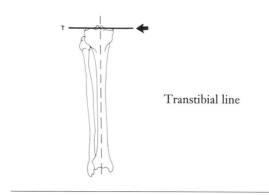

Transtibial line

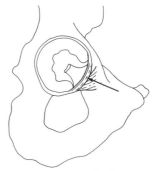

Transverse acetabular ligament

around a patient's waist to permit assistance by a therapist or other aide in the patient's transfer.

Transient (trans'shent) (adj.)   Short-lived.

Transient Ischemic Attack (trans'shent/is-kēm'ik/ah-tak') (n.)   A short-lived interruption in cerebral blood flow causing temporary interruption of neurologic function. Recovery of function is usually complete. Also known as a **Ministroke**. Abbreviated **TIA**.

Transitional Vertebra (trans-zish'un-al/ver'te-brah) (n.)   A vertebra whose structure features some of the characteristics of both of two adjacent spinal regions. Such vertebrae are usually found at the junctions of the various major divisions of the spine, most frequently at the thoracolumbar and the lumbosacral areas. For example, the first lumbar may have rudimentary ribs articulating with the transverse processes. The fifth lumbar may be partially sacralized or the first sacral segment may become partially lumbarized in the same manner.

Translation (trans-lā'shun) (n.)   The motion of a rigid body in which a straight line through the body is shifted but remains parallel to its initial position. The unit of measure is meters (feet).

Translocation (trans"lō-kā'shun) (n.)   The displacement of a part along a transverse axis.

Transplant (trans-plant) (v.)   1. To transfer from one part to another. 2. (n.) Graft; the material transferred from one part to another.

Transtibial Line (trans-tib'ē-al/līn) (n.)   A line joining the most superior aspects of the medial and lateral tibial plateau surfaces. It intersects the axis of the tibia (anatomic or mechanical) at approximately 88 degrees.

Transverse (trans-vers') (adj.)   Cutting across the long axis of a structure or part.

Transverse Acetabular Ligament (trans-vers'/as"ĕ-tab'u-lar/lig'ah-ment) (n.)   The ligament that connects the open inferior bony portions of the acetabular rim.

Transverse Arch of the Foot (trans-vers'/arch/of/the/foot) (n.)   The transverse hollow on the inner

part of the sole of the foot, in the line of the tarso-metatarsal articulations.

Transverse Arch Of The Hand (trans-vers'/arch/ov/the/hand) (n.)   The transverse hollow on the palmar side of the hand, in the line of the neck of the metacarpals.

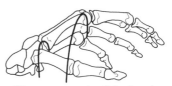

Transverse arch of the hand

Transverse Carpal Ligament (trans-vers'/kar'pal/lig'ah-ment) (n.)   The ligament that connects the wrist bones on the palmar side, forming the roof of the carpal tunnel.

Transverse Foramen (trans-vers'/fo-rā'men) (n.)   The passage in either transverse process of a cervical vertebra that, in the upper six vertebrae, transmits the vertebral vessels.

Transverse Fracture (trans-vers'/frak'chur) (n.)   A fracture line at a right angle to the longitudinal axis of the broken bone.

Transverse Hemimelia (n.)   See **Hemimelia Transverse**.

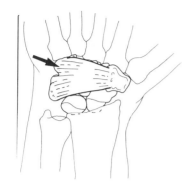

Transverse carpal ligament

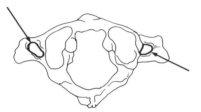

Transverse foramen

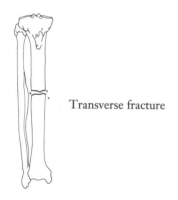

Transverse fracture

Transverse Humeral Ligament (trans-vers'/hu'mer-al/lig'ah-ment) (n.) The ligament that crosses the bicipital groove and prevents dislocation of the long head of the biceps from the groove.

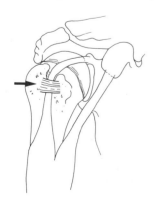

Transverse humeral ligament

Transverse Ligament of the Knee (trans-vers'/lig'ah-ment/of the knee) (n.) The ligament that connects the anterior portions of the medial and lateral menisci of the knee.

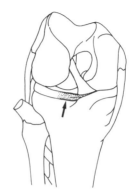

Transverse ligament

Transverse Lines of Park (trans-vers'/linz/of/park) (n.) See **Harris Lines**.

Transverse Myelitis (trans-vers'/mi"e-li'tis) (n.) An inflammatory process of the spinal cord that mimics the appearance of a transverse cord lesion. It affects an entire cross-section of the cord but over a limited distance. Also known as **Transverse Myelopathy**.

Transverse Process (trans-vers'/pros'es) (n.) A bony process projecting from the base of the neural arch of the vertebra at the junction of the pedicle and the lamina. It is used for muscle attachment.

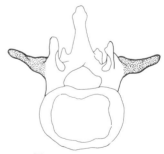

Transverse process

Transverse Tarsal Joint (trans-verz/tahr'sal/joint) (n.) The midtarsal joint with articulations between the talus and the navicular bones and the calcaneus and cuboid. See **Chopart's Joint**.

Trapeze (trah-pēz) (n.) A metal triangle or a short horizontal bar suspended by two ropes or chains above a bed or chair, providing a handhold for a patient rising or changing position.

Trapezium (trah-pe'ze-um) (n.) One of the carpal bones of the wrist, articulating with the scaphoid proximally and the first metacarpal distally.

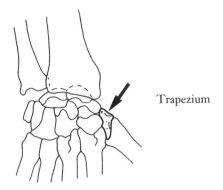

Trapezium

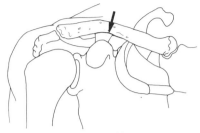

Trapezoid line

Trapezius Muscle (trah-pē′zē-us/mus′el) (n.) See **Muscle**.

Trapezoid (trap′-e-zoid) (n.) One of the carpal bones of the wrist, articulating with the second metatarsal bone distally, the scaphoid proximally, and the trapezium and capitate bones on either side.

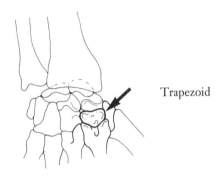

Trapezoid

Trapezoid Ligament (trap′e-zoid/lig-ah-ment) (n.) A ligament that, with the conoid ligament, forms the coracoclavicular ligaments that bind the clavicle to the coracoid process of the scapula. The trapezoid portion restrains the forward movement of the clavicle.

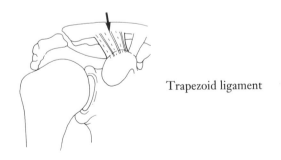

Trapezoid ligament

Trapezoid Line (trap′e-zoid/līn) (n.) The area on the inferior surface of the clavicle, near its lateral extremity, to which the trapezoid ligament attaches. Synonym: **Trapezoid Ridge**.

Trauma (traw′mah) (n.) A physical wound or injury to living tissue caused by an extrinsic agent.

Traumatic (traw-mat′ik) (adj.) Of or pertaining to trauma.

Traumatic Myositis Ossificans (traw-mat′ik/mi″o-si′tis/os″ĭ-fi-kanz″) (n.) See **Myositis Ossificans**.

Traumatic Neurosis (traw-mat′ik/nu-rō′sis) (n.) A neurosis whose onset immediately follows an occurrence perceived as traumatic.

Tread (tred) (n.) In shoe terminology, the weight-bearing surface of a sole between the shank and the forepart.

Treatment (trēt′ment) (n.) The care of a patient or the attempt to control or eliminate a disease.

Tremors (trem′orz) (n.) A series of involuntary, rhythmic, purposeless, oscillatory movements of the body or limbs, resulting from alternate contractions of agonist and antagonist groups of muscles that have reciprocal innervation. Tremors are recognized clinically by the movements they produce, which can be recorded by such mechanical or electrical transducers as accelerometers.

Trench Foot (trench/foot) (n.) A disorder of the feet, resembling frostbite, due to prolonged exposure to water and circulatory disturbance due to cold constriction, dampness, and inaction. It was prevalent during the World Wars among soldiers who were in the trenches in winter but was first described by Larry, Napoleon's chief surgeon, who encountered it during the Crimean War.

Trendelenburg Double Test (tren-del′en-berg/dub″l/test) (n.) A clinical test of competence of the valves in varicose veins of the legs. With the patient initially supine, empty the veins by raising the limb and stroking the varicose veins in a cephalad direction. Apply digital pressure over the termination of the long saphenous vein, and with the pressure maintained, ask the patient to stand. Maintain the pressure for at least 30 seconds. Consider the test positive if filling of the veins occurs during the period of digital compression, suggesting an incompetency of the communicating veins that connect the deep and the superficial sets.

Trendelenburg Gait (tren-del′en-berg/gāt) (n.) A walk resulting from a disturbance in the function of the hip abductors. During stance phase of the involved side, the pelvis cannot be stabilized and therefore drops on the side of the swinging lower limb. To compensate for a Trendelenburg gait, the patient avoids the drop of the pelvis by lateral trunk bending to the side of the supporting limb (i.e., the involved side). A waddling gait results when such compensatory trunk bending occurs bilaterally. Also known as **Gluteus Medius Gait** or **Lurch**.

Trendelenburg Position (tren-del′en-berg/po′zish-un) (n.) With the patient supine on a table, tilt the table so that the patient's head is lower than the foot. The patient's knees are flexed at the break in the table to avoid strain across the lower back.

Trendelenburg Single Test (tren-del′en-berg/sing′g′l/test) (n.) A clinical test used to evaluate the competence of the superficial set of veins. With the patient supine, empty the veins by raising the limb and stroking the varicose veins in a celphalad direction. Apply pressure over the termination of the long saphenous vein by placing a tourniquet on the proximal portion of the thigh. Ask the patient to stand. Release the tourniquet. If the saphenous vein fills rapidly from above, the test is positive, indicating incompetence of the valves.

Trendelenburg Test (tren-del′en-berg/test) (n.) A method used to evaluate the competence of the hip abductor muscles. Stand behind the patient and observe the dimples overlying the posterior superior iliac spines. Normally, when the patient bears weight evenly on both legs, these dimples appear level. Ask the patient to stand first on one leg, then the other. The test is positive when the opposite pelvis drops. Normally, the contralateral side of the pelvis is maintained in elevation by contraction of the strong ipsilateral hip abductor muscles.

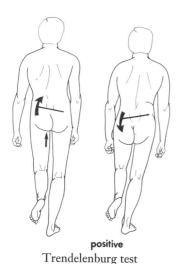

positive
Trendelenburg test

Treponema (trep″ō-nē-mah) (n.) Genus of motile, gram-negative spirochetes from the family Trepo-

nemataceae. Best observed under darkfield illumination or immunofluorescence.

Trevor's Disease (tre-vorz/di-zēz′) (n.) See **Fairbank's Disease**.

Triad (trī′ad) (n.) A group of three united or closely associated structures or three symptoms or effects that occur together.

Triage (trē′ahzh) (n.) The sorting of medical patients according to their relative priority for treatment. During a disaster, patients are divided into three groups: (1) the highest priority is assigned to those who need treatment in order to survive; (2) those who will recover without treatment; (3) the lowest priority is assigned to those who cannot be expected to survive even with treatment.

Triangular Bandage (trī-ang′gū-lar/ban′dij) (n.) A piece of material cut or folded into a triangular shape and used as an arm sling or to hold dressings in place.

Triangular Bone (tri-ang′gu-lar/bōn) (n.) See **Triquetrum**.

Triangular Fibrocartilage Complex (trī-ang′gu-lar/fī″brō-kar′ti-lij/kom′pleks) (n.) A cartilaginous structure in the ulnocarpal space of the wrist that also provides stability to the distal radioulnar joint. It is a homogeneous-appearing structure consisting of a nondissectable articular disk and a meniscal homolog and is confluent with dorsal and volar ligamentous structures. Abbreviated **TFCC**.

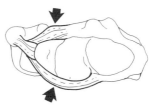

Triangular fibrocartilage complex

Triangular Sign (trī-ang′gu-lar/sīn) (n.) A radiographic marker used for the diagnosis of an early slip of the capital femoral epiphysis. In the normal adolescent hip, a portion of the diaphysis of the neck inferomedially is intraarticular and overlays the posterior wall of the acetabulum as seen on the AP view, creating a dense triangular appearance. In most cases of slipped epiphysis this dense triangle is lost, as that portion of the neck translocates lateral to the acetabulum.

Triangular Space (trī-ang′gu-lar/spās) (n.) An anatomic space bounded by the subscapularis and teres minor muscles superiorly, the teres major muscles inferiorly, and the long head of the triceps muscles laterally.

Triangulation (trī-ang″gu-lā′shun) (n.) The principle of successful arthroscopic surgery in which an instrument is inserted through a portal distinct from that through which the arthroscope passes and is placed into the optical field of the arthroscope. For

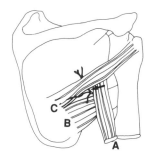

Triangular space.
A, Triceps, long head;
B, Teres major;
C, Teres minor.

adequate visualization and orientation, the projected tips of the instrument and the arthroscope should form the apex of a triangle.

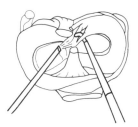

Triangulation

Triaxial Hinge (trī′aks-ē-al/hing) (n.)   A type of semiconstrained total elbow replacement prosthesis.

Triceps Crutch (trī′seps/kruch) (n.)   A crutch ending with a cuff at about mid-arm level.

Triceps Muscle (trī′seps/mus′el) (n.)   See **Muscle.**

Triceps Reflex (trī′seps/re′fleks) (n.)   A muscle stretch reflex in the upper extremity. Elicit this reflex by tapping the triceps tendon just above its insertion on the olecranon process of the ulna. The response is one of contraction of the triceps muscle, with extension of the forearm. The sensory and motor innervations are through the sixth through eighth cervical segment but primarily C7.

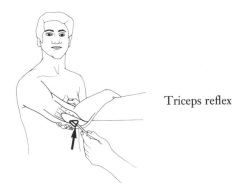

Triceps reflex

Triceps Surae Reflex (trī′seps/su′re/re′fleks) (n.) See **Achilles Reflex.**

Trigger Finger (trig′er/fing′ger) (n.)   A painful snapping and locking of the finger in marked flexion. Commonly found in the thumb, ring, and long fingers. It is caused by nodular swellings and stenosis of the flexor tendon sheath at the level of the metacarpo phalangeal joint. On unclenching the fist, the affected finger at first remains bent. Then, overcoming the resistance, it suddenly straightens (triggers). Definitive treatment is surgical division of the flexor tendon sheath at the level of the A1 pulley.

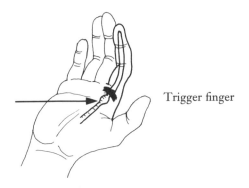

Trigger finger

Trigger Thumb (trig′er/thum) (n.)   A trigger finger affecting the thumb.

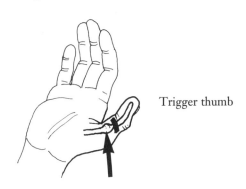

Trigger thumb

Trigger Point (trig′er/point) (n.)   A localized area in muscle tissue that, when palpated, causes pain over an area removed from the stimulus site. Usually, the patient will dramatically withdraw from the examiner on palpation of one of those points. Trigger points can be anesthetized by topical or local anesthesia in order to relieve symptoms.

Trilateral Orthosis (tri′lat′er-al/or-thō′sis) (n.)   A lower extremity orthosis used in the treatment of Legg-Calvé-Perthes disease. It is so named because the lateral wall of the plastic thigh brim is cut away distal to the greater trochanter to reduce adduction-generated forces. It consists of an ischial weight-bearing plastic brim, a single medial upright bar, and a spring-loaded shoe attachment. A contra lateral shoe lift is needed with the brace.

Trillat Procedure (trē′-jah/pro-sē′jur) (n.)   A surgical technique described for the treatment of recurrent anterior shoulder dislocation in which an osteotomy is performed at the base of the coracoid and the coracoid is then displaced laterally and distally. This is more commonly called the **Helfet Bristow Procedure**.

Trimalleolar Fracture (trī-mal-ē′-ō-lar/frak′chur) (n.) Designation of an ankle fracture in which the fracture involves the medial and lateral as well as the posterior malleolus of the tibia.

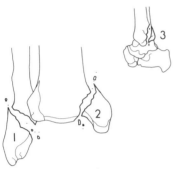

Trimalleolar fracture

Triphalangeal Thumb (tri″fah-lan′jē-al/thum) (n.) Any congenital abnormality of the thumb in which the first digit has three phalanges. There are three types: (1) thumbs with a delta-shaped phalanx, (2) thumbs with three relatively normal-shaped phalanges of excess length, and (3) hands with five normal-appearing fingers and no true thumb.

Triplane Fracture (trī-plān′/frak′chur) (n.) A fracture of the distal tibia, seen in the late immature skeleton, whose fracture lines are visualized in three planes—in cross-section, coronal, and sagittal planes. Triplane fractures may have two to four fragments. The classic three-fragment fracture is composed of the anterolateral portion of the distal tibial epiphysis, the remainder of the epiphysis with an attached posterolateral spike of the distal tibial-metaphysis, and the remainder of the metaphysis and the tibial shaft. The mechanism of injury is planter flexion and external rotation.

Triple Arthrodesis (trip″l/ar″thro-dē′sis) (n.) A surgical procedure consisting of fusion of the subtalar, calcaneocuboid, and talonavicular joints.

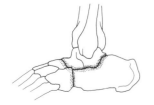

Triple arthrodesis

Triple Innominate Osteotomy (trip″l/i-nom′i-nāt/ os″te-ot′ō-mē) (n.) A corrective osteotomy for hip dysplasia that frees the acetabulum by dividing the ischium, the superior pubic ramus, and the ilium superior to the acetabulum. After the acetabulum is repositioned, it is stabilized by a bone graft and pins. Also known as **Steel Osteotomy**.

Tripod Cane (trī′pod/kān) (n.) A cane with three tips. Synonym: **Three-Point Cane**.

Tripod Drag-to Gait (trī′pod/drag-to/gāt) (n.) A walk in which the feet are dragged forward together after the crutches have been advanced. If crutches are advanced together, this is called the tripod simultaneous-crutch gait; if advanced separately, the tripod alternate-crutch gait.

Tripod Gait (trī′pod/gāt) (n.) A gait, using crutches (or rarely, canes), in which the feet always remain close together and behind the crutches. Thus the feet form one part of a tripod, and the crutches the other two.

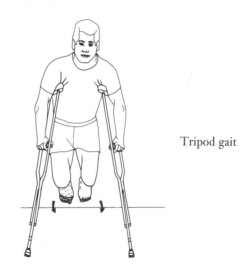

Tripod gait

Trippier's Amputation (trip″e-āz/am″pu-tā′shun) (n.) An amputation of the foot through the calcaneus. Rarely performed.

Triquetrum (trī-kwe′trum) (n.) One of the carpal bones of the wrist that articulates with the ulna proximally and with the pisiform, hamate, and lunate within the carpus. Synonym: **Triquetral Bone** or **Triangular Bone**.

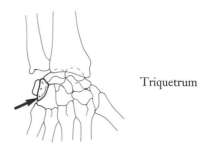

Triquetrum

Triradiate Cartilage (trī-rā′de-āt/kar′ti-lij) (n.) The cartilage in the hemipelvis of the immature skeleton where the primary ossification centers of the ilium, ischium, and pubis meet. See **Y Cartilage**.

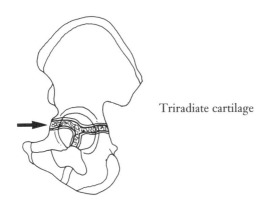

Triradiate cartilage

Trocar (trō′kar) (n.) A sharp instrument used to enter a body cavity such as a joint.

Trochanter (trō-kan′ter) (n.) Either of the two bony protuberances that project from below the neck of the femur; known as the greater and lesser trochanters.

Trochanteric (trō″kan-ter′ik) (adj.) Of or pertaining to a trochanter.

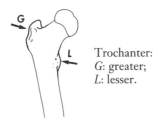

Trochanter:
G: greater;
L: lesser.

Trochanteric Bursitis (trō″kan-ter′ik/ber-sī′tis) (n.) An inflammatory process in the bursa overlying the greater trochanter of the proximal femur.

Trochanteric Height (trō″kan-ter′ik/hīt) (n.) A term that describes the height of the tip of the greater trochanter relative to the femoral head on an AP radiograph of the pelvis. Divide the head into four quadrants. If the trochanter is at the level of the middle of quadrant 2, give it the numerical value of 2.0; if it is halfway between quadrants 2 and 3, the value is 2.5 and so on. An imaginary fifth quadrant is placed above quadrant 4.

Trochlea (trōk′lē-ah) (n.) 1. An anatomic part that serves as a pulley. 2. Specifically, the medial articular surface of the distal humerus through which the articular surface of the proximal ulna glides through flexion and extension of the elbow.

Trochlear Groove (trōk′lē-ar/grūv) (n.) The patel-

lar articular surface on the anterior aspect of the distal femur.

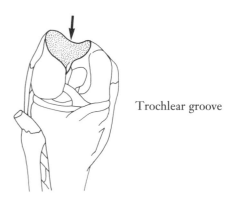

Trochlear groove

Tronzo Classification (trahn′-zo/klas″sĭ-fĭ-ka′shun) (n.) A classification of intertrochanteric hip fractures presumably based on the reduction potential. These are divided into Types 1 through 5 as follows:
Type 1: Incomplete fractures.
Type 2: Noncomminuted fractures in which both trochanters are fractured, with or without displacement.
Type 3: Comminuted fractures in which the lesser trochanter fracture is large. These are so-called unstable fractures, with the beak of the inferior neck displaced into the medullary cavity of the shaft.
Type 4: Comminuted fractures with displacement of the spike of the inferior neck medial to the shaft.
Type 5: Any fracture with reverse obliquity.

Tropocollagen (tro″po-kol′ah-jen) (n.) The basic molecular unit of collagen, composed of three polypeptide chains assembled into a triple helix.

Tropomyosin (tro″po-mī′ō-sin) (n.) Filamentous proteins with a molecular weight of about 70,000 that are attached to each troponin molecule. They lie along the grooves in the double helix of actin.

Troponin (tro′po-nin) (n.) In the structure of muscle myofilaments, a globular protein in spaces between the two strands of actin subunits.

Trotter Bulge Sign (trot′-er/bulj/sīn) (n.) Clinical technique to detect the presence of small knee effusions. Milk the medial aspect of the knee firmly upward two or three times to displace any fluid. Then press on top of the knee just behind the lateral margin of the patella. Watch for a bulge of returning fluid medial to the patella.

Trough Line (trof/līn) (n.) A radiographic sign of posterior shoulder dislocation characterized by two parallel lines located on the medial aspect of the humeral head. One line represents the medial cortex of the humeral head, the other, the margin of a trough-like impaction fracture.

Trousseau's Sign (trū-sōz′/sīn) (n.) A clinical sign of tetany. Compress the arm by squeezing or constricting it with a tourniquet or blood pressure cuff. Involuntary tonic spasm of the hand indicates a positive result. Maintain inflation of the cuff for a full 4 minutes before concluding that the result is negative.

True Pelvis (trū/pel′vis) (n.)   The part of the pelvis inferior to the iliopectineal lines. Compare to **False Pelvis**.

Trunk (trunk) (n.)   1. The main or primary part of a blood vessel, lymph vessel, or nerve before branches arise from it. 2. The torso, or main part of the body; excludes the head and extremities.

Tubercle (tū′ber-k′l) (n.)   1. A well-circumscribed, elevated solid prominence on the surface of an anatomic part, such as skin or bone or on a mucous membrane. In bone, these elevations usually serve as an originating point for muscles or ligaments. See **Tuberosity**. 2. A granulomatous lesion due to infection with *Mycobacterium tuberculosis*.

Tuberculosis (tū-ber″ku-lō′sis) (n.)   A necrotizing bacterial infection caused by *Mycobacterium tuberculosis*. Clinical manifestations are seen shortly after exposure as primary tuberculosis or after a variable latency period. Although pulmonary affection is most common, lesions may affect bone, kidneys, meninges, or other tissues and organs. Historically referred to as **Consumption**. Abbreviated **TB**.

Tuberosity (tū″be-ros′i-tē) (n.)   A large bony projection or protuberance. Usually serves as an attachment for tendons, e.g., greater and lesser tuberosities of the humerus, and tibial tuberosity.

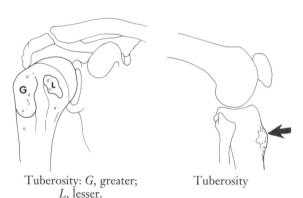

Tuberosity: *G*, greater; *L*, lesser.   Tuberosity

Tubular Plates (tū′bu-lar/plātz) (n.)   Metallic plates used in the internal fixation of bone whose profile is circular: either semitubular, one-third tubular, or one-quarter tubular. These plates are thin, self-compressing, and easily deformable. The holes for screws are oval, allowing for eccentric screw placement.

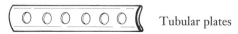

Tubular plates

Tuck Position (tuk/pō-zish′un) (n.)   Kneeling with feet in plantar flexion, buttocks on heels, trunk com-

pletely flexed, and head close to knees. The position also may be maintained with the subject on his or her side.

Tuft (tuft) (n.)   The terminal end of the distal phalanx.

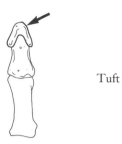

Tuft

Tumor (tū′mor) (n.)   Any abnormal growth in or on a part of the body. It may be benign or malignant. Synonym: **Neoplasm**.

Tumor Registry (tū-mor/rej′is-trē) (n.)   Repository of data, drawn from medical records, on the incidence of cancer and personal characteristics, treatment, and treatment outcomes of cancer patients.

Tumoral Calcinosis (tū′mor-al/kal″si-nō′sis) (n.)   A rare condition primarily affecting black people in which calcium salts are deposited in painless localized masses in the soft tissues around joints. It is characterized by single or multiple lobulated cystic masses containing chalky material.

Tunica (tū′ni-kah) (n.)   A covering, coat, lining, or layer of an organ or part (e.g., a layer of the wall of a blood vessel).

Tunica Adventitia: 1. An outer layer of various tubular structures. 2. The outer connective tissue coat of an organ, where it is not covered by a serous membrane.

Tunica Externa: An outer layer.

Tunica Intima: The innermost layer of a blood or lymph vessel.

Tunica Media: The middle coat of a blood or lymph vessel, composed of varying amounts of smooth muscle and elastic tissue.

Tunica Mucosa: 1. Mucous membrane. 2. A mucous membrane lining.

Tunica Serosa: A membrane lining the external walls of the body cavities and reflected over the surfaces of protruding organs. It secretes a watery exudate.

Tunnel (tun′el) (n.)   A passageway of varying length through a solid body, completely enclosed except for an open entrance and exit. An example is the carpal tunnel.

Tunnel View (tun′el/vū) (n.)   A frontal view of the knee obtained with the knee in 60 degrees of flexion. It allows demonstration of the posterior aspect of the medial and lateral femoral condyles, the intercondylar notch, the tibial spines, and the tibial plateau.

Tunneling Resorption (tun′el-ing/rē-sorp′shun) (n.)   A histologic characteristic of bone affected by hyperparathyroidism in which there is a dissecting resorption of trabeculae creating a tunnel-like appearance. The apices of these tunnels are lined by osteoclasts, usually with some fibrosis noted behind these resorbing cells.

Turco Procedure (tur'-kō/pro-se'jur) (n.) A technique for a one-stage posteromedial release of soft tissue intended for children aged 6 to 12 months with a residual clubfoot deformity after conservative treatment.

Turf Toe (terf/tō) (n.) A sprain of the first metatarsophalangeal joint so named because of its prevalence in football players. The mechanism of injury is believed to be forced hyperextension of the joint when the foot is in equinus and the toe is fixed to the ground.

Turnbuckle Cast Technique (tern'-buk-l/kast/tek-nēk') (n.) See **Risser Cast**.

Turner's Syndrome (tur'nerz/sin'drōm) (n.) An X chromosome abnormality in which there is an absence of one X chromosome and a karyotype of only 45 chromosomes. Typically, these patients have short stature, webbing of the neck, an increasing carrying angle at the elbow, and often, scoliosis.

Turret Exostosis (tur'-et/ek"sos-tō'sis) (n.) A smooth, dome-shaped extracortical mass of bone lying beneath the extensor apparatus on the middle or proximal phalanx of a finger. The lesion develops posttraumatically when subperiosteal new bone formation occurs as a hematoma ossifies. Clinically, this mass limits excursion of the extensor apparatus, thus limiting flexion of the interphalangeal joints distal to the lesion.

Turyn's Sign (tū'rinz/sīn) (n.) A clinical sign in sciatica. It is a modification of the basic sciatic stretch test in which only the great toe, instead of the entire foot and ankle, is dorsiflexed while the patient lies supine with both legs extended. Pain results when sciatic nerve involvement is extensive because stretching of the nerve occurs through its connection into the great toe.

Twitch (twich) (n.) A single muscular contraction in response to a single stimulus.

Two-Point Discrimination Test (too-point/dis-krim'i-nā'shun/test) (n.) A test of skin sensibility that determines whether the patient can discriminate between the pressure of one or two points and the minimum distance at which two points touching the skin are recognized. Set the points 10 mm apart and progressively narrow them as accurate responses are obtained, making sure that the pressure from the test instrument does not produce an ischemic area on the skin. When applying two points, make contact simultaneously, with the line between the points following the longitudinal axis of the extremity. To perform the test, ask the patient to close his or her eyes and indicate if he or she feels one or two points. Compare the minimal distance discerned to that of the contralateral extremity. The usual distance for two-point recognition is 3 to 5 mm over the volar pulp tip of the fingers, 7 to 10 mm over the volar pulp tip of the toes and the base of the palm, 10 to 20 mm over the dorsum of the hand or foot, and 40 mm below the elbow or below the knee. In 1958, Moberg first popularized the two-point discrimination test as an objective method for determining the functional value of sensibility in the hand. Also known as **Moberg's Test**.

Two-Point Gait (too-point/gāt) (n.) A walk in which the right foot and left-sided support (such as a crutch or cane) are advanced together, and then the left foot moves with the right-sided support.

Tyloma Molle (tī-lo'mah/mō'le) (n.) See **Soft Corn**.

U

UCL Abbreviation for Ulnar Collateral Ligament.

U-Figure (u-fig'ūr) (n.) A radiographic landmark seen on an AP projection of the pelvis. It is a U-shaped density composed of a fairly straight line created medially by the flat, parasagittal surface of the ilium and laterally by a semicircular line created by the wall of the acetabulum and an inferior connecting line that corresponds to the semicylindrical cortex of the acetabular notch. Also known as the **Radiographic U** or the **Teardrop**.

UHMWP Abbreviation for ultra high molecular weight polyethylene.

Ulcer (ul'ser) (n.) An irregularly shaped excavation of the skin, mucous membrane, or other surface, that is accompanied by an inflammation of adjacent tissue. Necrotic tissue discharging from its surface is termed a slough.

Ullman's Sign (ul'manz/sīn) (n.) A radiographic finding in spondylolisthesis. On a lateral radiograph

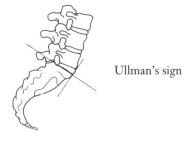

Ullman's sign

of the lumbosacral spine, a line drawn upward from the anterior surface of the sacrum perpendicular to its superior surface normally lies at or in front of the anteroinferior angle of the fifth lumbar body. In spondylolisthesis, this perpendicular line intersects the slipped vertebral body of L5.

Ulna (ul′nah) (n.) The medial bone of the forearm. Proximally, it has an olecranon and coronoid process that articulate with the distal humerus at the elbow. There is also a radial notch to accommodate articulation with the radial head. Distally, it terminates in a cone-shaped styloid process. It articulates distally with the radius to create the distal radioulnar joint, and indirectly with the carpus.

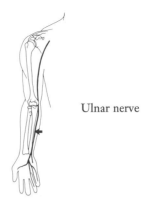

Ulnar nerve

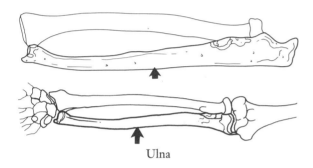

Ulna

Ulnar Collateral Ligament (ul′nar/kŏ-lat′er-al/lig′ah-ment) (n.) Any ligament of the upper extremity on the ulnar or medial side of a joint that resists valgus stress. An example is the ulnar collateral ligament of the elbow or metacarpophalangeal joint of the thumb. Abbreviated as **UCL**.

Ulnar Deviation (ul′nar/dē″vē-ā′shun) (n.) 1. Refers to the position of the hand relative to the wrist in which the hand is directed ulnarly. 2. Any abnormal angulation of the carpus or digits in an ulnar or medial direction. Compare to **Radial Deviation**.

Ulnar Drift (ul′nar/drift) (n.) A deformity of the fingers and wrist most frequently in rheumatoid arthritis in which the carpus or digits tend to deviate medially.

Ulnar Minus Variance (ul′nar/mī′nus/var′ē-ans) (n.) A variation in the anatomy of the forearm bones when there is a relatively short ulna. This is determined by comparing the level of the distal radial and ulnar articular surfaces on an AP radiograph of the wrist.

Ulnar Nerve (ul′nar/nerv) (n.) A terminal nerve of the brachial plexus. It supplies motor power to the intrinsic muscle of the hand and muscles on the ulnar side of the forearm, as well as sensation to the little finger and half of the ring finger.

Ulnar Nerve Palsy (ul′nar/nerv/pawl′zē) (n.) Any paralysis, partial or complete, of the ulnar nerve. It is often used to refer to a low ulnar nerve palsy, which classically results in a clawing of the ring and

little fingers as the metacarpophalangeal joints hyperextend from the unopposed action of the extrinsic extensors, and the interphalangeal joints cannot be extended because of paralysis of the intrinsic muscles.

Ulnar Tunnel Syndrome (ul-nar′/tun-el/sin-drōm) (n.) A compression neuropathy of the ulnar nerve within Guyon's canal at the wrist. The exact level of compression determines whether symptoms are motor, sensory, or both. Compression just distal to the tunnel, usually caused by a ganglion, affects the deep branch of the nerve that supplies most of the intrinsic muscles of the hand. A number of other factors may cause pressure on the ulnar nerve: true or false aneurysms of the ulnar artery, thromboses of the ulnar artery, fractures of the hamate with hemorrhages, lipoma, and aberrant muscles.

Occasionally in rheumatoid disease, carpal tunnel and ulnar tunnel syndromes both develop in the same hand. Treatment consists of exploration of the ulnar nerve at the wrist and the removal of any ganglion or other cause of compression.

Ulnar Tunnel (ul′nar/tun′el) (n.) See **Guyon's Canal**.

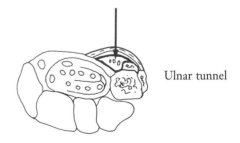

Ulnar tunnel

Ulnar Variance (ul′nar/var′ē-ans) (n.) The relative lengths of the ulna and radius as determined on an AP wrist roentgenogram. Compare the heights of the distal articular surfaces. Zero or neutral variance indicates both bones are equal in length. Positive variance designates an ulna that extends distal to the radius; negative variance refers to an ulna that does not extend as far as the radius.

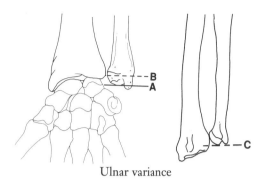

Ulnar variance

Ultimate Load (ul'tĭ-māt/lōd) (n.)   The largest load a structure can sustain without failure. The unit of measure is newtons (poundforce) if the load is a force, and newton meters (foot poundforce) if the load is a torque or moment.

Ultimate Tensile Strength (ul'ti-mat/ten'sīl/strenth) (n.)   The load a material can withstand in a single application without breaking.

Ultrahigh Molecular Weight Polyethylene (ul'tra-hī/mō'lek'ū-lar/wāt/pol"ē-eth'i-lēn) (n.)   A plastic formed from the polymerization of ethylene. It is a viscoelastic material that is highly wear-resistant and has limited flexibility under loading conditions. It is commonly used in the design of components of prosthetic joint implants, such as the plastic cups of total hip arthroplasties.

Ultrasonography (ul"trah-son-og'rah-fē) (n.)   A radiographic technique in which deep structures of the body are visualized by recording the reflection of ultrasonic waves.

Ultrasound (ul'trah-sownd) (n.)   1. A physical agent used in the treatment of chronic and acute pain. It is produced by a crystal that vibrates rapidly when exposed to an electrical current. The transducer generates a pressure wave at frequencies of more than 20,000 cycles per second. The vibrations are then transmitted to the patient via a coupling agent, such as water, mineral oil, or transmission gel. Resolution and penetration of the beam are determined by the frequency of oscillations of the transducer. Increasing the frequency generally results in increased resolution but decreased penetration of the body tissues. 2. The use of ultrasonic energy for the purpose of studying alterations of anatomic structure. See **Ultrasonography**. 3. Sound waves that vibrate at frequencies beyond the hearing power of the human ear (above about 20,000 Hz).

Ultrastructure (ul'trah-struk"chur) (n.)   A structure visible only under an ultramicroscope or an electron microscope.

Umbaü Zone (um'-bow/zōn) (n.)   An osteolytic area

in the diaphysis of a bone resembling a pseudofracture. See **Looser Lines**.

Uncinate Process (un'si-nāt/pros'es) (n.)   1. A hook-like projection of the hamate bone of the carpus. 2. A bone projection from the lateral superior surface of the last 5 cervical vertebrae. See **Uncovertebral Joint**.

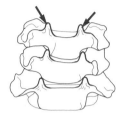

Uncinate process

Unconscious (un-kon'shus) (adj.)   Psychologic functions of which an individual is not aware.

Unconsciousness (un-kon'shus-nes) (n.)   An imprecise term used to describe impaired consciousness.

Unconstrained Prosthesis (un-kon'strānd/pros-thē'sis) (n.)   Any implant for arthroplasty that has no or minimal inherent stability; stability therefore depends on the patient's own intact ligaments and other soft-tissue structures. These require minimal bone resection for implantation and are more appropriately known as surface replacement prostheses. Unconstrained prostheses have been designed for knee, elbow, shoulder, and other joint arthroplasties.

Uncovertebral Joints of Luschka (un"ko-ver'te-bral/jointz/of/lush'kah) (n.)   Amphiarthrodial joints beginning between C2-C3 and extending to the level of C6-C7. They are formed between the uncus of the lower vertebrae and the lateral inferior surfaces of the vertebrae above, and form posterolateral articulations between the cervical vertebrae. Synonym: **Luschka's Joint**.

Underarm Crutch (un'der-arm/kruch) (n.)   An axillary crutch.

Ungual (ung'gwal) (adj.)   Of or pertaining to the nails.

Unguent (ung'gwent) (n.)   An ointment.

Unguis Incarnatus (ung'gwis/in-kar'na-tus) (n.)   See **Ingrown Toenail**.

Uni   Prefix for one.

Unicameral Bone Cyst (u"ni-kam'er-al/bōn/sist) (n.)   A benign bone cyst. It is a solitary cavity within the bone that contains serous fluid and is lined by a thin fibrous membrane. These are usually diagnosed during the first two decades of life and arise in the metaphysis of tubular bones, often in the proximal end of the humerus and the proximal end of the femur. The lesion is radiolucent and central within the metaphysis and can appear elongated in the direction of the shaft. The most common clinical presentation is a pathologic fracture. In most cases minimal displacement follows the fracture, which usually heals rapidly. The traditional treatment of this lesion has been curettage and bone grafting; more recent successful treatment has been achieved with intralesional steroid injections. Also known as a **Solitary Bone Cyst or a Simple Bone Cyst.**

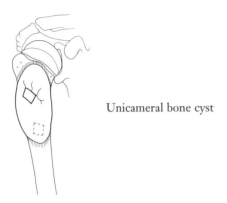

Unicameral bone cyst

Unicompartmental Knee Replacement (u″ni-kom″ part-men′tal/nē/rē′plās-ment) (n.) A design for knee arthroplasty in which only one compartment, either medial or lateral, is replaced. It is intended for use in patients whose arthritic changes are restricted to one compartment of the knee. Also known as **Hemiarthroplasty of the Knee.**

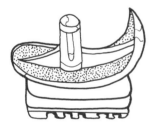

Unicompartmental knee replacement

Unilateral (u″ni-lat′er-al) (adj.) Affecting only one side.

Unilateral Bar (u″ni-lat′er-al/bar) (n.) A congenital

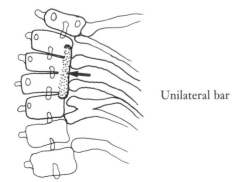

Unilateral bar

scoliosis that results from a unilateral failure of segmentation of the posterior elements of two or more vertebrae on one side.

Union (ūn′yun) (n.) The successful result of healing of a fracture in which the previously separated bone ends have become firmly united by newly formed bone.

Unit Vector (u′nit/vek′tor) (n.) A mathematical quantity used to define a direction. It has magnitude and direction.

United States Pharmacopeia (United/States/fahr″ mah-ko-pē′ah) (n.) The pharmacopeia officially recognized by the United States Food, Drug, and Cosmetics Act. Abbreviated as **USP.** It is a compendium that classifies drugs and other medical preparation.

Universal Endoprosthesis (u″ni-ver′sal/en″do-pros-thē′sis) (n.) See **Bateman Endoprosthesis.**

Unna's Paste Boot (ū′nahz/pāst/boot) (n.) A bandage impregnated with gelatin, zinc oxide, and glycerin paste. It is applied in alternate layers on the leg to create a semirigid boot. It is used for the treatment of venous leg ulcers, ankle sprains, and edema. Also known as an **Unna Boot** or **Soft Cast.**

Unstable (un-stā′bl) (adj.) 1. Without inherent stability. 2. This term is used in orthopaedics to refer to either joints with ligamentous damage or bone deficiency that create a tendency for the joint to subluxate. 3. It can also refer to a fracture that is difficult to maintain reduced in an adequate alignment.

Unstable Fracture (un-stā′bl/frak′chur) (n.) A fracture that cannot be easily maintained in satisfactory alignment after reduction. These fractures often require operative intervention and internal or external fixation of the fracture. Example: **Bennett's Fracture,** or **Unstable Hip Fracture.**

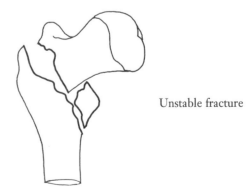

Unstable fracture

Untidy Hand Injury (un-tī′dē/hand/in′ju-rē) (n.) A wound whose skin edges are usually multiple, jagged, and irregular. Tendons and nerves may be exposed, and are sometimes severed. These injuries are usually caused by presses, power saws, or other machinery. Compare with **Tidy Hand Injury.**

Upper (up'er) (n.)   In shoe terminology, the portion above the sole. It consists of an anterior section, the vamp, and a posterior section, known as the quarters.

Upper Brachial Plexus Paralysis (up'er/brā'kē-al/plek'sus/pah-ral'i-sis) (n.)   See **Erb-Duchenne Paralysis**.

Upper Extremity (up'er/eks-trem'i-te) (n.)   The upper limb, including the humerus, forearm bones, carpus and fingers, and the surrounding soft tissues.

Upper Limb Orthoses (up'er/lim/or-thō'sēs) (n.)   Orthotic devices for the upper extremity.

Upper Limb Prostheses (up'er/lim/pros-thē'ses) (n.)   Prosthetic devices for the upper extremity.

Upper Motor Neuron (up'er/mo'tor/nū'ron) (n.)   Any efferent neuron whose cell body is in the motor cortex of the brain and that connects with the motor nuclei of the brainstem and the anterior horns of the spinal cord to create the pyramidal tracts.

Upper Motor Neuron Lesion (up'er/mo'tor/nū'ron/lē'zhun) (n.)   An injury to the cell body or axon of an upper motor neuron. It results in spastic paralysis of the muscle involved, hyperactive deep reflexes (but diminished or absent superficial reflexes), little or no muscle atrophy, and pathologic reflexes and signs. Lesions may be located in the cerebral cortex, cerebral peduncles, brainstem, or spinal cord and may be due to various causes.

Upright (up'rīt) (n.)   The part of an orthosis or prosthesis that is designed to reinforce the device, provide rigidity, maintain shape, or support another part.

Uracil (ū'rah-sil) (n.)   A pyrimidine component of nucleotides and nucleic acids.

Urethritis (ū"re-thrī'tis) (n.)   Any inflammatory process of the urethra, including infections. Urethritis is part of the classic triad of the clinical presentation of Reiter's syndrome: urethritis, iritis, and arthritis.

Uric Acid (ū'rik/as-id) (n.)   The final product of purine metabolism. It is formed by the actions of the enzyme xanthine oxidase on xanthine and hypoxanthine.

Uricosuric Agents (ū"ri-ko-sū'rik/ā'jents) (n.)   Any chemical agent that results in increased urinary excretion of uric acid. These drugs are used to reduce hyperuricemia associated with the development of gouty arthritis.

Urinary Tract Infection (u'ri-ner"ē/trakt/in-fek'shun) (n.)   The presence of significant numbers of pathogenic microorganisms anywhere within the urinary tract. It is ordinarily detected by examination and culture of the urine.

Urokinase (ū"ro-kī'nās) (n.)   A proteinase, similar to streptokinase, that may be used in the treatment of arterial emboli.

Urticaria (ūr"ti-kār'ē-ah) (n.)   A vascular reaction pattern characterized by the appearance of transient erythematous or whitish swellings in the skin or mucous membranes; these swellings represent localized areas of edema called wheals.

U-Shaped Coaptation Splint (u-shāp'd/ko"ap-tā'shun/splint) (n.)   See **Sugar Tong Splint**.

USP   Abbreviation for United States Pharmacopeia, a book that classifies drugs and other medical preparations.

Utilization Review Committee (u"til-i-zā'shun/rē'vū/kom'it-ē) (n.)   The committee composed of medical staff members whose purpose is to evaluate the appropriateness of a hospital's admissions, its medical and support services, and a patient's length of stay.

Uveitis (u-vē-ī-tis) (n.)   Any inflammatory process of the uveal tract of the eye, including the iris, the ciliary body, and the choroid. This may be seen in arthritides associated with inflammatory bowel disease.

V

V Fracture (v/frak'chur) (n.)   A type of fracture shaped like a V.

V Osteotomy (V/os"te-ot'ō-mē) (n.)   Any cut through bone made with two converging limbs that create a "V" shape.

Vaccine (vak'sēn) (n.)   A suspension of dead or living organisms that is injected or ingested to produce a state of immunity.

Vacuole (vak'u-ōl) (n.)   A small, usually spherical cellular organelle bounded by a membrane and containing fluid, solid matter, or both.

Vacuum Phenomenon (vak'u-um/fe-nom'e-non) (n.)   1. A term applied to the radiographic shadow of gas density in a joint. 2. It is commonly used to indicate the presence of an air shadow within an intervertebral disk on a roentgenogram. This is indicative of underlying disk degeneration.

Valgus (val'gus) (n.)   Angulation, bending, or twisting away from the midline of the body. Opposite of varus.

Valgus Stress Test (val'gus/stres/test) (n.)   See **Abduction Stress Test**.

Valleix Points (vahl-lāz/points) (n.)   In patients with lumbosacral radiculopathy, these are points of tenderness along the sciatic nerve and its branches. They occur between the ischial tuberosity and the

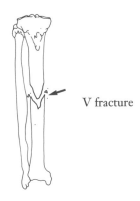

V fracture

greater trochanter, at the center of the posterior aspect of the thigh, just lateral to the middle of the popliteal space, at the middle of the calf, and just behind the medial malleolus. Synonym: **Puncta Dolorosa**.

Vallois Lumbar Index (vahl'-wah/lum'bar/in'deks) (n.) A numerical index described by Vallois and Lozarthes that relates the height of the posterior border of a vertebral body to its anterior body by the following ratio:

$$\frac{\text{Height of posterior border of body}}{\text{Height of anterior border of body}} \times 100$$

They found the average lumbar index to be 89 in 500 normal spines, 83 in 41 spines with spondylolysis, and 76 in 65 spines with spondylolisthesis. Also known as **Lumbar Index**.

Valsalva Maneuver (val-sal'vah/mah-nū'ver) (n.) The increase of intrathoracic pressure due to forcible exhalation against the closed glottis (e.g., coughing, sneezing, or yawning).

Vamp (vamp) (n.) In shoe terminology, the anterior or forepart of the upper.

Van der Hoeve's Disease (vahn-der-hōvz/di'zēz') (n.) One of the many eponyms under which osteogenesis imperfecta has been discussed in the past.

Van Neck's Disease (vahn-neks/di'zēz') (n.) A radiographic asymmetry of the ischiopubic synchondrosis seen in children just prior to its fusion. Its irregular bubbly appearance may or may not be associated with regional clinical signs.

Vanzetti's Sign (vahn-tset'ēz/sīn) (n.) In patients with a clinical scoliosis due to sciatica, the pelvis is always horizontal in spite of scoliosis. In other lesions associated with scoliosis, the pelvis is usually inclined.

Variable Resistance (va'rē-ah-b'l/re-zis'tans) (n.) Changes in the effective torque a load places on a muscle during contraction, either through mechanical or electronic means or through the effects of gravity and the movement of the limbs.

Varicose Vein (var'i-kōs/vān) (n.) An abnormally dilated, tortuous vein, usually seen in the leg. It is caused by increased intraluminal pressure and, to a

lesser extent, by loss of support of the vessel wall. Synonyms: **Phlebectasia**, **Venous Aneurysm**.

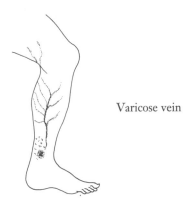

Varicose vein

Varney Harness (var'-nē/har'nes) (n.) An immobilizing device used in the treatment of acromioclavicular joint dislocations.

Varus (va'rus) (n.) Angulation, bending, or twisting toward the midline of the body. Opposite of **Valgus**.

Varus Derotation Osteotomy (va'rus/dē'rō-tā'shun/os"te-ot'ō-mē) (n.) A popular proximal femoral osteotomy used in the treatment of congenital dislocation of the hip. It is indicated when simple internal rotation of the femur is insufficient to stabilize the hip and abduction of the thigh is necessary to obtain adequate position of the femoral head in the acetabulum. This should be evaluated roentgenographically.

Vascular (vas'kū-lar) (adj.) Pertaining to blood vessels.

Vascularization (vas"ku-lar-i-zā'shun) (n.) The formation of new blood vessels.

Vascularized Graft (vas'kū-lar"īz'd/graft) (n.) Any bone or soft tissue flap that retains its vascularity either through a pedicle or a free flap whose vascularity is reestablished with microsurgical techniques.

Vasculitis (vas"ku-li'tis) (n.) Inflammation of a vessel. Synonym: **Angiitis**.

Vasoconstriction (vās"ō-kon'strik'shun) (n.) Narrowing or decrease in the lumen of blood vessels.

Vasodilatation (vās"ō-di-la-tā'shun) (n.) Widening or increasing in the lumen of blood vessels.

Vastus Intermedius Muscle (vas'tus/in"ter-mē'de-us/mus'el) (n.) See **Muscle**.

Vastus Lateralis Muscle (vas'tus/lat"er-a'lis/mus'el) (n.) See **Muscle**.

Vastus Medialis Muscle (vas'tus/mē"de-a'lis/mus'el) (n.) See **Muscle**.

Vastus Medialis Obliquis Muscle (vas'tus/mē"de-a'lis/ob-li'kwus/mus'el) (n.) See **Muscle**.

Vater (va'ter) (n.) An association of congenital anomalies that consist of vertebral segmentation and fusion abnormalities, anal atresia, tracheoesophageal fistula, esophageal atresia, renal abnormalities, and radial ray deficiencies.

Vector (vek'tor) (n.)   1. Anything that possesses both magnitude and direction. It can be represented as a straight line of appropriate length and direction. 2. A living carrier that transmits an infectious agent from one individual or species to another susceptible individual or species. The vector itself is not affected by the disease.

Vein (vān) (n.)   A vessel that carries blood toward the heart. Anatomic name: **Vena**.

Velcro (vel'kro) (n.)   A textile fastener consisting of two interlocking layers, one with tiny hooks, the other with loops. The two surfaces are closed by simple pressure and are easily pulled apart.

Velocity (ve-los'i-tē) (n.)   The rate of change of a point's position with respect to a coordinate system. Its magnitude is called speed, and its velocity may be linear or angular, depending on the type of motion. Therefore, the unit of measure is meters per second (feet per second) or radians per second.

Velpeau Bandage (vel-pō/ban'dij) (n.)   An immobilizing bandage that fixes the arm against the side, with the forearm flexed at an angle of greater than 90 degrees, resting across the body. The bandage envelops the shoulder, arm, forearm, and hand.

Vena Cava (vē'nah/ka'vah) (n.)   Either of the two main veins that convey blood from other veins to the right atrium of the heart.

Venipuncture (vēn'i-punk"tūr) (n.)   Surgical puncture of a vein.

Venogram (vē'nō-gram) (n.)   **Phlebogram**.

Venography (vē'nog'rah-fē) (n.)   A radiographic method of demonstrating venous structures and their course after intravenous injection of opaque media.

Ventral (ven'tral) (adj.)   Of or pertaining to the anterior surface.

Verruca (ve-rū'kah) (n.)   A common viral infection of the skin. Synonym: **Wart**.

Version (ver'zhun) (n.)   Inclination or tilt.

Vertebra (ver'te-brah) (n.)   1. One of the bony segments of the spinal column. In humans, there are usually 33 segments—7 cervical, 12 thoracic, 5 lumbar, 5 sacral, and 4 coccygeal vertebrae. Each vertebra typically consists of a body, or centrum. An arch of bone, the neural arch, arises from the body to enclose a cavity, the vertebral canal, through which the spinal cord passes. The arch bears one posterior spinous process and two transverse processes, which provide anchorage for muscles, and four articular processes, with which adjacent vertebrae articulate. Individual vertebrae are bound together by ligaments and intervertebral disks.

Vertebra Plana (ver'te-brah/plā'nah) (n.)   An extremely flat vertebra.

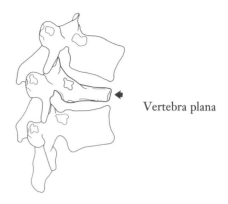

Vertebra plana

Vertebra Prominens (ver'te-brah/prom'i-nens) (n.)   The seventh cervical vertebra. The spinous process of C_7 is much longer than the one above, making it more prominent.

Vertebral (ver'te-bral) (adj.)   Of or pertaining to a vertebra or vertebrae.

Vertebral Arch (ver'te-bral/arch) (n.)   An arch formed by the paired pedicles and laminae of a vertebra. It comprises the posterior part of a vertebra. Together with the anterior part, or body, it encloses the vertebral foramen through which the spinal cord passes.

Vertebral Artery Syndrome (ver'te-bral/ar'ter-ē/ sin'drōm) (n.)   A condition with symptoms and signs of muscular inadequacy in the posterior cranial circulation, caused by spondylotic comprise of the vertebral artery.

Vertebral Body (ver'te-bral/bod'ē) (n.)   A short, cylindrical column of bone forming the anterior aspect of a vertebra.

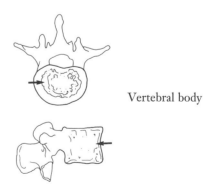

Vertebral body

Vertebral Canal (ver'te-bral/kah-nal) (n.)   A canal, formed by the foramina of the vertebrae, that contains the spinal cord and its meninges. The canal is formed by the posterior aspect of the vertebral body, the medial portion of the pedicles, and the anterior surface of the laminae.

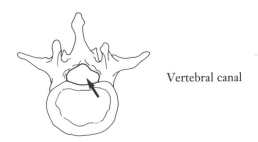

Vertebral canal

Vertebral Column (ver'te-bral/kol'-um) (n.) The flexible supporting column of the axial skeleton composed of vertebrae separated by intervertebral disks and bound together by ligaments. Synonym: **Spinal Column.**

Vertebral End-Plates (ver'te-bral/end/plātz) (n.) The superior and inferior plates of cortical bone of the vertebral body, adjacent to the intervertebral disk.

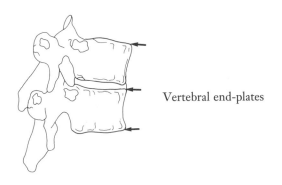

Vertebral end-plates

Vertebral Growth Plate (ver'te-bral/grōth/plat) (n.) The cartilaginous surface covering the top and bottom of a vertebral body in the immature skeleton. It is responsible for the linear growth of the vertebra.

Vertebral Lamina (ver'te-bral/lam'i-nah) (n.) One of the paired dorsal parts of the vertebral arch connected to the pedicles of the vertebra.

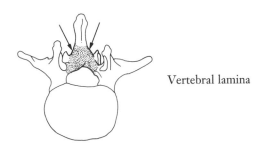

Vertebral lamina

Vertebral Notching (ver'te-bral/noch'ing) (n.) Notches, seen radiographically both superiorly and inferiorly in the preadolescent vertebral body, that

receive the epiphyseal ring. They are of no pathologic significance.

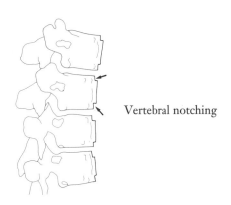

Vertebral notching

Vertebral Osteomyelitis (ver'te-bral/os"te-ō-mi"e-lī'tis) (n.) Infection in the bony structures of the spine.

Vertebral Pedicle (ver'te-bral/ped'i-k'l) (n.) One of the paired parts of the vertebral arch that connects a lamina to the vertebral body. They are constructed of tubular bone.

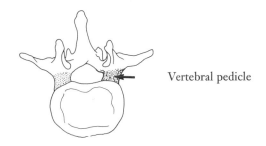

Vertebral pedicle

Vertebral Ring Apophyses (ver'te-bral/ring/ah-pof'i-sēz) (n.) Secondary ossification centers that develop in the cartilaginous end-plates of the vertebral bodies. Because they are thicker in the periphery, they appear ringlike with early ossification.

Vertebral Syndrome (ver'te-bral/sin'drōm) (n.) See **Putti's Syndrome.**

Vertex (ver'teks) (n.) The summit or top, especially the top of the head.

Verticle Shear (ver'ti-k'l/shēer) (n.) A description of the mechanism of injury that may produce unstable pelvic fractures when the disruption force is applied along a vertical axis. The affected hemipelvis is usually displaced cephalad.

Vesicle (ves'i-kl) (n.) 1. Any small sac or hollow structure containing fluid. 2. A circumscribed, elevated fluid-filled skin lesion. Vesicles larger than 0.5 cm in diameter are termed "bullae."

Vibratory White Finger (vi'brah-tor"ē/hwīt/fing'ger) (n.) A disorder of the hands, resembling Raynaud phenomenon, associated with workers exposed to occupational vibration caused by the use of chain saws, electric hand-held tools, and other machines. Synonyms: **White Finger**, **VWF**, **Vibration-Induced White Finger**, and **Raynaud Phenomenon of Occupational Origin**.

Vicryl (vī′kril) (n.) A brand name of an absorbable, braided, synthetic suture material.

Viet's Test (vyets/test) (n.) See **Jugular Compression Test**.

Villus (vil′lus) (n.) A projection from the surface, usually a mucous membrane or a synovial membrane.

Vinculum (ving′kū-lum) (n.) A connecting or restricting bandlike structure that usually connects a relatively fixed part to a moveable part.

Vinculum Breve (ving′kū-lum/brā-vē) (n.) The short v. tendinum that runs in the most distal aspect of the flexor sheath.

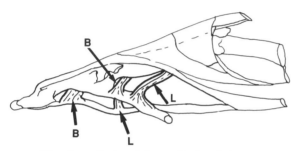

Vinculum: *B*, vincula breve; *L*, vincula longa.

Vinculum Longum (ving′kū-lum/long′gum) (n.) The longer, narrow vinculum in the more proximal aspect of the flexor sheath.

Vinculum Tendinum (ving′kū-lum/ten′dĭ-num) (n.) Collective term for v. breve and v. longum that conducts blood vessels to the flexor tendons of the digits. They arise from the internal surface of the flexor sheath.

Vinke Tongs (vin-kē/tongs) (n.) Tongs used to exert traction on the skull, as in surgery for fractures or cervical vertebrae.

Virchow's Triad (fir′kōz/tri′ad) (n.) Thrombus formation resulting from a combination of vascular injury, activation of blood coagulation, and venous stasis.

Virulence (vir′ū-lens) (n.) The capacity of a microorganism to produce disease.

Virus (vī′rus) (n.) A submicroscopic infective organism composed of nucleic acid and protein. It is an obligate parasite, replicating only within a living host cell.

Viscera (vis′er-ah) (n.) Collective term for the internal organs of an animal.

Viscoelastic Stability (vis′kō-ē-las-tic/stah-bil′i-tē)

(n.) Stability in which the application of a critical load is rate-dependent as well as dependent on the geometric and material properties of the structure.

Viscoelasticity (vis′kō-ē-las-tis′i-tē) (n.) The biomechanical property of a material to show rate-dependent sensitivity to the effect of loading. Elastic properties determine the maximum deformity; viscous properties determine how long it will take to be maximally deformed.

Viscosity (vis′kos′i-tē) (n.) 1. The resistance of a substance to flowing. 2. The property of materials to resist loads that produce shear. Viscosity is defined as the ratio of shearing stress to shearing strain rate or shearing stress to velocity gradient. It is commonly represented by η (eta) or μ (mu). The units of measure are newton seconds per square meter (poundforce per square foot) and poise (1 poise = 0.1 newton seconds per square meter).

Visual Method of Smith (vizh′u-al/meth′ud/of/smith) (n.) An evaluation technique in cubitus varus. With the patient's elbows in 90 degrees of flexion, examine posteriorly and draw three points: at the tip of the olecranon, at the medial epicondyle, and at the lateral epicondyle. Compare both elbows to determine the presence or absence of medial tilt.

Vitallium (vi-tāl′ē-um) (n.) A proprietary name for a cobalt-chromium-molybdenum alloy.

Vitamin (vi′tah-min) (n.) Any of a class of unrelated organic substances that cannot be synthesized by an organism but are essential in minute quantities for normal growth and function. Vitamins contribute to the formation of coenzymes and, therefore, to the action of cellular enzymes.

Vitamin C (vi′tah-min/C) (n.) A water-soluble vitamin that plays an important role in collagen synthesis. Possible other functions in the regulation of iron storage and tyrosine metabolism, for example, are not as well defined. Vitamin C deficiency results in scurvy.

Vitamin D (vi′tah-min/D) (n.) A fat-soluble vitamin that plays an integral part in calcium and phosphate metabolism and therefore in bone homeostasis. Vitamin D is manufactured in human skin when F-dehydrocholesterol is exposed to ultraviolet light. Further metabolic conversions are made in the liver and kidney. Endogenous Vitamin D is cholecalciferol, or Vitamin D_3. Dietary Vitamin D is ergocalciferol, or Vitamin D_2.

Vitamin D Deficiency (vi′tah-min/D/de-fish′en-sē) (n.) The disease state that results from insufficient Vitamin D. In children, rickets occurs; in adults, this results in oseteomalacia. See **Rickets** and **Osteomalacia**.

Vitamin D-Resistant Rickets (vi′tah-min/D/re-zis′tant/rik′ets) (n.) Any acquired or genetic condition that results in rickets not responsive to ordinary treatment with doses of Vitamin D. These disorders are generally classified into the following three types: (1) phosphate diabetes, (2) vitamin D–dependent rickets, and (3) end-organ insensitivity. Patient management depends on the etiology of the metabolic disturbance.

Vitamin K (vi'tah-min/K) (n.)   A fat-soluble vitamin that has a critical role in maintaining the function of clotting factors.

VMO   Abbreviation for Vastus Medialis Obliquis.

Volar (vō-lar) (adj.)   Referring to the palm of the hand or, less commonly, the sole of the foot.

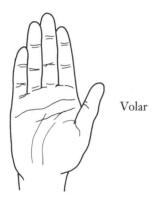

Volar

Volar Plate (vō'lar/plāt) (n.)   A dense, fibrocartilaginous ligament found on the volar aspect of the metacarpophalangeal and interphalangeal joints. Owing to the nature of its attachments, it deepens the articular surface of the phalanx and actually serves as part of the articular contact. Laterally, it is continuous with the collateral ligaments and the deep transverse metacarpal ligaments at the metacarpophalangeal joints. Also known as **Palmar Plate**.

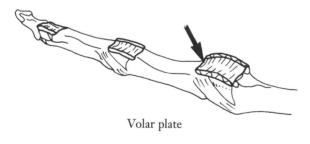

Volar plate

Volar Splint (vō'lar/splint) (n.)   A support to immobilize the bones and/or joints of the upper extremity. The splint can be temporarily applied to the palmar surface of the hand or the anterior (volar) surface of the extremity.

Volkmann's Canals (fōlk-mahnz/kah-nalz') (n.)   In the structure of cortical bone, the lateral branches of the Haversian canals that allow blood vessels to communicate between osteons. See **Haversian System**.

Volkmann's Contracture (fōlk'mahnz/kon-trak'tūr)

(n.)   The paralytic contractures that result from ischemia in an extremity. This is due to injury to the soft tissues of part or all of an extremity, causing ischemia in the muscles and nervous structures. Compartment syndrome is probably the most common cause of Volkmann's contractures. Acute Volkmann's contracture is more accurately known as an acute compartment syndrome. The clinical appearance of an established Volkmann's contracture depends on the degree of tissue injury. For the purpose of planning treatment, an established contracture is classified as mild, moderate, or severe. See **Compartment Syndrome**. Also known as **Volkmann's Ischemic Contracture** and **Volkmann's Paralysis**.

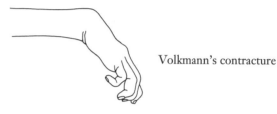

Volkmann's contracture

Volkmann's Deformity (fōlk'mahnz/de-for'mi-tē) (n.)   Congenital tibiotarsal dislocation. Also known as **Congenital Talus Luxation**.

Volkmann's Paralysis (fōlk'mahnz/pah-ral'i-sis) (n.)   See **Volkmann's Contracture**.

Voltaren (vol-tar'en) (n.)   A proprietary brand of diclofenac sodium, a nonsteroidal, anti-inflammatory drug.

Voluntary Hospital System (vol'un-tār"ē/hos'pit'l/sis'tem) (n.)   Nationwide complex of autonomous, self-established, and self-supported private nonprofit and investor-owned hospitals in the United States.

Von Frey Pressure Test (von-frā/presh'ur/test) (n.)   A test for tactile gnosis. Apply a series of monofilaments of varying thickness and stiffness perpendicular to the body surface being examined. Increase the pressure until the monofilament bends. A patient with normal sensibility of an extremity can recognize pressure between 2.36 and 2.83 mg. First standardized by Von Frey in 1898.

Von Lackum's Transection Cast (von-lahk-umz/tran-sek'shun/kast) (n.)   A casting system that corrects a scoliotic curve by applying external corrective forces.

Von Recklinghausen's Disease (von-rek-ling-how-zenz/di-zēz') (n.)   See **Neurofibromatosis**.

Von Rosen Line (von/ro-zen/līn) (n.)   A radiographic sign of congenital dislocation of the hip. Take an AP radiograph of the pelvis with the legs abducted 45 degrees and internally rotated 25 degrees. Draw a line along the midshaft of the femur. In a normal hip this will bisect the edge of the acetabulum and intersect with the midline at the lumbosacral area. In a subluxated or dislocated hip, it will bisect the anterior superior iliac spine.

Von Rosen Splint (von/rō′-zen/splint) (n.) A rigid but malleable device made of flexible metal and covered by soft padding used in the management of developmental dysplasia of the hip (congenital dislocation of the hip). It is H-shaped, with the crossbar extended on each side. See **Rosen Splint**.

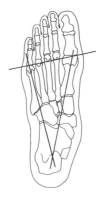

Von Weber's triangle

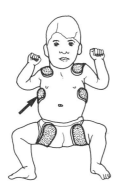

Von Rosen splint

Von Weber's Triangle (von/web′-erz/tri-ang′g′l) (n.) A triangle on the sole of the foot formed by lines connecting the head of the first metatarsal, the head of the fifth metatarsal, and the center of the undersurface of the heel.

Von Willebrand's Disease (von-vil-e-brahndz/di-zēz′) (n.) A congenital hemorrhagic disorder that has an autosomal dominant mode of inheritance. There is a deficiency of Factor VIII and a prolonged bleeding time due to inadequate plasma concentration of von Willebrand's protein. The protein is essential for normal platelet aggregation.

Voorhoeve's Disease (for-hev-ez/di-zēz′) (n.) A rare bone dysplasia of unknown etiology. It is usually an incidental radiographic finding in a patient who is asymptomatic but has had a roentgen study for another condition. It is typified by linear striations in the metaphysis extending into the diaphysis of long bones. The foot and ankle may occasionally be affected. Also known as **Osteopathia Striata**.

Vrolik's Disease (frō-liks/di-zēz′) (n.) One of the many eponyms under which Osteogenesis Imperfecta has been discussed in the past.

VTED Abbreviation for Venous Thromboembolic Disease.

V-Y Plasty (V-Y/plas′tē) (n.) Any operative technique for soft tissue in which a "V"-shaped incision is made and then converted to a "Y" shape at the time of closure to allow increased exposure, to release contracture, and to improve soft-tissue coverage. A variety of techniques for muscle, skin, and joint capsule have been described.

W

Waddell's Nonorganic Physical Signs (wah-delz′/non′-or-gan′-ik/fiz′-i-kel/sīnz) (n.) The standardization of a group of nonphysical signs seen in low back pain. These include 1) a large area of tenderness, 2) nondermatomal sensory loss, 3) simulation test, 4) distraction test, and 5) overreaction.

Waddell's Triad (wah-delz′/trī′ad) (n.) A femoral fracture associated with head and thoracic injury that is caused by an automobile and pedestrian accident.

Wadding (wad′-ing) (n.) The bit of material contained within a shotgun shell. Made of jute and hair, it is compressed with a binding agent. It is irritating to tissues and results in a severe inflammatory reaction if not removed when shotgun injuries are debrided.

Waddling Gait (wad-ling/gāt) (n.) A walk pattern in which there is an exaggerated alternation of lateral trunk flexion on each step toward the side of the supporting lower limb. This may be noted in bilateral congenital dislocation of the hip, progressive muscular dystrophy, and other deficiencies of the hip abductors.

Wadsworth Approach (wads′-werth/ah-prōch′) (n.) An extended posterolateral surgical approach to the elbow joint used when extensive exposure of the region is needed.

Wagner Apparatus (wag′-ner/ap-′e-rā′-tis) (n.) An external fixation device designed for use in limb-lengthening procedures. It consists of two telescoping square rods with a worm gear that connects percutaneous Schanz screws anchored in the ends of the long bone that is being lengthened.

Wagner Technique of Limb Lengthening (wägner/tek-nēk′/of/lim/len′-then-ng) (n.) A surgical technique for diaphyseal lengthening. It involves a transverse osteotomy in the shaft of either the femur or the tibia at the mid-diaphyseal level. This is then distracted continuously by percutaneous Schanz screws anchored in the proximal and distal metaphyseal regions. These screws are attached with a Wagner apparatus that consists of two telescoping square rods with a worm gear.

Wagon Wheel Fracture (wag′-en/wēl/frak′-chur) (n.) An outdated term for a fracture of the distal femoral epiphysis. It is named for the mechanism of injury in which the lower leg is caught in the spokes of a revolving wheel while the thigh is held against the vehicle.

Wagstaffe Fracture (wag′-staf/frak′-chur) (n.) A vertical fracture of the anterior margin of the distal fibula. The fragment includes the insertions of the anterior tibiofibular and talofibular ligaments.

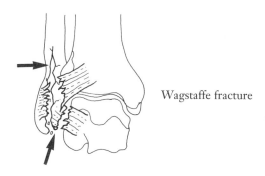

Wagstaffe fracture

Waist (wāst) (n.) In shoe terminology, the smallest dimension in girth between the ball and the instep.

Wake-up Test (wāk/up/test) (n.) A technique for intraoperative spinal cord monitoring during spinal surgery. In this test, anesthesia is lightened during surgery to allow the patient to be alert enough to actively move the extremities in response to commands. This test monitors motor function only. See **Stagnara Wake-up Test**. Compare to **Ankle Clonus Test**.

Waldenstrom's Overlap Sign (wahl′-den-stremz/ō′-ver-lap/sīn) (n.) A normal radiographic finding in the hip in which on an AP radiograph a crescentic shadow is formed by the overlapping of the femoral head on the posterior lip of the acetabulum. This shadow may be disrupted in cases of congenital dysplasia of the hip or in an inflammatory hip process when the femoral head is pushed laterally by an effusion or synovitis.

Walker (wal′-ker) (n.) 1. An individual capable of ambulation with or without assistive devices. 2. A four-legged frame with supports for the hands designed to aid the user in standing and ambulating. There are a number of walkers available:

Casterwalker: A walker in which the four legs are fitted with casters.
Folding Walker: A walker that can be folded for easy stowing and transportation.
Hemiwalker: Walker–cane combination.
Pick-up Walker: Also known as a walkerette. This is a lightweight, four-footed device.
Reciprocal Walker: A walkerette or pick-up walker is articulated in such a way that either side can be moved independently.

Walker Mureloch Wrist Sign (wal′-ker/mūr′-lok/rist/sīn) (n.) Because of the long fingers and thin forearms in patients with Marfan syndrome, an overlap of the patient's thumb and little finger is noted when the opposite wrist is grasped.

Walking (wal′-king) (n.) The process of body movement by foot. See **Ambulation**, **Gait**.

Walking Cast (wal′king/kast) (n.) Any lower extremity cylindrical cast in which the wearer may bear weight for ambulation. A rubber walking heel or a cast boot is applied to the sole of the cast to prevent slipping.

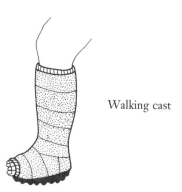

Walking cast

Walking Cycle (wal′-king/sī′-kl) (n.) See **Gait Cycle**.

Wall (wal) (n.) In shoe terminology, the medial and lateral perimeter of the forepart, or last, of the shoe. It comprises the relatively straight sides around the periphery.

Wallerian Degeneration (waw-ler′-ē-an/dē-jen′-e-rā′-shun) (n.) The secondary degeneration of a neuron that occurs distal to the point of injury.

Wallerian Law (waw-ler′-ē-an/law) (n.) In nerve physiology, the principle that states if the sensory fibers of a spinal nerve are divided proximal to the level of the ganglion, the fibers peripheral to the injury will not degenerate, whereas those that remain connected to the spine will degenerate.

Walther's Fracture (vahl′-terz/frak′-chur) (n.) A transverse ischioacetabular fracture in which the fracture line passes through the ischial ramus and terminates in the ilium near the sacroiliac joint. The entire medial wall of the acetabulum is displaced and tilted inward. When healed, this fracture resembles a unilateral Otto-pelvis.

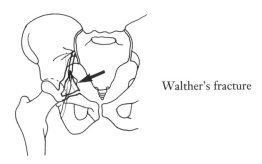

Walther's fracture

Ward (ward) (n.) A hospital room designed and equipped to house more than four inpatients.

Ward's Triangle (wardz/trī'-ang'-gl) (n.) A small area in the neck of the femur that contains only thin and loosely arranged bony trabeculae. It is formed between the trabeculae of the primary and secondary compressive groups and the primary tensile group.

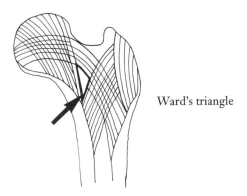

Ward's triangle

Warfarin Sodium (war'-fā-rin/sō'dē-um) (n.) The generic name for Coumadin, a commonly used oral anticoagulation agent.

Warm Springs Crutch (wărm/springz/kruch) (n.) A variety of the Canadian crutch.

Wart (wart) (n.) The common name for verruca.

Wartenberg's Oriental Prayer Sign (wawr'-ten-bergz/or'ē-en'-tal/prār/sīn) (n.) A clinical test for median nerve function. The patient is asked to extend and adduct the four fingers of each hand and to keep the thumb extended. The patient then raises both hands in front of the face so that they are side-by-side in the same plane, with the tips of the thumbs and the fingers touching. If there is paralysis of the abductor pollicis brevis, the thumbs will not meet when the index fingers touch.

Wartenberg's Sign (wor'-ten-bergz/sīn) (n.) A clinical sign of lower ulnar nerve paralysis. The fifth finger assumes an abducted position, and the patient is unable to adduct the extended little finger to the extended ring finger.

Wartenberg's Syndrome (wor'-ten-bergz/sin'-drōm) (n.) An isolated neuritis of the superficial radial nerve. Also known as **Cheiralgia Paraesthetica.**

Watkins Technique (wat'-kinz/tek-nēk) (n.) A surgical technique for posterolateral spinal fusion in which the facet joints, pars interarticularis, and the bases of the transverse processes are fused with chip grafts; then a layer graft is placed across the transverse processes.

Watson-Jones Approach (wat'-son/jōnz/a-prōch) (n.) An anterolateral surgical approach to the hip. This technique uses the intermuscular plane between the tensor fascia lata and gluteus medius muscles.

Watson-Jones Arthrodesis (wat'-son/jōnz/ar-throd'-ē-sis) (n.) An extra-articular technique for shoulder arthrodesis.

Watson-Jones Tenodesis (wat'-son/jōnz/te-nōd'-ē-sis) (n.) A surgical procedure for the reconstruction of chronic instability of the lateral ankle. In this technique, the peroneus brevis tendon is used to reconstruct both the calcaneofibular and anterior talofibular ligaments.

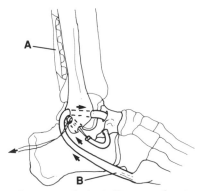

Watson-Jones tenodesis. **A,** Peroneus brevis tendon resected; **B,** peroneus brevis tendon.

Wear (wār) (n.) The loss of material from solid surfaces due to mechanical abrasion.

Weaver & Dunn Procedure (wē-ver/dun/pro-sē'-jer) (n.) Surgical reconstruction of an acromioclavicular dislocation in which the acromial end of the coracoacromial ligament is used to tether the lateral clavicle after its distal end is excised.

Weaver's Bottom (wē-verz/bot'-om) (n.) Ischiogluteal bursitis.

Web (web) (n.) The area at the base of the digits of the hands or feet that connects two adjacent digits. The web primarily consists of skin and subcutaneous tissue but also has muscle, fascia, and joint capsule within it. Frequently, the region beneath the skin is referred to as the web space. These are numbered from one through four, starting at the space between the first and second digits.

Web Space (web/spās) (n.)   See **Web**.

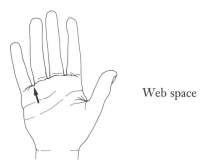

Web space

Web Space Infection (web/spās/in-fek'-shun) (n.) An infection of the hand located in one of the fat-filled spaces just proximal to the superficial transverse ligament at the level of the metacarpophalangeal joints. The patient presents with swelling in the web space that usually points dorsally, even if the infection begins palmarward. Both a dorsal and a palmar incision are usually required for adequate drainage. Also known as a **Collar Button Abscess**.

Webbed Finger (webd/fing'ger) (n.) A congenital condition in which adjacent fingers and abnormally connected by excess skin and subcutaneous tissue at their bases.

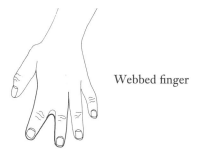

Webbed finger

Webbed Toe (webd/tō) (n.) A usually congenital condition in which toes are abnormally connected by excess tissue at their bases.

Weber Classification System (web'er/klas'si-fi-ka'-shun/sis'-tem) (n.) A modification of the Salter-Harris classification of epiphyseal injuries that adds extra- and intra-articular designations.

Weber Frame (web'er/frām) (n.) An external frame designed for the skeletal traction of femur fractures in which the hip is placed in 90 degrees of flexion and 20 degrees of abduction. Radiographs taken with the patient in the frame allow measurement of femoral anteversion in order to evaluate and correct rotation to prevent malalignment in traction.

Weber Two-Point Discrimination Test (web'-er/ tū/point/dis-krim-i-nā'-shun/test) (n.)   A clinical test used to determine whether the patient can discriminate between being touched with one or two points and what the minimum distance is at which the two points touching the skin are recognized. This test is used mostly to determine the level of sensitivity in the fingertips. See related term, **Moberg's Technique** and **Two-Point Discrimination Test**.

Webril (web-ril) (n.)   A proprietary brand of soft, lint-free cotton bandage available in various widths and thickness; used mostly as padding under a cast.

Weck Knife (wek/nīf) (n.)   A surgical instrument that uses to-and-fro motions of a blade to harvest a small skin graft.

Wedge (wej) (n.)   1. In shoe terminology, a piece of leather tapered to a thin edge that is used to elevate one side of sole or heel. 2. A term used to describe removing a wedge-shaped portion of plaster from a cast and then reapproximating the plaster in order to connect angulation at a fracture site that is already casted.

Wedge Fracture (wej/frak'chur) (n.)   A descriptive term for an anterior compression fracture of a vertebra that results from a flexion injury.

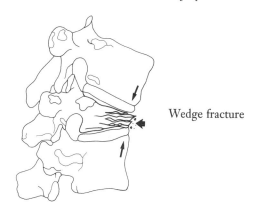

Wedge fracture

Wedge Graft (wej/graft) (n.)   A descriptive term for a triangular piece of full-thickness bone graft removed from the iliac crest.

Wedge Index (wej/in'-deks) (n.)   A radiographic measurement used to evaluate the degree of angulation in compression fractures of the vertebrae. A lateral roentgenogram of the spine is examined, and measurements of the anterior and posterior heights of the involved vertebra as well as the vertebra above and below the level of injury are reported as a "wedge index."

Wedge Osteotomy (wej/os'-tē-ot'-ō-mē) (n.)   Any surgical procedure in which a triangular piece of bone is resected to effect correction of an angular deformity of that bone.

Wedge-Shaped Vertebra (wej/shāpt/ver'-te-bra) (n.)   A vertebra that has a short anterior vertical height compared with its posterior height. Wedge-shaped vertebrae occur frequently in patients with osteoporosis of the spine, and secondary to fractures.

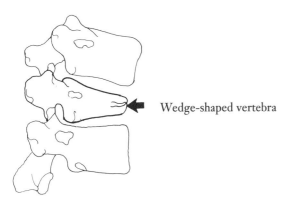

Wedge-shaped vertebra

Weight (wāt) (n.) The product of the force of gravity times the mass of a body.

Weight-Bearing (wāt/bār'-ing) (adj.) Refers to an extremity, joint, or other surface through which the weight of the body is carried.

Weight-Bearing Cast (wāt/bār'-ing/kast) (n.) Any short or long leg cast intended to bear a patient's weight.

Weight-Relieving Calipers (wāt/re-lēv'-ing/kal'-i-perz) (n.) A type of lower extremity orthosis that transfers the load of weight-bearing from the leg onto the ischium.

Well-Leg Traction (wel-leg/trak'-shun) (n.) A technique for the nonoperative treatment of hip fractures that involves the bilateral casting of the lower limbs using the normal limb for countertraction. This allows the patient to be moved from the bed to the chair and eliminates the need for skeletal traction. Synonym: **Roger Anderson Well Leg Traction**.

Welt (welt) (n.) In shoe terminology, a narrow strip of leather used to unite by stitching the upper innersole and the outersole of a shoe.

Werdnig-Hoffmann Disease (verd'-nig/hof'-man/di-zēz') (n.) An infantile form of spinal muscular atrophy. This is a congenital neuromuscular disorder inherited as an autosomal recessive disease. It is characterized by progressive, widespread weakness due to degeneration of the anterior horn cells of the spinal cord. In the infantile form, the disorder is usually diagnosed during the first years of life; death usually occurs within 4 to 5 years. Synonym: **Infantile Spinal Muscular Atrophy**.

West Point View (west/point/vyōō) (n.) A radiographic technique for imaging the shoulder joint. This is a modified axillary view in which a tangential view of the anteroinferior rim of the glenoid is obtained. The patient is placed prone on the x-ray table with the shoulder abducted. The cassette is placed superior to the shoulder and the beam is centered in the axilla, which is tilted 25 degrees downward from

the horizontal and 25 degrees medially from the midline. A positive finding confirms that the patient has an unstable shoulder joint.

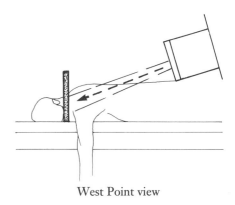

West Point view

Wet-to-Dry-Dressing (wĕt/to/drī/dres'-ing) (n.) A gentle mechanical method of wound debridement. Several layers of meshed gauze dressings are applied to an open wound, with the inner layer moistened at the time of application. The proteinaceous secretions of the wound then diffuse from the moist dressing into the outer dry dressing. The dressing is removed when it is dry so that all adherent material can be removed and thereby debrided with the dressing change.

Wheelchair (wēl'-chār') (n.) A chair mounted on wheels for the transportation of an occupant who is incapable of ambulation. It may be manually or electronically propelled by the occupant or by another individual.

Whiplash (wip'-lash) (n.) A colloquial term for an injury in which the cervical spine is unexpectedly and violently forced or whipped in one direction and then suddenly in the opposite direction. This is often seen in automobile collisions. The syndrome is characterized by neck pain, headache, and tenderness of the occipitonuchal-paravertebral muscles. A loss of normal cervical lordosis of the cervical spine associated with posterior joint strain of the cervical vertebrae may result.

Whirlpool Baths (wirl'-pūl/bath) (n.) A form of hydrotherapy.

White Cane (wīt/kān) (n.) A cane used by a blind person. Its white color has traditionally informed others of its user's condition. The cane is not used to bear or transfer weight.

Whiteside Technique (wītsīd/tek-nēk') (n.) A measurement of intracompartmental tissue pressures. In this simple technique, a mercury manometer is used within a closed tube system to determine the pressure needed to overcome the pressure within a closed compartment into which a needle is placed and a minute amount of saline is injected.

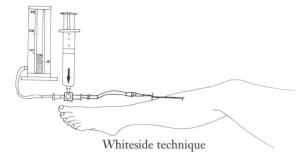

Whiteside technique

Whitman Arch Support (wit/man/ārch/sup-port′) (n.) A metal arch support for a shoe with a medial flange under the longitudinal arch and lateral flange at the heel; it ends just proximal to the metatarsal heads.

Wiberg's angle (wī-bergz/ang′-ǵl) (n.) A radiographic measurement used to evaluate the hip for subluxation in congenital hip dysplasia or developmental dysplasia of the hip. The angle is formed between Perkin's horizontal line (**B**) and a line drawn from the center of the ossified nucleus of the femoral head (**C**) to the most lateral ossified margin of the roof of the acetabulum (**E**). This angle should be at least 20 degrees. Also known as **Center Edge** or a **CE Angle**.

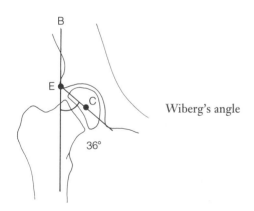

Wiberg's angle

Width (width) (n.) In shoe terminology, the dimension across the ball area of the last or shoe at its widest point.

Wilkins Classification (wil′-kinz/klas″sĭ-fĭ-ka′-shun) (n.) A classification system for pediatric radial neck fractures.

Wilkins Syndrome (wil′-kinz/sin′drōm) (n.) The chronic form of the cast syndrome in which the distal third of the duodenum is compressed by the superior mesenteric artery. See **Cast Syndrome**.

Williams Brace (wil′-yamz/brās) (n.) The commonly used name for a lumbosacral extension-lateral control orthosis that maintains the spine in a slightly flexed position. It is composed of pelvic and thoracic bands joined by a pair of pivotable lateral uprights

and an elastic abdominal support with a pad. It provides a three-point force system consisting of posteriorly directed forces from the abdominal support and anteriorly directed forces from the pelvic and thoracic bands.

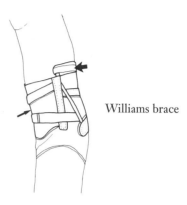

Williams brace

Williams Flexion Exercises (wil′-yumz/flek′-shun/ek′-ser-sīz′-ez) (n.) A series of flexion exercises used in the treatment of lower back problems. The original program consisted of four exercises: partial sit-up in the hook-lying position to strengthen the abdominal muscles; gluteal setting with an anterior pelvic tilt; knees-to-chest raises; and stretching the hip flexors in the standing lunge position. These exercises have been altered through the years, and currently about a dozen variations of flexion exercises exist.

Wilmington Brace (wil-ming-ton/brās) (n.) A type of custom-made thoracolumbosacral orthosis used in the treatment of scoliosis. The jacket is made of orthoplast and opens anteriorly.

Wilson Fracture (wil′son/frak′chur) (n.) A fracture of the volar plate of the middle phalanx of a finger.

Wilson Frame (wil′son/frām) (n.) An adjustable padded frame upon which a patient lies in the prone position during spinal surgery. Adjustments allow the creation of lordosis or kyphosis while keeping the abdomen or chest free of the operative table.

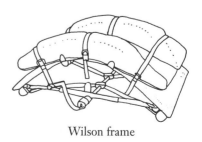

Wilson frame

Wilson Plate (wil′-son/plāt) (n.) A curved metal plate that attaches to the spinous processes of the vertebra. It is used to internally fix the vertebrae during spine fusion.

Wilson's Sign (wil'-sons/sīn) (n.) A nonspecific sign that suggests a diagnosis of osteochondritis of the knee. With the patient supine, the affected knee is flexed to a right angle and the leg is internally rotated fully. The knee is then gradually extended; at approximately 30 degrees of flexion, the patient will complain of pain over the anterior aspect of the medial femoral condyle. The pain is relieved on external rotation of the leg.

Wiltsie Technique (wilt-sē/tek-nēk') (n.) A technique for posterolateral spinal fusion in which the sacrospinalis muscle is split longitudinally and the laminae are included in the fusion, along with the facet joints and articular processes.

Wimberger's Sign (wim'-ber-gerz/sīn) (n.) A radiographic finding in children with scurvy. Owing to radiolucency of the epiphysis in conjunction with an unaffected calcification front of the cartilage, an eggshell appearance or "ringed epiphysis" is seen in the long bones.

Winchester Syndrome (win'-ches-ter/sin'drōm) (n.) An extremely rare type of idiopathic osteolysis inherited with an autosomal recessive pattern. The carpotarsal osteolysis is associated with joint contractures, short stature, osteoporosis, corneal clouding, skin lesions, and normal kidneys. Also known as **Type V Idiopathic Osteolysis**.

Window (win'-dō) (n.) A term used to describe an opening created in a bone or cast.

Windshield Wiper Sign (wind'-shēld/wī'-per/sīn) (n.) A radiographic sign indicating loosening and motion of an intramedullary implant, such as a prosthetic implant or an intramedullary nail. Owing to the to-and-fro motion of the implant, there is an endosteal reaction around the shaft of the prosthesis and local bony erosion at the tip of the prosthesis or nail.

Windswept Deformity (wind'-swept/dē-for'-mi-tē) (n.) A descriptive term for the condition in which a valgus deformity in one knee is associated with a varus deformity in the opposite knee.

Winged Scapula (wing'ed/skap'ū-lah) (n.) Prominence of the vertebral border of the scapula. This border is unable to remain close to the ribs during

shoulder motion because of weakness of the serratus anterior muscle or long thoracic nerve paralysis.

Wingfield Frame (wing-fēld/frām) (n.) A device for the gradual closed reduction of congenital hip dysplasia. It is no longer used.

Winograd Technique (win'-o-grad/tek'-nēk) (n.) A surgical technique for the partial removal of the nail-plate and matrix in the treatment of ingrown toenails in the late stage of abscess or in the granulation stage.

Winquist and Hansen Classification (win-kwist/han-sen/klas"sǐ-fǐ-ka'shun) (n.) A classification system for femoral shaft fractures. The fractures are designated as segmental in nature or graded I through IV, based on the degree of comminution and remaining cortical contact. This classification will determine the correct method of fixation.

Winter Anterior Osteotomy (win'-ter/an-ter'-ē-or/os'-te-ot'-ō-mē) (n.) A surgical technique for anterior spinal fusion that is used in the correction of congenital kyphosis.

Winter Formula (win'ter/form-ū-la) (n.) A calculation derived from standard growth tables that approximates the potential shortening of the spine that would result from spinal fusion in an immature skeleton. It is calculated as centimeters of shortening = 0.07 number of segments fused per number of years of growth remaining.

Wire (wīr) (n.) A narrow, flexible strand or rod made of metal.

Wiring (wīr'ing) (n.) The process of using wires for the internal fixation of bone-to-bone or tendon-to-bone. More formally known as a wire fixation.

WNL Abbreviation for "within normal limits."

Wolf Skin Graft (wolf/skin/graft) (n.) A full-thickness free skin graft (0.030 inches thick).

Wolff's Law (wolfs/law) (n.) A principle stating that bone responds dynamically to stress and strain by altering its internal architecture.

Wood Screw (wod/skrū) (n.) A screw type that has a sharp point but is tapered to that point. The neck portion is unthreaded and a preliminary drill hole is not needed. These screws are unsuitable for use in cortical bone because they tend to split it.

Woodward Technique (wod-ward/tek-nēk') (n.) Surgical repair of congenital elevation of the scapula in which the origin of the trapezius muscle is moved to a more inferior position on the spinous processes, which also moves the scapula to a more inferior position.

Work (wurk) (n.) The amount of energy required to move a body from one position to another. Biomechanically, this is defined as the product of the force applied times the distance moved in the direction of force. The unit of measurement for work is newton-meters or joules (foot poundforce).

Wormian Bones (worm'-ē-an/bōnz') (n.) The name

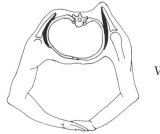

Winged scapula

given to the multiple centers of ossification seen in the skull that are associated with skeletal disorders, most commonly osteogenesis imperfecta.

Wound (woond) (n.) 1. A break or trauma to the structure of an organ or tissue that is the result of a mechanical force. Examples include bruises, tears, lacerations, punctures, and burns. 2. A surgical incision.

Wound and Skin Isolation (woond/and/skin/ī'-sō-lā'shun) (n.) Patient care techniques intended to prevent transmission of pathogens from an open wound or the skin surface to another patient. Also known as **Wound-to-Skin Precautions**.

Woven Bone (wō'ven/bōn) (n.) The immature bone seen during development, in fracture callus, osteogenic tumors, and conditions in which the rate of bone formation is rapid. Histologically, the collagen matrix is disordered and irregularly "woven," reminiscent of the threads in fabric.

Wright's Test (rītz/test) (n.) A clinical test that is used in the diagnosis of thoracic outlet syndrome. The patient is seated with both arms hanging at his or her sides and the examiner standing behind. Then the arm is passively moved through an arc of 180 degrees while palpating the radial pulse. The test is positive if there is a point where the pulse diminishes or disappears entirely. The level of this change is also noted.

Wrinkle Test (rin'-kel/test) (n.) A clinical test that is useful in assessing the intactness of peripheral nerve function. If innervated skin is immersed in water for a period, wrinkling occurs. If the skin is de-nervated, wrinkling will not occur. See O'Rain Wrinkle Test.

Wrisberg's Ligament (rīs'-bergz/lig'-ah-ment) (n.) The posterior lateral meniscofemoral ligament of the knee. When it is present, it traverses posterior to the posterior cruciate ligament. Synonym: **Meniscofemoral Ligament**.

Wrist (rist) (n.) The articulation between the forearm and the hand. It is composed of the distal radioulnar, radiocarpal, and ulnocarpal joints.

Wrist Drop (rist/drop) (n.) The inability to extend the wrist and the metacarpophalangeal joints owing to paralysis of the long finger extensors and the wrist extensor muscles secondary to radial nerve palsy.

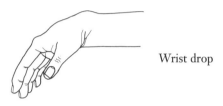

Wrist drop

Wryneck (rī'nek) (n.) A contracted state of the muscles of the neck, causing a twisting of the neck and malposition of the head. The chin is typically pointed in one direction, and the head is tilted toward the other direction. It is usually associated with unilateral spasm of the sternocleidomastoid muscle. See **Torticollis**.

X

X Chromosome (x/krō'mō-sōm) (n.) One of the sex chromosomes. Females have two X chromosomes; males have one X and one Y chromosome. Genes carried on this chromosome are called X-linked or sex-linked.

Xanthoma (zan-thō'mah) (n.) A benign, tumorlike lesion of histiocytic origin. It appears as soft, yellow nodule, papule, or plaque, usually found within the dermis or tendons but occasionally in other tissues of the body. The lesions are characterized histologically by the presence of histiocytic foam cells. Occasionally, giant cells containing lipid substances are also present.

Xenograft (zēn'ō-graft) (n.) A graft of tissue transplanted between animals of different species. Synonym: **Heterograft**.

Xeroform (zē'rō/form) (n.) A proprietary brand of nonadherent wound dressing. It is composed of fine mesh gauze impregnated with bismuth tribromophenate.

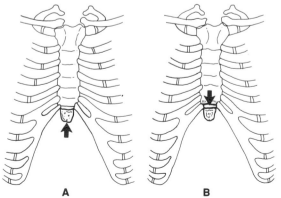

A, Xiphoid process; **B**, xiphoid-sternal junction

Xeroradiography (zē″rō-rā″dē-og′rah-fē) (n.) A technique of producing radiographs by a photoelectric-dry electrostatic process using selenium plates. The main advantage over conventional radiography is the resulting edge enhancement that demonstrates abrupt changes in density between adjoining areas. The major disadvantage is the higher radiation exposure necessary.

Xerography (ze-rog′rah-fe) (n.) See **Xeroradiography**.

Xiphoid Process (zīf′oid/pro′ses) (n.) The pointed process of cartilage supported by a core of bone at the lowermost section of the sternum. It does not articulate with any ribs. Also known as **Ensiform Process** or **Cartilage, Xiphisternum**. See **Sternum**.

X-Ray (eks′rā) (n.) Electromagnetic radiation of very short wavelength. Synonym: **Roentgen Ray**.

X-Ray Microscope (eks′rā/mī′krō-skōp) (n.) A microscope in which x-rays replace light. The resulting image is usually reproduced on film.

Xylocaine (zī′lō-kān) (n.) A proprietary name for Lidocaine. A local anesthetic agent.

Y

Y Cartilage (y/kar′ti-lij) (n.) A descriptive name for the triradiate cartilage of the growing pelvis. See **Triradiate Cartilage**.

Y Chromosome (y/krō′mō-sōm) (n.) One of the sex-linked chromosomes. Males have one Y and one X chromosome. Females have two X and no Y chromosomes.

Y Coordinate (y/ko-or′di-nit) (n.) One of the radiographic signs of congenital dislocation of the hip. This line is drawn from the femoral head to the sacrum, perpendicular to Perkins line. In congenital dislocation of the hip, it will be displaced superiorly. Also called **Ponseti's Y Line**.

Y Fracture (y/frak′chur) (n.) A term used to describe the appearance of fracture lines in relation to the long axis of the broken bone. It is most commonly used to describe intra-articular fractures with this pattern.

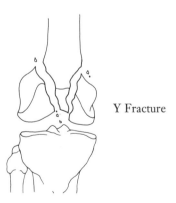

Y Fracture

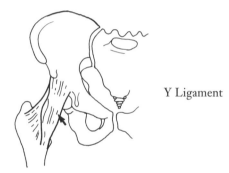

Y Ligament

Y Ligament (y/lig′ah-ment) (n.) See **Bigelow's Ligament** and the **Ileofemoral Ligament**.

Y Line (y-līn) (n.) See **Hilgenreiner's Line**.

Yergason Chair Test (yer′-ga-son/chār/test) (n.) A clinical test for the evaluation of disorders of the sacroiliac joint. While extending a hand for him or her to grasp, ask the patient to step onto a chair, which you support firmly with your hand. Then, still holding his or her hand, ask the patient to step down, and push slightly through the forearm so that he or she steps down unexpectedly, producing a very slight jar transmitted through the weight-bearing extremity. Next, change hands and repeat the procedure with the patient's opposite leg. A patient with sacroiliac joint disease will have pain in stepping down on the affected side. The "sacroiliac malingerer," however, will step down hard on the foot of the "affected side" without pain.

Yergason's Supination Sign (yer-ga-sonz/soo″pi-nā′ shun/sīn) (n.) A clinical test for tenosynovitis of the biceps tendon. Flex the patient's elbow to 90 degrees and pronate the forearm. Hold the patient's wrist to resist supination; then ask the patient to actively supinate. Pain localized in the bicipital groove may indicate the presence of tendinitis in the long head of the biceps or synovitis of its tendon sheath. A painful snap along the bicipital groove is diagnostic of biceps tendon subluxation.

Yield Point (yēld/point) (n.) In biomechanics, the point on the stress-strain curve where the material begins to yield. Further loading after this point results in permanent deformation.

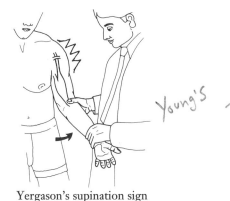

Yergason's supination sign

Yield Strain (yēld/strān) (n.) The amount of defor-

mation that a material can sustain before nonelastic deformation begins.

Yield Stress (yēld/stres) (n.) The amount of load per unit area that a material can sustain before nonelastic deformation occurs.

Young Modulus (yung/mod″u-lus) (n.) The slope of the elastic region fo a stress-strain curve that is a measure of the material's stiffness. It is obtained by dividing the stress by the strain at any point in this region of the curve. Stiffer materials have higher moduli. Also known as **Elastic Modulus**.

Y-V Plasty (y-v/plas′tē) (n.) A surgical technique for obtaining increased soft-tissue coverage, for example, in the release of constricting digital bands. A Y-shaped incision in skin or soft tissue is converted to a V-shape at the time of closure.

Y-Y Line (y-y/līn) (n.) See **Hilgenreiner's Line**.

Z

Z Foot (z/fut) (n.) A descriptive term for a clubfoot in which the association of metatarsus adductus with a relaxed valgus in the hind foot gives the foot a "Z" shape.

Zancolli Capsuloplasty (zahn-kō-lē/kap′su-lo-plas″tē) (n.) A surgical procedure for intrinsic paralysis of fingers, using a capsulodesis to stabilize the metacarpophalangeal joint.

Zausmer Scale (zowz′-mer/skāl) (n.) A rating scale for the evaluation and determination of the quality of motor performance in children with neuromuscular disorders:

O: No attempt has been made.

T: An attempt has been made, thus expressing a certain amount of motivation and understanding of the test situation. However, the additional motivation, understanding, or capacity to perform the act is still missing.

TT: A higher level of motivation and perseverence has been attained. However, the patient still shows the lack of capacity to achieve, even partially, the goal.

P: In this category the quality of performance is analyzed. Complete independence has not yet been reached; the patient performs partially; correctness, coordination, and rhythm have not yet been attained. The pattern is executed poorly.

F: Independence has been reached without assistance. The patient fully achieves the goal. The quality of performance has improved, but is not yet consistently good.

G: Endurance and speed are stressed, and there are a great number of repetitions and greater speed. The patient shows consistent correctness, coordination, and rhythm—a good pattern.

N: While the preceding grade (G) expressed a still-existing need and possibility for growth and perfection in all areas of the performance, the N represents the top grade for the performance expected at a given age.

Z-Band (z-band) (n.) A sharply defined line that is the termination of one group of filaments seen in the ultrastructure of striated muscle. It is found in the center of a relatively light band of moderate width, the isotrophic band, and it forms the boundary of a sarcomere. The "Z" is an abbreviation for Zwischenscheibe. Also known as **Z Line**, **Krause's Membrane**, **Telophragma**, **Amici's** or **Intermediate Disk**.

Zero Position (ze′ro/pō′zish-un) (n.) The starting position for range-of-motion and other tests at which every joint is considered at point zero. The zero position most generally accepted is synonymous with the position.

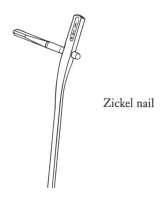

Zickel nail

Zickel Nail (zik′-l/nāl) (n.) An intramedullary femoral nail designed for fixation of subtrochanteric femur fractures. The apparatus consists of a tapered intramedullary rod with a tunnel in its proximal portion. A triflanged nail is placed into the femoral head and neck through this tunnel, and then locked with a set screw. This apparatus is designed to permit early mobilization and ambulation. Developed by Robert Zickel of New York.

Zickel Supracondylar Device (zik′-l/soo″prah-kon′di-lar/de-vīs′) (n.) An intramedullary device for the fixation of supracondylar femur fractures. It is composed of two fairly flexible, curved, intramedullary rods that have angulated tunnels in the condylar ends through which cancellous screws are inserted.

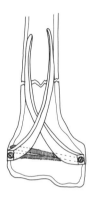

Zickel supracondylar device

Zielke Instrumentation (zīlkē/in″strū-men-tā′shun) (n.) A System for anterior internal fixation of the spine. With this system, a solid, flexible rod is used instead of a cable.

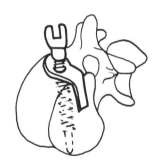

Zielke instrumentation

Ziemssen's Motor Points (zēm′senz/mo′tor/points) (n.) The entrance points of motor nerves into muscles. In the therapeutic application of electrical stimulation, this should be the point of application of stimulation to the muscle.

Zinc Oxide (zingk/ok′sīd) (n.) A mild astringent used in the treatment of various skin conditions.

Z-Line (z-/lin) (n.) See **Z-Band**.

Zone of Provisional Calcification (zōn/of/prō-vizh′un-al/kal″si-fi-kā′shun) (n.) One of the histologic zones of the cartilaginous component of the physeal plate. It is the bottom of the hypertrophic zone in which the initial calcification of the matrix occurs. It may be defined radiographically as a thin, white, radiodense line.

Z-Plasty (z-plas′tē) (n.) A surgical technique for the transfer of two interdigitating triangular flaps of skin, used for reduction of tension lines. Its name derives from the fact that, drawn out on the skin, the three limbs of the flaps have the overall shape of a Z. Geometrically, the Z-plasty consists of a central or longitudinal limb, or arm, and two-sided limbs, or arms. The three limbs must be equal in length, with their overall length varying to fulfill the specific requirement. The angles may vary widely, but their usual size is 60 degrees.

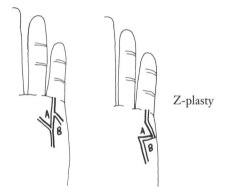

Z-plasty

Zygapophyseal (zi″gapō-fiz′ē-al) (adj.) Of or pertaining to the lateral articulating joints of the spine.

ISBN 0-397-51311-9

90000